D1757935

Lung Transplantation

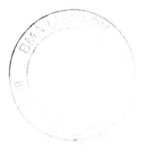

Epigraph

Difficulty in breathing with limited life span to breathing easy with extended life following lung transplantation.

—Ganesh Raghu

I dedicate this book to all the donors and recipients of lung transplantation and to the caregivers and families of pre- and post-lung transplant patients.

—Ganesh Raghu

The capacity to help others is a blessing. I dedicate this book to those who donated life to others and to those who, by their heroic decision to donate the organs of their loved ones, gifted new life to others.

—Roberto G. Carbone

Preface

Management of advanced or end-stage nonmalignant lung diseases is always challenging to the pulmonary specialist as the path of the breath of life for patients with lung diseases comes to an end with no further medical treatments to extend life. The frustrations and sense of despair that the patient, their loved ones, families, friends, caregivers, and physicians are confronted with are significant.

While many patients unfortunately succumb to advanced lung diseases, new horizons have opened up for patients suffering from end-stage lung disease, thanks to pioneers including Cooper, Pearson, and Viganò, by making lung transplantation a reality to these patients, who are otherwise healthy. Since the advent of lung transplantation, nearly 6000 patients have received lung transplantations between 1988 and 1995, increasing progressively to 17,715 bilateral lung transplantations between 2005 and 2010, with a statistically significant ($p < 0.0001$) smaller risk of rejection compared to the preceding period considered. Indeed, lung transplantation has evolved into standard of care for these patients, with improved quality of life and enhanced survival for patients with idiopathic pulmonary fibrosis (IPF), cystic fibrosis, etc.

Indeed, lung transplantation is a potential option for the patient who has reached advanced stages, but, unfortunately, it is not an option for all patients who have reached advanced stages and for whom there are no further medical treatment interventions to stabilize their lung problems. The general pulmonologist needs to be aware of the indications and contraindications of lung transplantation as well as of post-lung transplant management, risks, complications, and outcomes in order to be able to help patients understand the complexity and benefits of lung transplantation as well as be prepared for the anticipated outcomes. Pulmonologists also must help patients improve and/or maintain their physical stability and overall fitness as possible while coping with advanced stages of diseases such as IPF, chronic obstructive pulmonary disease (COPD), cystic fibrosis, pulmonary hypertension, pulmonary sarcoidosis, interstitial pneumonia associated with connective tissue diseases such as systemic sclerosis, rheumatoid arthritis, and polymyositis, and other orphan lung diseases.

This is the first book to discuss all aspects of lung transplantation and is intended to equip the general pulmonologist/physician worldwide with all the necessary tools, awareness, and knowledge to help patients with management of advanced stages, preparation for lung transplantation, and care post-lung transplantation. This book also serves as a clinical guide to refer appropriate patients early for consideration for lung transplantation worldwide.

We have organized the chapters into four broad parts and have leading global experts who have written on the different topics pertinent to medical, surgical, psychological, and social aspects of lung transplantation. Additionally, we have summarized the history of lung transplantation and discussed the immunological aspects and epigenetic changes with vascular injury after lung transplantation.

The first part discusses eligibility criteria including specific evaluation, timing for listing, indications and contraindications for lung transplantation, pretransplant considerations, psychosocial patient evaluation, and lung allocation score, in combination with the impact of new revisions and successive outcome. A particular emphasis is given to lung transplantation with regard to COPD, cystic fibrosis, and interstitial lung diseases with pulmonary fibrosis.

Issues related to the donor lung with detailed consideration of immunology, physiology, epigenetics, and surgical treatment are discussed in the second part.

The third part discusses medical management of the lung transplantation recipient including cellular and humeral rejection, prevention of viral and nonviral infection, lung allograft dysfunction, and complications such as bronchiolitis obliterans pneumonia, gastro-esophageal reflux, and essential topics including bronchoscopy, imaging, and lung rejection pathology.

Finally, the last part highlights directions for the future to bridge the gaps in the field of lung transplantation.

We are very grateful to all the leading experts in the field for agreeing to discuss their expertise in their chapters and for their contribution to this book dedicated to lung transplantation.

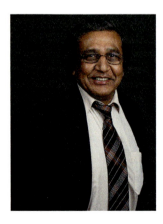

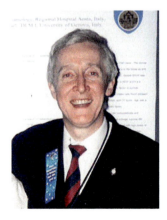

Ganesh Raghu   Roberto G. Carbone
Seattle, WA, USA   Genoa, Italy

Contents

Contributors

Ali Abedi, MSc, MD Department of Pulmonary and Critical Care Medicine, University of Texas Health San Antonio, San Antonio, TX, USA

Jitesh Ahuja, MBBS, MD Department of Radiology, University of Washington Medical Center, Seattle, WA, USA

Shahnaz Ajani, MD Division of Pulmonary, Allergy, Critical Care, and Sleep Medicine, Emory University Hospital, Emory University School of Medicine, Emory Transplant Center, Atlanta, GA, USA

Giovanni Bottino, MD Department of Medicine, University of Genoa—DIMI, Genoa, Italy

Roberto G. Carbone, MD, FCCP Department of Internal Medicine, University of Genoa, Genoa, Italy

Martin R. Carby, MBBS, BSc, FRCP Transplant Unit, Harefield Hospital, Royal Brompton and Harefield NHS Foundation Trust, London, UK

Department of Cardiothoracic Transplantation, Harefield Hospital, Harefield, UK

Richard N. Channick, MD Division of Pulmonary and Critical Care Medicine, Department of Medicine, Massachusetts General Hospital, Boston, MA, USA

Paul A. Corris, MBBS, FRCP Department of Respiratory Medicine, Freeman Hospital and Institute of Cellular Medicine, Newcastle University, Newcastle Upon Tyne, UK

Andrea Maria D'Armini, MD Department of Cardiothoracic and Vascular Surgery, University of Pavia, School of Medicine, Foundation IRCCS Policlinico San Matteo, Pavia, Italy

Idoia Gimferrer, MD, PhD, D(ABHI) Department of Immunogenetics/HLA, Bloodworks Northwest, Seattle, WA, USA

Valentina Grazioli, MD Department of Cardiothoracic and Vascular Surgery, University of Pavia, School of Medicine, Foundation IRCCS Policlinico San Matteo, Pavia, Italy

Reed Hall, PharmD Pharmacy, University Hospital—University Health System, San Antonio, TX, USA

Steven Kenneth Huang, MD Department of Pulmonary and Critical Care Medicine, University of Michigan, Ann Arbor, MI, USA

Hardeep Singh Kalsi, MBBS, IBSc(Hons), MRCP Transplant Unit, Harefield Hospital, Royal Brompton and Harefield NHS Foundation Trust, London, UK

Department of Cardiothoracic Transplantation, Harefield Hospital, Harefield, UK

Siddhartha G. Kapnadak, MD Division of Pulmonary and Critical Care Medicine, University of Washington Medical Center, Seattle, WA, USA

Shaf Keshavjee, MD, MSc, FRCSC, FACS Division of Thoracic Surgery, Toronto General Hospital, University Health Network, Toronto, ON, Canada

Toronto Lung Transplant Program, Toronto General Hospital, University Health Network, University of Toronto, Toronto, ON, Canada

Robert M. Kotloff, MD Department of Pulmonary Medicine, Cleveland Clinic, Cleveland, OH, USA

Erika D. Lease, MD Division of Pulmonary, Critical Care, and Sleep Medicine, University of Washington, Seattle, WA, USA

Deborah Jo Levine, MD Department of Pulmonary and Critical Care Medicine, University of Texas Health Science Center San Antonio, San Antonio, TX, USA

Andrea Mariscal, MD Division of Thoracic Surgery, Toronto General Hospital, University Health Network, Toronto, ON, Canada

Toronto Lung Transplant Program, Toronto General Hospital, University Health Network, University of Toronto, Toronto, ON, Canada

Gerard J. Meachery, MB BCh (HONS), FRCP, FRCP Department of Respiratory Medicine, Freeman Hospital, Newcastle Upon Tyne, UK

Keith C. Meyer, MD, MS Department of Medicine, University of Wisconsin School of Medicine and Public Health, Madison, WI, USA

Assaf Monselise, MD Departments of Dermatology and Internal Medicine, Clalit Health Services, Tel-Aviv, Israel

Michael S. Mulligan, MD Department of Surgery, University of Washington, Seattle, WA, USA

Karen A. Nelson, PhD, D(ABHI) Department of Immunogenetics/HLA, Bloodworks Northwest, Seattle, WA, USA

Brant K. Oelschlager, MD Division of General Surgery, Department of Surgery, University of Washington Medical Center, Seattle, WA, USA

M. Patricia George, MD Department of Medicine, National Jewish Health, Denver, CO, USA

Carlos A. Pellegrini, MD, FACS Department of Surgery, University of Washington, Seattle, WA, USA

Sudhakar Pipavath, MD Department of Radiology, University of Washington Medical Center, Seattle, WA, USA

Matthew R. Pipeling, MD Division of Pulmonary, Allergy and Critical Care Medicine, University of Pittsburgh School of Medicine, Pittsburgh, PA, USA

Francesco Puppo, MD Department of Internal Medicine, University of Genoa, Genoa, Italy

Ganesh Raghu, MD, FCCP, FACP Division of Pulmonary, Critical Care, and Sleep Medicine, Department of Medicine University of Washington, Seattle, WA, USA

Center for Interstitial Lung Disease, ILD, Sarcoid and Pulmonary Fibrosis Program, University of Washington Medicine, Seattle, WA, USA

Scleroderma Clinic, University of Washington Medicine, Seattle, WA, USA

Anja C. Roden, MD Department of Laboratory Medicine and Pathology, Mayo Clinic Rochester, Rochester, MN, USA

Pablo Gerardo Sanchez, MD, PhD Division of Cardiothoracic Surgery, Department of Surgery, University of Washington, Seattle, WA, USA

Thomas M. Soeprono, MD Department of Psychiatry, University of Washington, Seattle, WA, USA

Henry D. Tazelaar, MD Department of Laboratory Medicine and Pathology, Mayo Clinic Arizona, Scottsdale, AZ, USA

Bart Vanaudenaerde, MSc, PhD Laboratory of Respiratory Diseases, Department of Clinical and Experimental Medicine, Katholieke Universiteit Leuven, Leuven, Belgium

Elly Vandermeulen, PhD Department of Clinical and Experimental Medicine, Katholieke Universiteit Leuven, Leuven, Belgium

Geert Verleden, MD, PhD, FERS Lung Transplantation Unit, University Hospital Gasthuisberg, Leuven, Belgium

Stijn Verleden, PhD, MSc Department of Clinical and Experimental Medicine, Katholieke Universiteit Leuven, Leuven, Belgium

Mario Viganó, MD Department of Cardiothoracic and Vascular Surgery, University of Pavia, School of Medicine, Foundation IRCCS Policlinico San Matteo, Pavia, Italy

Robin Vos, MD, PhD Laboratory of Respiratory Diseases, Department of Clinical and Experimental Medicine, Katholieke Universiteit Leuven, Leuven, Belgium

Lung Transplant and Respiratory Intermediate Care Unit, Department of Respiratory Medicine, University Hospitals Leuven, Leuven, Belgium

Dustin M. Walters, MD Department of Thoracic and Cardiovascular Surgery, University of Virginia, Charlottesville, VA, USA

Keith M. Wille, MD Department of Medicine, Pulmonary, Allergy, and Critical Care Medicine, University of Alabama at Birmingham, Birmingham, AL, USA

Alison S. Witkin, MD Division of Pulmonary and Critical Care Medicine, Department of Medicine, Massachusetts General Hospital, Boston, MA, USA

Robert B. Yates, MD Department of Surgery, Northwest Hospital and Medical Center, University of Washington Medicine, Seattle, WA, USA

Martin R. Zamora, MD Division of Pulmonary Sciences and Critical Care Medicine, University of Colorado, Aurora, CO, USA

Part I

General Principles and Considerations for Lung Transplantation

The History of Lung Transplantation

Andrea Maria D'Armini, Valentina Grazioli,
and Mario Viganò

Milestones in Transplantation History

"… if there is a father of heart and lung transplantation.
then Demikhov certainly deserves this title" (C. Barnard).

The miracle of Cosmas and Damian (martyrs, 287 A.D.) depicted the first evidence of transplantation. According to tradition, these martyrs grafted the leg from a barely deceased Ethiopian onto a Caucasian patient, in order to replace his ulcerated leg. See Fig. 1.1.

In modern times, Vladimir P. Demikhov (Moscow) (Fig. 1.2a), a Russian physiologist, presented the first important stimulus in developing transplantation science: he transplanted a dog head onto the neck of another dog in 1940, and this dog survived for several days [1]. Furthermore, he performed the first lung transplantation (right inferior lobe) on a dog, and the dog survived for 7 days; it died from a pneumothorax due to a bronchial suture dehiscence [1]. Demikhov continued these attempts at transplantations in dogs (Fig. 1.2b). The complication which doomed his first lung transplant attempt became the main challenge in his following attempts; simultaneously, Demikhov

A. M. D'Armini · V. Grazioli (✉) · M. Viganò
Department of Cardiothoracic and Vascular Surgery, University of Pavia, School of Medicine, Foundation IRCCS Policlinico San Matteo, Pavia, Italy
e-mail: darmini@smatteo.pv.it

demonstrated that bronchial arteries and nerves are unnecessary in the lung function of the recipient [1].

Alexis Carrel (University of Chicago) (Fig. 1.3) is another important pioneer in the lung transplantation field. His innovations in surgical techniques, mainly in end-to-end anastomosis (for which he received the Nobel Prize in 1912), allowed the beginning of a new era dedicated to whole organ transplantations [2]. In 1907, Carrel and C.C Guthrie (University of Chicago) performed a heterotopic heart-lung transplantation on the neck of a cat; it died 3 days later, probably from an acute rejection [3, 4].

In 1954, Joseph E. Murray (Massachusetts) performed the first human kidney transplantation on twins in order to avoid rejection problems. This experience established the first evidence of the feasibility of transplants applied to human [5]. The most important landmark in lung transplantation history was the first human single-lung transplantation performed in 1963 by the pioneer James D. Hardy (University of Mississippi) [2]. Four years later, Christiaan Barnard (University of Cape Town) (Fig. 1.4) realized the first human-to-human heart transplantation [2].

However, despite these and other achievements and promising results, lung transplantation developed with delay when compared to transplantation of other organs such as the heart, kidney, and liver. This was due mainly to the lung's frailty, to the major exposure to infections

G. Raghu, R. G. Carbone (eds.), *Lung Transplantation*, https://doi.org/10.1007/978-3-319-91184-7_1

Fig. 1.1 The Healing of Justinian by Saint Cosmas and Saint Damian. Fra Angelico (circa 1438–1440) (Source: https://commons.wikimedia.org/wiki/File:Fra_Angelico_-_The_Healing_of_Justinian_by_Saint_Cosmas_and_Saint_Damian_-_WGA00519.jpg. Fra Angelico [Public domain], via Wikimedia Commons)

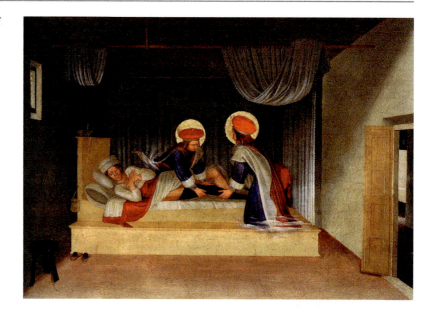

Fig. 1.2 (**a**) Vladimir Demikhov (1916–1998) (Source: ITAR-TASS News Agency/Alamy Stock Photo). (**b**) The last dog head transplant performed by Dr. Demikhov (Source: Bundesarchiv, Bild 183–61478-0004/Weiß, Günter/CC-BY-SA 3.0)

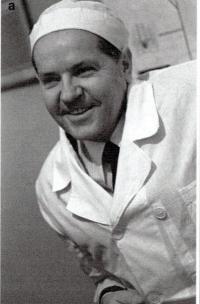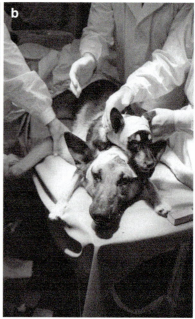

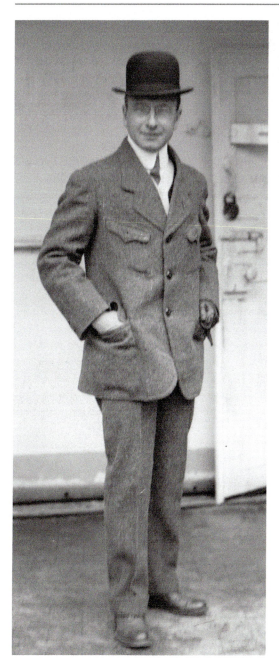

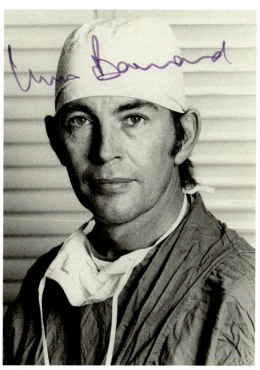

Fig. 1.4 Dr. Christiaan Barnard (1922–2001) (Used with permission of University Stamp Co., Inc./University Archives, Westport, CT, USA)

from the external world, and to the absence of systemic bronchial connections after the transplantation [2].

The Pre-Hardy First Human Lung Transplant Era: Lessons Learned from Animal Models of Lung Transplantation

In 1950, Henri Metras (Marseille) described an innovative experiment concerning the venous anastomosis of a lung transplantation in a dog involving the pulmonary veins with the left atrium cuff [6]. He also demonstrated the possibility of preserving the bronchial arterial

Fig. 1.3 Dr. Alexis Carrel (1873–1944) in 1912 (Source: https://commons.wikimedia.org/wiki/File:Alexis_Carrel_ (1912).jpg#filelinks. Forms part of George Grantham Bain Collection, Library of Congress. Public Domain)

support with a connection to the subclavian artery. Furthermore, he was the first to succeed in allotransplantation [6].

In 1950, Vittorio Staudacher (Milan) compared allotransplantation and autotransplantation in dogs in order to better investigate the physiopathology of rejections [7]. In the same manner, A. A. Juvenelle (Buffalo University) attempted reimplantation (autotransplantation) in canine models for physiological studies [8]. This study would be continued later in 1953 by W. B. Neptune (Philadelphia), who conducted canine experiments on bronchial anastomosis and investigated post-transplant dehiscence and the resulting recipient death. He proved that the use of adrenocorticotropic hormone (ACTH) actually improved survival [9]. In 1954, Creighton A. Hardin and C. F. Kittle (Kansas) established the functional capacity of a lung allotransplant.

They also demonstrated that the use of cortisone could efficiently increase the survival of the recipient [10].

Nevertheless, despite these advancements, the main issue still being debated was the role of hilar vascular and nerve structures [11]. Table 1.1 lists the most important stages of this phase: the grafted lung has normal functional pattern if part of the recipient lung remains in place, and the autonomic nerves are important for pulmonary function. However, there is no explanation regarding the reduction of lung function posttransplantation [11].

Finally, immunosuppressive therapy received attention through the work of David A. Blumenstock in 1961 (New York) and James D. Hardy in 1963 (Mississippi) [12, 13], specifically concerning the possible use of cortisone, ACTH, total body irradiation, and splenectomy.

Table 1.1 Lessons from animal models of lung transplantation

Author/Study	Year	Lesson
Bogardus (Washington)[a]	1958	Normal grafted lung function if part of recipient lung remains in place
Faber and Beattle (Chicago) [b]	1958	
Nigro (Chicago)[c]	1962	Importance of autonomic nerves for lung function
Yeh (Georgia)[d]	1962	
Hardy (Mississippi)[e]	1963	
Haglin (Minneapolis)[f]	1963	Experiments on baboons prove normal functional lung and increase survival with respect to surveys realized on dogs. The same conclusion is reached also when recipient pneumonectomies are performed. This demonstrated that the rule of autonomic nerve in lung function is species-specific

[a]Borgadus GM. An Evaluation in Dogs of the Relationship of Pulmonary, Bronchial, and Hilar Adventitial Circulation to the Problem of Lung Transplantation. Surgery. 1958;43:849–856

[b]Faber LP, Beaitie EJ Jr. Respiration Following Lung Denervation. Surg Forum. 1958;9:383–385

[c]Nigro SL, Evans RH, Benfield JR, Gago O, Fry WA, Adams WE. Physiologic Alterations of Cardiopulmonary Function in Dogs Living one and one-Half Years on Only a Reimplanted Right Lung. J Thorac Cardiovasc Surg. 1963;46:598–605

[d]Yeh TJ, Ellison LT, Ellison RG. Functional Evaluation of the Autotransplanted Lung in the Dog. Am Rev Resp Dis. 1962;86:791–797.

[e]Shumway SJ, Shumway NE. Thoracic Transplantation. Part I. Historical Background. Cambridge, MA: Blackwell Science;1995

[f]Haglin J, Telander RL, Muzzall RE, Kiser JC, Strobel CJ. Comparison of Lung Autotransplantation in the Primate and Dog. Surg Forum. 1963;14:196–198

Lessons from the First Human Lung Transplantation by Hardy

In 1963, James D. Hardy (Fig. 1.5) performed the first human lung transplantation on a prisoner affected by lung central carcinoma with nodal metastases; the left graft lung was harvested from a man who died of massive acute myocardial infarction [11, 14]. Immunosuppressive therapy, consisting of azathioprine, cortisone, and cobalt irradiation of the thymic region, was also administered [11, 14]. The patient survived for 18 days, and the death was ascribed to kidney failure and malnutrition [11, 14].

From 1963 to 1973, several lung transplantation attempts were performed, but with little success. Indeed, only sporadic experiments showed significant results, such as the one by Fritz Derom in 1968 (Belgium), who reported a 10-month posttransplantation survival [15].

In 1970, Frank J. Veith (New York) confirmed the feasibility of single-lung transplantation [16]. However, several troublesome issues still existed: the unadapted immunosuppression and consequent graft rejection, the infection problems, and, finally,

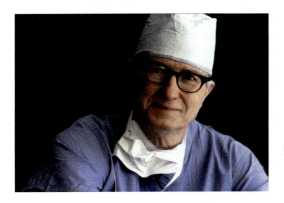

Fig. 1.5 Dr. James D. Hardy (1918–2003): "…research became a vital part of my professional life…." (Used with permission of the University of Mississippi. Medical Center. Source: https://www.umc.edu/uploadedImages/UMCedu/Content/Administration/Institutional_Advancement/Public_Affairs/News_and_Publications/Press_Releases/2013/2013-06-10/Hardy%20in%20Scrubs.jpg)

the maldistribution of ventilation and perfusion in the grafted lung [16]. Subsequently, the anastomosis dehiscence problem became the main topic.

From 1963 to 1983, many laboratories focused their studies on [11]:

1. *Pulmonary denervation*: Based on Haglin's work (Minneapolis, 1963), S. Nakae (Texas Southwestern) conducted studies in 1967 testing the efficiency of lung transplantation on rhesus monkeys, dogs, and cats; only rhesus monkeys had normal pattern lung ventilation after the transplantation [17]. He tested different techniques on four categories of animals from different species: mediastinal denervation with tracheal transaction and reanastomosis onto dogs, cats, and rhesus monkeys. The fourth group consisted of dogs that underwent total mediastinal denervation [17]. The conclusion of his work was that humans and primates have a different respiratory reflex compared to dogs, and, for this reason, they have a normal functional lung pattern after lung transplantation [17].

2. *Pulmonary vascular physiology after lung transplantation:* Several studies up until 1960 had underlined the frequency of pulmonary hypertension after lung transplantation and ligation of the contralateral pulmonary artery [18–20]. This problem was mainly due to venous anastomosis obstruction. In order to prevent this complication, Frank J. Veith and K. Richards introduced the concept of left atrium cuff in 1970 [21].

3. *Dehiscence of bronchial anastomosis*: This complication was the focal point of interest of the "Toronto Lung Transplantation Group," the main thoracic surgical center in Toronto, founded by F. Griff Pearson in 1968 (Fig. 1.6) and later directed by Joel D. Cooper (Fig. 1.7). It was Joel D. Cooper who in 1978 first performed a right lung transplantation in a 19-year-old man who was ventilator-dependent and affected by pulmonary failure due to inha-

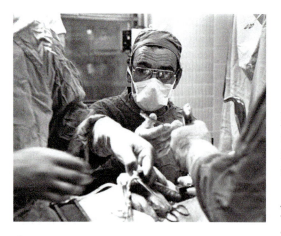

Fig. 1.6 Dr. F. Griff Pearson (1926–2016). Removal of kidneys, donor for lung transplant (Used courtesy of University Health Network Archives, Toronto, Canada)

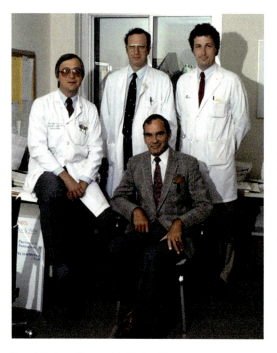

Fig. 1.7 Drs. Thomas Todd, Joel Cooper, Alec Patterson, and Griffith Pearson (seated). Toronto General Hospital Division of Thoracic Surgery (1987) (Used with permission of Joel D. Cooper, MD, FACS, Chief of Thoracic Surgery, Department of Surgery, University of Pennsylvania Health System)

lation injuries sustained during a home fire [22]. A veno-venous extracorporeal membrane oxygenator (ECMO) was previously positioned and maintained for few days after the transplant [22]. The patient survived for 17 days and died from bronchial anastomosis dehiscence [22]. The autopsy reported circumferential area of necrosis, poor healing of pulmonary artery, and atrium anastomosis [22].

Due to the results of the Toronto Centre experiments and different trials from similar groups, the human transplant program was temporarily interrupted in order to assess the bronchial anastomosis in laboratory studies [2, 11].

The 1970s to the Early 1990s: The Bronchial Anastomosis Era—Lung Transplantation Dilemma

In 1981, M. Goldberg (Toronto Group) first evaluated the combined use of cortisone and azathioprine after lung transplantation in canine models and reported bronchial anastomosis damage associated with this technique; later, he analyzed these drugs separately in order to underline the sensitivity of bronchial dehiscence to steroids [23]. Another study compared the use of different immunosuppression drugs in dogs: in the first group, dogs were treated with a combination of steroid and azathioprine; in the second group, only cyclosporine A was used; the third control group was composed of untreated dogs [24]. This analysis revealed that the correct regimen for healing anastomosis for dogs was with cyclosporine A [24].

At this time, important efforts were focused on finding a method providing bronchial arterial blood flow to the anastomosis site. R. M. Stone in 1966 (Toronto Group) demonstrated the restoration of bronchial circulation in only 4 weeks in dogs following a primary phase of cyanosis, edema, and secretion retention mainly due to irregular bronchial mucosa blood supply [25].

In 1970, N. L. Mills (New York) proposed the connection of the left bronchial artery and the intercostal arteries to the aorta as an alternative solution for left lung transplantation [26]. The control group of dogs without reimplantation evidenced more postoperative complications, such as ulcerations, poor healing anastomosis, and stenosis [26].

F. Griff Pearson (Toronto), using angiography in 1970, demonstrated the bronchial artery reconstruction after 4 weeks from lung asportation and reimplantation in dog models, thanks to the connection of the bronchial arterial channels into the bronchial wall [27]. This result was also successively confirmed by J. J. Rabinovich (Moscow) through left inferior lung lobe autotransplantation [28].

In 1977, Stanley S. Siegelman (New York) analyzed allotransplantation versus autotransplantation/reimplantation in canine models in a manner that was different from previous studies [29]. He noticed that, during the second week after the transplant, an arterial network develops around the bronchial anastomosis and that, after 31 days, a copious arterial pattern is generally present behind the anastomosis [29]. Furthermore, he announced that no correlation existed between the possible regeneration of bronchial flow and bronchial anastomosis dehiscence: some animals with bronchial flow restoration had bronchial dehiscence in any case, but the opposite situation was also observed [29].

Hence, the cause of the lung transplantation dilemma could be attributed to two different sources: the immunosuppression therapy and the correlated rejection. With Goldberg's study in mind, O. Lima and Joel D. Cooper (Toronto) introduced the omentopexy technique in 1982: using an omental pedicle appropriately vascularized and able to avoid infections, the bronchial anastomosis was reinforced and its healing facilitated [30].

After all these experimental results, the Toronto Lung Transplantation Group restarted its attempts of lung transplantation in humans.

The Successful Lung Transplantation Era: From the Mid-1990s to the Present

In 1982, Bruce A. Reitz and Norman E. Shumway (Fig. 1.8) performed the first three heart-lung transplantations in humans at the University of Stanford [31]. The three recipients were affected by primary pulmonary hypertension,

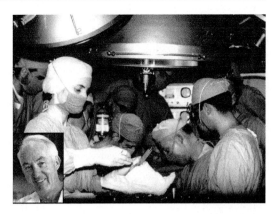

Fig. 1.8 Dr. Norman E. Shumway (1923–2006) (inset and at patient's left) performing the first adult US heart transplant with Dr. Edward Stinson, January 7, 1968 (Source: http://bulletin.facs.org/wp-content/uploads/2012/05/Shumway.jpg. Used with permission of the American College of Surgeons, Chicago, IL, USA)

Eisenmenger's syndrome, and transposition of the great vessels, respectively. In all the cases, cyclosporine A was the immunosuppression therapy: it became the primary agent for immunosuppression [31]. It was generally associated with azathioprine or mycophenolate, followed by induction therapy with basiliximab. The survival range of these three attempts was from 12 h to 23 days [31]. The Stanford Group underlined the importance of preserving the vagus nerves and the left recurrent laryngeal nerve during recipient dissection [31].

In 1982, the Toronto Group performed a right lung transplantation on a patient with respiratory failure due to an accidental paraquat poisoning; the left lung also ended up being transplanted [32]. However, paraquat induced generalized myopathy which caused the patient's death 3 months later [32]. The selection criteria of the recipient came under scrutiny, and, at this time, only patients affected by idiopathic pulmonary fibrosis and end-stage disease without important comorbidities and who were not ventilator-dependent could be treated by transplantation [2].

November 7, 1983, marked the beginning of the successful lung transplantation era with a right lung transplant in a patient who survived for nearly 5 years: the bronchial anastomosis was performed using omentopexy, and immunosuppression with azathioprine, cyclosporine, and steroid was introduced [2, 33]. After nearly 5 years, the patient died from transbronchial biopsy complications [2, 33].

For patients affected by cystic fibrosis or chronic obstructive pulmonary diseases (COPD) with bilateral impairment, a heart-lung transplant was at this point under consideration [2, 11]. However, there were several areas of concern: heart transplant was unnecessary; heart or/and lung rejection could develop simultaneously or separately; postoperative follow-up was more complicated; a right heart dysfunction could be reversible after lung transplantation [2, 11].

In light of these concerns, J. H. Dark introduced, in 1986, the en bloc double-lung transplantation with distal tracheal anastomosis, pulmonary artery anastomosis at the main pulmonary artery level, and venous anastomosis with the left atrium cuff [34]. This procedure was complicated due to the necessity of the cardiopulmonary bypass but also due to the possible tracheal anastomosis dehiscence [2]. Consequently, the Toronto Group introduced the sequential bilateral lung transplant, implanting each lung separately with transverse bilateral thoracosternotomy incision [2].

With regard to bronchial anastomosis, Joel D. Cooper in 1987 described the use of an interrupted or running sutures with Prolene® (Ethicon, Somerville, NJ, USA) for the cartilaginous portion and interrupted sutures with Vicryl® (Ethicon, Somerville, NJ, USA) for the membranous portion (the "end-to-end bronchus anastomosis") associated with the omentopexy by the omental mobilization with a small upper abdominal midline incision and its placement in subxiphoid position [35]. The omentopexy was successively abandoned in place of local tissue used to surround bronchial anastomosis [2].

J. H. Calhoon and J. K. Trinkle introduced the "telescoped bronchus anastomosis": a running suture for the posterior and membranous part of the bronchus and an interrupted figure-of-eight suture for the anterior portion [36]. Considering that generally there is some size discrepancy between the two bronchial stumps, the anastomosis telescopes one ring [36], and the donor bronchus was invaginated into the recipient bronchus by one or two cartilaginous rings [37]. This new technique did not use

omentopexy, avoided the laparotomy, and reduced surgical time [36].

E. S. Garfein described the superiority of the end-to-end bronchus anastomosis versus the telescoped one in 2001: a higher incidence of anastomotic complications was seen for the telescoped versus the end-to-end anastomosis, in particular ischemia, dehiscence, and severe stenosis [37]. At this point, certain centers adopted the end-to-end anastomosis, and others adopted the telescoped one, with the range of complications slightly higher for the telescoped anastomosis [37].

In 2002, C. Schröder introduced a modified intussuscepting technique to avoid complications (malacia, granulation tissue, or subcritical stenosis) that still remained with end-to-end or telescoped anastomosis [38]. The modified technique uses a running suture for the membranous portion, just three U stitches (at 0°, 90°, and 180°) and two or three figure-of-eight sutures in between; it allows for an improved coaptation of the bronchial walls and reduces the ledge of the bronchus that protrudes into the lumen of the other one [38].

At this juncture, new issues arose: the selection of donor and recipient; the best timing for transplant and allocation system, lung preservation, and immunosuppression; and the diagnosis of/therapy for rejection [2]. Lung transplantation at this time was indicated for all end-stage pulmonary diseases [39]: pulmonary vascular diseases, obstructive lung pathologies, and restrictive lung diseases.

In 1990, Stanford University performed the first lung transplant from a living donor: a 45-year-old mother donated a third of her right lung to substitute for the whole right lung of her 12-year-old daughter affected by bronchopulmonary dysplasia [40]. This option was not accepted as a rule due to the high risk to the pulmonary reserve of the donor [41]. However, the lack of organ donors imposed the introduction of best lung preservation strategies [41]: as reported by Thomas M. Egan (Fig. 1.9), "improved methods for preservation will increase the supply of suitable lungs…efficient use of donor organs remains of paramount importance" [39]. In the beginning, the Toronto Group used hypothermic cold saline solution before adopting the Euro-Collins solution to rinse lungs [2]. Later, S. Fujimura demonstrated the preservation of dog lungs for more

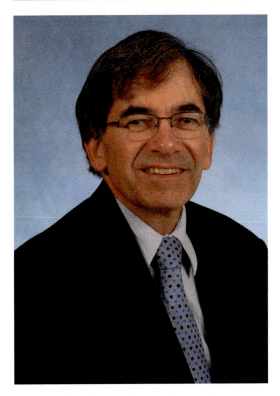

Fig. 1.9 Dr. Thomas M. Egan (Source: https://www.med. unc.edu/ct/images/Egan%20photo%202%202-11.jpg. Used with permission of University of North Carolina Health Care)

than 24 h with a low-potassium dextran solution [2, 39]. This became known as the "Fujimura solution" and was used in the following years to flush lungs during the preservation period [2, 39].

Changes in the Allocation of Donor Lung to Recipient in 1986: Allocation Prioritized Based on Severity of the Recipient Status Rather Than the Order of Listing

In 1986, the Health Resources and Services Administration (HRSA) in the United States introduced the Organ Procurement and Transplantation Network (OPTN) to create a connection between the solid organ donation organizations and the transplantation system [42]. Prior to this, the United Network for Organ Sharing (UNOS) operated the OPTN, under a contract with the HRSA [42]. The Scientific Registry for Transplant Recipients

(SRTR) with the OPTN supported the scientific and clinical status of solid organ transplant in the United States [42]. In 1990, the donor lung allocation system was based on ABO match and cumulative time on the waiting list; first, the candidate was placed into the donor service area of the donor hospital and thereafter into an area 500 nautical miles distant from this hospital [42]. In 1998, the "final rules" of the allocation system based on clinical criteria and medical urgency were drafted, with the purpose of sharing organs and reducing the number of deaths on the waiting list [43]. Finally, in 2005, a new system of allocation was created by the OPTN, the Lung Allocation Score (LAS): a donor priority was assigned based on a score calculated using the waiting list survival (urgency criteria) and the 1-year survival after transplant; this score has been regularly updated; is still in use in the United States, Germany, and the Netherlands; and is used by the Eurotransplant Program when the match is outside of the donor's country [2].

Information sharing internationally in the field of heart and lung transplant became mandatory at this point in order to improve knowledge in this field; therefore, in 1981, Norman E. Shumway founded the International Society for Heart and Lung Transplantation (ISHLT), a voluntary registry and data sharing organization and a source for classifications and guidelines that are still used to this day [2].

In 1993, the ISHLT introduced the concept of bronchiolitis obliterans syndrome (BOS) as a chronic allograft dysfunction in order to address post-lung transplantation dysfunction [2]. Recently, restrictive allograft syndrome was recognized as a new form of chronic lung rejection [2]. Regarding immunosuppression therapy, the associated use of calcineurin inhibitor, steroid, and either azathioprine or mycophenolate mofetil has continued as a drug strategy after lung transplantation [2].

At this point, the topic of bronchial artery revascularization after lung transplantation was being revisited, and it is important to mention several developments. Since H. H. J. Schreinemakers [44, 45], who reemphasized the possible role of bronchial ischemia in airway healing impairment and previously described the use of an intercostobronchial artery pedicle [46], different attempts were subsequently published. L. Couraud described the possible use of a vein graft [47, 48].

In 1993, R. C. Daly and Magdi H. Yacoub described the possible use of the left internal thoracic artery in double-lung transplantation to obtain an immediate revascularization of the whole tracheobronchial tree [49]. In 1994, they showed analogous data concerning the single-lung transplantation [45]. In 1996, M. A. Norgaard highlighted the convincing results of the correlation between the healing bronchial airway and bronchial artery revascularization and the long-term patency of the mammary artery [50]. Lastly, the wide experience of Copenhagen Group showed the use of mammary artery for single-/double-lung transplantation or heart-lung transplant [48, 51].

The entire role and long-term outcome of bronchial revascularization should be confirmed by future multicenter studies [52].

In order to increase the donor organ number, different strategies have been introduced, such as extending donor criteria and/or using deceased cardiac donors (DCD) [53]. The field of normothermic ex vivo lung perfusion (EVLP) developed in response to questionable and injured lungs in order to expand donor criteria [53]. The first report of nor-mothermic ex vivo organ experiences was described by Alexis Carrel and C. A. Lindbergh in 1935 [53, 54], while the first EVLP was presented by D. W. Jirsch in 1970 [55]. However, these experiences failed due to the loss of the lung alveolar-capillary barrier, the onset of edema, and the vascular resistance increase during EVLP [53]. The Steen Solution (XVIVO Perfusion, Göteborg, Sweden) was introduced as lung perfusion to maintain the fluid in the intravascular space and supply nutrients for pulmonary homeostasis [56–58]. At this juncture, the main issue was the duration of the preservation period, which was less than 60 min. Hence, in 2008, the Toronto Group introduced a new EVLP method in order to extend this time to longer than 12 h and, thus, gain time to assess, recondition, and repair the donor lungs [53, 59]. Actually, the Toronto method is the one most used for the EVLP: it consists of creating an optimal environment for the donor lung operation, a protective ventilation setting without circuit-induced injuries (using flow parameter to prevent mechanical shear stress), and adopting a perfusate with a chemical composition appropriate for homeostasis [53]. See Fig. 1.10.

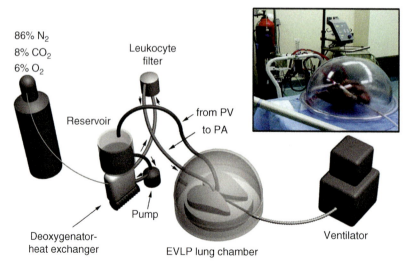

Fig. 1.10 Cypel ex vivo lung circuit. EVLP normothermic lung circuit allowing both functional assessment and repair. Note insert's red tank indicating a hypoxic gas. For more information see Cypel M, Liu M, Rubacha M, Yeung JC, Hirayama S, Anraku M, Sato M, Medin J, Davidson BL, de Perrot M, Waddell TK, Slutsky AS, Keshavjee S. Functional repair of human donor lungs by IL-10 gene therapy. Sci Transl Med. 2009;Oct 28:1(4):4ra9; and Steen S, Ingemansson R, Eriksson L, Pierre L, Algotsson L, Wierup P, Liao Q, Eyjolfsson A, Gustafsson R, Sjöberg T. First human transplantation of a nonacceptable donor lung after reconditioning ex vivo. Ann Thorac Surg. 2007;83(6):2191–4 (Used with permission of Dr. James G. Chandler and the American College of Surgeons, from http://bulletin.facs.org/2012/01/sanctity-2/#.WqBgCGrwaM9)

Despite the controversy that emerged at the beginning of DCD attempts due to the frailty of the donor lungs, there were reports of successes; starting with one first reported in 1995 by R. B. Love [60], later attempts also confirmed positive results, as demonstrated by G. I. Snell in 2008 [61] and successive ones by Jeremie Reeb [62] and Marcelo Cypel [63]. Thus, a new category of lung donor developed: the uncontrolled donation after circulatory determination of death donor (uDCDD) associated with the use of EVLP. Good postoperative outcomes have been reported [53, 64, 65].

References

1. Demikhov VP. Experimental transplantation of vital organs. New York: Consultants Bureau; 1962.
2. Vigneswaran W, Garrity E, Odell J. Lung transplantation: principles and practice. General topics. History of lung transplantation. Boca Raton: CRC Press; 2015.
3. Carrel A, Guthrie CC. Anastomosis of blood vessels by the patching method and transplantation of kidney (classical article reprinted from JAMA 1906;47:1648-51). Yale J Biol Med. 2001;74:243–7.
4. Carrel A. The surgery of blood vessels, etc. Bull John Hopkins Hosp. 1907;18:18–28.
5. Murray JE, Merril JP, Harrison JH. Kidney transplantation between seven pairs of identical twins. Ann Surg. 1958;148:343–57.
6. Metras H. Note preliminare sur la greffe totale du pumon chez le chien. Proc Acad Sci (Paris). 1950;231:1176–8.
7. Staudacher V, Bellinazzo P, Pulin A. Primi rilievi su tentativi di reimpianti autoplastici e di trapianti omoplastici dei lobi pulmonari. Chirurgia (Milano). 1959;5:233–27.
8. Juvenelle AA, Citret C, Wiles CE, Stewart JD. Pneumonectomy with replantation of the lung in the dog for physiologic study. J Thorac Surg. 1951;21:111–5.
9. Neptune WB, Weller R, Bailey CP. Experimental lung transplantation. J Thorac Surg. 1953;26:275–89.
10. Hardin CA, Kittle CE. Experiences with transplantation of the lung. Science. 1954;119:97–8.
11. Shumway SJ, Shumway NE. Thoracic transplantation. Part I. Historical background. Blackwell Science: Cambridge; 1995.
12. Blumenstock DA, Collin JA, Thomas ED, Ferrebee JW. Homotransplants of the lung in dogs. Surgery. 1962;51:541–5.
13. Hardy JD, Eraslan S, Dalton ML Jr, Alican F, Turner MD. Re-implantation and homotransplantations of the lung: laboratory studies and clinical potential. Ann Surg. 1963;157:707–18.
14. Hardy JD, Webb WR, Dalton ML, Walker GR. Lung homotransplantations in man. JAMA. 1963;186:1065–74.
15. Derom F, Barbier F, Ringoir S, Versieck J, Rolly G, Berzsenyi G, Vermeire P, Vrints L. Ten month survival after lung homotransplantations in man. J Thorac Cardiovasc Surg. 1971;61:835–46.
16. Veith FJ. Lung transplantation. Ann Thorac Surg. 1970;9:580–3.
17. Nakae S, Webb WR, Theodorides T, Sugg WL. Respiratory function following cardiopulmonary denervation in dog, cat, and monkey. Surg Gynecol Obstet. 1967;125:1285–92.
18. Yeh TJ, Ellison LT, Ellison RG. Functional evaluation of the autotransplanted lung in the dog. Am Rev Resp Dis. 1962;86:791–7.
19. Linberg EJ, Demetriades A, Armstrong BW, Konsuwan N. Lung reimplantation in the dog. JAMA. 1961;178:486–7.
20. Blumenstock DA, Kahn DR. Replantation and transplantation of the canine lung. J Surg Res. 1961;1:40–7.
21. Veith FJ, Richards K. Improved technic for canine lung transplantation. Ann Surg. 1970;171:553–8.
22. Nelems JMB, Rebuck AS, Cooper JD, Goldberg M, Halloran PF, Vellend H. Human lung transplantation. Chest. 1980;78:569–73.
23. Lima O, Cooper JD, Peters WJ, Ayabe H, Townsend E, Luk SC, Goldberg M. Effects of methylprednisolone and azathioprine on bronchial healing following lung autotransplantation. J Thorac Cardiovasc Surg. 1981;82:211–5.
24. Goldberg M, Lima O, Morgan E, Ayabe HA, Luk S, Ferdman A, Peters WJ, Cooper JD. A comparison between cyclosporin A and methylprednisolone plus azathioprine on bronchial healing following canine lung autotransplantation. J Thorac Cardiovasc Surg. 1983;85:821–6.
25. Stone RM, Ginsberg RJ, Colapinto RF, Pearson FG. Bronchial artery regeneration after radical hilar stripping. Surg Forum. 1966;17:109–10.
26. Mills NL, Boyd AD, Gheranpong C, Spencer FC. The significance of bronchial circulation in lung transplantation. J Thorac Cardiovasc Surg. 1970;60:866–74.
27. Pearson FG, Golberg M, Stone RM, Colapinto RF. Bronchial arterial circulation restored after reimplantation of canine lung. Can J Surg. 1970;13:243–50.
28. Rabinovich JJ. Re-establishment of bronchial arteries after experimental lung lobe autotransplantation. J Thorac Cardiovasc Surg. 1972;64:119–26.
29. Siegelman SS, Hagstrom JWC, Koerner SR, Veith FJ. Restoration of bronchial artery circulation after canine lung allotransplantation. J Thorac Cardiovasc Surg. 1977;73:792–5.
30. Lima O, Goldberg M, Peters WJ, Ayabe H, Townsend E, Cooper JD. Bronchial omentopexy in canine lung transplantation. J Thorac Cardiovasc Surg. 1982;83:418–21.

31. Reitz BA, Wallwork JL, Hunt SA, Pennock JL, Billingham ME, Oyer PE, Stinson EB, Shumway NE. Heart-lung transplantation: successful therapy for patients with pulmonary vascular disease. N Engl J Med. 1982;306:557–64.
32. Toronto Lung Transplant Group. Sequential bilateral lung transplantation for Paraquat poisoning. J Thorac Cardiovasc Surg. 1985;89:734–42.
33. Toronto Lung Transplant Group. Unilateral lung transplantation for pulmonary fibrosis. N Engl J Med. 1986;314:1140–5.
34. Dark JH, Patterson GA, Al-Jilaihawi AN, Hsu H, Egan TM, Cooper JD. Experimental en bloc double-lung transplantation. Ann Thorac Surg. 1986;42(4):394–8.
35. Cooper JD, Pearson FG, Patterson GA, Todd TR, Ginsberg RJ, Goldberg M, DeMajo WA. Technique of successful lung transplantation in humans. J Thorac Cardiovasc Surg. 1987;93(2):173–81.
36. Calhoon JH, Grover FL, Gibbons WJ, Bryan CL, Levine SM, Bailey SR, Nichols L, Lum C, Trinkle JK. Single lung transplantation. Alternative indications and technique. J Thorac Cardiovasc Surg. 1991;101(5):816–24.
37. Garfein ES, Ginsberg ME, Gorenstein L, McGregor CC, Schulman LL. Superiority of end-to-end versus telescoped bronchial anastomosis in single lung transplantation for pulmonary emphysema. J Thorac Cardiovasc Surg. 2001;121(1):149–54.
38. Schröder C, Scholl F, Daon E, Goodwin A, Frist WH, Roberts JR, Christian KG, Ninan M, Milstone AP, Loyd JE, Merrill WH, Pierson RN III. A modified bronchial anastomosis technique for lung transplantation. Ann Thorac Surg. 2003;75(6):1697–704.
39. Egan TM, Kaiser LR, Cooper JD. Lung transplantation. Curr Probl Surg. 1989;26:673–751.
40. Goldsmith MF. Mother to child: first living donor lung transplant. JAMA. 1990;264:2724.
41. American Thoracic Society, Medical Section of the American Lung Association. Lung transplantation. Report of the ATS workshop on lung transplantation. American Thoracic Society, Medical Section of the American Lung Association. Am Rev Respir Dis. 1993;147:772–6.
42. Egan TM, Murray S, Bustami RT, Shearon TH, McCullough KP, Edwards LB, Coke MA, Garrity ER, Sweet SC, Heiney DA, Grover FL. Development of the new lung allocation system in the United States. Am J Transplant. 2006;6:1212–27.
43. Health Resources and Services Administration (HRSA), Department of Health and Human Services (HHS). Organ procurement and transplantation network. Final Rule. Fed Regist. 2013;78:40033–42.
44. Schreinemakers HHJ, De Leyn PRJ, Marcus M, Wouters P, Moerman F, Flameng W, Lerut A, Cooper J. Role of bronchial arteries in lung function. Ann Thorac Surg. 1992;54:395–7.
45. Daly RC, McGregor CG. Routine immediate direct bronchial artery revascularization for single-lung transplantation. Ann Thorac Surg. 1994;57:1446–52.
46. Schreinemakers HH, Weder W, Miyoshi S, Harper BD, Shimokawa S, Egan TM, McKnight R, Cooper JD. Direct revascularization of bronchial arteries for lung transplantation: an anatomical study. Ann Thorac Surg. 1990;49:44–53.
47. Couraud L, Baudet E, Martigne C, Roques X, Velly JF, Laborde N, Dubrez J, Clerc F, Dromer C, Vallieres E. Bronchial revascularization in double-lung transplantation: a series of 8 patients. Bordeaux Lung and Heart-Lung Transplant Group. Ann Thorac Surg. 1992;53:88–94.
48. Pettersson G, Nørgaard MA, Arendrup H, Brandenhof P, Helvind M, Joyce F, Stentoft P, Olesen PS, Thiis JJ, Efsen F, Mortensen SA, Svendsen UG. Direct bronchial artery revascularization and en bloc double lung transplantation—surgical techniques and early outcome. J Heart Lung Transplant. 1997;16:320–33.
49. Daly RC, Tadjkarimi S, Khaghani A, Banner NR, Yacoub MH. Successful double-lung transplantation with direct bronchial artery revascularization. Ann Thorac Surg. 1993;56:885–92.
50. Nørgaard MA, Olsen PS, Svendsen UG, Pettersson G. Revascularization of the bronchial arteries in lung transplantation: an overview. Ann Thorac Surg. 1996;62:1215–21.
51. Nørgaard MA, Efsen F, Arendrup H, Olsen PS, Svendsen UG, Pettersson G. Surgical and arteriographic results of bronchial artery revascularization in lung and heart lung transplantation. J Heart Lung Transplant. 1997;16:302–12.
52. Pettersson GB, Yun JJ, Nørgaard MA. Bronchial artery revascularization in lung transplantation: techniques, experience, and outcomes. Curr Opin Organ Transplant. 2010;15:572–7.
53. Reeb J, Cypel M. Ex vivo lung perfusion. Clin Transpl. 2016;30(3):183–94.
54. Carrel A, Lindbergh CA. The culture of whole organs. Science. 1935;81:621–3.
55. Jirsch DW, Fisk RL, Couves CM. Ex vivo evaluation of stored lungs. Ann Thorac Surg. 1970;10(2):163–8.
56. Steen S, Sjoberg T, Pierre L, Liao Q, Eriksson L, Algotsson L. Transplantation of lungs from non-heart beating donor. Lancet. 2001;357:825–9.
57. Steen S, Liao Q, Wierup PN, Bolys R, Pierre L, Sjöberg T. Transplantation of lungs from non-heart-beating donors after functional assessment ex vivo. Ann Thorac Surg. 2003;76(1):244–52.
58. Steen S, Ingemansson R, Eriksson L, Pierre L, Algotsson L, Wierup P, Liao Q, Eyjolfsson A, Gustafsson R, Sjöberg T. First human transplantation of a nonacceptable donor lung after reconditioning ex vivo. Ann Thorac Surg. 2007;83(6):2191–4.
59. Cypel M, Yeung JC, Hirayama S, Rubacha M, Fischer S, Anraku M, Sato M, Harwood S, Pierre A, Waddell TK, de Perrot M, Liu M, Keshavjee S. Technique for prolonged normothermic ex vivo lung perfusion. J Heart Lung Transplant. 2008;27(12):1319–25.

60. Love RB, Stringham JC, Chomiak PN, Warner T, Pellett JR, Mentzer RM. Successful lung transplantation using a non-heart-beating donor [abstract]. J Heart Lung Transplant. 1995;14:S88.

61. Snell GI, Levvey BJ, Oto T, McEgan R, Pilcher D, Davies A, Marasco S, Rosenfeldt F. Early lung transplantation success utilizing controlled donation after cardiac death donors. Am J Transplant. 2008;8(6):1282–9.

62. Reeb J, Keshavjee S, Cypel M. Expanding the lung donor pool: advancements and emerging pathways. Curr Opin Organ Transplant. 2015;20(5): 498–505.

63. Cypel M, Levvey B, Van Raemdonck D, Erasmus M, Dark J, Love R, Mason D, Glanville AR, Chambers D, Edwards LB, Stehlik J, Hertz M, Whitson BA, Yusen RD, Puri V, Hopkins P, Snell G, Keshavjee S, International Society for Heart and Lung Transplantation. International Society for Heart and Lung Transplantation donation after Circulatory Death Registry Report. J Heart Lung Transplant. 2015;34(10):1278–82.

64. Egan TM. Lung transplant from an uncontrolled donation after circulatory determination of death donor: moving to other countries. Am J Transplant. 2016;16(4):1051–2.

65. Egan TM, Requard JJ. Uncontrolled donation after circulatory determination of death donors (uDCDDs) as a source of lungs for transplant. Am J Transplant. 2015;15(8):2031–6.

Single- and Bilateral Lung Transplantation: Indications, Contraindications, Evaluation, and Requirements for Patients to Be Considered Eligible

Gerard J. Meachery and Paul A. Corris

Abbreviations

BLT	Bilateral lung transplant
BMI	Body mass index
CF	Cystic fibrosis
CHDAPAH	Congenital heart disease-associated pulmonary arterial hypertension
COPD	Chronic obstructive pulmonary disease
CPB	Cardiopulmonary bypass
CT	Computed tomography
CTEPH	Chronic thromboembolic pulmonary hypertension
DLCO	Diffusing capacity for carbon monoxide
ECLS	Extracorporeal lung support
ECMO	Extracorporeal membrane oxygenation
FEV1	Forced expiratory volume in one second
FVC	Forced vital capacity
HLT	Heart-lung transplant
ILD	Interstitial lung disease
IPAH	Idiopathic pulmonary arterial hypertension
IPF	Idiopathic pulmonary fibrosis
ISHLT	International Society for Heart and Lung Transplantation
LAD	Lung assist device
LAS	Lung allocation score
LLLT	Living lobar lung transplantation
NSIP	Non-specific interstitial pneumonitis
NTM	Non-tuberculous mycobacteria
NYHA FC	New York Heart Association Functional Class
PAH	Pulmonary arterial hypertension
PH	Pulmonary hypertension
SLT	Single-lung transplant
SSc	Systemic sclerosis
UIP	Usual interstitial pneumonitis
UNOS	United Network for Organ Sharing
US	United States

G. J. Meachery (✉)
Department of Respiratory Medicine,
Freeman Hospital,
Newcastle Upon Tyne, UK
e-mail: gerard.meachery@nuth.nhs.uk

P. A. Corris
Department of Respiratory Medicine, Freeman Hospital and Institute of Cellular Medicine, Newcastle University, Newcastle Upon Tyne, UK
e-mail: paul.corris@ncl.ac.uk

Introduction

Despite significant advances in pharmacological and remedial therapies, there remains a large proportion of patients with end-stage lung disease who require lung transplantation as a definitive method of treatment to enhance life expectancy and improve health-related quality of life. Multiple factors determine the suitability of potential lung transplant recipients. Solid organ lung transplantation is indicated for patients with medically and/or surgically refractory end-stage lung disease when expected survival is anticipated to be limited. While the major limitation to the number of transplants performed is primarily the lack of availability of suitable organ donors, cogent to successful outcome is the patient selection process. Despite recognized variation in patient selection processes between transplant centers, the principal goal is the evaluation and identification of individuals who fulfill criteria of end-stage lung disease and who are deemed potentially suitable candidates based on strict eligibility criteria and rigorous assessment.

The overall evaluation process aims to define the relevant disease characteristics and attempt to individualize the predicted trajectory of disease activity to inform timing of intervention and maximize potentially successful outcomes. This task is inherently challenging given the heterogeneity of the disease processes leading to end-stage lung disease and the lack of reliable predictive models and evidence-based practice in informing the selection process and potential outcomes. Strategies to inform clinical decision-making worldwide have recently led to an updated consensus statement by the International Society for Heart and Lung Transplantation [1] that endeavors to assist physicians in rationalizing the referral process of suitable individuals for lung transplantation.

Key Requirements to Consider Candidacy for Lung Transplantation (Fig. 2.1)

When considering referring an individual for a lung transplant assessment, it is important to be cognizant of the absolute contraindications that would halt the patient selection process immediately. Once the referring clinician has excluded absolute general contraindications to lung transplantation, the next step is to define the candidate's suitability from a respiratory viewpoint. This involves rigorous evaluation of the individual's disease burden, confirmation of refractory disease, and assessment of their fitness for transplantation (Table 2.1).

Next in the patient selection process is the identification of relative contraindications including identification of comorbidities [2] that may impact negatively on outcome while balancing against potential benefit. A risk-benefit profile is constructed. This involves extensive blood tests; functional and radiological investigations; screening for malignancy, infection, and autoimmune disease; and a dental review. In addition, it is imperative to assess adherence to complete cessation of substance abuse or dependency and assess an individual's ability to comply with self-care behaviors demanded of such a complex regime of medical care. Additional specialist consultations may be warranted pending the underlying cause of lung disease or in those patients deemed as higher-risk candidates (Table 2.1). Such preliminary assessments are part of a rigorous screening process to ensure appropriate patient selection while identifying any areas (both clinical and psychosocial [3]) that may benefit from targeted interventional strategies [4].

The lung allocation score (LAS), devised by the United Network for Organ Sharing (UNOS), in 2005, is a numerical score based on the concept of "net transplant benefit," with those in greatest need and expected to derive most benefit receiving a maximum score of 100 [5]. Implementation of the LAS in the USA has significantly impacted on the patient selection process [6–8] and has led to the transplantation of older and sicker individuals [9], most notably patients with idiopathic pulmonary fibrosis [6, 10, 11]. While increasing LAS predicts reduced survival in lung transplant recipients [12, 13], its implementation has impacted on the number of procedures performed and waiting list deaths and resulted in a paradigm shift in recipient diagnosis and perhaps a small but significant increase in 1-year survival [14]. However, its translation into clinical practice has been associated with increasing resource use [15], and further evaluation of its merit worldwide is ongoing.

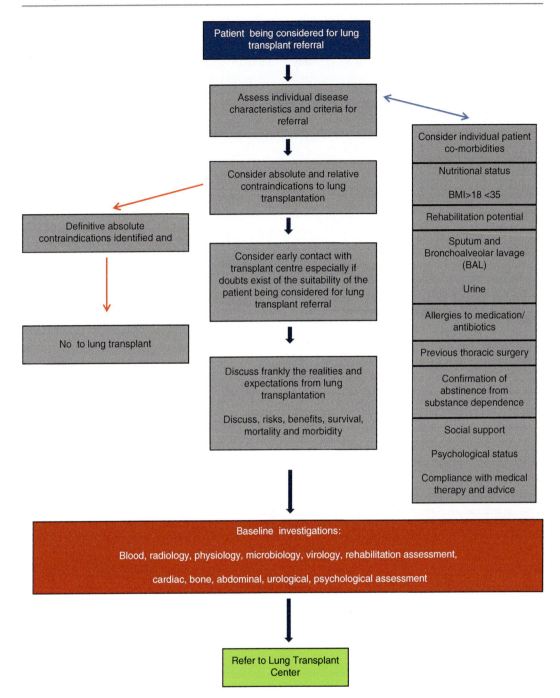

Fig. 2.1 Lung transplant referral pathway

Table 2.1 Key investigations and assessments to appraise patient suitability for lung transplantation

Blood profile	Full blood count
	Coagulation screen
	Urea, electrolytes, creatinine
	Glomerular filtration rate (GFR)
	Glucose
	Liver function
	Bone profile
	Magnesium, phosphate
	Lipid profile
	Thyroid function
	Blood group
	HLA antibodies
	Serum panel-reactive antibody (PRA) status
	Autoimmune screen
	Prostate-specific antigen (PSA)
Pulmonary function tests	Spirometry, lung volumes, diffusion capacity
	Maximal inspiratory and expiratory pressures
	Arterial blood gas analysis
Functional exercise assessment	6-min walk test (6MWT)
Cardiac functional assessment	Electrocardiogram
	Echocardiogram
	Coronary angiography
	[a]Right heart catheter studies
	[a]Cardiopulmonary exercise test
Microbiology	Sputum
	Urine
	Swabs for methicillin-resistant Staphylococcus aureus
	Hepatitis serology
	HIV serology
	Epstein-Barr serology
	Cytomegalovirus serology
	Varicella zoster serology
Radiology assessment	Chest radiograph
	Chest computed tomography
	Differential perfusion lung scan
Additional assessments	Bone mineral density
	Nutritional assessment
	Dental assessment
	Psychology profile
	Physiotherapy
	Exercise rehabilitation program
	Ambulatory oxygen assessment
	[b]Others

[a]Pulmonary arterial hypertension
[b]Consideration for appropriate specialty referral should be made in light of each patient's individual assessment. These would include, but not limited to, (a) cardiology referral and further cardiac imaging, e.g., cardiac MRI if there is concern of cardiac ventricular function, (b) gastroenterology where applicable if there are concerns of underlying gastrointestinal disease or malignancy, (c) urology referral for renal calculi or unexplained recurrent urinary tract infection, and (d) neurology referral, particularly in patients with pre-existing neurological disorders, e.g., epilepsy

Absolute Contraindications

There are several absolute contraindications to lung transplantation which include:

1. Severe liver or renal impairment (synthetic function of liver and creatinine clearance <50 mL/min with preserved cardiac output)
2. Heart failure with reduced systolic function
3. Active and ongoing nicotine dependence
4. Active and ongoing substance abuse and dependence (including alcohol and narcotics)
5. Progressive neuromuscular disease
6. Active malignancy (within the past 2 years) with the exceptions of skin basal cell carcinoma and squamous cell carcinoma
7. Remote history (within the past 5 years) of the following malignancies: breast carcinoma (stage 2+), extracapsular renal cell carcinoma, colonic carcinoma (Duke A+), and malignant melanoma level III+)

In such instances conventional tumor markers may not always be sensitive or specific to the presence of occult malignancy and may simply reflect end-stage lung disease, such as in IPF [16]. Hence, monitoring of CEA levels confers no additional benefit on prediction of survival posttransplant nor the presence or development of malignancy [17].

Relative Contraindications

Relative contraindications to lung transplantation are primarily comorbidities (but not exclusively) that are deemed to potentially impact on long-term outcome. It is these relative contraindications that may benefit most from targeted interventional strategies prior to active patient listing. Although older patients often have a poorer outcome post-lung transplant, due to increasing comorbidities, increased age alone does not infer recipient ineligibility. Older patients (over 65 years old) often require more extensive investigations due to the recognized potential to develop comorbidities of the central nervous system, cardiovascular system, and peripheral vascular system and risk of malignancy prior to consideration for transplantation [18–21].

Medical comorbidities such as poorly controlled diabetes mellitus, hypertension, arteriosclerosis, epilepsy, peptic ulcer disease, gastroesophageal reflux disease, and chronic venous obstruction are only contraindications to lung transplantation if they result in end-organ damage and should be optimally treated preoperatively [1]. In the setting of coronary artery disease, candidates may warrant coronary revascularization preoperatively to maximize their potential for a good long-term outcome. The use of corticosteroids no longer prohibits active transplant listing; however, it should always be endeavored to either discontinue or minimize the daily dosage (ideally to less than 20 mg/day).

Severe symptomatic osteoporosis confers significant morbidity posttransplantation due to the increased risk of fractures and reduced health-related quality of life, and targeted therapy to preserve bone mass and improve bone density should be implemented prior to transplantation [22–29]. In addition body mass index (BMI) should be regulated with targeted weight gain in the case of cachexia to achieve and sustain a minimum BMI of 18.0 kg/m^2 and maintained weight loss in the case of obesity (Class I; BMI 30.0–34.9 kg/m^2) as both factors have been associated with poorer outcomes posttransplant, albeit if only in the short term in the case of preoperative obesity [30].

Chronic viral infections such as hepatitis B and C (HCV) and HIV are considered relative contraindications to lung transplantation. In such instances, stabilized disease on appropriate treatment without significant end-organ sequelae may be deemed suitable for transplantation [1]. Despite conflicting evidence on lung transplant outcome [31, 32], in the era of interferon-based therapy, 5-year survival rates in HCV-seropositive patients would appear identical to HCV-seronegative patients [33, 34]. Similarly HIV patients, compliant on combined antiretroviral therapy, with stable HIV disease and undetectable HIV RNA are considered suitable candidates; yet the long-term outcomes have yet to be fully elucidated [35, 36].

Other chronic infections such as multidrug-resistant *Mycobacterium abscessus*, *Burkholderia cenocepacia*, and *Burkholderia gladioli* do not absolutely preclude transplantation if the infection is adequately treated preoperatively and the presumption that sufficient control can be achieved postoperatively. However, in practice, many centers do not offer lung transplantation to these candidates due to the recognized associated poorer outcomes and survival. Hence, it is recommended that patients colonized by these organisms are best assessed by centers with the demonstrable expertise of their management to improve a candidate's transplant chances and outcome. It is also imperative that patients and their family are aware of the significant increased risk and poorer health outcomes with infection or colonization with these organisms [37, 38].

Another relative contraindication and potential concern is chronological age as lung transplant recipients over 70 years of age have a poorer outcome [39]. While some lung transplant programs strictly adhere to the 70-year age cutoff for consideration of lung transplantation (with a cutoff of 65 years in certain transplant centers), other programs assess the chronological age on a case-by-case basis determined by the overall health, fitness, and motivation of the 70+ years potential recipient. Indeed, over the past 15 years, survival in this advanced age group has reported improving outcomes [40].

With the advent of new antifibrotic agents—pirfenidone and nintedanib—that are indicated for the treatment of idiopathic pulmonary fibrosis (IPF) to decrease the rate of disease progression and thus appropriate to be used for the patient tolerating the medication, while waiting for lung transplantation, there are no data to consider the use of these agents as absolute or relative contraindication for lung transplantation [41–44]. A recent observational study in a small number of patients documented no adverse effects of lung transplantation in patients who were on antifibrotic agents at the time of lung transplantation and follow-up of 1 year [45].

While the indications and contraindications are in general accepted by most if not all lung transplant programs, variations and policies of the individual lung transplant programs may vary and are tailored to their individual program.

Choice of Lung Transplant Operative Procedure

Bilateral Lung Transplant (BLT) Versus Single-Lung Transplant (SLT)

Bilateral lung transplantation (BLT) is consistently indicated in patients with evidence of chronic suppurative lung disease (such as cystic fibrosis (CF)- and non-CF-related bronchiectasis) or evidence of chronic colonization with microorganisms deemed a high peri- and/or postoperative deleterious infective risk. However, in a patient with a rapidly declining respiratory status, single-lung transplantation is often considered, particularly when balancing between the critical and urgent medical need, with the challenge of donor organ shortages.

Variation between centers on the choice of transplant operation remains. BLT is often the surgical procedure of choice in patients with preexistent idiopathic pulmonary arterial hypertension and right ventricular dysfunction, to reduce the risk of primary graft dysfunction that may negatively impact on survival. BLT is also considered in patients with congenital heart disease-associated pulmonary arterial hypertension where the primary cardiac defect is assessed as suitable to undergo corrective surgery during the lung transplant procedure. The registry of the International Society for Heart and Lung Transplantation (ISHLT) reports that the percentage of bilateral lung transplant procedures have consistently risen worldwide, accounting for in excess of 70% of all lung transplant procedures [46]. The evolution of this practice can be accounted by historical reports of survival benefit of bilateral lung transplant recipients compared to single-lung transplant recipients, even accounting for selection bias [47–49].

The technique of single-lung transplantation and subsequently of bilateral sequential lung transplantation was pioneered by Joel Cooper's group in Toronto with the SLT procedure first successfully performed in 1983. SLT is associated with less morbidity and mortality compared with other transplant procedures, has shorter operating times, is performed without extracorporeal support, and generally has shorter waiting times for a single donor organ [50–52]. Outcomes following SLT in cases of secondary pulmonary hypertension associated with advanced lung disease remain controversial. Meyer and colleagues systematically reviewed the outcomes of 279 consecutive SLT recipients, stratified by mean pulmonary artery pressure, attending a single transplant center. The findings suggest that primary graft dysfunction and long-term survival did not differ significantly between patient groups, advocating that SLT is safe in patients with pulmonary hypertension associated with advanced lung disease. Moreover, Schaffer and colleagues has shown that the disease process and procedure choice may impact on graft survival with BLT demonstrated to confer a survival advantage, over SLT in patients with IPF but not COPD [53]. These findings are in stark contrast to historical reports in the pre-LAS era, when BLT for COPD had reported better outcomes over SLT.

Moreover the results for SLT in patients who were selected on their suitability for this procedure on the basis of a lack of evidence for bacterial or fungal colonization in the pretransplant period (suggesting that the native lung to be left intact would not confer a posttransplant infective risk) or a lack of evidence for true bronchiectasis with impaired sputum clearance (and not just a descriptive radiological reference to traction bronchiectasis seen in pulmonary fibrosis patients) as well as various reports of adjusted analyses finding no statistically significant differ-

ence in survival in IPF patients who received BLT or SLT suggest that the widespread drift toward performing BLT in all patients should be challenged [47, 54–58]. This point is particularly important to highlight when donor shortage continues to mitigate the restriction in the number of patients that can be transplanted or when only a single lung is available from a donor for transplantation to a recipient at high risk of mortality on the transplant waiting list. The data supporting the value of SLT in older recipients and SLT in the presence of secondary pulmonary hypertension (WHO Group 3 disease) demonstrate that the presence of pulmonary hypertension alone in this setting should not have a primary influence in mandating a decision to proceed with BLT. Finally, data from a national cohort study in the UK demonstrated that survival immediately posttransplantation was not significantly different for BLT or SLT in patients with pulmonary fibrosis (referred to as the diffuse parenchymal lung disease or DPLD group of patients in this study). Not surprisingly this study showed waiting list mortality was at the highest risk for pulmonary fibrosis patients compared to patients with COPD who were at lower risk than all other patient groups, with pulmonary fibrosis patients having a better chance of survival from listing if they are listed for SLT (Box 2.1) [59].

Box 2.1 Summary Box for Choice of Transplant Operation: Bilateral Lung Transplant Versus Single Lung Transplant

Indications for BLT
Bilateral suppurative disease such as CF, bronchiectasis
COPD with large bilateral ventilated bullae
COPD with bilateral evidence of bronchiectasis
IPF with regular bacterial or fungal isolates from sputum
Group 1 pulmonary arterial hypertension
Indications for consideration of SLT
IPF with or without PAH and negative sputum microbiology
Elderly COPD patients without bilateral bullae or bronchiectasis

Heart-Lung Transplantation (HLT)

Heart-lung transplantation (HLT) first performed successfully by the transplant group in Stanford in 1981 [60] heralded a new era in surgical treatment options for selected patients with severe end-stage lung disease. In more recent times, the continued limitations imposed by the shortage in suitable donor organs have necessitated a focus of this limited transplant resource. HLT is considered mainly for patients with irreparable complex congenital heart defects with associated Eisenmenger's syndrome and pulmonary arterial hypertension, patients with severe end-stage lung disease with significant coronary artery disease that cannot be remedied by percutaneous coronary arterial revascularization, as well as a selected group of patients that have severe intrinsic left ventricular dysfunction and/or severe right ventricular diastolic dysfunction with concomitant end-stage lung disease [61].

Size Reduction Lung Transplant (Including Cadaveric Bilateral Lobar Lung Transplantation, Cadaveric Split Lung Transplantation, Peripheral Resection Size Reduction Lung Transplantation, Living Lobar Lung Transplantation)

The scarcity of suitable lung donors adds to the challenge of successfully obtaining suitably sized donors for pediatric and small lung transplant recipients. Innovative approaches have been developed in operative techniques to utilize lungs from larger-sized donors to be surgically reduced in size for an appropriate smaller recipient. The Vienna University transplant group reported their experience with cadaveric split lung transplantation, lobar transplantation, and peripheral resection size reduction lung transplantation. This group reported no statistically significant difference between the standard lung transplant group and the size reduction transplant group in terms of surgical complications, bronchial healing, and postoperative bleeding. Three-month survival was 85.2% in the size-reduced transplant group compared to a survival of 92.9% in the standard lung transplant group [62]. Further reports from other centers have lent support to this strategy that provides additional opportunities to optimize the utilization of a scarce resource in smaller-sized recipients [63]. Living lobar lung transplantation (LLLT) is performed as a bilateral sequential lung transplant procedure in the recipient, in most cases utilizing a clam shell approach to gain surgical access to the thorax. In all cases, it is expected that hyperinflation of the lobar lung grafts associated with expected remodeling of the thoracic cage will eventually lead to gradual filling of the pleural space [64–68].

Intraoperative Extracorporeal Lung Support (ECLS)

The routine use of intraoperative extracorporeal support in bilateral lung transplantation varies considerably between centers and surgical operators. The most commonly used modality is cardiopulmonary bypass (CPB). The argument for the use of extracorporeal support is advocated by the intention to avoid uncontrolled reperfusion of the lung that has been implanted first as well as providing intraoperative cardiac and circulatory stability. Increasingly, the utilization of extracorporeal membrane oxygenation (ECMO) has gained favor with the added advantage of avoiding full heparinization and consequent reduction of blood products and reduction in bleeding risk. However, as opposed to CPB which allows the surgeon to perform a bilateral pneumonectomy of the recipients' diseased lungs before implantation of the donor lungs, the use of ECMO requires a sequential pneumonectomy and implantation approach. There is increasing advocacy to continue with immediate posttransplant ECMO support particularly in patients with pulmonary hypertension [62, 69].

Pre-lung Transplant Extracorporeal Lung Support (ECLS) as a Strategy for Mechanical Bridging to Lung Transplantation

This is a limited and expensive therapeutic strategy for a carefully selected lung transplant candidate that requires significant commitment by the transplant and intensive care teams and is associated with a considerable resource burden. Patient selection has to be interrogated and reviewed very carefully by the teams involved, to responsibly set out with frank discussions, the clear parameters, intentions, goals, and strict adherence on withdrawal criteria if a transplant does not occur and the patient continues to deteriorate despite this intervention. The intention to proceed down this treatment pathway is to prolong the life expectancy of a lung transplant recipient as an inpatient in the pretransplant period, in order to maximize their chances of survival by stabilizing their deteriorating critical respiratory state in order to remain eligible to receive a potential lung transplant from a suitable donor [70]. The modern era of ECLS systems have had much more encouraging results compared to early experience with high complication and mortality rates [71, 72] that have advocated the increasing utilization of this strategy in carefully selected patients residing within experienced centers. The goal in the current era is to apply ECLS systems that allow a patient to be awake, extubated, and ambulant and to actively rehabilitate while awaiting a lung transplant. Despite the increased risk of bleeding, hemolysis, infection, neurological events, multi-organ failure, and the potential limitations to maintain physical conditioning, there are encouraging reports to support the use of modern ECLS strategies in providing clinical stability in patients with critical respiratory failure and potentially improving posttransplant outcomes while reducing lung transplant waiting list mortality.

Newer ECLS systems avoid the deleterious effects of mechanical ventilation such as ventilator-associated lung injury, ventilator-associated pneumonia, sedation (with or without paralysis), intubation, and progressive muscle deconditioning [70, 73–81]. ECLS is not advised for patients with multi-organ dysfunction, evidence of sepsis or septic shock, severe arterial occlusive disease, heparin-induced thrombocytopenia, prior history of prolonged mechanical ventilation, advanced age, and obesity [1]. ECLS is also not advised in patients who present acutely with advanced respi-

ratory failure, placed on mechanical ventilation without prior evaluation for transplant suitability by a transplant team, and generally is associated with poorer outcomes. In mechanically ventilated patients, even though some centers report favorable outcomes posttransplantation, limited results have not advocated extensive use of this route as a pathway toward successful lung transplantation [75, 82–85].

Novalung (XENIOS, Heilbronn, Germany) Lung Assist Device (LAD)

The application of the pumpless Novalung interventional lung assist device (LAD) as a method to mechanically bridge patients with refractory hypercapnic respiratory failure who would otherwise die from progressive lung disease has gained recognition of its usefulness in this clinical setting [69, 70]. In carefully selected patients, experiencing acute clinical decompensation from progressive cardiogenic shock associated with advanced pulmonary arterial hypertension refractory to medical therapy, the utilization of this device in a novel manner has been advocated as a bridge to lung transplantation. In this situation, the device is used as a low-resistance mechanical shunt device, effectively performing as a vascular connection between the pulmonary arterial trunk and the left atrium. The descriptive notion is of a mechanical "mimic" to a functioning septostomy effectively unloading the severe pulmonary arterial pressures on the right ventricle to the left atrium in a very similar fashion to an atrial septostomy [85, 86].

Disease-Specific Considerations for Potential Lung Transplant Candidates: Optimizing Timing for Referral and Listing for Lung Transplantation

Timing of referral and listing for lung transplantation are intimately dependent on disease-specific predictors of survival [1, 4, 87]. A myriad of clinical, laboratory, and functional measures are used to predict early mortality and inform the decision-making process (Table 2.1). This section outlines the indications for transplantation and predictors of survival among the prevailing lung diseases indicated for lung transplantation [1, 4]. Chapters 3 and 4 elaborate on the issues associated with consideration of lung transplantation for obstructive lung diseases and interstitial and rare lung diseases, respectively.

Cystic Fibrosis (CF) (Fig. 2.2a–c)

A general working principle applies to all cystic fibrosis (CF) patients potentially being considered for referral for lung transplantation who have a predicted 2-year survival of <50% with functional limitations classified as New York Heart Association Class III or IV. However, attempts to objectively and accurately predict the survival characteristics for CF patients are complex and challenging. In part, this can be attributed to the advances in dedicated, personalized, and increasingly complex CF care, the multisystemic involvement of pulmonary and extrapulmonary CF-related disease, and the unique CF sputum microbiology. In addition, issues of intravenous access, antimicrobial allergies, and psychosocial challenges confer additional layers of complexity in dealing with posttransplant CF patients who have undergone major thoracic surgery and being actively immunosuppressed.

There is not a single accurate predictive denominator that can confer a confident trajectory of the survival characteristics of any one CF patient. An early report by Kerem and colleagues [88] defined that a FEV1 <30% of predicted was associated with a 2-year mortality rate of approximately 40% in men and 55% in women. Subsequently, several other prognostic factors of early mortality for patients with CF without lung transplantation have been identified [89–95]. These included age, height, FEV1, respiratory microbiology, number of hospitalizations, and home intravenous antibiotic usage as significant predictors of 2-year mortality [89]; and FEV1<30% [91] predicted only when the $PaCO_2$ was >50 mmHg [90]. Liou and colleagues [96], utilizing a Cystic Fibrosis Foundation database, developed a 5-year survival model which predicted poorer survival outcome in CF patients who were female, suffered from diabetes mellitus, and had increasingly frequent exacerbations and those patients that were colonized with *B. cepacia* infection [97, 98].

Factors at assessment that have been demonstrated to negatively impact on 90-day and long-term survival post-lung transplantation include the presence of a lower left ventricular ejection fraction [99], pulmonary arterial hypertension and impaired pulmonary arterial compliance [100–102], and poor exercise tolerance [103]. Notably, caution needs to be employed on the accuracy and limitations of bedside echocardiography in the estimation of pulmonary arterial systolic pressure [104]. Modern CF care places strong emphasis on maintaining appropriate nutrition [105]. Increasing clinical need for nutritional supplementation requirements is

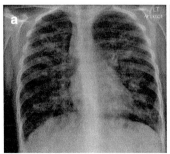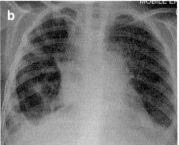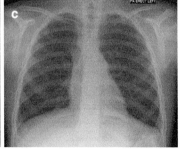

Fig. 2.2 (**a**) Chest X-ray of a pediatric CF patient showing fibrocystic lung parenchymal changes prior to transplant; (**b**) chest X-ray 36-day post-bilateral sequential upper lobar lung transplant with large hydropneumothorax (black arrow) filling the residual thoracic cavity; (**c**) chest X-ray showing full inflation of the lobar lung transplant into the thoracic cavity 171 days posttransplantation

reported to have a dramatic effect on reduced survival in CF patients [90, 106]. Additional factors that contribute to the unique complexity and concern in assessing CF patients for lung transplantation are the implications of the presence of *Burkholderia cepacia complex (BCC)* and *non-tuberculous mycobacteria (NTM)* in CF sputum culture. These organisms require complex medical management approaches in treatment regimens pretransplantation, and in certain centers, conclusive evidence of the presence of these organisms in patients are considered absolute contraindications to lung transplantation. Recent evidence-based recommendations for the investigation and management of *NTM* disease in CF patients have been devised to optimize their clinical status [107].

B. cepacia Complex (BCC) in Patients with Cystic Fibrosis

BCC encompasses 17 closely related species of *Burkholderia cepacia* bacteria [108] (also referred to as genomovars [109, 110]) that individually exhibit variable pathogenicity [111–113]. It is recognized that preoperative CF patients infected with *B. cepacia complex* experience a more rapid decline in respiratory status cogent to increased mortality rates [114, 115]. In particular, patients infected preoperatively with *B. cenocepacia* experience poorer outcomes post-lung transplantation [116, 117]. Hence many lung transplant centers have concluded that these patients present an unacceptably high risk of morbidity and mortality [116] and as a result are not offered lung transplantation as a therapeutic modality. However, this is in contrast to patients infected with *non-B. cenocepacia BCC* species; these patients do not represent an increased risk of mortality perioperatively compared with other CF patients and hence should be considered for assessment and potential listing on condition that the other assessment criteria are satisfactory to the standards and protocols employed by individual lung transplant centers [1, 37]. Therefore it is critically important that all CF patients' sputum microbiology being considered for lung transplantation are stringently assessed for the presence of *B. cepacia* species [118].

Non-tuberculous Mycobacteria (NTM) in Patients with Cystic Fibrosis

There is an increasing burden of positive sputum cultures of *non-tuberculous mycobacteria (NTM)* in CF patients, presenting a uniquely complex challenge to CF centers and lung transplant centers. From a lung transplant perspective, the reported literature is largely based on case series [119, 120]. The treatment regime for *NTM* and specifically in *M. abscessus* involves multiple complex antimicrobial regimes administered often both intravenously and enterally for a prolonged time period with a significant side effect profile. It is recommended by the ISHLT consensus group [1] that CF patients infected with *M. abscessus* under consideration for lung transplant referral must be able to tolerate the optimal therapeutic regime prior to lung transplant listing and that inability to tolerate the treatment regime or progressive pulmonary and/or extrapulmonary disease is a contraindication to lung transplantation. In this era, all patients with CF being referred for consideration of lung transplantation should be evaluated for the presence of *NTM* disease and if confirmed definitively, should commence treatment according to the CF unit's guidelines before being referred for lung transplant assessment or listing. The transplantation of patients with *M. abscessus* is a significant undertaking by any transplant center, and it is advisable that careful evaluation is performed in a center with significant experience in this specific area of transplantation.

These compilations of studies highlight many variables to be considered in a CF patient for the key point reiterated in all these studies is that FEV1 alone is not a sufficient predictor of early mortality in CF patients being considered for lung transplantation and hence cannot be utilized as a single data point to consider a CF patient for referral and listing. Indeed in practice, there is recognition by CF centers and lung transplant centers that the variable characteristics of individual CF patients require a broader evaluation and interrogation of all the factors outlined to assist a multidisciplinary transplant team with the necessary experience and expertise to decide if a patient has reached the time to be considered for referral and aid the transplant centers in their decisions toward listing and transplanting the appropriate patient [1] (Table 2.1).

Therefore, defining specific criteria to predict timing for referral and listing of CF patients for lung transplantation remains challenging as the course of the disease is highly variable and heterogeneous. In addition, individual transplant centers will need to take into consideration the unique challenges presented by their own unit protocols and the limitations placed by local and national waiting times for transplantation. The final decision to list and transplant a CF patient is a result of a detailed, thorough, and comprehensive evaluation which takes into account as far as possible the individual and general predictive clinical variables according to best practice available to ultimately confer a survival benefit to the selected patients. There must be continued scrutiny and evaluation of these clinical characteristics that influence survival of CF patients and potential future predictive models. These points, however, cannot compensate for an early referral of an increasingly complex group of patients combined with enhanced communication and working part-

nerships between different CF centers and the lung transplant center. Late referrals of CF patients or indeed any group of end-stage respiratory patients place unrealistic expectations of a patient being assessed within an acceptable timeframe to achieve the goals that may be necessary before listing, and transplantation can occur with a confident prediction of a positive outcome and survival benefit [116]. In the current era of improved CF survival with the emphasis on dedicated CF multidisciplinary care, CF microbiology and new CF therapeutics, the final common pathway inevitably will lead to lung transplantation as a realistic consideration for a proportion of these patients.

Interstitial Lung Disease (ILD) (Fig. 2.3a–d)

While interstitial lung disease (ILD) exhibits the least favorable outcome among the common lung

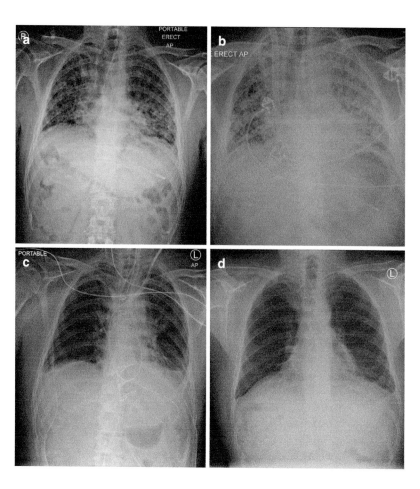

Fig. 2.3 (a) Chest X-ray of a 48-year-old male patient with severe interstitial lung disease; (b) chest X-ray demonstrating worsening pulmonary infiltrates, placed on extracorporeal lung support with Avalon catheter in situ; (c) chest X-ray of the same patient, day 1 post-bilateral lung transplant via sternotomy; (d) chest X-ray at day 26 post-bilateral lung transplant on discharge from the ward

diseases designated for lung transplantation, recent changes to donor lung appropriation have significantly increased lung transplant rates among this group of patients. Yet, despite this, mortality rates remain high among waiting list ILD transplant candidates. Combined with the refractory nature of disease, the lack of effective therapies and poor prognosis in patients with ILD, early consideration and referral for transplantation is imperative.

Consensus guidelines [1] for the appropriate timing of referral and listing in patients with ILD are summarized in Table 2.2. Variables affecting the timing of referral include progressive and dis-

Table 2.2 Timing of referral and consideration for lung transplantation

CF	FEV1 <30% predicted PaCO$_2$ of >50 mmHg or 6.6 kPa and/or PaO$_2$ <60 mmHg or 8 kPa 6MWT <400 m Advanced disease with a rapidly declining FEV1 despite optimal medical therapy—especially young female CF patients Increasing frequency of exacerbations with a clinical decline Respiratory failure requiring noninvasive ventilation Increasing antibiotic requirements and antibiotic resistance Increasing burden of disease with extended antibiotic therapy and poor recovery from exacerbations Worsening nutritional status and increasing nutritional supplementation and accessory feeding regimes Development of a pneumothorax Life-threatening hemoptysis Infection with *Burkholderia cepacia complex* or *non-tuberculous mycobacteria (NTM)* Complex CF patient with associated liver disease, diabetes Development of pulmonary hypertension (in the absence of a hypoxic exacerbation)
ILD	Radiological or histopathological evidence of usual interstitial pneumonitis (UIP) or fibrosing non-specific pneumonitis (NSIP), irrespective of lung function Forced vital capacity (FVC) of <80% of predicted or diffusion capacity for carbon monoxide (DLCO) of <40% predicted Decline in FVC ≥10% in a 6-month follow-up Decline in DLCO <40% predicted Oxygen desaturation <88% or distance <250 m on a 6MWT >50 m decline in 6MWT over a 6-month period Oxygen requirement at rest or on exertion Failure of attempted medical therapy to decrease the rate of progression of disease Evidence of pulmonary hypertension as defined by mean PA pressure Survivor of acute exacerbation of IPF pneumothorax Functional limitation and dyspnea directly related to decline in lung disease Increasing hospitalization with respiratory failure or complications directly related to the underlying lung disease
COPD	PaCO$_2$ of >50 mmHg or 6.6 kPa and/or PaO$_2$ <60 mmHg or 8 kPa FEV1 <25% predicted ªBODE index ≥7 Progressive lung disease with three of more exacerbations, worsening respiratory failure after maximal medical therapy, oxygen therapy, and pulmonary rehabilitation Progressive lung disease despite attempts at endoscopic or surgical lung volume reduction Patient not a candidate to for lung volume reduction Development of a pneumothorax Respiratory failure requiring noninvasive ventilation Previous episode of invasive ventilation Evidence of right heart failure with moderate to severe pulmonary hypertension Increasing hospitalization with respiratory failure or complications directly related to the underlying lung disease

(continued)

Table 2.2 (continued)

PH	NYHA Class III or IV symptoms of dyspnea
	Pericardial effusion
	Worsening 6MWT <350 m
	Escalating use of targeted combination therapy for pulmonary arterial hypertension
	Hemoptysis
	Syncope
	Signs of progressive right heart failure
	Worsening respiratory failure
	Cardiac index <2 L/min/m^2
	Right atrial pressure >15 mmHg

CF cystic fibrosis, *ILD* interstitial lung disease, *PH* pulmonary hypertension, *FEV1* forced expiratory volume in one second, *FVC* forced vital capacity, *DLCO* diffusing capacity for carbon monoxide, *PaO₂* oxygen tension, *PaCO₂* partial pressure of arterial carbon dioxide tension, *6MWT* 6-min walk test, *NYHA* New York Heart Association

Data from Weill D, Benden C, Corris PA, Dark JH, Davis RD, Keshavjee S, et al. A consensus document for the selection of lung transplant candidates: 2014—an update from the Pulmonary Transplantation Council of the International Society for Heart and Lung Transplantation. The Journal of Heart and Lung Transplantation. 2015;34(1):1–15

[a](Modified) BODE score: composite score of body mass index (B), airway obstruction as a measure of percentage predicted FEV1 (O), dyspnea (D), and exercise capacity (E); a higher score indicating more severe disease and worse survival [110]

abling dyspnea secondary to parenchymal disease, limiting functionality, oxygen dependency (at rest or on exertion), radiological or histopathological evidence of fibrosing non-specific interstitial pneumonitis (NSIP) or usual interstitial pneumonitis (UIP), and in the case of inflammatory ILD, no improvement or decline in clinical parameters including dyspnea, oxygen needs, and/or pulmonary function despite a maximum trial of appropriate, targeted medical therapy. In addition, abnormal pulmonary function including FVC less than 80% predicted or DLCO less than 60% predicted would be indicative of need to introduce the concept and/or early referral for transplantation evaluation and discuss timing for listing and optimal candidacy of lung transplantation. The decision to proceed to listing of a candidate with ILD for lung transplantation encompasses a core set of prognostic tests suggesting rapid decline in pulmonary function, over an ensuing 6-month interval. These include a reduction in FVC ≥10% or DLCO (≥15%); oxygen desaturation <88% or absolute reduction on performance in the 6MWT (<250 m on 6MWT or >50 m decline in 6MWT over 6 months); the development of pulmonary hypertension or hospitalization secondary to acute exacerbation; and development of a spontaneous pneumothorax in a patient with severe lung function impairment or who has demonstrated progressive decline in respiratory status.

Chronic Obstructive Pulmonary Disease (COPD)

COPD encompasses a group of clinical and pathologic entities, resulting in airway obstruction, and includes the chronic lung diseases of emphysema and chronic bronchitis [121]. COPD is associated with significant morbidity and mortality. It is the leading cause of respiratory disease in the UK, the third leading cause of death in the USA and the fourth leading cause of death worldwide [122]. COPD is the most common indication for lung transplantation and accounts for up to 38% of all procedures performed worldwide [123]. Referral of COPD patients for lung transplantation [123] should be considered in the context of relentless disease progression despite optimization of pharmacological, oxygen, and rehabilitation therapies. Associated quantifiable criteria indicating appropriate timing of referral include a body mass index (BMI), obstruction, dyspnea, and exercise capacity (BODE) [124] index of 5–6; drop in FEV1 <25% predicted, PaCO₂ >50 mmHg or 6.6 kPa and/or PaO₂ <60mmHg or 8 kPa; a patient with significant progressive bullous lung disease; and/or a patient not suitable for endoscopic or surgical lung volume reduction strategies. Further deterioration in a single clinical parameter mitigates consideration for candidate listing. Clinical criterion for lung transplant listing includes proven factors that negatively impact on survival in patients with COPD and includes an increase in BODE index (≥7), further reduction in FEV1 to <15 to 20% predicted, moderate to severe pulmonary hypertension ("cor pulmonale"), and a single severe exacerbation associated with acute hypercapnic respiratory failure or three or more severe exacerbations over the preceding 12 months [123].

Pulmonary Arterial Hypertension (PAH)

Lung transplantation is the only therapeutic option available for selected patients with pulmonary arterial hypertension (PAH) that are deteriorating from the condition being refractory to maximal medical and optimal pulmonary vasodilator treatment. Prior to the introduction of targeted pulmonary vasodilator therapy, PAH was associated with a dramatically reduced survival reported in patients with adverse prognostic markers found on right heart catheterization, namely, a cardiac index less than 2 L/min/m², a right atrial pressure (RAP) of 20 mmHg or higher, and/or a pulmonary artery systolic pressure of 85 mmHg or higher [125]. However, the medical therapeutic strategies for patients with a diagnosis of PAH have advanced considerably since the introduction of systemic prostanoid therapy which demonstrated improvement in pulmonary hemodynamics, functional capacity, and 5-year survival rates [126–130]. This alongside the availability of treatment modalities that include endothelin receptor antagonists, phosphodiesterase inhibitors, and atrial septostomy [131, 132] with the introduction of goal-directed combination therapy introduced early in the disease course has proven efficacious in the management of this difficult condition [1, 126–129, 133–150]. These strategies have proven to be efficacious in most cases with good treatment responses but have altered the timeline for referral and listing for lung transplantation in this group of patients and indeed in patients with other causes of pulmonary hypertension. The improved medical management of patients with PAH has been associated with a reduction in the number of patients requiring lung transplantation for PAH [151, 152]. In the pre-prostanoid era, functional capacity is measured by the 6-min walk distance served as a strong predictor of mortality, and this assessment remains a critical parameter for PAH patients in terms of their response to treatment as well as timing for referral and listing for transplantation [126, 127, 153, 154]. The long-term effects and the uncertainty of sustained medical benefit is an area that continues to be under close review particularly when decisions need to be made on deciding the timing for referral and listing for transplantation, and there remains considerable variation in practice between transplant centers for this particular disease spectrum.

It is critically important to identify the prognostic features in patients with PAH that can predict a progressive decline and death without transplantation. The confirmation of the diagnosis, optimization of treatment strategies, and monitoring of treatment response are crucial indicators for the pulmonary hypertension teams in terms of timing the decision to move forward with a lung transplant assessment and listing. A general consideration is to refer patients with PAH for assessment when the patients remain in NYHA Class III or present in NYHA Class IV despite optimal pulmonary vasodilator therapy, a low or declining 6-min walk test (<350 m) and/or with a predicted survival of 2 years which is less than 50%. Further hemodynamic parameters that predict a poor outcome in PAH patients include a cardiac index of <2 L/min/m², mean right atrial pressure >15 mmHg, and mean pulmonary artery pressure >55 mmHg [155, 156]. Since the implementation of LAS for lung transplantation in the USA, transplantation for idiopathic PAH (IPAH) patients has remained worryingly low, with IPAH patients demonstrating low LAS scores and yet having increased mortality rates on the transplant waiting list [157] reinforcing concerns that the LAS model was underestimating the mortality risk in patients with IPAH. This likely reflected that the previous LAS model utilized a 6-min walk distance of 150 ft that was inappropriately low in IPAH patients to predict survival and did not factor in the cardiopulmonary hemodynamic analysis and assessment of right ventricular function.

Analysis from the US Registry to Evaluate Early and Long-term PAH Disease Management (REVEAL) [158, 159] has identified many additional factors associated with increased mortality in the PAH patients group: NYHA Functional Class IV, male gender with age >60 years, increased pulmonary vascular resistance (PVR), PAH associated with portal hypertension, and a family history of PAH [158, 160, 161]. Additional factors associated with increased mortality in PAH patients include NHYA Functional Class III, increased mean right atrial pressure, decreased resting systolic blood pressure or an elevated heart rate, decreased 6-min walk distance, increased brain natriuretic peptide, renal insufficiency, PAH associated with connective tissue disease, decreased DLCO, and the presence of a pericardial effusion. Even though this registry did not reflect the transplant waiting list population, it provided important points to consider when evaluating a deteriorating patient with IPAH. Appeals to these concerns and subsequent revision to the LAS effective from February 2015 include the following points specific for IPAH patients: a cardiac index <2 L/min/m^2, CVP >7 mmHg, a rise in creatinine, a rise in bilirubin, the 6-min walk test as a continuous variable if <1200 ft, and the reduced impact of oxygen utilization [162–166].

Bilateral lung transplantation is the recommended procedure of choice in IPAH, and with careful early postoperative management, there is an expected satisfactory recovery of the right ventricle following bilateral lung transplantation cogent to improved long-term survival benefit compared to single-lung transplantation [167–169]. Due to the limited availability of heart-lung blocs, heart-lung transplantation in IPAH is rarely a clinical option.

Special Considerations for PAH

Congenital Heart Disease-Associated Pulmonary Arterial Hypertension

The option of heart-lung transplantation is an option reserved for patients with complex congenital heart disease-associated pulmonary arterial hypertension (CHDAPAH) or highly selected patients with severe IPAH and severe right ventricular dysfunction. Patients with CHDAPAH have a preferable prognosis on transplant waiting lists compared to patients with IPAH [170, 171]. Other therapeutic options are bilateral lung transplant with concurrent surgical repair of the underlying cardiac defects [1].

Chronic Thromboembolic Pulmonary Hypertension (CTEPH)

In patients with chronic thromboembolic pulmonary hypertension (CTEPH), pulmonary thromboendarterectomy is the favored treatment of choice where the appropriate expertise is available. The procedure confers a significant survival benefit without the added complication of requiring long-term immunosuppressive therapy [172, 173].

Connective Tissue Disease-Associated PAH

The disease most associated with this form of PAH is systemic sclerosis (SSc) which characteristically can develop into severe PAH associated with a rapid clinical decline and increased mortality. The nature of this systemic connective tissue disease can involve vasculitic features with major organ involvement [174] that may preclude lung transplantation being a realistic therapeutic option. One key feature of SSc is the presence of esophageal dysmotility and gastroparesis [175]. This a major concern due to the risk of gastric aspiration, pneumonia, and the adverse effect on the lung allograft [176–181]. Previous reports from Saggar [182] and Sottile [183] reported similar survival rates compared with other patients with ILD. However, Saggar and colleagues reported increased rates of acute rejection [182], while the incidence of freedom from bronchiolitis obliterans syndrome (BOS) was similar between both groups [182, 183]. However, many centers continue to exercise a high degree of caution in assessing this group of patients. In general, highly selected patients with SSc and PAH can be considered on a case-by-case basis with a careful evaluation of the activity of the systemic vasculitic features as well as close scrutiny and assessment of esophageal function [184]. However, the presence of severe esophageal dysmotility with no realistic or satisfactory prevention of aspiration risk by gastric fundoplication will in general preclude a patient from undergoing lung transplantation.

Additional Considerations and Special Lung Transplant Circumstances

Lung Re-transplantation

Lung re-transplantation accounts for a very small percentage of lung transplants performed worldwide. The criteria used to assess and select candidates for lung transplantation are largely extended in principle to potential candidates being considered for lung re-transplantation. Careful consideration must be applied stringently particularly with regard to the presence of comorbid disease and particular attention to the presence of significant renal dysfunction [185, 186]. The surgical options for re-transplant candidates may be either single- or bilateral lung transplants. Patients who were previous recipients of single-lung transplants can be considered for a contralateral single-lung transplant with the option of avoiding removal of the previous lung allograft. However, very careful consideration and investigation of the potential infective risk of the retained lung allograft must be undertaken [185]. The trend generally has been toward undertaking bilateral lung re-transplantation. Survival outcomes appear to favor patients re-transplanted for BOS and patients who are more than 2 years following initial lung transplant [186–188]. There are also ethical considerations that inevitably arise when offering lung re-transplantation in an era where organ donation remains a vastly limited resource with deaths on waiting lists for first time lung transplant candidates.

Summary/Conclusions

Lung transplantation remains a great challenge for the future with expanding knowledge and treatment options for patients with advanced lung disease, clinical trials of potential new therapies, improving strategies to expand the utilization of donor organs, and the prospect of improving transplant survival with research into the prevention and treatment of lung allograft dysfunction. Alongside the advent of greater access to online information, it is imperative that referring teams are up to date on the realistic prospects, expectations, survival characteristics, and risks involved with lung transplantation in terms of managing the expectations of patients with severe end-stage lung disease. It is important that the referring physicians and members of the transplant team maintain a good working partnership and present realistic expectations to their patients, and the patients' relatives and care providers, of the realities involved in preparation and assessment for lung transplantation; the life while on the waiting list; the regime of medication, treatment, and follow-up after transplantation; as well as a frank discourse on the morbidity, risks, survival facts and mortality associated with lung transplantation. This realistic outlook and facts are couched together with the real benefits that can be enjoyed by a majority of patients who derive a definitive survival benefit from lung transplantation and a potential expectation to improve their quality of life for an unspecified period of time.

References

1. Weill D, Benden C, Corris PA, Dark JH, Davis RD, Keshavjee S, et al. A consensus document for the selection of lung transplant candidates: 2014—an update from the Pulmonary Transplantation Council of the International Society for Heart and Lung Transplantation. J Heart Lung Transplant. 2015;34(1):1–15.
2. Barrios JMV, Montero JR, Luna FS. Comorbidities impacting on prognosis after lung transplant. Arch Bronconeumol. 2014;50(1):25–33.
3. Smith PJ, Blumenthal JA, Trulock EP, Freedland KE, Carney RM, Davis RD, et al. Psychosocial predictors of mortality following lung transplantation. Am J Transplant. 2016;16(1):271–7.
4. Glanville AR, Estenne M. Indications, patient selection and timing of referral for lung transplantation. Eur Respir J. 2003;22(5):845–52.
5. Egan TM, Murray S, Bustami RT, Shearon TH, McCullough KP, Edwards LB, et al. Development of the new lung allocation system in the United States. Am J Transplant. 2006;6(5p2):1212–27.

6. Lingaraju R, Blumenthal NP, Kotloff RM, Christie J, Ahya VN, Sager JS, et al. Effects of lung allocation score on waiting list rankings and transplant procedures. J Heart Lung Transplant. 2006;25(9):1167–70.

7. Kozower BD, Meyers BF, Smith MA, De Oliveira NC, Cassivi SD, Guthrie TJ, et al. The impact of the lung allocation score on short-term transplantation outcomes: a multicenter study. J Thorac Cardiovasc Surg. 2008;135(1):166–71.

8. Egan TM, Kotloff RM. Pro/Con debate: lung allocation should be based on medical urgency and transplant survival and not on waiting time. Chest J. 2005;128(1):407–15.

9. Kotloff RM, Thabut G. Lung transplantation. Am J Respir Crit Care Med. 2011;184(2):159–71.

10. Martinez FJ, Safrin S, Weycker D, Starko KM, Bradford WZ, King TE, et al. The clinical course of patients with idiopathic pulmonary fibrosis. Ann Intern Med. 2005;142(12_Part_1):963–7.

11. Lynch JP, Huynh RH, Fishbein MC, Saggar R, Belperio JA, Weigt SS. Idiopathic pulmonary fibrosis: epidemiology, clinical features, prognosis, and management. Semin Respir Crit Care Med. 2016;37(3):331–57.

12. Russo MJ, Iribarne A, Hong KN, Davies RR, Xydas S, Takayama H, et al. High lung allocation score is associated with increased morbidity and mortality following transplantation. Chest J. 2010;137(3):651–7.

13. Liu V, Zamora MR, Dhillon GS, Weill D. Increasing lung allocation scores predict worsened survival among lung transplant recipients. Am J Transplant. 2010;10(4):915–20.

14. Egan TM, Edwards LB. Effect of the lung allocation score on lung transplantation in the United States. J Heart Lung Transplant. 2016;35(4):433–9.

15. Maxwell BG, Mooney JJ, Lee PHU, Levitt JE, Chhatwani L, Nicolls MR, et al. Increased resource use in lung transplant admissions in the lung allocation score era. Am J Respir Crit Care Med. 2015;191(3):302–8.

16. Fahim A, Crooks MG, Wilmot R, Campbell AP, Morice AH, Hart SP. Serum carcinoembryonic antigen correlates with severity of idiopathic pulmonary fibrosis. Respirology. 2012;17(8):1247–52.

17. Hadjiliadis D, Tapson VF, Davis RD, Palmer SM. Prognostic value of serum carcinoembryonic antigen levels in patients who undergo lung transplantation. J Heart Lung Transplant. 2001;20(12):1305–9.

18. Christie JD, Edwards LB, Aurora P, Dobbels F, Kirk R, Rahmel AO, et al. The Registry of the International Society for Heart and Lung Transplantation: twenty-sixth official adult lung and heart-lung transplantation report—2009. J Heart Lung Transplant. 2009;28(10):1031–49.

19. Tomaszek SC, Fibla JJ, Dierkhising RA, Scott JP, Shen K-HR, Wigle DA, et al. Outcome of lung transplantation in elderly recipients. Eur J Cardiothorac Surg. 2011;39(5):726–31.

20. Thabut G, Ravaud P, Christie JD, Castier Y, Fournier M, Mal H, et al. Determinants of the survival benefit of lung transplantation in patients with chronic obstructive pulmonary disease. Am J Respir Crit Care Med. 2008;177(10):1156–63.

21. Fischer S, Meyer K, Tessmann R, Meyer A, Gohrbandt B, Simon A, et al. Outcome following single vs bilateral lung transplantation in recipients 60 years of age and older. Transplant Proc. 2005;37(2):1369–70.

22. Aris RM, Neuringer IP, Weiner MA, Egan TM, Ontjes D. Severe osteoporosis before and after lung transplantation. Chest J. 1996;109(5):1176–83.

23. Tschopp O, Boehler A, Speich R, Weder W, Seifert B, Russi EW, et al. Osteoporosis before lung transplantation: association with low body mass index, but not with underlying disease. Am J Transplant. 2002;2(2):167–72.

24. Aris RM, Lester GE, Renner JB, Winders A, Denene Blackwood A, Lark RK, et al. Efficacy of pamidronate for osteoporosis in patients with cystic fibrosis following lung transplantation. Am J Respir Crit Care Med. 2000;162(3):941–6.

25. Shane E, Silverberg SJ, Donovan D, Papadopoulos A, Staron RB, Addesso V, et al. Osteoporosis in lung transplantation candidates with end-stage pulmonary disease. Am J Med. 1996;101(3):262–9.

26. Braith RW, Conner JA, Fulton MN, Lisor CF, Casey DP, Howe KS, et al. Comparison of alendronate vs alendronate plus mechanical loading as prophylaxis for osteoporosis in lung transplant recipients: a pilot study. J Heart Lung Transplant. 2007;26(2):132–7.

27. Munro PE, Holland AE, Bailey M, Button BM, Snell GI. Pulmonary rehabilitation following lung transplantation. Transplant Proc. 2009;41(1):292–5.

28. Caffarelli C, Gonnelli S, Pitinca MDT, Francolini V, Fui A, Bargagli E, et al. Idiopathic pulmonary fibrosis a rare disease with severe bone fragility. Intern Emerg Med. 2016;11(8):1087–94.

29. Tabarelli W, Bonatti H, Tabarelli D, Eller M, Müller L, Ruttmann E, et al. Long term complications following 54 consecutive lung transplants. J Thorac Dis. 2016;8(6):1234.

30. Culver DA, Mazzone PJ, Khandwala F, Blazey HC, DeCamp MM, Chapman JT, et al. Discordant utility of ideal body weight and body mass index as predictors of mortality in lung transplant recipients. J Heart Lung Transplant. 2005;24(2):137–44.

31. Carreno MC, Piedad UG, Maite L, Andrés V, Francisca P, Cesar B, et al. Hepatitis C virus infection after lung transplantation: dim prognosis. J Heart Lung Transplant. 2001;20(2):224.

32. Cotler SJ, Jensen DM, Kesten S. Hepatitis C virus infection and lung transplantation: a survey of practices. J Heart Lung Transplant. 1999;18(5):456–9.

33. Fong T-L, Cho YW, Hou L, Hutchinson IV, Barbers RG, Herrington CS. Outcomes after lung transplantation and practices of lung transplant programs in the United States regarding hepatitis C seropositive recipients. Transplantation. 2011;91(11):1293–6.

34. Doucette KE, Weinkauf J, Jackson K, Lein D. Survival following lung transplantation is not

impacted by hepatitis C infection. Am J Transplant. 2012;12(S3):27–542.

35. Kern RM, Seethamraju H, Blanc PD, Sinha N, Loebe M, Golden J, et al. The feasibility of lung transplantation in HIV-seropositive patients. Ann Am Thorac Soc. 2014;11(6):882–9.

36. Morabito V, Grossi P, Lombardini L, Ricci A, Trapani S, Peritore D, et al. Solid organ transplantation in HIV+ recipients: Italian experience. Transplant Proc. 2016;48(2):424–30.

37. De Soyza A, Meachery G, Hester KLM, Nicholson A, Parry G, Tocewicz K, et al. Lung transplantation for patients with cystic fibrosis and Burkholderia cepacia complex infection: a single-center experience. J Heart Lung Transplant. 2010;29(12):1395–404.

38. Olland A, Falcoz P-E, Kessler R, Massard G. Should cystic fibrosis patients infected with Burkholderia cepacia complex be listed for lung transplantation? Interact Cardiovasc Thorac Surg. 2012;13(6):631–4.

39. Bruckner BA, Motomura T, Kaleekal TS, Jyothula SS, Scheinin S, Bunge RR, et al. Clinical outcomes in elderly lung transplant recipients 70 years and older. J Heart Lung Transplant. 2013;32(4):S266–S7.

40. Hayanga AJ, Aboagye JK, Hayanga HE, Morrell M, Huffman L, Shigemura N, et al. Contemporary analysis of early outcomes after lung transplantation in the elderly using a national registry. J Heart Lung Transplant. 2015;34(2):182–8.

41. Nathan SD, Albera C, Bradford WZ, Costabel U, Du Bois RM, Fagan EA, et al. Effect of continued treatment with pirfenidone following clinically meaningful declines in forced vital capacity: analysis of data from three phase 3 trials in patients with idiopathic pulmonary fibrosis. Thorax. 2016;71(5):429–35.

42. Raghu G, Rochwerg B, Zhang Y, Garcia CAC, Azuma A, Behr J, et al. An official ATS/ERS/JRS/ALAT clinical practice guideline: treatment of idiopathic pulmonary fibrosis. An update of the 2011 clinical practice guideline. Am J Respir Crit Care Med. 2015;192(2):e3–19.

43. Richeldi L, du Bois RM, Raghu G, Azuma A, Brown KK, Costabel U, et al. Efficacy and safety of nintedanib in idiopathic pulmonary fibrosis. N Engl J Med. 2014;370(22):2071–82.

44. Kolb M, Richeldi L, Behr J, Maher TM, Tang W, Stowasser S, et al. Nintedanib in patients with idiopathic pulmonary fibrosis and preserved lung volume. Thorax. 2017;72(4):340–6.

45. Delanote I, Wuyts WA, Yserbyt J, Verbeken EK, Verleden GM, Vos R. Safety and efficacy of bridging to lung transplantation with antifibrotic drugs in idiopathic pulmonary fibrosis: a case series. BMC Pulm Med. 2016;16(1):156.

46. Stehlik J, Edwards LB, Kucheryavaya AY, Aurora P, Christie JD, Kirk R, et al. The Registry of the International Society for Heart and Lung Transplantation: twenty-seventh official adult heart transplant report—2010. J Heart Lung Transplant. 2010;29(10):1089–103.

47. Thabut G, Christie JD, Ravaud P, Castier Y, Brugière O, Fournier M, et al. Survival after bilateral versus single lung transplantation for patients with chronic obstructive pulmonary disease: a retrospective analysis of registry data. Lancet. 2008;371(9614):744–51.

48. Thabut G, Christie JD, Ravaud P, Castier Y, Dauriat G, Jebrak G, et al. Survival after bilateral versus single-lung transplantation for idiopathic pulmonary fibrosis. Ann Intern Med. 2009;151(11):767–74.

49. Kaiser LR, Pasque MK, Trulock EP, Low DE, Dresler CM, Cooper JD. Bilateral sequential lung transplantation: the procedure of choice for double-lung replacement. Ann Thorac Surg. 1991;52(3):438–46.

50. Groui TLT. Unilateral lung transplantation for pulmonary fibrosis. N Engl J Med. 1986;314:1140–5.

51. Paoletti L, Whelan TPM. Lung transplantation for interstitial lung disease. Current Respiratory Care Reports. 2014;3(3):96–102.

52. Mal H, Andreassian B, Pamela F, Duchatelle J-P, Rondeau E, Dubois F, et al. Unilateral lung transplantation in end-stage pulmonary emphysema1• 2. Am Rev Respir Dis. 1989;140:797.

53. Schaffer JM, Singh SK, Reitz BA, Zamanian RT, Mallidi HR. Single-vs double-lung transplantation in patients with chronic obstructive pulmonary disease and idiopathic pulmonary fibrosis since the implementation of lung allocation based on medical need. JAMA. 2015;313(9):936–48.

54. Keating D, Levvey B, Kotsimbos T, Whitford H, Westall G, Williams T, et al. Lung transplantation in pulmonary fibrosis: challenging early outcomes counterbalanced by surprisingly good outcomes beyond 15 years. Transplant Proc. 2009;41(1):289–91.

55. Mason DP, Brizzio ME, Alster JM, McNeill AM, Murthy SC, Budev MM, et al. Lung transplantation for idiopathic pulmonary fibrosis. Ann Thorac Surg. 2007;84(4):1121–8.

56. De Oliveira NC, Osaki S, Maloney J, Cornwell RD, Meyer KC. Lung transplant for interstitial lung disease: outcomes for single versus bilateral lung transplantation. Interact Cardiovasc Thorac Surg. 2012;14(3):263–7.

57. Nwakanma LU, Simpkins CE, Williams JA, Chang DC, Borja MC, Conte JV, et al. Impact of bilateral versus single lung transplantation on survival in recipients 60 years of age and older: analysis of United Network for Organ Sharing database. J Thorac Cardiovasc Surg. 2007;133(2):541–7.

58. Taylor DO, Edwards LB, Boucek MM, Trulock EP, Aurora P, Christie J, et al. Registry of the International Society for Heart and Lung Transplantation: twenty-fourth official adult heart transplant report—2007. J Heart Lung Transplant. 2007;26(8):769–81.

59. Titman A, Rogers CA, Bonser RS, Banner NR, Sharples LD. Disease-specific survival benefit of lung transplantation in adults: a national cohort study. Am J Transplant. 2009;9(7):1640–9.

60. Reitz BA, Wallwork JL, Hunt SA, Pennock JL, Billingham ME, Oyer PE, et al. Heart-lung transplan-

tation: successful therapy for patients with pulmonary vascular disease. N Engl J Med. 1982;306(10):557–64.

61. Christie JD, Edwards LB, Kucheryavaya AY, Benden C, Dobbels F, Kirk R, et al. The Registry of the International Society for Heart and Lung Transplantation: twenty-eighth adult lung and heart-lung transplant report—2011. J Heart Lung Transplant. 2011;30(10):1104–22.

62. Aigner C, Mazhar S, Jaksch P, Seebacher G, Taghavi S, Marta G, et al. Lobar transplantation, split lung transplantation and peripheral segmental resection-reliable procedures for downsizing donor lungs. Eur J Cardiothorac Surg. 2004;25(2):179–83.

63. Inci I, Schuurmans MM, Kestenholz P, Schneiter D, Hillinger S, Opitz I, et al. Long-term outcomes of bilateral lobar lung transplantation. Eur J Cardiothorac Surg. 2013;43(6):1220–5.

64. Barr ML, Starnes VA. Living lobar lung transplantation. Adult chest surgery. 2nd ed. New York: McGraw Hill; 2013.

65. Spray TL, Mallory GB, Canter CB, Dulleston CB. Pediatric lung transplantation: indications, techniques and early results. J Thorac Cardiovasc Surg. 1994;107:990–1000.

66. Starnes VA, Barr ML, Cohen RG, Hagen JA, Wells WJ, Horn MV, et al. Living-donor lobar lung transplantation experience: intermediate results. J Thorac Cardiovasc Surg. 1996;112(5):1284–91.

67. Couetil J-PA, Tolan MJ, Loulmet DF, Guinvarch A, Chevalier PG, Achkar A, et al. Pulmonary bipartitioning and lobar transplantation: a new approach to donor organ shortage. J Thorac Cardiovasc Surg. 1997;113(3):529–37.

68. Artemiou O, Birsan T, Taghavi S, Eichler I, Wisser W, Wolner E, et al. Bilateral lobar transplantation with the split lung technique. J Thorac Cardiovasc Surg. 1999;118(2):369–70.

69. Fischer S, Hoeper MM, Tomaszek S, Simon A, Gottlieb J, Welte T, et al. Bridge to lung transplantation with the extracorporeal membrane ventilator Novalung in the veno-venous mode: the initial Hannover experience. ASAIO J. 2007;53(2):168–70.

70. Strueber M. Bridges to lung transplantation. Curr Opin Organ Transplant. 2011;16(5):458–61.

71. Diaz-Guzman E, Hoopes CW, Zwischenberger JB. The evolution of extracorporeal life support as a bridge to lung transplantation. ASAIO J. 2013;59(1):3–10.

72. Strueber M. Extracorporeal support as a bridge to lung transplantation. Curr Opin Crit Care. 2010;16(1):69–73.

73. Cypel M, Yeung JC, Machuca T, Chen M, Singer LG, Yasufuku K, et al. Experience with the first 50 ex vivo lung perfusions in clinical transplantation. J Thorac Cardiovasc Surg. 2012;144(5):1200–7.

74. de Perrot M, Granton JT, McRae K, Pierre AF, Singer LG, Waddell TK, et al. Outcome of patients with pulmonary arterial hypertension referred for lung transplantation: a 14-year single-center experience. J Thorac Cardiovasc Surg. 2012;143(4):910–8.

75. de Perrot M, Granton JT, McRae K, Cypel M, Pierre A, Waddell TK, et al. Impact of extracorporeal life support on outcome in patients with idiopathic pulmonary arterial hypertension awaiting lung transplantation. J Heart Lung Transplant. 2011;30(9):997–1002.

76. Javidfar J, Bacchetta M. Bridge to lung transplantation with extracorporeal membrane oxygenation support. Curr Opin Organ Transplant. 2012;17(5):496–502.

77. Toyoda Y, Bhama JK, Shigemura N, Zaldonis D, Pilewski J, Crespo M, et al. Efficacy of extracorporeal membrane oxygenation as a bridge to lung transplantation. J Thorac Cardiovasc Surg. 2013;145(4):1065–71.

78. Shafii AE, Mason DP, Brown CR, Vakil N, Johnston DR, McCurry KR, et al. Growing experience with extracorporeal membrane oxygenation as a bridge to lung transplantation. ASAIO J. 2012;58(5):526–9.

79. Hoopes CW, Kukreja J, Golden J, Davenport DL, Diaz-Guzman E, Zwischenberger JB. Extracorporeal membrane oxygenation as a bridge to pulmonary transplantation. J Thorac Cardiovasc Surg. 2013;145(3):862–8.

80. Bittner HB, Lehmann S, Rastan A, Garbade J, Binner C, Mohr FW, et al. Outcome of extracorporeal membrane oxygenation as a bridge to lung transplantation and graft recovery. Ann Thorac Surg. 2012;94(3):942–50.

81. Fuehner T, Kuehn C, Hadem J, Wiesner O, Gottlieb J, Tudorache I, et al. Extracorporeal membrane oxygenation in awake patients as bridge to lung transplantation. Am J Respir Crit Care Med. 2012;185(7):763–8.

82. MacLaren G, Combes A, Bartlett RH. Contemporary extracorporeal membrane oxygenation for adult respiratory failure: life support in the new era. Intensive Care Med. 2012;38(2):210–20.

83. Gottlieb J, Warnecke G, Hadem J, Dierich M, Wiesner O, Fühner T, et al. Outcome of critically ill lung transplant candidates on invasive respiratory support. Intensive Care Med. 2012;38(6):968–75.

84. Vermeijden JW, Zijlstra JG, Erasmus ME, van der Bij W, Verschuuren EA. Lung transplantation for ventilator-dependent respiratory failure. J Heart Lung Transplant. 2009;28(4):347–51.

85. Strueber M, Hoeper MM, Fischer S, Cypel M, Warnecke G, Gottlieb J, et al. Bridge to thoracic organ transplantation in patients with pulmonary arterial hypertension using a pumpless lung assist device. Am J Transplant. 2009;9(4):853–7.

86. Taylor K, Holtby H. Emergency interventional lung assist for pulmonary hypertension. Anesth Analg. 2009;109(2):382–5.

87. Hook JL, Lederer DJ. Selecting lung transplant candidates: where do current guidelines fall short? Expert Rev Respir Med. 2012;6(1):51–61.

88. Kerem E, Reisman J, Corey M, Canny GJ, Levison H. Prediction of mortality in patients with cystic fibrosis. N Engl J Med. 1992;326(18):1187–91.

89. Mayer-Hamblett N, Rosenfeld M, Emerson J, Goss CH, Aitken ML. Developing cystic fibrosis lung transplant referral criteria using predictors of 2-year mortality. Am J Respir Crit Care Med. 2002;166(12):1550–5.

90. Augarten A, Akons H, Aviram M, Bentur L, Blau H, Picard E, et al. Prediction of mortality and timing of referral for lung transplantation in cystic fibrosis patients. Pediatr Transplant. 2001;5(5):339–42.

91. Milla CE, Warwick WJ. Risk of death in cystic fibrosis patients with severely compromised lung function. Chest J. 1998;113(5):1230–4.

92. Aurora P, Wade A, Whitmore P, Whitehead B. A model for predicting life expectancy of children with cystic fibrosis. Eur Respir J. 2000;16(6): 1056–60.

93. Vizza CD, Yusen RD, Lynch JP, Fedele F, Alexander Patterson G, Trulock EP. Outcome of patients with cystic fibrosis awaiting lung transplantation. Am J Respir Crit Care Med. 2000;162(3):819–25.

94. Sharma R, Florea VG, Bolger AP, Doehner W, Florea ND, Coats AJS, et al. Wasting as an independent predictor of mortality in patients with cystic fibrosis. Thorax. 2001;56(10):746–50.

95. Emerson J, Rosenfeld M, McNamara S, Ramsey B, Gibson RL. Pseudomonas aeruginosa and other predictors of mortality and morbidity in young children with cystic fibrosis. Pediatr Pulmonol. 2002;34(2):91–100.

96. Liou TG, Adler FR, FitzSimmons SC, Cahill BC, Hibbs JR, Marshall BC. Predictive 5-year survivorship model of cystic fibrosis. Am J Epidemiol. 2001;153(4):345–52.

97. Fauroux B, Hart N, Belfar S, Boulé M, Tillous-Borde I, Bonnet D, et al. Burkholderia cepacia is associated with pulmonary hypertension and increased mortality among cystic fibrosis patients. J Clin Microbiol. 2004;42(12):5537–41.

98. Alexander BD, Petzold EW, Reller LB, Palmer SM, Davis RD, Woods CW, et al. Survival after lung transplantation of cystic fibrosis patients infected with Burkholderia cepacia complex. Am J Transplant. 2008;8(5):1025–30.

99. Tonelli AR, Fernandez-Bussy S, Lodhi S, Akindipe OA, Carrie RD, Hamilton K, et al. Prevalence of pulmonary hypertension in end-stage cystic fibrosis and correlation with survival. J Heart Lung Transplant. 2010;29(8):865–72.

100. Andersen KH, Schultz HHL, Nyholm B, Iversen MP, Gustafsson F, Carlsen J. Pulmonary hypertension as a risk factor of mortality after lung transplantation. Clin Transplant. 2016;30(4):357–64.

101. Scarsini R, Prioli MA, Milano EG, Castellani C, Pesarini G, Assael BM, et al. Hemodynamic predictors of long term survival in end stage cystic fibrosis. Int J Cardiol. 2016;202:221–5.

102. Galiè N, Humbert M, Vachiery J-L, Gibbs S, Lang I, Torbicki A, et al. 2015 ESC/ERS Guidelines for the diagnosis and treatment of pulmonary hypertension. Eur Heart J. 2016;37(1):67–119.

103. Manika K, Pitsiou GG, Boutou AK, Tsaoussis V, Chavouzis N, Antoniou M, et al. The impact of pulmonary arterial pressure on exercise capacity in mild-to-moderate cystic fibrosis: a case control study. Pulm Med. 2012;2012:252345.

104. Mourani PM, Sontag MK, Younoszai A, Ivy DD, Abman SH. Clinical utility of echocardiography for the diagnosis and management of pulmonary vascular disease in young children with chronic lung disease. Pediatrics. 2008;121(2):317–25.

105. Stallings VA, Stark LJ, Robinson KA, Feranchak AP, Quinton H, Clinical Practice Guidelines on Growth and Nutrition Subcommittee, et al. Evidence-based practice recommendations for nutrition-related management of children and adults with cystic fibrosis and pancreatic insufficiency: results of a systematic review. J Am Diet Assoc. 2008;108(5):832–9.

106. Efrati O, Mei-Zahav M, Rivlin J, Kerem E, Blau H, Barak A, et al. Long term nutritional rehabilitation by gastrostomy in Israeli patients with cystic fibrosis: clinical outcome in advanced pulmonary disease. J Pediatr Gastroenterol Nutr. 2006;42(2):222–8.

107. Floto RA, Olivier KN, Saiman L, Daley CL, Herrmann J-L, Nick JA, et al. US Cystic Fibrosis Foundation and European Cystic Fibrosis Society consensus recommendations for the management of non-tuberculous mycobacteria in individuals with cystic fibrosis. Thorax. 2016;71(Suppl 1):i1–22.

108. Leitão JH, Sousa SA, Ferreira AS, Ramos CG, Silva IN, Moreira LM. Pathogenicity, virulence factors, and strategies to fight against Burkholderia cepacia complex pathogens and related species. Appl Microbiol Biotechnol. 2010;87(1):31–40.

109. Coenye T, Vandamme P, Govan JRW, LiPuma JJ. Taxonomy and identification of the Burkholderia cepacia complex. J Clin Microbiol. 2001;39(10):3427–36.

110. Mahenthiralingam E, Baldwin A, Vandamme P. Burkholderia cepacia complex infection in patients with cystic fibrosis. J Med Microbiol. 2002;51(7):533–8.

111. Parke JL, Gurian-Sherman D. Diversity of the Burkholderia cepacia complex and implications for risk assessment of biological control strains. Annu Rev Phytopathol. 2001;39(1):225–58.

112. Mahenthiralingam E, Urban TA, Goldberg JB. The multifarious, multireplicon Burkholderia cepacia complex. Nat Rev Microbiol. 2005;3(2):144–56.

113. Mahenthiralingam E, Vandamme P. Taxonomy and pathogenesis of the Burkholderia cepacia complex. Chron Respir Dis. 2005;2(4):209–17.

114. Schaedel C, De Monestrol I, Hjelte L, Johannesson M, Kornfält R, Lindblad A, et al. Predictors of deterioration of lung function in cystic fibrosis. Pediatr Pulmonol. 2002;33(6):483–91.

115. Egan TM, Detterbeck FC, Mill MR, Bleiweis MS, Aris R, Paradowski L, et al. Long term results of lung transplantation for cystic fibrosis. Eur J Cardiothorac Surg. 2002;22(4):602–9.

116. Meachery G, De Soyza A, Nicholson A, Parry G, Hasan A, Tocewicz K, et al. Outcomes of lung transplantation for cystic fibrosis in a large UK cohort. Thorax. 2008;63(8):725–31.

117. De Soyza A, Morris K, McDowell A, Doherty C, Archer L, Perry J, et al. Prevalence and clonality of

Burkholderia cepacia complex genomovars in UK patients with cystic fibrosis referred for lung transplantation. Thorax. 2004;59(6):526–8.

118. Nash EF, Coonar A, Kremer R, Tullis E, Hutcheon M, Singer LG, et al. Survival of Burkholderia cepacia sepsis following lung transplantation in recipients with cystic fibrosis. Transpl Infect Dis. 2010;12(6):551–4.

119. Qvist T, Pressler T, Høiby N, Katzenstein TL. Shifting paradigms of nontuberculous mycobacteria in cystic fibrosis. Respir Res. 2014;15(1):41.

120. Lobo LJ, Chang LC, Esther CR, Gilligan PH, Tulu Z, Noone PG. Lung transplant outcomes in cystic fibrosis patients with pre-operative Mycobacterium abscessus respiratory infections. Clin Transplant. 2013;27(4):523–9.

121. Guirguis-Blake JM, Senger CA, Webber EM, Mularski RA, Whitlock EP. Screening for chronic obstructive pulmonary disease: evidence report and systematic review for the US Preventive Services Task Force. JAMA. 2016;315(13):1378–93.

122. Mannino DM, Kiri VA. Changing the burden of COPD mortality. Int J Chron Obstruct Pulmon Dis. 2006;1(3):219–33.

123. Lane CR, Tonelli AR. Lung transplantation in chronic obstructive pulmonary disease: patient selection and special considerations. Int J Chron Obstruct Pulmon Dis. 2015;10:2137.

124. Celli BR, Cote CG, Marin JM, Casanova C, Montes de Oca M, Mendez RA, et al. The body-mass index, airflow obstruction, dyspnea, and exercise capacity index in chronic obstructive pulmonary disease. N Engl J Med. 2004;350(10):1005–12.

125. D'Alonzo GE, Barst RJ, Ayres SM, Bergofsky EH, Brundage BH, Detre KM, et al. Survival in patients with primary pulmonary hypertension: results from a national prospective registry. Ann Intern Med. 1991;115(5):343–9.

126. Sitbon O, Humbert M, Nunes H, Parent F, Garcia G, Hervé P, et al. Long-term intravenous epoprostenol infusion in primary pulmonary hypertension: prognostic factors and survival. J Am Coll Cardiol. 2002;40(4):780–8.

127. McLaughlin VV, Shillington A, Rich S. Survival in primary pulmonary hypertension the impact of epoprostenol therapy. Circulation. 2002;106(12):1477–82.

128. Conte JV, Gaine SP, Orens JB, Harris T, Rubin LJ. The influence of continuous intravenous prostacyclin therapy for primary pulmonary hypertension on the timing and outcome of transplantation. J Heart Lung Transplant. 1998;17(7):679–85.

129. Robbins IM, Christman BW, Newman JH, Matlock R, Loyd JE. A survey of diagnostic practices and the use of epoprostenol in patients with primary pulmonary hypertension. Chest J. 1998;114(5):1269–75.

130. Hoeper MM, Barberà JA, Channick RN, Hassoun PM, Lang IM, Manes A, et al. Diagnosis, assessment, and treatment of non-pulmonary arterial hypertension pulmonary hypertension. J Am Coll Cardiol. 2009;54(1s1):S85–96.

131. Condliffe R, Kiely DG, Gibbs JSR, Corris PA, Peacock AJ, Jenkins DP, et al. Improved outcomes in medically and surgically treated chronic thromboembolic pulmonary hypertension. Am J Respir Crit Care Med. 2008;177(10):1122–7.

132. Trulock EP. Lung transplantation and atrial septostomy for pulmonary arterial hypertension. In: Hill NS, Farber HW, editors. Contemporary cardiology: pulmonary hypertension. New York: Springer; 2008. p. 383–403.

133. Galiè N, Ghofrani HA, Torbicki A, Barst RJ, Rubin LJ, Badesch D, et al. Sildenafil citrate therapy for pulmonary arterial hypertension. N Engl J Med. 2005;353(20):2148–57.

134. Ghofrani HA, Seeger W, Grimminger F. Imatinib for the treatment of pulmonary arterial hypertension. N Engl J Med. 2005;353(13):1412–3.

135. Galiè N, Rubin LJ, Hoeper MM, Jansa P, Al-Hiti H, Meyer GMB, et al. Treatment of patients with mildly symptomatic pulmonary arterial hypertension with bosentan (EARLY study): a double-blind, randomised controlled trial. Lancet. 2008;371(9630):2093–100.

136. Oudiz RJ, Galiè N, Olschewski H, Torres F, Frost A, Ghofrani HA, et al. Long-term ambrisentan therapy for the treatment of pulmonary arterial hypertension. J Am Coll Cardiol. 2009;54(21):1971–81.

137. Rosenkranz S. Pulmonary hypertension: current diagnosis and treatment. Clin Res Cardiol. 2007;96:527–41.

138. Macchia A, Marchioli R, Tognoni G, Scarano M, Marfisi R, Tavazzi L, et al. Systematic review of trials using vasodilators in pulmonary arterial hypertension: why a new approach is needed. Am Heart J. 2010;159(2):245–57.

139. Barst RJ, Gibbs JSR, Ghofrani HA, Hoeper MM, McLaughlin VV, Rubin LJ, et al. Updated evidence-based treatment algorithm in pulmonary arterial hypertension. J Am Coll Cardiol. 2009;54(1s1):S78–84.

140. Galiè N, Manes A, Negro L, Palazzini M, Reggiani MLB, Branzi A. A meta-analysis of randomized controlled trials in pulmonary arterial hypertension. Eur Heart J. 2009;30(4):394–403.

141. Ghofrani H-A, Galiè N, Grimminger F, Grünig E, Humbert M, Jing Z-C, et al. Riociguat for the treatment of pulmonary arterial hypertension. N Engl J Med. 2013;369(4):330–40.

142. Pulido T, Adzerikho I, Channick RN, Delcroix M, Galiè N, Ghofrani H-A, et al. Macitentan and morbidity and mortality in pulmonary arterial hypertension. N Engl J Med. 2013;369(9):809–18.

143. Hoeper MM, Leuchte H, Halank M, Wilkens H, Meyer FJ, Seyfarth HJ, et al. Combining inhaled iloprost with bosentan in patients with idiopathic pulmonary arterial hypertension. Eur Respir J. 2006;28(4):691–4.

144. Hoeper MM, Markevych I, Spiekerkoetter E, Welte T, Niedermeyer J. Goal-oriented treatment and combination therapy for pulmonary arterial hypertension. Eur Respir J. 2005;26(5):858–63.

145. Simonneau G, Barst RJ, Galie N, Naeije R, Rich S, Bourge RC, et al. Continuous subcutaneous infusion of treprostinil, a prostacyclin analogue, in patients with pulmonary arterial hypertension: a double-blind, randomized, placebo-controlled trial. Am J Respir Crit Care Med. 2002;165(6):800–4.

146. Galié N, Badesch D, Oudiz R, Simonneau G, McGoon MD, Keogh AM, et al. Ambrisentan therapy for pulmonary arterial hypertension. J Am Coll Cardiol. 2005;46(3):529–35.

147. Rubin LJ, Badesch DB, Barst RJ, Galiè N, Black CM, Keogh A, et al. Bosentan therapy for pulmonary arterial hypertension. N Engl J Med. 2002;346(12):896–903.

148. Sitbon O, Humbert M, Jaïs X, Ioos V, Hamid AM, Provencher S, et al. Long-term response to calcium channel blockers in idiopathic pulmonary arterial hypertension. Circulation. 2005;111(23):3105–11.

149. Galiè N, Brundage BH, Ghofrani HA, Oudiz RJ, Simonneau G, Safdar Z, et al. Tadalafil therapy for pulmonary arterial hypertension. Circulation. 2009;119(22):2894–903.

150. Tapson VF, Gomberg-Maitland M, McLaughlin VV, Benza RL, Widlitz AC, Krichman A, et al. Safety and efficacy of IV treprostinil for pulmonary arterial hypertension: a prospective, multicenter, open-label, 12-week trial. Chest J. 2006;129(3):683–8.

151. Galiè N, Corris PA, Frost A, Girgis RE, Granton J, Jing ZC, et al. Updated treatment algorithm of pulmonary arterial hypertension. J Am Coll Cardiol. 2013;62(25 Suppl):D60–72.

152. Baldi F, Fuso L, Arrighi E, Valente S. Optimal management of pulmonary arterial hypertension: prognostic indicators to determine treatment course. Ther Clin Risk Manag. 2014;10:825–39.

153. Launay D, Sitbon O, Hachulla E, Mouthon L, Gressin V, Rottat L, et al. Survival in systemic sclerosis-associated pulmonary arterial hypertension in the modern management era. Ann Rheum Dis. 2013;72(12):1940–6. https://doi.org/10.1136/annrheumdis-2012-202489.

154. Miyamoto S, Nagaya N, Satoh T, Kyotani S, Sakamaki F, Fujita M, et al. Clinical correlates and prognostic significance of six-minute walk test in patients with primary pulmonary hypertension: comparison with cardiopulmonary exercise testing. Am J Respir Crit Care Med. 2000;161(2):487–92.

155. Lordan JL, Corris PA. Pulmonary arterial hypertension and lung transplantation. Expert Rev Respir Med. 2011;5(3):441–54.

156. Woods PR, Taylor BJ, Frantz RP, Johnson BD. A pulmonary hypertension gas exchange severity (PH-GXS) score to assist with the assessment and monitoring of pulmonary arterial hypertension. Am J Cardiol. 2012;109(7):1066–72.

157. Chen H, Shiboski SC, Golden JA, Gould MK, Hays SR, Hoopes CW, et al. Impact of the lung allocation score on lung transplantation for pulmonary arterial hypertension. Am J Respir Crit Care Med. 2009;180(5):468–74.

158. Benza RL, Miller DP, Barst RJ, Badesch DB, Frost AE, McGoon MD. An evaluation of long-term survival from time of diagnosis in pulmonary arterial hypertension from the REVEAL Registry. Chest J. 2012;142(2):448–56.

159. Badesch DB, Raskob GE, Elliott CG, Krichman AM, Farber HW, Frost AE, et al. Pulmonary arterial hypertension: baseline characteristics from the REVEAL Registry. Chest J. 2010;137(2):376–87.

160. Benza RL, Miller DP, Gomberg-Maitland M, Frantz RP, Foreman AJ, Coffey CS, et al. Predicting survival in pulmonary arterial hypertension insights from the registry to evaluate early and long-term pulmonary arterial hypertension disease management (REVEAL). Circulation. 2010;122(2):164–72.

161. Benza RL, Gomberg-Maitland M, Miller DP, Frost A, Frantz RP, Foreman AJ, et al. The REVEAL Registry risk score calculator in patients newly diagnosed with pulmonary arterial hypertension. Chest J. 2012;141(2):354–62.

162. Valapour M, Skeans MA, Heubner BM, Smith JM, Hertz MI, Edwards LB, et al. OPTN/SRTR 2013 annual data report: lung. Am J Transplant. 2015;15(S2):1–28.

163. Orens JB, Estenne M, Arcasoy S, Conte JV, Corris P, Egan JJ, et al. International guidelines for the selection of lung transplant candidates: 2006 update—a consensus report from the Pulmonary Scientific Council of the International Society for Heart and Lung Transplantation. J Heart Lung Transplant. 2006;25(7):745–55.

164. Kreider M, Highland K. Pulmonary involvement in Sjögren syndrome. Semin Respir Crit Care Med. 2014;35(2):255–64.

165. Kreider M, Hadjiliadis D, Kotloff RM. Candidate selection, timing of listing, and choice of procedure for lung transplantation. Clin Chest Med. 2011;32(2):199–211.

166. Gottlieb J. Lung transplantation for interstitial lung diseases and pulmonary hypertension. Semin Respir Crit Care Med. 2013;34(3):281–7.

167. Christie JD, Edwards LB, Kucheryavaya AY, Benden C, Dipchand AI, Dobbels F, et al. The Registry of the International Society for Heart and Lung Transplantation: 29th adult lung and heart-lung transplant report—2012. J Heart Lung Transplant. 2012;31(10):1073–86.

168. Toyoda Y, Thacker J, Santos R, Nguyen D, Bhama J, Bermudez C, et al. Long-term outcome of lung and heart-lung transplantation for idiopathic pulmonary arterial hypertension. Ann Thorac Surg. 2008;86(4):1116–22.

169. Fadel E, Mercier O, Mussot S, Leroy-Ladurie F, Cerrina J, Chapelier A, et al. Long-term outcome of double-lung and heart–lung transplantation for

pulmonary hypertension: a comparative retrospective study of 219 patients. Eur J Cardiothorac Surg. 2010;38(3):277–84.

170. Hopkins WE, Ochoa LL, Richardson GW, Trulock EP. Comparison of the hemodynamics and survival of adults with severe primary pulmonary hypertension or Eisenmenger syndrome. J Heart Lung Transplant. 1996;15(1 Pt 1):100–5.

171. Charman SC, Sharples LD, McNeil KD, Wallwork J. Assessment of survival benefit after lung transplantation by patient diagnosis. J Heart Lung Transplant. 2002;21(2):226–32.

172. D'Armini AM, Cattadori B, Monterosso C, Klersy C, Emmi V, Piovella F, et al. Pulmonary thromboendarterectomy in patients with chronic thromboembolic pulmonary hypertension: hemodynamic characteristics and changes. Eur J Cardiothorac Surg. 2000;18(6):696–702.

173. McNeil K, Dunning J. Chronic thromboembolic pulmonary hypertension (CTEPH). Heart. 2007;93(9):1152–8.

174. McMahan ZH, Hummers LK. Systemic sclerosis—challenges for clinical practice. Nat Rev Rheumatol. 2013;9(2):90–100.

175. Savarino E, Bazzica M, Zentilin P, Pohl D, Parodi A, Cittadini G, et al. Gastroesophageal reflux and pulmonary fibrosis in scleroderma: a study using pH-impedance monitoring. Am J Respir Crit Care Med. 2009;179(5):408–13.

176. Shitrit D, Amital A, Peled N, Raviv Y, Medalion B, Saute M, et al. Lung transplantation in patients with scleroderma: case series, review of the literature, and criteria for transplantation. Clin Transplant. 2009;23(2):178–83.

177. Schachna L, Medsger TA, Dauber JH, Wigley FM, Braunstein NA, White B, et al. Lung transplantation in scleroderma compared with idiopathic pulmonary fibrosis and idiopathic pulmonary arterial hypertension. Arthritis Rheum. 2006;54(12): 3954–61.

178. Mertens V, Blondeau K, Van Oudenhove L, Vanaudenaerde B, Vos R, Farre R, et al. Bile acids aspiration reduces survival in lung transplant recipients with BOS despite azithromycin. Am J Transplant. 2011;11(2):329–35.

179. Robertson AGN, Ward C, Pearson JP, Corris PA, Dark JH, Griffin SM. Lung transplantation, gastroesophageal reflux, and fundoplication. Ann Thorac Surg. 2010;89(2):653–60.

180. D'Ovidio F, Mura M, Tsang M, Waddell TK, Hutcheon MA, Singer LG, et al. Bile acid aspiration and the development of bronchiolitis obliterans after lung transplantation. J Thorac Cardiovasc Surg. 2005;129(5):1144–52.

181. D'Ovidio F, Singer LG, Hadjiliadis D, Pierre A, Waddell TK, de Perrot M, et al. Prevalence of gastroesophageal reflux in end-stage lung disease candidates for lung transplant. Ann Thorac Surg. 2005;80(4):1254–60.

182. Saggar R, Khanna D, Furst DE, Belperio JA, Park GS, Weigt SS, et al. Systemic sclerosis and bilateral lung transplantation: a single centre experience. Eur Respir J. 2010;36(4):893–900.

183. Sottile PD, Iturbe D, Katsumoto TR, Connolly MK, Collard HR, Leard LA, et al. Outcomes in systemic sclerosis-related lung disease following lung transplantation. Transplantation. 2013;95(7):975.

184. Diamond JM, Lee JC, Kawut SM, Shah RJ, Localio AR, Bellamy SL, et al. Clinical risk factors for primary graft dysfunction after lung transplantation. Am J Respir Crit Care Med. 2013;187(5):527–34.

185. Kawut SM. Lung retransplantation. Clin Chest Med. 2011;32(2):367–77.

186. Novick RJ, Stitt LW, Al-Kattan K, Klepetko W, Schäfers H-J, Duchatelle J-P, et al. Pulmonary retransplantation: predictors of graft function and survival in 230 patients. Ann Thorac Surg. 1998;65(1):227–34.

187. Brugiere O, Thabut G, Castier Y, Mal H, Dauriat G, Marceau A, et al. Lung retransplantation for bronchiolitis obliterans syndrome: long-term follow-up in a series of 15 recipients. Chest J. 2003;123(6):1832–7.

188. Strueber M, Fischer S, Gottlieb J, Simon AR, Goerler H, Gohrbandt B, et al. Long-term outcome after pulmonary retransplantation. J Thorac Cardiovasc Surg. 2006;132(2):407–12.

Pretransplant Considerations in Patients with Obstructive Lung Disease: COPD, Lymphangioleiomyomatosis, Cystic Fibrosis, and Non-CF Bronchiectasis

3

Shahnaz Ajani and Robert M. Kotloff

Introduction

Pulmonary diseases characterized by progressive and irreversible airflow obstruction include chronic obstructive pulmonary disease (COPD), lymphangioleiomyomatosis (LAM), cystic fibrosis (CF), and non-CF bronchiectasis. Despite advances in treatment of these diseases, all have the potential to progress to a far-advanced and life-threatening stage, prompting consideration of lung transplantation as a therapeutic option. Since 1995, over 18,000 lung transplants have been performed for COPD (including alpha-1 antitrypsin-associated emphysema), over 7800 procedures for CF, and over 1300 for non-CF bronchiectasis [1]. Despite this extensive experience, questions remain about the appropriate timing of transplantation in the natural history of these disorders, the true survival benefits of transplantation, and, in the case of COPD, the best

procedure to perform. Similar questions arise when considering transplantation for patients with LAM, a rare obstructive lung disease for which only 500 transplants have been performed to date.

This chapter will explore the available literature with the goal of offering an evidence- and/or consensus-based assessment of issues related to the pretransplant evaluation and management of patients with obstructive lung disorders.

Chronic Obstructive Pulmonary Disease (COPD)

Prior to the institution of the lung allocation score (LAS), COPD was the most frequent indication for lung transplantation. Organs were allocated on a time-based system such that individuals who accrued the most time on the waiting list were given priority for the organ. This favored COPD patients who, because of the more indolent natural history of their disease, were able to accrue time, whereas individuals with more rapidly progressive diseases such as idiopathic pulmonary fibrosis (IPF) and CF were more likely to become too ill for transplantation or die while waiting. The LAS system allocates lungs preferentially on the basis of medical urgency and predicted survival benefit of transplantation,

S. Ajani
Division of Pulmonary, Allergy, Critical Care, and Sleep Medicine, Emory University Hospital, Emory University School of Medicine, Emory Transplant Center, Atlanta, GA, USA
e-mail: shahnaz.ajani@emory.edu

R. M. Kotloff (✉)
Department of Pulmonary Medicine, Cleveland Clinic, Cleveland, OH, USA
e-mail: kotlofr@ccf.org

© The Author(s) 2018
G. Raghu, R. G. Carbone (eds.), *Lung Transplantation*, https://doi.org/10.1007/978-3-319-91184-7_3

without consideration of time accrued. Since institution of the LAS in the United States in 2005, individuals with COPD have comprised less and less of the lung transplant waiting list, falling to a low of 32.6% in 2014. This group of individuals also has the lowest mortality rate while on the list [2].

Prognostic Factors and Implications for Timing of Listing

Recent studies have demonstrated that the natural history of COPD is often quite indolent, with a majority of patients demonstrating minimal decline in lung function over a 3–5-year period of observation [3, 4]. Long-term survival is possible for many patients with advanced COPD, and, consequently, it is often difficult to decide when lung transplantation should be offered.

Many factors have been associated with increased mortality in individuals with COPD including older age [5–8], low 6-min walk distance [9, 10], low FEV1 [6, 8, 11], low diffusion capacity [7], pulmonary hypertension [7, 12], concurrent heart failure [13], low BMI [5, 8, 14, 15], hyperinflation [5], dyspnea [6, 9, 16], low PaO_2 [16], frequent exacerbations [6, 17], and hypercapnia [8]. However, these factors are of limited utility in defining the prognosis of an individual patient and, in particular, in determining whether the risk of short-term mortality is sufficiently high to justify transplantation. More recently, the multidimensional BODE (*B*ody mass index, airflow *O*bstruction, *D*yspnea, and *E*xercise capacity) index was developed to help predict mortality in those with COPD [18]. The BODE index score ranges from 0 to 10, with a higher score indicating higher risk of death. The index has been prospectively validated and shown to be a better predictor of risk of death than FEV1 alone. The highest quartile (BODE score of 7–10) was shown to be associated with a mortality rate of 80% at 4 years, thus identifying a subset of patients for whom the disease poses an imminent threat to survival. In addition to using the BODE score as a static predictor of survival,

the predictive utility of serial measurements of the BODE index has been demonstrated [19]. In this regard, an increase in BODE score of greater than 1 point over a 6–24-month period of observation was associated with a twofold increase in mortality.

Another approach to the question of timing of transplantation has been to determine characteristics of patients most likely to derive a survival benefit. This approach considers not only the likelihood of survival without transplantation but also the predicted outcome following transplantation. One of the first studies to address this issue was conducted by Hosenpud and colleagues, who reviewed outcomes of all patients listed for lung transplant in the United States between January 1, 1992, and December 31, 1994. They found that survival on the waiting list was significantly higher for those with emphysema compared to CF and idiopathic pulmonary fibrosis. They also noted that for the emphysema patients, a survival benefit of transplantation could not be demonstrated at any time during the 2-year follow-up period. Notably, they assumed a constant death rate while on the waiting list, which may have underestimated waitlist mortality for this group [20]. This study was also performed prior to introduction of the LAS system and therefore at a time when patients were placed on the waiting list even before they were deemed in imminent need of transplantation, again biasing in favor of waitlist survival.

A more recent study utilizing the large United Network for Organ Sharing (UNOS) database containing 8182 COPD patients listed for lung transplantation between 1986 and 2004 identified subsets of patients with COPD that appeared to derive a survival benefit from transplantation [21]. The likelihood of a survival benefit was greater in those undergoing bilateral lung transplantation (BLT) rather than single-lung transplantation (SLT). In this regard, approximately 45% of patients would gain a survival benefit of at least 1 year by undergoing BLT compared to only 22% who would derive such a benefit if SLT were employed. In addition to procedure type, FEV_1 was a major determinant of the survival benefit. As an example, nearly 80% of patients with an FEV1 <16% but only 11% of those with an FEV1 >25% were predicted to gain at least a year of life with BLT. Other factors associated with survival benefit (gain >1 year) were systolic pulmonary artery pressure (>40 mmHg), BMI (<20), exercise capacity (walk distance ≥150 ft), functional status (class III), need for continuous mechanical ventilation or supplemental oxygen, and absence of diabetes.

Lahzami and colleagues utilized the BODE index to generate predicted survival without transplantation for 54 COPD patients and compared this to actual posttransplantation survival of this cohort. They found that a survival advantage at 4 years after transplant was expected only for those with a BODE ≥7 [22].

Based on a review of the literature and on consensus opinion, the most recent International Society for Heart and Lung Transplantation (ISHLT) consensus guidelines recommend listing individuals with COPD for lung transplantation when at least one of the following is present [23]:

- BODE index ≥7
- FEV1 <15–20% predicted
- Three or more severe exacerbations during the preceding year
- One severe exacerbation with acute hypercapnic respiratory failure
- Moderate to severe pulmonary hypertension

Patients with advanced COPD who do not meet these criteria may still benefit from referral to a transplant center for initial consultation. Early referral permits the patient and family members to meet the transplant team and learn about the benefits as well as considerable risks and commitments of transplantation at a time when the patient is not under pressure to make an immediate decision about evaluation and listing. It also allows the transplant team to identify and address factors that might compromise the future candidacy of the patient, such as ongoing smoking, extremes of weight, poor functional status, severe osteoporosis, excessive corticosteroid use, and coronary artery disease.

Comorbidities Affecting Transplant Suitability

Malnutrition

Poor nutritional status is prevalent among patients with advanced COPD and is associated with a poor prognosis [5, 8, 14, 15]. Notably, malnutrition, indicated by hypoalbuminemia or low BMI, has been associated with increased mortality following lung transplantation [24–26]. In light of its adverse effects on both pre- and posttransplantation mortality, malnutrition should be aggressively addressed in patients being considered for lung transplantation, with interventions ranging from high-calorie oral supplements to placement of a gastrostomy tube for supplemental enteral feeding.

Osteoporosis

Another frequently encountered comorbidity in individuals with COPD is osteoporosis. Although related in part to steroid exposure, COPD itself has been shown to be an independent risk factor for low bone mineral density [27, 28]. Patients with COPD have been found to have the lowest bone mineral density when compared to fibrotic lung disease and sarcoidosis [29]. All patients being considered for lung transplantation should undergo DEXA scanning, and those found to have osteopenia or osteoporosis should be aggressively treated to minimize the risk of further bone demineralization and resultant fractures.

Debility

Functional disability is another feature of advanced COPD. Contributing factors include reduced physical activity, corticosteroid myopathy, and systemic effects of COPD on peripheral muscle function. Six-minute walk testing has been the predominant means by which functional status of lung transplant candidates has been assessed. Recently, Singer and colleagues employed the Short Physical Performance Battery, an available frailty instrument that emphasizes physical functioning, to assess candidates awaiting lung transplantation [30]. These investigators found an association between increasing frailty scores and risk of delisting or death while awaiting transplantation. In order to mitigate these risks, and to optimize the candidate's functional status in preparation for transplantation, enrollment in a pulmonary rehabilitation program is strongly encouraged.

Role of Lung Volume Reduction Surgery (LVRS) as a Bridge to Transplant

LVRS is a palliative surgical option for a subset of COPD patients with advanced, upper lobe-predominant emphysema who meet criteria for this procedure. The National Emphysema Treatment Trial documented improved exercise capacity and, in some subgroups, improved survival for individuals with emphysema who underwent LVRS [31]. For select patients with advanced emphysema, there is the option of offering LVRS first, reserving transplantation for failure to respond to LVRS or to subsequent functional decline after a period of sustained improvement. Successful LVRS can postpone the need for transplantation for up to several years, and the associated improvement in functional and nutritional status can optimize the patient's suitability as a transplant candidate [32–35].

Prior LVRS can lead to formation of pleural adhesions, which can pose technical challenges to the surgeon at the time of transplantation. It may be necessary to leave residual native lung tissue and visceral pleura behind, particularly to protect the recurrent laryngeal and phrenic nerves [32]. Published reports of posttransplant outcomes for patients who previously underwent LVRS paint a somewhat conflicting picture. Senbaklavaci and colleagues found that "successful" LVRS prior to transplant (defined as a 20% or greater increase in FEV1) was associated with a significant improvement in pretransplant BMI and a reduced perioperative mortality rate following lung transplantation [33]. Nathan and colleagues found no difference in the need for reoperation, index hospital length of stay, or mortality following transplantation between individuals who had previously undergone

LVRS and those who had not [36]. In contrast, Shigemura and colleagues noted an increase in operative time, incidence of postoperative bleeding requiring re-exploration, and ICU length of stay for individuals who had previously undergone LVRS; however, no difference in survival was noted [37]. Similarly, Burns and colleagues reported an increased transfusion requirement related to perioperative pleural bleeding compared to a matched cohort without antecedent LVRS. Despite this, there was no significant difference in survival rates or long-term pulmonary function between the two groups [34]. Backhus and colleagues documented longer operative time and hospital length of stay for individuals who had previously undergone LVRS. Although no difference in 30-day mortality was noted, 1-, 5-, and 10-year survival was lower in individuals who had undergone LVRS prior to transplant when compared to individuals who had undergone transplant alone [38].

Choice of Lung Transplant Procedure for COPD

SLT was for many years the preferred procedure for patients with COPD. Beginning in 2006, however, BLT replaced SLT as the procedure most commonly employed for COPD patients, and currently approximately three-quarters of the transplants performed for this patient population are BLTs [1]. Factors that have influenced the debate about the preferred procedure include survival differences, functional outcomes, native lung complications, donor organ scarcity, and center-specific preferences.

Survival
Studies demonstrating superior long-term survival associated with BLT compared to SLT for COPD recipients have served as the principal impetus behind the preferential employment of BLT over the past decade. Meyer and colleagues analyzed a cohort of 2260 adult lung transplant recipients with COPD entered into the ISHLT registry [39]. They demonstrated superior survival associated with BLT in recipients under the

age of 60 years but were unable to demonstrate a difference in survival in older recipients. Thabut and colleagues subsequently performed an analysis of almost 10,000 COPD patients in the ISHLT registry transplanted between 1987 and 2006 [21]. Consistent with the previous study, they demonstrated a survival advantage associated with BLT; median survival following BLT was 6.4 years vs. 4.5 years following SLT. Again, a survival advantage for BLT could not be confirmed in recipients over the age of 60 years. A recent study calls into question whether these findings apply in the post-LAS era, which has resulted in changes in the demographics and clinical characteristics of recipient populations. Examining outcomes of transplants performed since LAS implementation in 2005 and controlling for confounders with propensity score analysis, Schaffer and colleagues found no difference in 5-year graft survival (a composite of death and graft failure requiring retransplantation) between SLT and BLT recipients [40].

Functional Outcomes

Lung function improves dramatically among COPD patients following both SLT and BLT; as expected, BLT recipients experience a greater magnitude of improvement. Following SLT, FEV1 typically increases to 40–60%, while the FEV1 typically exceeds 80% predicted following BLT [41–43]. This difference in FEV1 is sustained over time. Exercise tolerance, as assessed by 6-min walk test (6MWT), also improves to a greater degree following BLT, though the disparity is less than that seen in relation to FEV1 [42, 43]. Notably, 6MWT distances are not adjusted for age. Since BLT patients are on average younger than those undergoing SLT, the differences in walk distance could reflect age-related rather than procedure-specific effects. Despite the differences in 6-min walk distance, studies have not demonstrated a significant difference in measures of daily physical activity between the two recipient populations [44, 45] nor have significant differences been noted in exercise performance as assessed by the age-adjusted parameter of maximum oxygen consumption [46, 47].

Complications Related to the Native Lung

Two native lung complications are unique to SLT recipients: lung cancer and native lung hyperinflation. Since essentially all patients undergoing lung transplantation for advanced COPD are former smokers, they are at increased risk for developing lung cancer. With rare exception, lung cancer is encountered in the remaining native lung following SLT. Dickson and colleagues performed a retrospective review of 131 consecutive SLT recipients and a control group of 131 consecutive BLT recipients matched for underlying disease; 75% of recipients in both groups had COPD [48]. Among the SLT recipients, 6.9% developed primary lung cancer, all in the native lung and all but one in patients with underlying COPD, compared with no cases in the BLT group. Numerous other studies have corroborated the finding of an increased risk of lung cancer in the native lung of COPD SLT recipients [49–52]. Data are conflicting as to whether factors related to transplantation (e.g., immunosuppression) confer additional risk for developing lung cancer or whether the incidence is comparable to that of the general population with similar risk factors. Although candidates for lung transplantation routinely undergo screening with chest computed tomography, this strategy results in the frequent detection of nodules ultimately proven to be benign and fails to detect native lung cancers that develop de novo after transplantation.

Native lung hyperinflation can occasionally complicate the immediate postoperative period of COPD patients following SLT. In a single-center case series, Weill and colleagues documented a 31% incidence of acute native lung hyperinflation in this patient population [53]. Although recipients with symptomatic native lung hyperinflation had longer lengths of stay, there was no difference in 30-day, 1-, 2-, or 3-year survival or in FEV_1 and 6-min walk distance at 1 year. Although risk factors have not been well defined, the combination of positive pressure ventilation and significant allograft edema serves to magnify the compliance differential between the two lungs and may predispose to this complication. The consequences of marked over distention of

the native lung are identical to those seen in association with tension pneumothorax: hypotension,
hypoxemia, and hypercapnia. The risk of acute
hyperinflation can be minimized by early extubation, which in uncomplicated cases can often be
performed at the completion of the surgical procedure. For patients who cannot be extubated and
who develop severe respiratory or hemodynamic
consequences of acute hyperinflation, replacement of the standard endotracheal tube with a
double-lumen tube permits selective application
of a low respiratory rate and prolonged expiratory time to facilitate more complete emptying of
the native lung.

More insidiously, up to 5% of SLT recipients
with COPD demonstrate progressive native lung
hyperinflation in the months to years following
transplantation, leading to allograft compression, diminished pulmonary function, increasing
oxygen requirements, and decreasing exercise
tolerance [54]. In select patients, native lung
hyperinflation can be successfully addressed
with lung volume reduction surgery [54–56] or
with bronchoscopic insertion of endobronchial
valves [57, 58].

Organ Allocation

An important consideration in the choice of procedure is organ availability. Despite the decrease
in the size of the active waiting list since the institution of the LAS system, and a modest increase
in the number of lung transplants performed
annually, approximately 1000 candidates remain
on the waiting list at the end of each calendar year
in the United States [59]. In the context of ongoing organ shortages, SLT provides greater access
to this limited resource. In a study utilizing statistical models, Munson and colleagues found that
a SLT strategy resulted in more patients transplanted and fewer waitlist deaths, with equivalent "total" posttransplant survival (incorporating
both the total number of patients transplanted and
the expected survival of each patient after transplantation) [60]. The model they employed was
sensitive to waitlist size, survival benefit from
BLT, and donor availability, which is subject to
regional variation. The authors acknowledged
that BLT would be an appropriate strategy in cir-

cumstances where waiting lists are short, donors
are common, and the survival advantage of BLT
is large but few if any transplant centers currently
possess these features.

Conclusions Regarding Choice of Procedure

The purported survival advantage associated with
BLT has now been called into question in the
post-LAS era. There may still be modest functional benefits to BLT, and this procedure spares
the recipient the complications associated with
maintaining a native lung in situ, though these
are relatively uncommon. These advantages for
the individual recipient must be weighed against
the collective benefits of maximizing organ allocation to the greatest number of recipients. In our
opinion, SLT is an appropriate option for patients
with COPD, and as a less rigorous surgical procedure, it is well suited for older and frailer patients.

Lymphangioleiomyomatosis (LAM)

LAM is a rare cystic lung disease almost exclusively affecting women, most often during child-
bearing years. It is characterized by abnormal
smooth muscle proliferation around the small
airways, lymphatics, and blood vessels of the
lung. LAM is an uncommon indication for transplant, accounting for only 1% of the total lung
transplant procedures performed worldwide
since 1995 [1]. Current 1-, 5-, and 10-year posttransplant survival rates for LAM recipients are
89%, 67%, and 47%, respectively [61]. These
rates compare favorable to survival rates of other
recipient populations. Although LAM has been
documented to occasionally recur in the allograft
[62–65], such recurrence is typically an incidental finding that, with rare exception [66], does not
compromise allograft function.

Timing of Listing

Although early retrospective cohort studies documented 10-year survival rates following diagnosis
of 20% or less, more recent data demonstrate that

close to 90% of patients with LAM are alive at 10 years [67]. It is anticipated that the recent introduction of sirolimus as a disease-stabilizing agent for progressive disease will further improve the prognosis. The evolving natural history of LAM complicates decisions about the appropriate time to list patients for transplantation. Additionally, prognostic parameters that can be used to identify high-risk patients in imminent danger of short-term mortality, and therefore in need of listing for transplantation, are limited. One registry study found that younger age at diagnosis, use of supplemental oxygen, and weight loss were independent predictors of time to death or transplantation [67]. In the absence of precise indices, patients with LAM are considered for listing when there is evidence of severe and progressive impairment in pulmonary function, functional status, and quality of life. Characteristics of LAM patients listed for transplantation can be gleaned from reviewing the published worldwide experience encompassing over 250 patients, with possible overlap of some patients between publications [62–66, 68]. The mean age at the time of transplantation was between 40 and 42 years, FEV1 ranged from 20 to 30% predicted, mean room air PaO_2 was 53–59 mmHg, and mean 6MWT distance was 702–826 ft. The Organ Procurement and Transplantation Network/United Network for Organ Sharing (OPTN/UNOS) database provides additional insight, having recorded 56 lung transplants for LAM in the United States between 2005 and 2011. Mean FEV1 for this group was 0.65 L (24% predicted), and mean 6MWT distance was 683 ft [61].

Special Considerations in Selection of LAM Patients

Pleural Disease
Many patients with LAM develop recurrent pneumothoraces or, less commonly, chylous effusions that require pleurodesis or pleurectomy for management. Prior performance of these procedures should not be viewed as a contraindication for lung transplantation but can pose challenges in explanting the lung(s). Pleural adhesions are encountered in 47–71% of LAM patients undergoing transplantation. In most but not all cases, this is a direct consequence of a prior pleural procedure. The reported frequency of moderate to severe intraoperative hemorrhage arising from this situation is 12–50%, with a need for repeat thoracotomy to control bleeding in up to 22% of these cases [62, 64, 65, 68]. The increased risk of bleeding does not translate into excessive early mortality, as evidenced by the excellent 1-year posttransplant survival rate achieved in the LAM population.

Angiomyolipoma
Renal angiomyolipomas are benign vascular tumors that are present in up to 50% of women with sporadic LAM and an even higher percentage of patients with LAM associated with underlying tuberous sclerosis. When large (>3 cm), they pose a risk of spontaneous rupture and bleeding and, rarely, may compromise renal function. Following lung transplantation, bleeding complications related to angiomyolipomas appear to be rare, occurring in <6% of patients with pretransplant lesions, though the length of follow-up in published series is limited [62, 63]. Survival of transplant recipients with and without renal angiomyolipomas is similar [65]. Based on this experience, renal angiomyolipomas are not considered a contraindication to transplantation as long as large lesions have been adequately addressed with embolization or medication, and renal function is not significantly compromised.

Sirolimus Use
Many LAM patients are now on sirolimus prior to transplantation due to its proven disease-stabilizing effects. Sirolimus is an antiproliferative agent and can impair surgical wound healing. It has been implicated as a cause of postsurgical wound dehiscence, including fatal bronchial anastomotic dehiscence [69, 70]. The half-life of sirolimus is 62 h. Although there are no data indicating how early to stop sirolimus prior to transplantation, at least 5–10 days would be necessary to permit full elimination of the drug. Since the timing of transplantation is unpredictable, many transplant centers require that patients

stop sirolimus at the time of listing. Given that waiting times for LAM patients are often prolonged, this strategy places the patient at risk for progressive decline in lung function prior to transplantation, with the attendant risks of death or delisting. Anecdotally, our center and others have transplanted several LAM patients maintained on sirolimus up to the time of transplant without encountering bronchial dehiscence in the early posttransplant period. An alternative strategy is to switch the patient at the time of listing to everolimus, an mTOR inhibitor that also appears to stabilize lung function in LAM patients [71]. This drug has a much shorter half-life than sirolimus, and blood levels would be expected to rapidly diminish in the first several days following transplantation. In a clinical trial of everolimus for treatment of idiopathic pulmonary fibrosis, five patients took the drug up to the day of lung transplantation; none developed bronchial dehiscence [72].

Choice of Procedure

Both SLT and BLT have been successfully performed in patients with LAM. The ISHLT Registry documents 500 transplants performed on LAM patients between 1995 and 2015; 70% of these were bilateral procedures [1]. BLT is associated with considerably higher posttransplant FEV1 (reported means 76–78% predicted) compared to SLT (reported means 53–54% predicted) [62, 65]. BLT also avoids the risk of native lung pneumothorax, reported to occur in 17–21% of single-lung recipients [62, 65]. In previous published reports, survival rates following SLT and BLT were similar [65, 66]. However, current statistics from the OPTN/UNOS registry suggest a trend toward more favorable survival following BLT. In this regard, 1-year survival rates for BLT and SLT are 91% vs. 86%, respectively, and 5-year survival rates are 71% vs. 60%, respectively [61].

In summary, both SLT and BLT are acceptable options for patients with LAM. At present, the choice of procedure should be individualized, taking into account technical challenges related to explanting the native lungs (in particular, in those who have undergone prior pleurodesis or pleurectomy), the ability of the patient to tolerate the more rigorous bilateral procedure, and the availability of organs in a particular region. Should BLT ultimately prove to confer superior survival, this would provide further justification for the preferred use of this procedure in suitable candidates.

Cystic Fibrosis (CF)

The projected median survival for children with CF born in 2010 is 39 years for females and 40 years for males [73]. Despite the dramatic improvement in survival over the last decades, the primary cause of death for patients with CF remains respiratory failure. CF was the underlying indication for 16% of lung transplants performed worldwide since 1995 and remains the third leading indication behind IPF and COPD [1, 2].

Prognostic Factors and Implications for Timing of Listing

The introduction of lung transplantation as a therapeutic option for treatment of advanced CF has stimulated efforts over the past several decades to more accurately predict the natural history of this disease in order to determine the appropriate time to list patients. Kerem and colleagues, in a landmark paper published in 1992, found that CF patients with a FEV1 less than 30% predicted had a 2-year mortality rate exceeding 50% [74]. Based on this study, an FEV1 <30% became the benchmark for referral for lung transplantation for this patient population. Subsequent studies documenting more favorable median survival rates associated with an FEV1 <30% have challenged the utility of this parameter in deciding when to refer [75–77]. A recent study from London, for example, demonstrated that the median survival for those with FEV1 less than 30% predicted improved from 1.2 years in 1990–1991 to 5.2 years in 2002–2003 [77].

Rather than using FEV1 as a static parameter, Rosenbluth and colleagues used rate of decline of FEV1 to determine appropriate timing for lung transplant referral [78]. They reported that younger age, malnutrition, and concurrent infection with both *Pseudomonas aeruginosa* and *Staphylococcus aureus* were risk factors for rapidly declining lung function. Use of their model permitted the identification of a subset of individuals with rapidly declining lung function; this strategy would have resulted in earlier referral for lung transplantation, possibly decreasing mortality in this group.

Six-minute walk test distance has been identified as an alternative functional parameter of prognostic import in predicting the natural history of CF. In a study of 286 CF patients in France, Martin and colleagues found that a 6-min walk distance $\leq$475 m was an independent predictor of death or transplantation [79]. Vizza and colleagues similarly found that shorter 6-min walk distance was associated with an increased risk of death on the transplant waiting list but a cutoff that reliably separated the patients who died from those still alive could not be identified [80].

Another approach has been to develop multivariate predictive models for mortality based on analysis of the comprehensive CF Foundation database. Liou and colleagues developed a 5-year survivorship model derived from data on 5800 patients in the CF Foundation Patient Registry and validated using data from an additional 5800 registry patients [81]. When applied to the validation cohort, this complex model predicted survival in superior fashion to the simpler model proposed by Kerem utilizing FEV1 alone. The authors found that higher FEV1%, higher weight-for-age z score, pancreatic sufficiency, and *Staphylococcus aureus* infection predicted increased survival. Increasing age, female gender, diabetes mellitus, *Burkholderia cepacia* infection, and a higher number of acute pulmonary exacerbations predicted decreased survival. Plugging these variables into a logistic regression equation allowed calculation of the probability of 5-year survival for a given patient. In a follow-up study, these same investigators employed their survivorship model as well as a model of

posttransplant survival to demonstrate that only those patients over the age of 18 years with a 5-year predicted survival of <50% and without *Burkholderia cepacia* airway infection or CF arthropathy were likely to derive a survival benefit from transplantation [82].

Mayer-Hamblett and colleagues utilized a larger cohort of 14,572 patients in the CF Foundation National Patient Registry to determine factors predictive of 2-year mortality [83]. They found that increasing age and height, lower FEV1, colonization with *Pseudomonas aeruginosa* or *Burkholderia cepacia*, more than two hospitalizations for pulmonary exacerbations annually, or more than two courses of home intravenous antibiotics annually were all associated with a higher odds ratio of dying within 2 years. In contrast to the findings of Liou, the authors found that the diagnostic accuracy of their multidimensional model incorporating these parameters was not significantly better than the simpler FEV1 criterion proposed by Kerem; both were much better at predicting who would survive 2 years than who would die.

In summary, no one predictive model has emerged that can be utilized to make definitive recommendations regarding appropriate timing for listing CF patients. The ISHLT consensus guidelines [23] recommend listing when any of the following are present:

- Chronic respiratory failure with PaO_2 <60 mmHg or $PaCO_2$ >50 mmHg
- Long-term noninvasive ventilation
- Pulmonary hypertension
- Frequent hospitalizations
- Rapid decline in lung function
- World Health Organization Functional Class IV

Implications of Airway Pathogens in Patient Selection

Chronic infection of the airways is a universal feature of CF and poses unique concerns in selecting CF patients for transplantation. The majority of adult CF patients are infected with

Pseudomonas aeruginosa by the time they are considered for lung transplantation [84]. While these organisms are often highly resistant, the impact of the resistance pattern on survival following transplantation appears to be small. Two single-center retrospective studies found that posttransplant survival of CF patients with pan-resistant *Pseudomonas aeruginosa* was similar to that of patients harboring sensitive strains [85, 86]. In contrast to these studies, Hadjiliadis and colleagues found that patients harboring pan-resistant organisms had lower, albeit still highly favorable, survival rates compared to patients with sensitive strains: 87% vs. 97% at 1 year and 58% vs. 86% at 5 years [87]. Taken in summary, these three studies suggest that patients with pan-resistant *Pseudomonas aeruginosa* should not be excluded from consideration for lung transplantation.

The situation is more complicated with respect to pretransplant infection with *Burkholderia cepacia complex*, encountered in approximately 4% of CF adults [84]. The name reflects the fact that *B. cepacia complex* is not a single entity but a heterogeneous collection of species (previously referred to as genomovars) with varying pathogenicity and impact on pre- and posttransplant outcomes. Infection with *B. cepacia complex*, and in particular with *B. cenocepacia*, has been associated with accelerated decline in lung function and excess mortality in individuals with CF [88–92]. Pretransplantation infection with *B. cepacia* also has an adverse impact on survival posttransplantation due to reemergence of this organism as a cause of lethal pulmonary and disseminated infections. Reports from multiple centers document 1-year survival rates in the range of 50–67% for patients with *B. cepacia* compared to 83–92% for those without [93, 94]. Using predictive models of pre- and posttransplant survival, Liou and colleagues reported that CF patients infected with *B. cepacia* do not derive a survival benefit from transplantation [82]. More recent studies have attributed the excessive posttransplant mortality specifically to *B. cenocepacia* and possibly to *B. gladioli* [95, 96]. In contrast, infection with other members of the *B. cepacia* complex does not appear to adversely impact posttransplant

survival. Although the majority of transplant centers now exclude candidates with *B. cenocepacia* from consideration for lung transplantation, many will consider candidates who harbor less virulent species.

Aspergillus species are isolated from pretransplant respiratory cultures in up to 50% of CF patients. Studies suggest that recovery of *Aspergillus* from preoperative sputum cultures in the CF population is not predictive of subsequent acquisition of deep-seated infection in the allografts, though there may be an increased risk of infection of the bronchial anastomosis [97, 98]. Some centers do choose to initiate antifungal therapy either prior to or at the time of transplantation for patients in whom aspergillus is recovered from sputum cultures. Recovery of aspergillus does not, however, represent a contraindication to transplantation.

Nontuberculous mycobacteria are isolated in up to 20% of CF patients referred for consideration of lung transplantation. The most common mycobacterium isolated is *Mycobacterium avium* complex; its presence does not adversely impact outcomes after lung transplantation. In contrast, pretransplant recovery of *Mycobacterium abscessus* has been associated with subsequent development of serious infections posttransplantation, albeit not conclusively with reduced survival [99, 100]. Although the recovery of nontuberculous mycobacteria in respiratory tract cultures is not considered a contraindication to transplantation, evidence of progressive pulmonary or extrapulmonary disease despite optimal therapy, or failure to tolerate such therapy, is [23].

Common Comorbidities

Malnutrition
Malnutrition is common in the CF population and has been shown in some studies to adversely affect the natural history of the disease [88, 101]. In a study utilizing the UNOS database, 42% of CF patients who underwent lung transplantation in the United States were underweight (BMI <18.5). Notably, this was associated with a 25% higher posttransplant mortality rate compared

to CF patients of normal weight range [26]. In light of this, attempts to aggressively correct nutritional deficiencies prior to transplantation appear justified. Strategies to accomplish this goal include the use of high-calorie oral supplements, nocturnal enteral supplementation using a percutaneously placed gastrostomy or jejunostomy tube, and parenteral alimentation.

Diabetes

CF-related diabetes is encountered in up to 50% of adults with CF and is associated with an increased mortality pretransplant [102–104]. Augmentation of the diabetic regimen may be required in the posttransplant period due to the hyperglycemic effects of corticosteroids and tacrolimus. However, the presence of CF-related diabetes does not appear to negatively impact outcomes after lung transplant [105, 106].

Osteoporosis

Patients with CF are particularly prone to loss of bone mineral density and development of osteoporosis. CF is characterized by increased levels of circulating cytokines, reduced sex hormone production, and pancreatic insufficiency with reduced intestinal absorption of calcium and vitamin D, all of which may contribute to the development of bone demineralization. Additionally, many CF patients have received glucocorticoids as part of their treatment regimen. A cross-sectional study of bone mineral density in lung transplant candidates and recipients demonstrated that CF patients, despite being younger in age, had significantly lower pre- and posttransplantation bone mineral density than patients with COPD and other lung diseases [107]. Seventy-five percent of the CF patients had bone mineral density at or below the fracture threshold prior to transplantation, compared to 45% of patients with COPD. Symptomatic fractures occurred in 15% of CF patients prior to transplantation and in 25% following transplantation. In order to minimize the risk that debilitating vertebral compression fractures could compromise the outcome of transplantation, CF patients should be screened for bone demineralization with DEXA scans. Those documented to

have osteopenia or osteoporosis should receive appropriate medical therapy aimed at minimizing further bone loss. Standard recommendations for maintaining bone mineral density in patients with CF include minimizing the use of systemic steroids, optimizing pancreatic enzyme replacement and diet to ensure adequate intake and absorption of fat-soluble vitamins and calcium, and promoting weight-bearing activity. Bisphosphonates have been demonstrated to be effective in stabilizing or improving bone mineral density in CF patients and should be initiated in the setting of significant bone demineralization [108, 109].

Sinusitis

Sinus disease is nearly universal in patients with CF and represents a reservoir for *Pseudomonas aeruginosa* following transplantation. As such, it was initially believed that prophylactic surgical drainage of the sinuses would be beneficial for lung transplant recipients. However, compelling data supporting surgical intervention are lacking. For example, a retrospective review of the experience at Stanford University found no benefit of routine pretransplant sinus surgery on posttransplant survival or the rate of recolonization of the allograft with *Pseudomonas aeruginosa* [110].

Liver Disease

Liver involvement is common in CF but leads to clinically overt cirrhosis in only 5% of patients. CF patients with advanced lung disease and concomitant cirrhosis have been successfully treated with combined lung (or heart-lung) and liver transplantation, with outcomes in experienced centers comparable to those achieved with lung transplantation alone [111]. For patients with well-compensated cirrhosis and preserved synthetic function, there are reports of successful short-term outcomes with lung transplantation alone, though this approach remains controversial [112, 113].

Non-CF Bronchiectasis

A number of disorders other than CF can also lead to extensive bronchiectasis potentially requiring lung transplantation, including quantitative and qualitative immunoglobulin deficiency states, primary ciliary dyskinesia, infection with non-tuberculous mycobacteria, and severe childhood pneumonias. Non-CF bronchiectasis accounts for approximately 3% of all lung transplants performed worldwide since 1995 [1]. Posttransplant outcomes approximate those of other recipient populations [114, 115].

Given the diverse etiologies and relatively small number of patients afflicted, it is not surprising that the natural history of non-CF bronchiectasis is not well defined. In deciding on the appropriate timing for listing these patients, the transplant community has generally utilized the guidelines established for CF patients [116]. Challenging this practice, however, is a recent analysis of the UNOS database that demonstrated significantly better waitlist survival for patients with non-CF bronchiectasis compared to patients with CF [117].

Patients with bronchiectasis due to quantitative or qualitative immunoglobulin deficiencies require lifelong immunoglobulin replacement therapy continuing into the posttransplant period. Patients presenting for lung transplant evaluation with "idiopathic" bronchiectasis should be screened with quantitative immunoglobulin levels and response to vaccine challenge to identify those who will need replacement therapy. Care of the potential transplant candidate with non-CF bronchiectasis is otherwise largely extrapolated from that employed for CF patients and includes systemic and inhaled antibiotics and airway clearance measures.

Summary

This chapter focused on COPD, LAM, CF, and non-CF bronchiectasis, four diseases that share a common pathophysiology of airflow obstruction and a propensity for some patients to advance to an incapacitating and life-threatening stage. Optimal utilization of transplantation for these challenging patient populations mandates a thorough appreciation of their natural history, prognostic factors, and accompanying comorbidities, all addressed in this chapter.

References

1. Yusen RD, Edwards LB, Dipchand AI, et al. The Registry of the International Society for Heart And Lung Transplantation: thirty-third official adult lung and heart-lung transplantation report—2016; focus theme: primary diagnostic indications for transplant. J Heart Lung Transplant. 2016;35:1170–84.
2. Valapour M, Skeans MA, Smith JM, et al. Lung. Am J Transplant. 2016;16(Suppl 2):141–68.
3. Vestbo J, Edwards LD, Scanlon PD, et al. Changes in forced expiratory volume in 1 second over time in COPD. N Engl J Med. 2011;365:1184–92.
4. Nishimura M, Makita H, Nagai K, et al. Annual change in pulmonary function and clinical phenotype in chronic obstructive pulmonary disease. Am J Respir Crit Care Med. 2012;185:44–52.
5. Budweiser S, Jorres RA, Riedl T, et al. Predictors of survival in COPD patients with chronic hypercapnic respiratory failure receiving noninvasive home ventilation. Chest. 2007;131:1650–8.
6. Esteban C, Quintana JM, Aburto M, et al. The health, activity, dyspnea, obstruction, age, and hospitalization: prognostic score for stable COPD patients. Respir Med. 2011;105:1662–70.
7. Hurdman J, Condliffe R, Elliot CA, et al. Pulmonary hypertension in COPD: results from the Aspire Registry. Eur Respir J. 2013;41:1292–301.
8. Yang H, Xiang P, Zhang E, et al. Is hypercapnia associated with poor prognosis in chronic obstructive pulmonary disease? A long-term follow-up cohort study. BMJ Open. 2015;5:e008909.
9. Golpe R, Perez-De-Llano LA, Mendez-Marote L, Veres-Racamonde A. Prognostic value of walk distance, work, oxygen saturation, and dyspnea during 6-minute walk test in COPD patients. Respir Care. 2013;58:1329–34.
10. Takigawa N, Tada A, Soda R, et al. Distance and oxygen desaturation in 6-min walk test predict prognosis in COPD patients. Respir Med. 2007;101:561–7.
11. Burrows B, Earle RH. Course and prognosis of chronic obstructive lung disease. A prospective study of 200 patients. N Engl J Med. 1969;280:397–404.
12. Andersen KH, Iversen M, Kjaergaard J, et al. Prevalence, predictors, and survival in pulmonary hypertension related to end-stage chronic obstructive pulmonary disease. J Heart Lung Transplant. 2012;31:373–80.
13. Boudestein LC, Rutten FH, Cramer MJ, Lammers JW, Hoes AW. The impact of concurrent heart failure on prognosis in patients with chronic obstructive pulmonary disease. Eur J Heart Failure. 2009;11:1182–8.
14. Cao C, Wang R, Wang J, Bunjhoo H, Xu Y, Xiong W. Body mass index and mortality in chronic obstructive pulmonary disease: a meta-analysis. PLoS One. 2012;7:e43892.
15. Marti S, Munoz X, Rios J, Morell F, Ferrer J. Body weight and comorbidity predict mortality in COPD

patients treated with oxygen therapy. Eur Respir J. 2006;27:689–96.

16. Coleta KD, Silveira LV, Lima DF, Rampinelli EA, Godoy I, Godoy I. Predictors of first-year survival in patients with advanced COPD treated using long-term oxygen therapy. Respir Med. 2008;102:512–8.

17. Soler-Cataluna JJ, Martinez-Garcia MA, Sanchez LS, Tordera MP, Sanchez PR. Severe exacerbations and Bode index: two independent risk factors for death in male COPD patients. Respir Med. 2009;103:692–9.

18. Celli BR, Cote CG, Marin JM, et al. The body-mass index, airflow obstruction, dyspnea, and exercise capacity index in chronic obstructive pulmonary disease. N Engl J Med. 2004;350:1005–12.

19. Martinez FJ, Han MK, Andrei AC, et al. Longitudinal change in the Bode index predicts mortality in severe emphysema. Am J Respir Crit Care Med. 2008;178:491–9.

20. Hosenpud JD, Bennett LE, Keck BM, Edwards EB, Novick RJ. Effect of diagnosis on survival benefit of lung transplantation for end-stage lung disease. Lancet. 1998;351:24–7.

21. Thabut G, Christie JD, Ravaud P, et al. Survival after bilateral versus single lung transplantation for patients with chronic obstructive pulmonary disease: a retrospective analysis of registry data. Lancet. 2008;371:744–51.

22. Lahzami S, Bridevaux PO, Soccal PM, et al. Survival impact of lung transplantation for COPD. Eur Respir J. 2010;36:74–80.

23. Weill D, Benden C, Corris PA, et al. A consensus document for the selection of lung transplant candidates: 2014—an update from the pulmonary transplantation council of the International Society for Heart and Lung Transplantation. J Heart Lung Transplant. 2015;34:1–15.

24. Chamogeorgakis T, Mason DP, Murthy SC, et al. Impact of nutritional state on lung transplant outcomes. J Heart Lung Transplant. 2013;32:693–700.

25. Baldwin MR, Arcasoy SM, Shah A, et al. Hypoalbuminemia and early mortality after lung transplantation: a cohort study. Am J Transplant. 2012;12:1256–67.

26. Lederer DJ, Wilt JS, D'ovidio F, et al. Obesity and underweight are associated with an increased risk of death after lung transplantation. Am J Respir Crit Care Med. 2009;180:887–95.

27. Vaquero-Barrios JM, Arenas-De Larriva MS, Redel-Montero J, et al. Bone mineral density in patients with chronic obstructive pulmonary disease who are candidates for lung transplant. Transplant Proc. 2010;42:3020–2.

28. Bon J, Fuhrman CR, Weissfeld JL, et al. Radiographic emphysema predicts low bone mineral density in a tobacco-exposed cohort. Am J Respir Crit Care Med. 2011;183:885–90.

29. Jastrzebski D, Lutogniewska W, Ochman M, et al. Osteoporosis in patients referred for lung transplantation. Eur J Med Res. 2010;15(Suppl 2):68–71.

30. Singer JP, Diamond JM, Gries CJ, et al. Frailty phenotypes, disability, and outcomes in adult candidates for lung transplantation. Am J Respir Crit Care Med. 2015;192:1325–34.

31. Fishman A, Martinez F, Naunheim K, et al. A randomized trial comparing lung-volume-reduction surgery with medical therapy for severe emphysema. N Engl J Med. 2003;348:2059–73.

32. Meyers BF, Yusen RD, Guthrie TJ, et al. Outcome of bilateral lung volume reduction in patients with emphysema potentially eligible for lung transplantation. J Thorac Cardiovasc Surg. 2001;122:10–7.

33. Senbaklavaci O, Wisser W, Ozpeker C, et al. Successful lung volume reduction surgery brings patients into better condition for later lung transplantation. Eur J Cardiothorac Surg. 2002;22:363–7.

34. Burns KE, Keenan RJ, Grgurich WF, Manzetti JD, Zenati MA. Outcomes of lung volume reduction surgery followed by lung transplantation: a matched cohort study. Ann Thorac Surg. 2002;73:1587–93.

35. Bavaria JE, Pochettino A, Kotloff RM, et al. Effect of volume reduction on lung transplant timing and selection for chronic obstructive pulmonary disease. J Thorac Cardiovasc Surg. 1998;115:9–17.

36. Nathan SD, Edwards LB, Barnett SD, Ahmad S, Burton NA. Outcomes of COPD lung transplant recipients after lung volume reduction surgery. Chest. 2004;126:1569–74.

37. Shigemura N, Gilbert S, Bhama JK, et al. Lung transplantation after lung volume reduction surgery. Transplantation. 2013;96:421–5.

38. Backhus L, Sargent J, Cheng A, Zeliadt S, Wood D, Mulligan M. Outcomes in lung transplantation after previous lung volume reduction surgery in a contemporary cohort. J Thorac Cardiovasc Surg. 2014;147:1678–83.E1.

39. Meyer DM, Bennett LE, Novick RJ, Hosenpud JD. Single vs bilateral, sequential lung transplantation for end-stage emphysema: influence of recipient age on survival and secondary end-points. J Heart Lung Transplant. 2001;20:935–41.

40. Schaffer JM, Singh SK, Reitz BA, Zamanian RT, Mallidi HR. Single- vs double-lung transplantation in patients with chronic obstructive pulmonary disease and idiopathic pulmonary fibrosis since the implementation of lung allocation based on medical need. JAMA. 2015;313:936–48.

41. Gaissert HA, Trulock EP, Cooper JD, Sundaresan RS, Patterson GA. Comparison of early functional results after volume reduction or lung transplantation for chronic obstructive pulmonary disease. J Thorac Cardiovasc Surg. 1996;111:296–306.

42. Pochettino A, Kotloff RM, Rosengard BR, et al. Bilateral versus single lung transplantation for chronic obstructive pulmonary disease: intermediate-term results. Ann Thorac Surg. 2000;70:1813–8.

43. Sundaresan SR, Shiraishi Y, Trulock EP, et al. Single or bilateral lung transplantation for emphysema? J Thorac Cardiovasc Surg. 1996;112:1485–95.

44. Bossenbroek L, Ten Hacken NH, Van Der Bij W, Verschuuren EA, Koeter GH, De Greef MH. Cross-sectional assessment of daily physical activity in chronic obstructive pulmonary disease lung transplant patients. J Heart Lung Transplant. 2009;28:149–55.
45. Gerbase MW, Spiliopoulos A, Rochat T, Archinard M, Nicod LP. Health-related quality of life following single or bilateral lung transplantation: a 7-year comparison to functional outcome. Chest. 2005;128:1371–8.
46. Levy RD, Ernst P, Levine SM, et al. Exercise performance after lung transplantation. J Heart Lung Transplant. 1993;12:27–33.
47. Williams TJ, Patterson GA, Mcclean PA, Zamel N, Maurer J. Maximal exercise testing in single and double lung transplant recipients. Am Rev Respir Dis. 1992;145:101–5.
48. Dickson RP, Davis RD, Rea JB, Palmer SM. High frequency of bronchogenic carcinoma after single-lung transplantation. J Heart Lung Transplant. 2006;25:1297–301.
49. Espinosa D, Baamonde C, Illana J, et al. Lung Cancer in patients with lung transplants. Transplant Proc. 2012;44:2118–9.
50. Grewal AS, Padera RF, Boukedes S, et al. Prevalence and outcome of lung cancer in lung transplant recipients. Respir Med. 2015;109:427–33.
51. Raviv Y, Shitrit D, Amital A, et al. Lung cancer in lung transplant recipients: experience of a tertiary hospital and literature review. Lung Cancer (Amsterdam, Netherlands). 2011;74:280–3.
52. Minai OA, Shah S, Mazzone P, et al. Bronchogenic carcinoma after lung transplantation: characteristics and outcomes. J Thorac Oncol. 2008;3:1404–9.
53. Weill D, Torres F, Hodges TN, Olmos JJ, Zamora MR. Acute native lung hyperinflation is not associated with poor outcomes after single lung transplant for emphysema. J Heart Lung Transplant. 1999;18:1080–7.
54. Reece TB, Mitchell JD, Zamora MR, et al. Native lung volume reduction surgery relieves functional graft compression after single-lung transplantation for chronic obstructive pulmonary disease. J Thorac Cardiovasc Surg. 2008;135:931–7.
55. Anderson MB, Kriett JM, Kapelanski DP, Perricone A, Smith CM, Jamieson SW. Volume reduction surgery in the native lung after single lung transplantation for emphysema. J Heart Lung Transplant. 1997;16:752–7.
56. Venuta F, De Giacomo T, Rendina EA, et al. Thoracoscopic volume reduction of the native lung after single lung transplantation for emphysema. Am J Respir Crit Care Med. 1997;156:292–3.
57. Crespo MM, Johnson BA, Mccurry KR, Landreneau RJ, Sciurba FC. Use of endobronchial valves for native lung hyperinflation associated with respiratory failure in a single-lung transplant recipient for emphysema. Chest. 2007;131:214–6.
58. Pato O, Rama P, Allegue M, Fernandez R, Gonzalez D, Borro JM. Bronchoscopic lung volume reduction in a single-lung transplant recipient with natal lung hyperinflation: a case report. Transplant Proc. 2010;42:1979–81.
59. Mccurry KR, Shearon TH, Edwards LB, et al. Lung transplantation in the United States, 1998-2007. Am J Transplant. 2009;9:942–58.
60. Munson JC, Christie JD, Halpern SD. The societal impact of single versus bilateral lung transplantation for chronic obstructive pulmonary disease. Am J Respir Crit Care Med. 2011;184:1282–8.
61. Shah RJ, Kotloff RM. Lung transplantation for obstructive lung diseases. Semin Respir Crit Care Med. 2013;34:288–96.
62. Benden C, Rea F, Behr J, et al. Lung transplantation for Lymphangioleiomyomatosis: the European experience. J Heart Lung Transplant. 2009;28:1–7.
63. Boehler A, Speich R, Russi EW, Weder W. Lung transplantation for Lymphangioleiomyomatosis. N Engl J Med. 1996;335:1275–80.
64. Pechet TT, Meyers BF, Guthrie TJ, et al. Lung transplantation for Lymphangioleiomyomatosis. J Heart Lung Transplant. 2004;23:301–8.
65. Reynaud-Gaubert M, Mornex JF, Mal H, et al. Lung transplantation for Lymphangioleiomyomatosis: the French experience. Transplantation. 2008;86:515–20.
66. Kpodonu J, Massad MG, Chaer RA, et al. The us experience with lung transplantation for pulmonary Lymphangioleiomyomatosis. J Heart Lung Transplant. 2005;24:1247–53.
67. Oprescu N, Mccormack FX, Byrnes S, Kinder BW. Clinical predictors of mortality and cause of death in Lymphangioleiomyomatosis: a population-based registry. Lung. 2013;191:35–42.
68. Machuca TN, Losso MJ, Camargo SM, et al. Lung transplantation for Lymphangioleiomyomatosis: single-center Brazilian experience with no Chylothorax. Transplant Proc. 2011;43:236–8.
69. Groetzner J, Kur F, Spelsberg F, et al. Airway anastomosis complications in De novo lung transplantation with Sirolimus-based immunosuppression. J Heart Lung Transplant. 2004;23:632–8.
70. King-Biggs MB, Dunitz JM, Park SJ, Kay Savik S, Hertz MI. Airway anastomotic dehiscence associated with use of Sirolimus immediately after lung transplantation. Transplantation. 2003;75:1437–43.
71. Goldberg HJ, Harari S, Cottin V, et al. Everolimus for the treatment of Lymphangioleiomyomatosis: a phase ii study. Eur Respir J. 2015;46:783–94.
72. El-Chemaly S, Goldberg HJ, Glanville AR. Should mammalian target of rapamycin inhibitors be stopped in women with Lymphangioleiomyomatosis awaiting lung transplantation? Expert Rev Respir Med. 2014;8:657–60.
73. Mackenzie T, Gifford AH, Sabadosa KA, et al. Longevity of patients with cystic fibrosis in 2000 to 2010 and beyond: survival analysis of the Cystic Fibrosis Foundation Patient Registry. Ann Intern Med. 2014;161:233–41.
74. Kerem E, Reisman J, Corey M, Canny GJ, Levison H. Prediction of mortality in patients with cystic fibrosis. N Engl J Med. 1992;326:1187–91.

75. Doershuk CF, Stern RC. Timing of referral for lung transplantation for cystic fibrosis: overemphasis on Fev1 may adversely affect overall survival. Chest. 1999;115:782–7.

76. Milla CE, Warwick WJ. Risk of death in cystic fibrosis patients with severely compromised lung function. Chest. 1998;113:1230–4.

77. George PM, Banya W, Pareek N, et al. Improved survival at low lung function in cystic fibrosis: cohort study from 1990 to 2007. BMJ. 2011;342:D1008.

78. Rosenbluth DB, Wilson K, Ferkol T, Schuster DP. Lung function decline in cystic fibrosis patients and timing for lung transplantation referral. Chest. 2004;126:412–9.

79. Martin C, Chapron J, Hubert D, et al. Prognostic value of six minute walk test in cystic fibrosis adults. Respir Med. 2013;107:1881–7.

80. Vizza CD, Yusen RD, Lynch JP, Fedele F, Alexander Patterson G, Trulock EP. Outcome of patients with cystic fibrosis awaiting lung transplantation. Am J Respir Crit Care Med. 2000;162:819–25.

81. Liou TG, Adler FR, Fitzsimmons SC, Cahill BC, Hibbs JR, Marshall BC. Predictive 5-year survivorship model of cystic fibrosis. Am J Epidemiol. 2001;153:345–52.

82. Liou TG, Adler FR, Huang D. Use of lung transplantation survival models to refine patient selection in cystic fibrosis. Am J Respir Crit Care Med. 2005;171(9):1053.

83. Mayer-Hamblett N, Rosenfeld M, Emerson J, Goss CH, Aitken M. Developing cystic fibrosis lung transplant referral criteria using predictors of 2-year mortality. Am J Respir Crit Care Med. 2002;166:1550–5.

84. Salsgiver EL, Fink AK, Knapp EA, et al. Changing epidemiology of the respiratory bacteriology of patients with cystic fibrosis. Chest. 2016;149:390–400.

85. Aris RM, Gilligan PH, Neuringer IP, Gott KK, Rea J, Yankaskas JR. The effects of Panresistant Bacteria in cystic fibrosis patients on lung transplant outcome. Am J Respir Crit Care Med. 1997;155:1699–704.

86. Dobbin C, Maley M, Harkness J, et al. The impact of pan-resistant bacterial pathogens on survival after lung transplantation in cystic fibrosis: results from a single large referral Centre. J Hosp Infect. 2004;56:277–82.

87. Hadjiliadis D, Steele MP, Chaparro C, et al. Survival of lung transplant patients with cystic fibrosis harboring Panresistant Bacteria other than Burkholderia Cepacia, compared with patients harboring sensitive Bacteria. J Heart Lung Transplant. 2007;26(8):834.

88. Courtney JM, Bradley J, Mccaughan J, et al. Predictors of mortality in adults with cystic fibrosis. Pediatr Pulmonol. 2007;42:525–32.

89. Courtney JM, Dunbar KE, Mcdowell A, et al. Clinical outcome of Burkholderia Cepacia complex infection in cystic fibrosis adults. J Cyst Fibros. 2004;3:93–8.

90. Fauroux B, Hart N, Belfar S, et al. Burkholderia Cepacia is associated with pulmonary hypertension and increased mortality among cystic fibrosis patients. J Clin Microbiol. 2004;42:5537–41.

91. Ledson MJ, Walshaw MJ. Burkholderia infection and survival in Cf. Thorax. 2005;60:439.

92. Zlosnik JE, Zhou G, Brant R, et al. Burkholderia species infections in patients with cystic fibrosis in British Columbia, Canada. 30 years' experience. Ann Am Thorac Soc. 2015;12:70–8.

93. Aris RM, Routh JC, Lipuma JJ, Heath DG, Gilligan PH. Lung transplantation for cystic fibrosis patients with Burkholderia Cepacia complex. Survival linked to genomovar type. Am J Respir Crit Care Med. 2001;164:2102–6.

94. Chaparro C, Maurer J, Gutierrez C, et al. Infection with Burkholderia Cepacia in cystic fibrosis: outcome following lung transplantation. Am J Respir Crit Care Med. 2001;163:43–8.

95. Alexander BD, Petzold EW, Reller LB, et al. Survival after lung transplantation of cystic fibrosis patients infected with Burkholderia Cepacia complex. Am J Transplant. 2008;8:1025–30.

96. Murray S, Charbeneau J, Marshall BC, Lipuma JJ. Impact of Burkholderia infection on lung transplantation in cystic fibrosis. Am J Respir Crit Care Med. 2008;178:363–71.

97. Paradowski LJ. Saprophytic fungal infections and lung transplantation-revisited. J Heart Lung Transplant. 1997;16:524–31.

98. Nunley DR, Ohori P, Grgurich WF, et al. Pulmonary aspergillosis in cystic fibrosis lung transplant recipients. Chest. 1998;114:1321–9.

99. Knoll BM, Kappagoda S, Gill RR, et al. Non-tuberculous mycobacterial infection among lung transplant recipients: a 15-year cohort study. Transpl Infect Dis. 2012;14:452–60.

100. Lobo LJ, Chang LC, Esther CR Jr, Gilligan PH, Tulu Z, Noone PG. Lung transplant outcomes in cystic fibrosis patients with pre-operative mycobacterium abscessus respiratory infections. Clin Transpl. 2013;27:523–9.

101. Aaron SD, Stephenson AL, Cameron DW, Whitmore GA. A statistical model to predict one-year risk of death in patients with cystic fibrosis. J Clin Epidemiol. 2015;68:1336–45.

102. Chamnan P, Shine BS, Haworth CS, Bilton D, Adler AI. Diabetes as a determinant of mortality in cystic fibrosis. Diabetes Care. 2010;33:311–6.

103. Hayes D Jr, Patel AV, Black SM, et al. Influence of diabetes on survival in patients with cystic fibrosis before and after lung transplantation. J Thorac Cardiovasc Surg. 2015;150:707–13.

104. Lewis C, Blackman SM, Nelson A, et al. Diabetes-related mortality in adults with cystic fibrosis. Role of genotype and sex. Am J Respir Crit Care Med. 2015;191:194–200.

105. Hofer M, Schmid C, Benden C, et al. Diabetes mellitus and survival in cystic fibrosis patients after lung transplantation. J Cyst Fibros. 2012;11:131–6.

106. Stephenson AL, Sykes J, Berthiaume Y, et al. Clinical and demographic factors associated with post-lung transplantation survival in individuals with cystic fibrosis. J Heart Lung Transplant. 2015;34:1139–45.

107. Aris RM, Neuringer IP, Weiner MA, Egan TM, Ontjes D. Severe osteoporosis before and after lung transplantation. Chest. 1996;109:1176–83.

108. Aris RM, Lester GE, Caminiti M, et al. Efficacy of alendronate in adults with cystic fibrosis with low bone density. Am J Respir Crit Care Med. 2004;169:77–82.

109. Aris RM, Lester GE, Renner JB, et al. Efficacy of Pamidronate for osteoporosis in patients with cystic fibrosis following lung transplantation. Am J Respir Crit Care Med. 2000;162:941–6.

110. Leung MK, Rachakonda L, Weill D, Hwang PH. Effects of sinus surgery on lung transplantation outcomes in cystic fibrosis. Am J Rhinol. 2008;22:192–6.

111. Grannas G, Neipp M, Hoeper MM, et al. Indications for and outcomes after combined lung and liver transplantation: a single-center experience on 13 consecutive cases. Transplantation. 2008;85:524–31.

112. Nash EF, Volling C, Gutierrez CA, et al. Outcomes of patients with cystic fibrosis undergoing lung transplantation with and without cystic fibrosis-associated liver cirrhosis. Clin Transpl. 2012;26:34–41.

113. Klima LD, Kowdley KV, Lewis SL, Wood DE, Aitken ML. Successful lung transplantation in spite of cystic fibrosis-associated liver disease: a case series. J Heart Lung Transplant. 1997;16:934–8.

114. Beirne PA, Banner NR, Khaghani A, Hodson ME, Yacoub MH. Lung transplantation for non-cystic fibrosis bronchiectasis: analysis of a 13-year experience. J Heart Lung Transplant. 2005;24: 1530–5.

115. Nathan JA, Sharples LD, Exley AR, Sivasothy P, Wallwork J. The outcomes of lung transplantation in patients with bronchiectasis and antibody deficiency. J Heart Lung Transplant. 2005;24:1517–21.

116. Orens JB, Estenne M, Arcasoy S, et al. International guidelines for the selection of lung transplant candidates: 2006 update—a consensus report from the Pulmonary Scientific Council f the International Society for Heart and Lung Transplantation. J Heart Lung Transplant. 2006;25:745–55.

117. Hayes D Jr, Kopp BT, Tobias JD, et al. Survival in patients with advanced non-cystic fibrosis bronchiectasis versus cystic fibrosis on the waitlist for lung transplantation. Lung. 2015;193:933–8.

Pretransplant Considerations in Patients with Pulmonary Fibrosis

4

Roberto G. Carbone, Assaf Monselise,
Keith M. Wille, Giovanni Bottino,
and Francesco Puppo

Abbreviations

6-MWT	6-minute walk test
ATS	American Thoracic Society
BOS	Bronchiolitis obliterans syndrome
COPD	Chronic obstructive pulmonary disease
DLCO	Diffusing capacity of CO
EMA	European Medicine Agency
ERS	European Respiratory Society
FDA	Food and Drug Administration
FPF	Familial pulmonary fibrosis
FVC	Forced vital capacity
GER	Gastroesophageal reflux
HRCT	High-resolution CT of the lung
ILD	Interstitial lung diseases
IPF	Idiopathic pulmonary fibrosis
ISHLT	International Society of Heart and Lung Transplantation
LVRS	Lung volume reduction surgery
NSIP	Non-specific interstitial pneumonia
NYHA	New York Heart Association
OSA	Obstructive sleep apnea
PAH	Pulmonary arterial hypertension
PAP	Pulmonary arterial pressure
PH	Pulmonary hypertension
QOL	Quality of life
RA	Rheumatoid arthritis
RHC	Right heart catheterization
SSc	Systemic sclerosis
UIP	Usual interstitial pneumonia

R. G. Carbone (✉)
Department of Internal Medicine, University of Genoa, Genoa, Italy

A. Monselise
Departments of Dermatology and Internal Medicine, Clalit Health Services, Tel-Aviv, Israel

K. M. Wille
Department of Medicine, Pulmonary, Allergy, and Critical Care Medicine, University of Alabama at Birmingham, Birmingham, AL, USA
e-mail: kwille@uabmc.edu

G. Bottino
Department of Medicine, University of Genoa—DIMI, Genoa, Italy

F. Puppo
Department of Internal Medicine, University of Genoa, Genoa, Italy
e-mail: puppof@unige.it

Introduction

The interstitial lung diseases (ILD) comprise a heterogeneous group of more than 200 acute and chronic pulmonary disorders which can be progressive, life-threatening diseases [1]. Idiopathic *pulmonary fibrosis* (IPF) is defined as a specific form of chronic, progressively fibrosing idiopathic interstitial pneumonia (IIP) of unknown cause associated with a high mortality rate. Men are more commonly affected than women by a ratio of 2:1, and median survival from diagnosis is about 3 years. Roughly 20–35% of patients previously

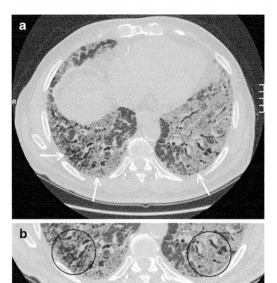

Fig. 4.1 (**a**, **b**) A 62-year-old male smoker with advanced-stage IPF. HRCT shows bilateral, multifocal, or diffuse areas of ground glass opacity and consolidation without pleural effusion (**a**, arrows). There is also honeycombing and traction bronchiectasis. The radiologic features of the lung are shown in magnification (**b**)

diagnosed with IPF instead have fibrotic non-specific interstitial pneumonia (NSIP), a newer ILD subgroup that can mimic IPF. The diagnostic criteria for IPF were revised in 2011 and include a UIP pattern on HRCT or lung biopsy. The diagnostic agreement for IPF among clinicians has notably improved with clinician-radiologist-pathologist case review and interaction [1, 2].

Survival is a critical important end point for assessing efficacy in IPF clinical trials. The mortality risk among elderly patients (≥66 years of age) with IPF is more than four times higher than that of younger patients (<58 years old) (Fig. 4.1a, b). Crucially, patients with progressive IPF—despite treatment with currently available antifibrotic therapy—should be considered for lung transplantation.

Interstitial Lung Diseases (ILD) and Timing of Transplant Referral

The International Society for Heart and Lung Transplantation (ISHLT) consensus document, published in January 2015, suggests that ILD patients undergo a transplant evaluation with the onset of clinical symptoms, such as dyspnea or functional limitation, or with a new oxygen requirement (at rest or during exertion). An FVC <80% or DLCO <40% predicted on pulmonary function testing should also prompt a transplant referral. Additionally, patients with histopathologic or radiologic features of usual interstitial pneumonitis (UIP) or fibrosing non-specific interstitial pneumonitis (NSIP) should be referred, regardless of lung function testing results. Finally, patients with inflammatory ILD and dyspnea, an oxygen requirement, and/or decreased lung function who fail to improve with medical therapy should be referred for lung transplantation [3].

Interstitial Lung Diseases (ILD) and Timing of Listing

The ISHLT considers the following to be poor prognostic factors for ILD and thus criteria for listing for lung transplantation: a decline in FVC ≥10% or DLCO ≥15%, oxygen desaturation <88% or distance <250 m on a 6-min walk (6MW) test or >50 m decline in 6MW distance over a 6-month period, pulmonary hypertension (PH) on right heart catheterization or 2D echocardiography, and hospitalization due to respiratory decline, pneumothorax, or acute exacerbations [3].

Medical Treatment for Idiopathic *Pulmonary Fibrosis* (IPF)

Treatment with the antifibrotic agents—nintedanib and pirfenidone—decreases the rate of FVC decline in IPF and thereby reduces disease progression, but these drugs do not halt or cure the disease.

The diagnostic and management guidelines were recently updated in 2015 to address newer recommendations based upon more recent IPF studies [4]. There are currently strong recommendations against the use of anticoagulation (warfarin), combination therapy with prednisone + azathioprine + N-acetylcysteine, the selective endothelin receptor antagonist ambrisentan, and the tyrosine kinase inhibitor imatinib. Macitentan and bosentan now have conditional (previously strong) recommendations against use, and sildenafil has a conditional recommendation against use. Pirfenidone and nintedanib, not addressed in the prior guideline, now have conditional recommendations for use in IPF. Use of pirfenidone or nintedanib [5, 6] should not delay referral for lung transplantation, and adjunctive measures such as pulmonary rehabilitation and supplemental oxygen therapy remain an essential part of IPF care. The use of these new antifibrotic agents is not a contraindication for lung transplant listing, and patients who are tolerating the medications and in whom the disease progression as measured by the rate of decline in FVC have slowed down may continue using these until the time of lung transplantation. Other therapeutic recommendations, for or against, are unchanged in the 2015 update. A summary of the newer recommendations is provided in Table 4.1.

Presently, IPF patients comprise the largest proportion of patients on the US transplant wait

Table 4.1 Comparison of recommendations in the 2015 and 2011 idiopathic pulmonary fibrosis (IPF) guidelines

Agent	2015 guideline	2011 guideline
New and revised recommendations		
Anticoagulation (warfarin)	Strong recommendation against use[a]	Conditional recommendation against use[b]
Combination prednisone + azathioprine + N-acetylcysteine	Strong recommendation against use[c]	Conditional recommendation against use[c]
Selective endothelin receptor antagonist (ambrisentan)	Strong recommendation against use[c]	Not addressed
Imatinib, a tyrosine kinase inhibitor with one target	Strong recommendation against use[a]	Not addressed
Nintedanib, a tyrosine kinase inhibitor with multiple targets	Conditional recommendation for use[a]	Not addressed
Pirfenidone	Conditional recommendation for use[a]	Conditional recommendation against use[b]
Dual endothelin receptor antagonists (macitentan, bosentan)	Conditional recommendation against use[c]	Strong recommendation against use[a]
Phosphodiesterase-5 inhibitor (sildenafil)	Conditional recommendation against use[a]	Not addressed
Unchanged recommendations		
Antiacid therapy	Conditional recommendation for use[b]	Conditional recommendation for use[b]
N-acetylcysteine monotherapy	Conditional recommendation against use[c]	Conditional recommendation against use[c]
Anti-pulmonary hypertension therapy for IPF-associated pulmonary hypertension	Reassessment of the previous recommendation was deferred	Conditional recommendation against use[b]
Lung transplantation: Single versus bilateral lung transplantation	Formulation of a recommendation for single versus bilateral lung transplantation was deferred	Not addressed

Used with permission of the America Thoracic Society and the AJRCCM Journal from Raghu G, Rochwerg B, Zhang Y, Garcia CA, Azuma A, Behr J, Brozek JL, Collard HR, Cunningham W, Homma S, Johkoh T, Martinez FJ, Myers J, Protzko SL, Richeldi L, Rind D, Selman M, Theodore A, Wells AU, Hoogsteden H, Schünemann HJ; American Thoracic Society; European Respiratory society; Japanese Respiratory Society; Latin American Thoracic Association. An Official ATS/ERS/JRS/ALAT Clinical Practice Guideline: Treatment of Idiopathic Pulmonary Fibrosis. An Update of the 2011 Clinical Practice Guideline. Am J Respir Crit Care Med. 2015 Jul 15;192(2): e3–19
[a]+ + + −, moderate confidence in effect estimates
[b]+ − − −, very low confidence in effect estimates
[c]+ + − −, low confidence in effect estimates. Reproduced from [3] with permission from the publisher

list, and the number of transplants for IPF patients has increased over time. However, OPTN data have shown that wait list mortality is higher for IPF patients compared to those on the wait list for other diagnoses. Studies have reported that 14–67% of IPF patients may die while awaiting transplantation [7]. It is therefore crucial to monitor these patients closely for worsening symptoms or clinical deterioration and intervene at the earliest opportunity.

Patients with IPF are at risk for several complications that may impact their transplant waiting list status and survival. An acute exacerbation of IPF (AE-IPF) has previously been defined by clinical and radiological features that include the subacute onset of dyspnea, bilateral ground glass changes on chest high-resolution computed tomography, and the absence of an identifiable etiology. The annual incidence of AE-IPF ranges from 5 to 15%. IPF patients with acutely worsening respiratory symptoms are often treated with corticosteroids and antimicrobials; however, there are few data to support the use of these therapies. Despite treatment, the short-term mortality of AE-IPF has been reported to be about 50% [8]. IPF patients are also at risk for other pulmonary disorders, including emphysema, lung cancer, and pulmonary hypertension. Other health risks include venous thromboembolism, coronary artery disease, congestive heart failure, gastroesophageal reflux disease, and sleep-disordered breathing [9]. Symptoms of anxiety and depression were observed in approximately 20% and 25% of IPF patients, respectively [10]. Early identification and treatment of the comorbidities associated with IPF may improve patient outcomes and prolong survival.

IPF patients who are evaluated for lung transplantation should enroll in pulmonary rehabilitation (PR) and maintain a regular exercise regimen after PR is completed. Rehabilitation appears to be safe for patients with IPF and leads to improvements in exercise capacity, dyspnea, and quality of life [11–13]. Adequate oxygenation should be maintained, and patients should be monitored routinely for hypoxemia at rest as well as upon exertion. Oxygen desaturation during sleep or exercise has been shown to predict survival in

IPF [14, 15]. Additional studies of the potential benefits of high oxygen delivery on the exercise capacity of IPF patients are underway [16]. Some lung transplant candidates who clinically deteriorate may, in rare instances, be supported by extracorporeal technology to bridge to transplantation; however, patients who become too sick for transplant are typically removed from the waiting list [17, 18]. As the wait list mortality for IPF patients remains high, early referral for palliative care should be encouraged for dying patients who are unable to have a transplant [19–22].

In summary, physicians should ensure an accurate diagnosis of IPF as per the 2011 criteria [1], be familiar with the potential benefits and limitations of antifibrotic therapy, provide patient education on the diagnosis and management of IPF, and consider early referral of patients for clinical trials. Patients awaiting for lung transplantation must participate in pulmonary rehabilitation, be ambulatory with supplemental oxygen, maintain weight less than BMI 30, and be seen at 2–3-month intervals to monitor overall health status, identify complications promptly and treat them appropriately, assure adequacy of supplemental oxygen during ambulation, and provide appropriate supportive measures and counseling at regular intervals. The LAS will need to be updated at every follow-up visit so that the patients are appropriately prioritized in the waiting list in centers/countries using LAS system.

Lung Transplantation for Idiopathic *Pulmonary Fibrosis* (IPF): Timing for Listing

Lung transplantation is considered for patients with progressive IPF refractory to antifibrotic therapy. In the United States, IPF became the leading indication for lung transplantation in 2007, when the number of transplants performed for IPF surpassed that for COPD. While transplant is the only intervention that may improve QOL and survival for IPF patients, 5-year survival following lung transplantation has remained approximately 50%, regardless of the transplant indication. The annual mortality rate following transplant is higher for IPF patients than for those with COPD. However, a multivariate analysis from a single-center study suggested that transplantation for IPF reduced the risk of death by 75%, after adjusting for potentially confounding variables [23, 24].

Key decisions that pertain to a potential lung transplantation candidate include the timing of transplant referral, whether criteria are met to proceed with listing for transplant, and whether single or bilateral lung transplantation should be performed. According to ISHLT guidelines, referral for transplantation should be considered for patients with a poor prognosis, defined as a 2–3-year predicted survival of less than 50% and/or class III–IV symptoms according to the New York Heart Association (NYHA) [25].

The ISHLT guidelines recommend that transplantation thresholds for IPF patients include >10% decline in FVC, DLCO <40% predicted, or desaturation below 88% on pulse oximetry during a 6-min walk test (6-MWT). However, there is no consensus as to whether FVC is equal or superior to 6-MWT in determining the transplant threshold; in fact, while parameters correlate, they may also worsen independently [26–29]. Also, the sensitivity and specificity of these indexes for determining the timing of transplant are quite low. More recently, scoring systems that combine functional parameters with radiologic imaging and clinical evaluation have been developed to better predict the clinical outcome of IPF and identify patients with a worse prognosis [26–29].

Potential candidates for transplantation should be carefully evaluated for contraindications before being placed on the waiting list for the procedure. The type of transplantation (single, bilateral, or heart-lung) should also be determined beforehand, as single lung transplantation is relatively simpler and better-tolerated by many IPF patients. Furthermore, bilateral lung transplantation has not been definitively shown to have a better survival outcome when compared to single lung transplantation for patients with IPF [30]. While there is considerable risk for complications, infection, and allograft rejection follow-

ing lung transplantation, recipients can achieve improved QOL and prolonged survival [30].

Comorbid Conditions

The recognition and management of comorbid conditions may benefit patients with advanced lung disease. The presence of pulmonary arterial hypertension (PAH), for example, correlates with a greater mortality risk in patients with UIP (Table 4.2) [31–33]. In a retrospective study of IPF patients undergoing pretransplantation right heart catheterization (RHC), Lettieri and colleagues [32] found that PAH, defined as a mean pulmonary artery pressure (mPAP) >25 mmHg, was present in 31.6% of patients. Additionally, higher mPAP correlated with a greater mortality risk, while FVC and DLCO did not. Nathan and colleagues [33] found that echocardiographic assessment of systolic pulmonary arterial pressure (PAP) was not sufficiently accurate for the evaluation of PAH, as nearly one-third of patients with normal systolic PAP by echocardiography in fact had PH by RHC. Unfortunately, randomized controlled trials to date have not shown that endothelin receptor antagonists (ERAs) benefit patients with IPF or other fibrosing lung disorders [34–39].

Acute respiratory deterioration is associated with an increased mortality risk for IPF patients. In many cases, the etiology is considered idiopathic, and an underlying cause—such as clinically apparent infection, left heart failure, or

Table 4.2 Pulmonary hypertension and risk of cor pulmonale

	Number in United States	% with PH	Number with PH: United States
IPF	*191.520*	*28%*	*53.626*
COPD	10 MIL	20–40%	2–4 MIL
OSA	7.6 MIL	20%	1.5 MIL
HFpEF	76 MIL	83%	63 MIL
CHF	5.8 MIL	10–60%	0.5–3.8 MIL
Sickle cell	100.000	10–30%	10–30 K
Total			*70 MIL*

pulmonary embolism—cannot be identified. These episodes of idiopathic acute deterioration are defined as acute exacerbations of IPF (AE-IPF) [40]. Typical features include worsening dyspnea, fever, cough, and flu-like symptoms. Patients may require mechanical ventilation due to severe hypoxemia and respiratory failure. The most commonly applied criteria for abnormal gas exchange include a PaO_2/FiO_2 ratio <225 and a decrease in PaO_2 by 10 mmHg or more over time [40]. Serum levels of KL-6 neutrophil elastase and lactate hydrogenase have been suggested as markers of AE-IPF [41].

Treatment with high-dose corticosteroids may resolve some acute exacerbations; however, clinical trials have failed to prove their efficacy, and short-term mortality following AE-IPF remains around 50% [8]. A recent pilot trial suggested specific treatments that reduce autoantibodies might also benefit some severely ill patients with AE-IPF [42].

Gastroesophageal reflux disease (GERD) occurs in over 80% of IPF patients and can also develop after lung transplantation. Transplant recipients should be promptly treated for GERD to reduce the risk of microaspiration and resulting bronchiolitis obliterans syndrome (BOS) (Fig. 4.2a, b) or allograft rejection [43]. Subclinical microaspiration of gastric contents—including food, salts, and trypsin—may in fact be a culprit in the development and progression of IPF. Furthermore, GERD and IPF play important roles in the pathogenesis of chronic bronchitis, bronchiectasis, diffuse panbronchiolitis, recurrent pneumonia, chronic cough, hoarseness, and asthma. Given the lack of effective treatment options for IPF, other management strategies, such as optimizing GERD therapy, should be considered to improve the outcomes of these patients [43]. Obstructive sleep apnea (OSA) syndrome occurs in over 80% of IPF patients, and coronary artery disease is found in over 25% [44, 45].

Heart-Lung Transplantation

Patients with both advanced heart and lung disease who are not candidates for heart or lung transplantation alone could be considered for combined heart-lung transplantation. Heart-lung transplantation is considered for patients with irreversible myocardial dysfunction, or congenital or irreversible defects of heart valves or chambers, combined with lung disease or severe PH. The presence of PH and/or an elevated pulmonary vascular resistance (PVR)—defined as PVR >3 Woods units or a transpulmonary pressure gradient >15 mmHg—is potential contraindications to isolated heart transplantation. A pretransplant vasodilator challenge can be considered for patients with pulmonary artery systolic pressure>50 mmHg, elevated PVR, or a

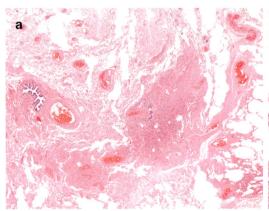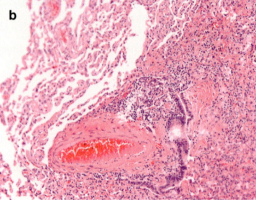

Fig. 4.2 (**a**, **b**) Obliterative bronchiolitis: acute and chronic inflammatory infiltrates within respiratory bronchioles, the interstitium, and adjacent alveoli, with luminal obliteration and organization of exudate. Sections were stained with hematoxylin and eosin, 10× (**a**) and 40× (**b**), respectively

transpulmonary pressure gradient >15 mmHg, as the risk of early right heart failure and death is increased in nonresponders following isolated heart transplant. Use of mechanical circulatory support may improve these parameters and enable some patients to undergo isolated heart transplantation. However, in the setting of PH associated with right ventricular failure, bilateral lung transplantation offers a similar or better outcome and less waiting time than combined heart-lung transplantation.

Pulmonary Vascular Diseases and Lung Transplantation

Systemic Sclerosis

Systemic sclerosis (SSc), also known as scleroderma, is a connective tissue disease characterized by small vessel vasculopathy, immune dysregulation with autoantibody production, and fibroblast dysfunction leading to tissue fibrosis [46] (Fig. 4.3). Pulmonary involvement, primar-

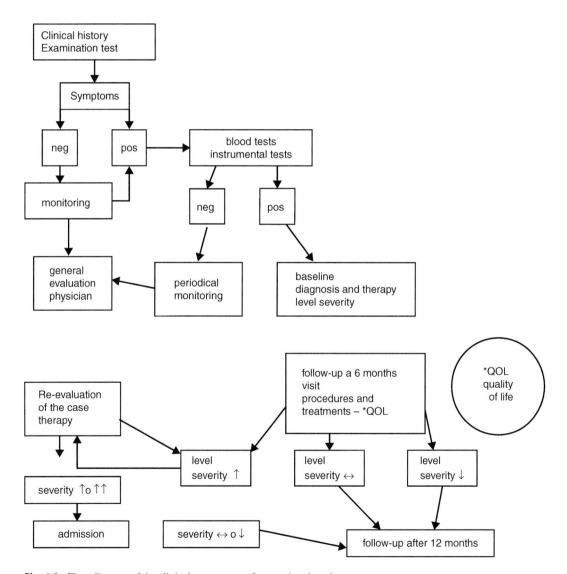

Fig. 4.3 Flow diagram of the clinical assessment of systemic sclerosis

ily as PH or ILD, can be a severe and life-threatening complication of systemic sclerosis (Box 4.1). The prevalence of ILD among SSc patients is around 40% [47, 48].

Box 4.1 Specific Contraindications for Lung Transplantation in Systemic Sclerosis

Worsening of extensive ILD [28] defined by a decline of FVC levels of >10% or DLCO levels of >15% despite an optimal medical approach of at least 6-month intravenous cyclophosphamide

DLCO <35% despite an optimal medical approach of at least 6-month intravenous cyclophosphamide

Coexistence of extensive ILD and PAH on right heart catheterization (whatever the value of mPAP)

Despite therapeutic advances, none of the current treatments are curative, and progressive ILD is now one of the leading causes of death in SSc patients [49] (Fig. 4.4a, b). As a result, lung transplantation is an important option for this subset of patients [50–55] (Box 4.2). The ISHLT, American Thoracic Society (ATS), and European Respiratory Society (ERS) published joint guidelines on the general indications and contraindications for lung transplantation [56]. However, in the absence of robust data, none of these guidelines specifically address the issue of lung trans-

plantation in the context of connective tissue disease. Consequently, the indications and timing of referral for lung transplantation for SSc patients are not as clearly defined, and case-by-case decisions are common. Lung transplantation should be considered in SSc patients with advanced ILD and a decline in FVC >10% or DLCO >15% predicted, despite maximal medical therapy that includes at least 6 months of intravenous cyclophosphamide. Coexisting PAH on RHC should also prompt a lung transplant referral. Transplant candidates should have a limited 2-year life expectancy and absence of systemic and extrapulmonary manifestations of SSc, such as digital ulcers (which can predispose to infection), renal insufficiency, significant cardiac abnormalities, and esophageal dysmotility [54, 57]. Potential exclusion criteria for transplant include esophageal dysmotility with uncontrolled gastroesophageal reflux, esophageal atonia or achalasia, upper gastrointestinal ulcer, and abnormal gastric emptying. Some reports suggest that gastroesophageal reflux might lead to BOS, and that BOS may be preventable by pH monitoring and anti-reflux surgery (fundoplication) before or after lung transplantation [58–60]. A French multidisciplinary working group [61] has proposed specific indications and contraindications for lung transplantation in patients with SSc. They suggest the immunosuppression regimen as presented in Box 4.3 for lung transplant recipients in this patient population.

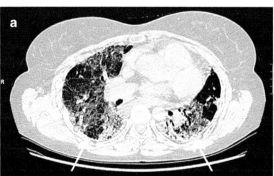 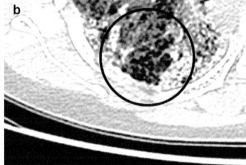

Fig. 4.4 (**a, b**) A 44-year-old non-smoking female with systemic sclerosis and end-stage IPF and histologically proven usual interstitial pneumonia (UIP). HRCT shows extensive reticular opacities in the lung bases and sub-pleural honeycombing with traction bronchiectasis and increased interlobular septal thickening, especially in the lower lobes (**a**, arrows). Honeycombing is shown with magnification in the enlarged detail (**b**)

Box 4.2 Criteria for Lung Transplantation in Absence of Contraindications for Patients with Systemic Sclerosis

1. Muscle
   - Uncontrolled active progressive inflammatory myopathy
   - Myopathy with diaphragm involvement
2. Digital ulcers
   - More than 1 severe episode/year despite optimal treatment
   - Active digital ulcer (temporary contraindication)
3. Gastrointestinal
   - Esophageal stricture
   - Active and severe upper gastrointestinal ulcerations
   - High grade dysplasia in a Barrett's esophagus
   - Gastroparesis
   - Chronic gastrointestinal bleeding
   - Involvement of the small intestine (malabsorption and pseudo-obstruction)
   - Colorectal involvement (pseudo-obstruction, diverticulitis, perforation)
4. Heart
   - Conduction and/or rhythm disturbances (symptomatic bradycardia, ventricular, and atrial tachycardia) must be managed prior to transplant but are not a contraindication
5. Kidney
   - Renal function should have been stable for 3 months except in the case of acute functional renal failure related to right ventricle dysfunction
   - Interval < 3 years between SSc and transplant
   - Increased risk of scleroderma renal crisis:
     (a) Diffuse systemic sclerosis evolving for less than 3 years since the first non-Raynaud sign/symptom
     (b) Rapidly progressive and severe cutaneous involvement (increase of more than 25% in Rodnan score within 6–12 months)
     (c) Corticosteroids >15 mg prednisone/day

Box 4.3 Immunosuppression Regimen for Lung Transplant Recipients with SSc

Bolus of 500 mg of methylprednisolone during the operation followed by 0.5 mg/kg/day of prednisone for 3 days and then progressively tapered

Tacrolimus 0.15 mg/kg/day in two divided doses to achieve a serum level of 10–5 ng/mL

Mycophenolate mofetil 1 g twice daily

If tacrolimus has to be delayed (because of impaired renal function), the anti-CD25 monoclonal antibody basiliximab 20 mg at day 0 and again at day 4 is recommended, followed by initiation of tacrolimus on postoperative day 4

Data from Launay D, Savale L, Berezne A, Le Pavec J, Hachulla E, Mouthon L, et al. Working Group on Heart/Lung transplantation in systemic sclerosis of the French Network on Pulmonary Hypertension. Lung and heart-lung transplantation for systemic sclerosis patients. A monocentric experience of 13 patients, review of the literature and position paper of a multidisciplinary working group. Presse Med. 2014;43:e345–63.

The potential for posttransplant complications among SSc patients excludes many of them from the procedure. In fact, United Network for Organ Sharing (UNOS) registry data indicate that only 186 of 25,260 (0.74%) total lung transplants performed from 1988 to 2013 were for patients with SSc. Moreover, guidelines regarding the choice of single or bilateral lung transplantation for patients with SSc do not exist. In general, bilateral transplantation is preferred for patients ≤60 years of age and/or with severe PAH, whereas single transplantation is preferred for patients ≥65 years of age [50]. While bilateral lung transplant recipients may have improved pulmonary function compared to single lung recipients, exercise performance has been shown to be similar for both groups [62, 63].

Despite the limited number of transplants performed for SSc, morbidity and mortality rates are similar to those reported for non-SSc ILD [64–72]. Survival is improved with early use of prostanoid therapy for SSc patients with ILD and PAH [28]. Unlike the idiopathic interstitial pneumonias, no survival difference has been observed between SSc patients with histological UIP and NSIP [73]. However, patients with extensive ILD on chest high-resolution computed tomography (HRCT), regardless of the histologic pattern, have a poorer prognosis and outcome compared to patients with limited ILD [73]. Early mortality posttransplant is commonly due to allograft failure, bacterial infection, cardiac events, and hemorrhagic stroke, whereas late mortality is more often due to respiratory failure, chronic rejection, infection, and pulmonary hypertension.

In conclusion and based on limited available data, lung transplantation may be a viable therapeutic option for carefully selected SSc patients with end-stage lung disease in the absence of severe renal failure, cardiac dysfunction, esophageal disease, or extensive skin involvement.

Rheumatoid Arthritis

Rheumatoid arthritis (RA) is a chronic multisystem disease characterized by (1) inflammatory synovitis causing cartilage damage and bone erosions and (2) extra-articular manifestations, including vasculitis, muscle atrophy, peripheral neuropathy, and pleuropulmonary involvement. ILD has been diagnosed using HRCT in approximately 20–30% of unselected RA populations; however, only about half of these patients develop respiratory symptoms [74, 75]. ILD represents the third leading cause of death in RA patients [76], and the limited therapeutic options available show modest benefit [77]. Therefore, the ISHLT guidelines suggest that lung transplantation should be considered for RA-ILD patients with quiescent disease [3]. However, there are limited survival and outcomes data for RA-ILD patients following lung transplantation. A recent study compared lung transplant outcomes for RA-ILD patients with IPF and scleroderma-associated ILD patients [78]. The investigators found that posttransplant survival at 1 year was similar among the three disease groups. Moreover, RA-ILD recipients had a marked improvement in QOL, mainly with regard to respiratory symptoms. As many RA-ILD patients have the UIP histological pattern and do not respond well to medical treatment, lung transplant referral should be considered for patients with stable disease, prior to oxygen dependence. Future clinical studies are needed to better define the role of lung transplantation for patients with RA-ILD.

Sarcoidosis

Studies in lung transplant recipients with sarcoidosis have reported 5-year posttransplant survival rates of approximately 50%, similar to outcomes reported for other respiratory disorders [79, 80]. However, data regarding graft outcomes are limited [79, 81, 82].

Still, there are very few lung transplants performed for sarcoid-related ILD compared to transplants performed for all other conditions. Statistics from the USA of admissions and deaths based on the International Classification of Diseases (ICD 9th ed., 2009) confirm this trend. In fact, out of a total of 3289 admissions for IPF and 7034 hospital admissions for sarcoidosis, approximately one-third and 85% of patients were less than 64 years of age, respectively. Transplant referral should be considered for sarcoid patients who present with advanced fibrocystic disease, where medical therapy or spontaneous resolution has failed. Guidelines also recommend referral for sarcoid patients with NYHA class 3–4 symptoms, hypoxemia at rest, PH, or right atrial pressure >15 mmHg; however, the optimal timing to list for transplantation is poorly defined due to the paucity of data regarding outcomes in this patient population.

Pulmonary Langerhans Cell Histiocytosis

Pulmonary Langerhans cell histiocytosis (PLCH), a rare bronchiolitis disorder, develops exclusively in young smokers [83, 84]. HRCT imaging may suggest the diagnosis, with the identification of nodules in a centrilobular distribution, cavitary nodules (thick-walled cysts), and/or thin-walled cysts, all typical findings of the disease (Fig. 4.5a, b) [85–90]. PLCH patients are commonly diagnosed with PH at the time of lung transplant referral, and PH occurs more frequently in advanced PLCH, as compared to other end-stage interstitial lung diseases [91, 92]. PLCH accounts for only 0.2% of all lung transplants [92].

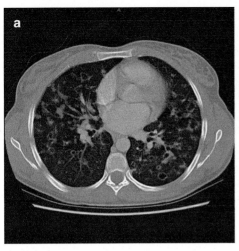
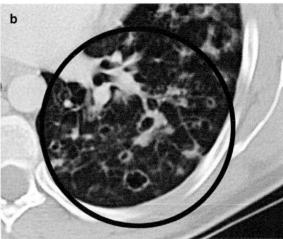

Fig. 4.5 (**a**, **b**) A 34-year-old male smoker with pulmonary Langerhans cell histiocytosis. HRCT shows diffuse cavities especially in the lower lungs with traction bronchiectasis (**a**). The reticular pattern is shown with magnification in the enlarged detail (**b**)

Acknowledgment We thank Maurilio Tavormina for the graphic design artwork.

References

1. Raghu G, Collard HR, Egan JJ, Martinez FJ, Behr J, Brown KK, et al. An official ATS/ERS/JRS/ALAT statement: idiopathic pulmonary fibrosis: evidence-based guidelines for diagnosis and management. Am J Respir Crit Care Med. 2011;183(6):788–824.
2. Wells AU. The revised ATS/ERS/JRS/ALAT diagnostic criteria for idiopathic pulmonary fibrosis (IPF)—practical implications. Respir Res. 2013;14 Suppl 1:S2.
3. Merha MR, Canter CE, Hnnan MM, Semigran MJ, Uber PA, Baran DE, et al. The 2016 International Society for Heart Lung Transplantation listing criteria for heart transplantation: a 10-year update 2016. J Heart Lung Transplant. 2016;35(1):1–23.
4. Wilson KC, Raghu G. The 2015 guidelines for idiopathic pulmonary fibrosis: an important chapter in the evolution of the management of patients with IPF. Eur Respir J. 2015;46:883–6.
5. King TE, Bradford WZ, Castro-Bernardini S, Fargan EA, Glaspole J, Glassberg MK, et al. A phase 3 trial of pirfenidone in patients with idiopathic pulmonary fibrosis. N Engl J Med. 2014;370(22):2083–92.
6. Richeldi L, du Bois RM, Raghu G, Azuma A, Brown KK, Costabel U, et al. Efficacy and safety of nintedanib in idiopathic pulmonary fibrosis. N Engl J Med. 2014;370(22):2071–82.
7. Kistler KD, Nalysnyk L, Rotella P, Esser D. Lung transplantation in idiopathic pulmonary fibrosis: a systematic review of the literature. BMC Pulm Med. 2014;14:139.
8. Ryerson CJ, Cottin V, Brown KK, Collard HR. Acute exacerbation of idiopathic pulmonary fibrosis: shifting the paradigm. Eur Respir J. 2015;46(2):512–20.
9. King CS, Nathan SD. Idiopathic pulmonary fibrosis: effects and optimal management of co-morbidities. Lancet Respir Med. 2017;5(1):72–84.
10. Lee YJ, Choi SM, Lee YJ, Cho YJ, Yoon HI, Lee JH, et al. Clinical impact of depression and anxiety in patients with idiopathic pulmonary fibrosis. PLoS One. 2017;12(9):e0184300.
11. Dowman L, Hill CJ, Holland AE. Pulmonary rehabilitation for interstitial lung disease. Cochrane Database Syst Rev. 2014;(10):CD006322.
12. Strookappe B, Elfferich M, Swigris J, Verschoof A, Veschakelen J, Knevel T, et al. Benefits of physical training in patients with idiopathic or end-stage sarcoidosis-related pulmonary fibrosis: a pilot study. Sarcoidosis Vasc Diffuse Lung Dis. 2015;32(1):43–52.
13. Tonelli R, Cocconcelli E, Lanini B, Romagnoli I, Florini F, Castaniere I, et al. Effectiveness of pulmonary rehabilitation in patients with interstitial lung disease of different etiology: a multicenter prospective study. BMC Pulm Med. 2017;17(1):130.
14. Kolilekas L, Manali E, Vlami KA, Lyberopoulos P, Triantafillidou C, Kagouridis K, et al. Sleep oxygen desaturation predicts survival in idiopathic pulmonary fibrosis. J Clin Sleep Med. 2013;9(6):593–601.
15. Triantafillidou C, Manali E, Lyberopoulos P, Kolilekas L, Kagouridis K, Gyftopoulos S, et al. The role of cardiopulmonary exercise test in IPF

prognosis. Pulm Med. 2013;2013:1. https://doi.org/10.1155/2013/514817.

16. Ryerson CJ, et al. High oxygen delivery to preserve exercise capacity in patients with idiopathic pulmonary fibrosis treated with Nintedanib. Methodology of the HOPE-IPF study. Ann Am Thorac Soc. 2016;13(9):1640–7.

17. Hoopes CW, Kukreja J, Golden J, Davenport DL, Diaz-Guzman E, Zwischenberger JB. Extracorporeal membrane oxygenation as a bridge to pulmonary transplantation. J Thorac Cardiovasc Surg. 2013;145(3):862–7; discussion 867–8.

18. Boling B, Dennis DR, Tribble TA, Rajagopalan N, Hoopes CW. Safety of nurse-led ambulation for patients on venovenous extracorporeal membrane oxygenation. Prog Transplant. 2016;26(2):112–6.

19. Bonella F, Wijsenbeek M, Molina-Molina M, Duck A, Mele R, Geissler K, et al. European IPF Patient Charter: unmet needs and a call to action for healthcare policymakers. Eur Respir J. 2016;47(2):597–606.

20. Sharp C, Lamb H, Jordan N, Edwards A, Gunary R, Meek P, et al. Development of tools to facilitate palliative and supportive care referral for patients with idiopathic pulmonary fibrosis. BMJ Support Palliat Care. 2017. pii: bmjspcare-2017-001330. [Epub ahead of print].

21. Lindell KO, Liang Z, Hoffman LA, Rosenzweig MQ, Saul MI, Pilewski JM, et al. Palliative care and location of death in decedents with idiopathic pulmonary fibrosis. Chest. 2015;147(2):423–9.

22. Liang Z, Hoffman LA, Nouraie M, Kass DJ, Donahoe MP, Gibson KF, et al. Referral to palliative care infrequent in patients with idiopathic pulmonary fibrosis admitted to an intensive care unit. J Palliat Med. 2017;20(2):134–40.

23. Thabut G, Mal H, Castier Y, Groussard O, Brugière O, Marrash-Chahla R, et al. Survival benefit of lung transplantation for patients with idiopathic pulmonary fibrosis. J Thorac Cardiovasc Surg. 2003;126(2):469–75.

24. Smits JM, Vanhaecke J, Haverich A, de Vries E, Smith M, Rutgrink E, et al. Three-year survival rates for all consecutive heart-only and lung-only transplants performed in Eurotransplant, 1997-1999. Clin Transpl. 2003:89–100.

25. Orens JB, Estenne M, Arcasoy S, Conte JV, Corris P, Egan JJ, et al. Pulmonary scientific Council of the International Society for heart and lung transplantation. International guidelines for the selection of lung transplant candidates: 2006 update—a consensus report from the Pulmonary Scientific Council of the International Society for Heart and Lung Transplantation. J Heart Lung Transplant. 2006;25:745–55.

26. Collard HR, King TE, Bartelson BB, Vourlekis JS, Schwarz MI, Brown KK. Changes in clinical and physiologic variables predict survival in idiopathic pulmonary fibrosis. Am J Respir Crit Care Med. 2003;168:538–42.

27. Flaherty KR, Mumford JA, Murray S, Kazerooni EA, Gross BH, Colby TV, et al. Prognostic implications of physiologic and radiographic changes in idiopathic interstitial pneumonia. Am J Respir Crit Care Med. 2002;168:543–8.

28. Du Bois RM, Weycker D, Albera C, Bradford WZ, Costabel U, Katashov A, et al. Ascertainment of individual risk of mortality for patients with idiopathic pulmonary fibrosis. Am J Respir Crit Care Med. 2011;184:459–66.

29. American Thoracic Society, American College of Chest Physicians. ATS/ACCP Statement on cardiopulmonary exercise testing. Am J Respir Crit Care Med. 2003;167:211–77.

30. Thabut G, Christie JD, Ravaud P, Castier Y, Dauriat G, Jebrak G, et al. Survival after bilateral versus single-lung transplantation for idiopathic pulmonary fibrosis. Ann Intern Med. 2009;151(11):767–74.

31. Carbone RG, Monselise A, Bottino G. Pulmonary hypertension in interstitial lung disease (Chapter 2). In: Baughman RP, Carbone RG, Bottino G, editors. Pulmonary arterial hypertension and interstitial lung diseases. New York: Humana Press; 2009.

32. Lettieri CJ, Nathan SD, Barnett SD, et al. Prevalence and outcomes of pulmonary arterial hypertension in advanced idiopathic pulmonary fibrosis. Chest. 2006;129:746–52.

33. Nathan SD, Shlobin OA, Barnett SD, et al. Right ventricular systolic pressure by echocardiography as a predictor of PH in IPF. Respir Med. 2008;102:1305–10.

34. Carbone R, Fireman E, Montanaro F, Musi M, Monselise A, Bottino G. Outcomes in interstitial lung diseases. Eur Respr J. 2005;26(Suppl 49):1807.

35. Nathan SD, Carbone RG. Pulmonary hypertension due to fibrotic lung disease: hidden value in a neutral trial. Am J Respir Crit Care Med. 2014;190(2):131–2.

36. Corte TJ, Keir GJ, Dimopoulos K, Howard L, Corris PA, Parfitt L, Foley C, Yanez-Lopez M, Babalis D, Marino P, Maher TM, Renzoni EA, Spencer L, Elliot CA, Birring SS, O'Reilly K, Gatzoulis MA, Wells AU, Wort SJ, BPHIT Study Group. Bosentan in pulmonary hypertension associated with fibrotic idiopathic interstitial pneumonia. Am J Respir Crit Care Med. 2014;190(2):208–17.

37. Raghu G, et al. ARTEMIS-IPFInvestigators. Treatment of idiopathic pulmonary fibrosis with ambrisentan: a parallel, randomized trial. Ann Intern Med. 2013;158:641–9.

38. King TE Jr, Behr J, Brown KK, du Bois RM, Lancaster L, de Andrade JA, et al. BUILD-1: a randomized placebo-controlled trial of bosentan in idiopathic pulmonary fibrosis. Am J Respir Crit Care Med. 2008;177:75–81.

39. Raghu G, et al. MUSIC Study Group. Macitentan for the treatment of idiopathic pulmonary fibrosis: the randomised controlled MUSIC trial. Eur Respir J. 2013;42:1622–32.

40. Collard HR, Moore BB, Flaherty KR, Brown KK, Kaner RJ, King TE, et al. Acute exacerbations of

idiopathic pulmonary fibrosis. Am J Respir Crit Care Med. 2007;76(7):636–43.

41. Yokoyama A, Kohno N, Hamada H, Sakatani M, Ueda E, Kondo K, et al. Circulating KL-6 predicts the outcome of rapidly progressive idiopathic pulmonary fibrosis. Am J Respir Crit Care Med. 1998;158:1680–4.

42. Donahoe M, Valentine VG, Chien N, Gibson KF, Raval JS, Saul M, et al. Autoantibody-targeted treatments for acute exacerbations of idiopathic pulmonary fibrosis. PLoS One. 2015;10(6):e0127771.

43. Savarino E, Carbone R, Marabotto E, Furnari M, Sconfienza L, Ghio M, et al. Gastro-oesophageal reflux and gastric aspiration in idiopathic pulmonary fibrosis patients. Eur Respir J. 2013;42(5):1322–31.

44. Nathan SD, Basavaraj A, Reichner C, Shlobin OA, Ahmad S, Kiernan J, et al. Prevalence and impact of coronary artery disease in idiopathic pulmonary fibrosis. Respir Med. 2010;104(7):1035–41.

45. Lancaster LH, Mason WR, Parnell JA, Rice TW, Loyd JE, Milstone AP, et al. Obstructive sleep apnea is common in idiopathic pulmonary fibrosis. Chest. 2009;136(3):772–8.

46. Gabrielli A, Avvedimento EV, Krieg T. Scleroderma. N Engl J Med. 2009;360:1989–2003.

47. Le Pavec J, Launay D, Mathai SC, Hassoun PM, Humbert M. Scleroderma lung disease. Clin Rev Allergy Immunol. 2011;40:104–16.

48. Hassoun PM. Lung involvement in systemic sclerosis. Presse Med. 2011;40:e3–17.

49. Steen VD, Medsger TA. Changes in causes of death in systemic sclerosis, 1972–2002. Ann Rheum Dis. 2007;66:940–4.

50. De Cruz S, Ross D. Lung transplantation in patients with scleroderma. Curr Opin Rheumatol. 2013;25:714–8.

51. Whelan TP. Lung transplantation for interstitial lung disease. Clin Chest Med. 2012;33:179–89.

52. Mouthon L, Bérezné A, Guillevin L, Valeyre D. Therapeutic options for systemic sclerosis related interstitial lung diseases. Respir Med. 2010;104(Suppl 1):S59–69.

53. Kubo M, Vensak J, Dauber J, Keenan R, Griffith B, McCurry K. Lung transplantation in patients with scleroderma. J Heart Lung Transplant. 2001;20:174–5.

54. Rosas V, Conte JV, Yang SC, Gaine SP, Borja M, Wigley FM, et al. Lung transplantation and systemic sclerosis. Ann Transplant. 2000;5:38–43.

55. Meyer KC, Raghu G, Verleden GM, Corris PA, Aurora P, Wilson KC, et al. The ISHLT/ATS/ERS BOS Task Force Committee. An International ISHLT/ATS/ERS clinical practice guideline: diagnosis and management of bronchiolitis obliterans syndrome. Eur Respir J. 2014;44:1479–503.

56. Pigula FA, Griffith BP, Zenati MA, Dauber JH, Yousem SA, Keenan RJ. Lung transplantation for respiratory failure resulting from systemic disease. Ann Thorac Surg. 1997;64:1630–4.

57. Shitrit D, Amital A, Peled N. Lung transplantation in patients with scleroderma: case series, review of the literature, and criteria for transplantation. Clin Transplant. 2009;23:178–83.

58. D'Ovidio F, Singer LG, Hadjiliadis D, Pierre A, Waddell TK, de Perrot M, et al. Prevalence of gastroesophageal reflux in end-stage lung disease candidates for lung transplant. Ann Thorac Surg. 2005;80:1254–60.

59. Fisichella PM, Reder NP, Gagermeier J, Kovacs EJ. Usefulness of pH monitoring in predicting the survival status of patients with scleroderma awaiting lung transplantation. J Surg Res. 2014;189:232–7.

60. Hoppo T, Jarido V, Pennathur A, Morrell M, Crespo M, Shigemura N, et al. Antireflux surgery preserves lung function in patients with gastroesophageal reflux disease and end-stage lung disease before and after lung transplantation. Arch Surg. 2011;146:1041–7.

61. Launay D, Savale L, Berezne A, Le Pavec J, Hachulla E, Mouthon L, et al. Working Group on Heart/Lung transplantation in systemic sclerosis of the French Network on Pulmonary Hypertension. Lung and heart-lung transplantation for systemic sclerosis patients. A monocentric experience of 13 patients, review of the literature and position paper of a multidisciplinary Working Group. Presse Med. 2014;43:e345–63.

62. Williams TJ, Patterson GA, McClean PA. Maximal exercise testing in single and double lung transplant recipients. Am Rev Respir Dis. 1992;145:101–5.

63. Patterson GA, Maurer JR, Williams TJ. Comparison of outcomes of double and single lung transplantation for obstructive lung disease. The Toronto Lung Transplant Group. J Thorac Cardiovasc Surg. 1991;101:623–32.

64. Bernstein EJ, Peterson ER, Sell JL, D'Ovidio F, Arcasoy SM, Bathon JM, Lederer DJ. Survival of adults with systemic sclerosis following lung transplantation: a nationwide cohort study. Arthritis Rheumatol. 2015;67:1314–22.

65. Volkmann ER, Saggar R, Khanna D, Torres B, Flora A, Yoder L, et al. Improved transplant-free survival in patients with systemic sclerosis-associated pulmonary hypertension and interstitial lung disease. Arthritis Rheumatol. 2014;66:1900–8.

66. Khan IY, Singer LG, de Perrot M, Granton JT, Keshavjee S, Chau C, et al. Survival after lung transplantation in systemic sclerosis. A systematic review. Respir Med. 2013;107:2081–7.

67. Sottile PD, Iturbe D, Katsumoto TR, Connolly MK, Collard HR, Leard LA, et al. Outcomes in systemic sclerosis-related lung disease after lung transplantation. Transplantation. 2013;95:975–80.

68. Saggar R, Khanna D, Furst DE, Belperio JA, Park GS, Weigt SS, et al. Systemic sclerosis and bilateral lung transplantation: a single centre experience. Eur Respir J. 2010;36:893–900.

69. Schachna L, Medsger TA Jr, Dauber JH, Wigley FM, Braunstein NA, White B, et al. Lung transplantation in scleroderma compared with idiopathic pulmonary fibrosis and idiopathic pulmonary arterial hypertension. Arthritis Rheum. 2006;54:3954–61.

70. Massad MG, Powell CR, Kpodonu J, Tshibaka C, Hanhan Z, Snow NJ, Geha AS. Outcomes of lung transplantation in patients with scleroderma. World J Surg. 2005;29:1510–5.
71. Kotloff RM, Thabut G. Lung transplantation. Am J Respir Crit Care Med. 2011;184:159–71.
72. Bouros D, Wells AU, Nicholson AG, Colby TV, Polychronopoulos V, Pantelidis P, et al. Histopathologic subsets of fibrosing alveolitis in patients with systemic sclerosis and their relationship to outcome. Am J Respir Crit Care Med. 2002;165:1581–6.
73. Goh NS, Desai SR, Veeraraghavan S, Hansell DM, Copley SJ, Maher TM, et al. Interstitial lung disease in systemic sclerosis: a simple staging system. Am J Respir Crit Care Med. 2008;177:1248–54.
74. Brown KK. Rheumatoid lung disease. Proc Am Thorac Soc. 2007;4:443–8.
75. Mc Donagh J, Greaves M, Wright AR, et al. High resolution computed tomography of the lungs in patients with rheumatoid arthritis and interstitial lung disease. Br J Rheumatol. 1994;33:118–22.
76. Olson AL, Swigris JJ, Sprunger DB, Fischer A, Fernandez-Perez ER, Solomon J, et al. Rheumatoid arthritis-interstitial lung disease-associated mortality. Am J Respir Crit Care Med. 2011;183:372–8.
77. Kelly C, Saravanan V. Treatment strategies for a rheumatoid arthritis patient with interstitial lung disease. Expert Opin Pharmacother. 2008;9:3221–30.
78. Yazdani A, Singer LG, Strand V, Gelber AC, Williams L, Mittoo S. Survival and quality of life in rheumatoid arthritis-associated interstitial lung disease after lung transplantation. J Heart Lung Transplant. 2014;33:514–20.
79. Taimeh Z, Hertz MJ, Shumway S, Pritzker M. Lung transplantation for pulmonary sarcoidosis. Twenty five years of experience in USA. Thorax. 2016;71(4):378–9.
80. Arcasoy SM, Christi JD, Pochettino A, Rosengard BR, Blumenthal NP, Bavaria JE, Kotloff RM. Characteristics and outcomes of patients with sarcoidosis listed for lung transplantation. Chest. 2001;120:673–80.
81. Wille KM, Gaggar A, Hajari AS, Leon KJ, Barney JB, Smith KH, et al. Bronchiolitis obliterans syndrome and survival following lung transplantation for patients with sarcoidosis. Sarcoidosis Vasc Diffuse Lung Dis. 2008;25(2):117–24.
82. Cai J, Mao Q, Ozawa M, Terasaki PI. Lung transplantation in the United States: 1990-2005 Clin Transpl. 2005:29–35.
83. Cordier JF, Johnson SR. Multiple cystic lung diseases. Eur Respir Mon. 2011;54:46–83.
84. Attili AK, Kazerooni EA, Gross BH, Flaherty KR, Myers JL, Martinez FJ. Smoking related interstitial lung disease: radiologic-clinical-pathologic correlation. Radiographics. 2008;28:1383–96.
85. Abbott GF, Rosado-de-Christenson MI, Franks TJ, Frazier AA, Galvin JR. From the archives of the AFIP: pulmonary Langerhans cell histiocytosis. Radiographics. 2004;24:821–41.
86. Leatherwood DI, Heitkamp DF, Emerson RE. Best cases from the AFIP: pulmonary Langerhans cell histiocytosis. Radiographics. 2007;27:265–8.
87. Moore AD, Godwin JD, Muller NL, Naidich DP, Hammar SP, Buschman DL, et al. Pulmonary histiocytosis X: comparison of radiographic and CT finding. Radiology. 1989;172:249–54.
88. Brauner MW, Grenier P, Mouelhi MM, Mompoint D, Lenoir S. Pulmonary histiocytosis X: evaluation with high-resolution CT. Radiology. 1989;172:255–8.
89. Brauner MW, Grenier P, Tijani K, Battesti JP, Valeyre D. Pulmonary Langerhans cell histiocytosis evolution of lesions on CT scans. Radiology. 1997;204:497–502.
90. Kim HJ, Lee KS, Johnkoh T, Tomiyama N, Lee HY, Han J, Kim TS. Pulmonary Langerhans cell histiocytosis in adults: high-resolution CT-pathology comparisons and evolutional changes at CT. Eur Radiol. 2011;21:1406–15.
91. Fartoukh M, Humbert M, Capron F, Maître S, Parent F, Le Gall C, et al. Severe pulmonary hypertension in histiocytosis X. Am J Respir Crit Care Med. 2000;161:216–23.
92. Dauriat G, Mal H, Tahbut G, Mornex JF, Bertocchi M, Tronc F, et al. Lung transplantation for pulmonary Langerhans' cell histiocytosis: a multicenter analysis. Transplantation. 2006;81:746–50.

Pulmonary Vascular Disease: Specific Evaluation and Timing for Listing Eligible Patients to Receive Lung Transplantation and Management of the Pre-lung Transplant Patient

5

Alison S. Witkin and Richard N. Channick

Abbreviations

6MWD	Six minute walk distance
APAH	Attributable pulmonary hypertension
CF	Cystic fibrosis
CHD	Congenital heart disease
COPD	Chronic obstructive pulmonary disease
DLT	Double-lung transplant
ECMO	Extracorporeal membrane oxygenation
FDA	Food and Drug Administration
IPF	Idiopathic pulmonary fibrosis
LAS	Lung allocation score
LT	Lung transplant
HLT	Heart/lung transplant
ILD	Interstitial lung disease
IPAH	Idiopathic pulmonary arterial hypertension
mPAP	Mean pulmonary artery pressure
NYHA	New York Heart Association
PAH	Pulmonary arterial hypertension
PASP	Pulmonary artery systolic pressure
PCH	Pulmonary capillary hemangiomatosis
PCWP	Pulmonary capillary wedge pressure
PH	Pulmonary hypertension
PPHN	Persistent pulmonary hypertension of the newborn
PTE	Pulmonary thromboendarterectomy
PVOD	Pulmonary veno-occlusive disease
PVR	Pulmonary vascular resistance
RHC	Right heart catheterization
SPH	Secondary pulmonary hypertension
TTE	Transthoracic echocardiogram
V/Q	Ventilation/perfusion
WHO	World Health Organization
WU	Woods units

A. S. Witkin (✉) · R. N. Channick
Division of Pulmonary and Critical Care Medicine, Department of Medicine, Massachusetts General Hospital, Boston, MA, USA
e-mail: aswitkin@partners.org; rchannick@mgh.harvard.edu

Introduction

Pulmonary arterial hypertension is characterized by progressive vasculopathy in the pulmonary arterial bed leading to right ventricular dysfunction and failure. Despite significant advances in medical therapy over the last several decades, lung transplantation remains a necessary treatment option for patients with severe and refractory disease. This chapter discusses the role of lung transplantation in the management of pulmonary

© The Author(s) 2018
G. Raghu, R. G. Carbone (eds.), *Lung Transplantation*, https://doi.org/10.1007/978-3-319-91184-7_5

hypertension as well as transplant-specific considerations, including the use of single versus dual lung transplant and the diminishing role of combined heart and lung transplantation.

Diagnosis of Pulmonary Hypertension

The earliest symptom of pulmonary hypertension (PH) is often dyspnea on exertion, but over time symptoms may become severe with development of edema, chest pain, syncope, and hemoptysis. Due to the non-specific nature of symptoms, diagnosis may be delayed for months or even years [1]. The initial evaluation of suspected PH focuses on noninvasive testing, including transthoracic echocardiogram (TTE) [2]. While TTE can demonstrate findings suggestive of pulmonary hypertension, such as an elevated estimated pulmonary artery systolic pressure (PASP) or right ventricular (RV) dilatation or hypokinesis, these findings lack the necessary sensitivity and specificity to confirm the diagnosis (Fig. 5.1a, b) [3, 4].

The diagnosis of PH requires right heart catheterization (RHC). PH is defined as an elevation in the mean pulmonary artery pressure (mPAP) to $\geq$25 mmHg on resting RHC. While any patient with an elevated mPAP is classified as having

PH, it is important to further distinguish between precapillary PH, which reflects pathology involving the pulmonary vascular bed and postcapillary PH, which indicates the presence of significant left heart disease. Precapillary PH is defined as a mPAP $\geq$25 mmHg with a pulmonary capillary wedge pressure (PCWP) $\leq$15 mmHg and a pulmonary vascular resistance (PVR) >3 WU. Postcapillary pulmonary hypertension is characterized by a PCWP >15 mmHg [5]. Patients may also have mixed disease with elevations in mPAP, PCWP, and PVR.

Classification of Pulmonary Hypertension

While confirming the diagnosis of PH with RHC is essential, it is also important to determine the etiology of PH, as this has significant implications for treatment and prognosis. The World Health Organization (WHO) classification system attempts to provide classification of disease based on both etiology and physiologic mechanism (Box 5.1). Lung transplant (LT) is primarily performed for patients with pulmonary arterial hypertension (PAH, WHO group 1), although smaller numbers are done for patients with chronic thromboembolic pulmonary hyperten-

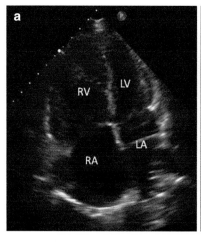
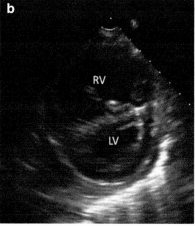
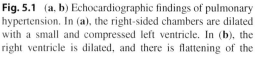

Fig. 5.1 (**a, b**) Echocardiographic findings of pulmonary hypertension. In (**a**), the right-sided chambers are dilated with a small and compressed left ventricle. In (**b**), the right ventricle is dilated, and there is flattening of the interventricular septum consistent with right-sided pressure and volume overload. Abbreviations: *RA* right atrium, *RV* right ventricle, *LA* left atrium, *LV* left ventricle

sion (CTEPH, WHO group 4) [6]. Additionally, patients receiving transplant for hypoxemic lung disease may have concurrent PH, and this needs to be considered in the transplant process.

Box 5.1 Classification of Pulmonary Hypertension from the Fifth World Symposium on Pulmonary Hypertension, Nice 2013. 1.2.1 and 1.2.2 List Genetic Mutations Associated with PAH

1. Pulmonary arterial hypertension
  1.1 Idiopathic PAH
  1.2 Heritable PAH
    1.2.1 BMPR2
    1.2.2. ALK-1, ENG, SMAD9, CAV1, KCNK3
    1.2.3 Unknown
  1.3 Drug and toxin induced
  1.4 Associated with:
    1.4.1 Connective tissue disease
    1.4.2 HIV infection
    1.4.3 Portal hypertension
    1.4.4 Congenital heart disease
    1.4.5 Schistosomiasis
1′. Pulmonary veno-occlusive disease and/or pulmonary capillary hemangiomatosis
1″. Persistent pulmonary hypertension of the newborn (PPHN)
2. Pulmonary hypertension due to left heart disease
  2.1 Left ventricular systolic dysfunction
  2.2 Left ventricular diastolic dysfunction
  2.3 Valvular disease
  2.4 Congenital/acquired left heart inflow/outflow tract obstruction and congenital cardiomyopathies
3. Pulmonary hypertension due to lung diseases and/or hypoxia
  3.1 Chronic obstructive pulmonary disease
  3.2 Interstitial lung disease
  3.3 Other pulmonary diseases with mixed restrictive and obstructive pattern
  3.4 Sleep-disordered breathing
  3.5 Alveolar hypoventilation disorders
  3.6 Chronic exposure to high altitude
  3.7 Developmental lung diseases
4. Chronic thromboembolic pulmonary hypertension (CTEPH)

5. Pulmonary hypertension with unclear multifactorial mechanisms
  5.1 Hematologic disorders: chronic hemolytic anemia, myeloproliferative disorders, splenectomy
  5.2 Systemic disorders: sarcoidosis, pulmonary histiocytosis, lymphangioleiomyomatosis
  5.3 Metabolic disorders: glycogen storage disease, Gaucher disease, thyroid disorders
  5.4 Others: tumoral obstruction, fibrosing mediastinitis, chronic renal failure, segmental PH

Used with permission of Elsevier from Simonneau G, Gatzoulis MA, Adatia I, et al. Updated clinical classification of pulmonary hypertension. J Am Coll Cardiol 2013;62:D34–41

Group 1 PAH consists of patients with idiopathic PAH, familial PAH, drug- and toxin-induced PAH, as well as PAH attributable to connective tissue diseases, HIV, portal hypertension, congenital heart disease, and schistosomiasis. Subtypes exist for pulmonary veno-occlusive disease (PVOD), pulmonary capillary hemangiomatosis (PCH), and persistent pulmonary hypertension of the newborn (PPHN) [2, 7]. PAH is a rare disease with an estimated prevalence of 10–52 cases per million [8]. Of patients with PAH, approximately 45% have idiopathic PAH (IPAH), and 50% have PAH attributable to other diseases (APAH), with the rest having PVOD, PCH, PPHN, or familial pulmonary hypertension. Of those with APAH, PAH associated with connective tissue disease or congenital heart disease are the most common attributable factors [9].

PH due to left heart disease (WHO group 2) includes patients with pulmonary hypertension due to left ventricular systolic and diastolic dysfunction as well as valvular heart disease. This is the most common type of pulmonary hypertension, and management focuses on treatment of the underlying cardiac disease [10, 11].

PH due to lung diseases and/or hypoxia (WHO group 3) includes patients with chronic obstructive pulmonary disease (COPD), interstitial lung disease (ILD), and sleep disordered breathing. While estimates vary between studies, over 30% of patients with COPD or ILD who are evaluated for LT have PH, as defined by mPAP $\geq$25 mmHg [12–15]. As in WHO group 2 disease, the primary focus is on treatment of the underlying disease with the use of pulmonary vasodilators limited to select patients under supervision of a PH expert [16].

Chronic thromboembolic pulmonary hypertension (WHO group 4) is a form of pulmonary hypertension in which an acute pulmonary embolism fails to undergo normal fibrinolysis causing chronic vascular obstruction. The ventilation/perfusion (V/Q) scan is the screening test of choice with pulmonary angiogram used for confirmatory testing [17–19]. As CTEPH is potentially curable with surgery, all patients with PH without significant underlying cardiac or pulmonary disease should be screened with a V/Q scan [2].

WHO group 5 represents pulmonary hypertension with unclear and/or multifactorial mechanisms. Although this is a heterogeneous group, this classification includes several pulmonary diseases that may be treated with LT such as sarcoidosis, pulmonary histiocytosis, and lymphangioleiomyomatosis [2].

Treatment of PAH

Over the last 30 years, the treatment of PAH has changed dramatically from primarily supportive with consideration of LT to the availability of multiple classes of disease-specific medications. The current treatment of PAH focuses on maximizing response to medical therapy while reserving surgical interventions such as balloon atrial septostomy and LT for patients with refractory disease and right heart failure (Fig. 5.2) [2, 20]. There are currently 14 therapies approved by the US Food and Drug Administration (FDA) for treatment of pulmonary hypertension (Table 5.1). Treatment options are available via oral, subcutaneous, intravenous, and inhaled routes.

The first medication approved for treatment of PAH was intravenous epoprostenol. Now there are medications available targeting three different molecular pathways: nitric oxide, prostacyclin, and endothelin; this allows for patients to be treated with double or triple therapy.

The AMBITION trial compared single-drug therapy using either ambrisentan or tadalafil to treatment with both of these medications in combination. The findings indicate a decrease in a composite clinical failure outcome that included death, hospitalization, and disease progression with combination therapy [21]. While early studies in PAH used improvement in 6-min walk distance (6MWD) as a marker of drug efficacy, more recent trials have used long-term, event-driven morbidity/mortality end points. This changing paradigm in PAH trials reflects evolution of PAH in general, from a universally fatal disease to one that is treatable and associated with long-term survival [21–23].

The advances in medical therapy have decreased the need for transplant for PAH. An analysis done following the approval of epoprostenol found that treatment with the medication was either able to delay or eliminate the need for LT [24]. While the majority of clinical trials are not powered to detect differences in mortality, there nonetheless appears to be a significant mortality benefit with medical treatment of PAH when data from multiple trials are pooled together [25, 26].

Despite significant advances in medical therapy, PAH remains a life-threatening disease for many patients. A registry including over 2000 patients with PAH found that, as of 2012, the estimated 5-year survival rate was 57% [27]. For patients who develop decompensated right heart failure despite maximum medical therapy, LT is the only viable treatment option (Fig. 5.2). Other procedural options include balloon atrial septostomy and the use of extracorporeal membrane oxygenation (ECMO) as a bridge to LT.

Atrial septostomy involves the creation of a connection between the right and left atria. This allows for flow of blood from the right to the left atrium and can assist with decompression of the

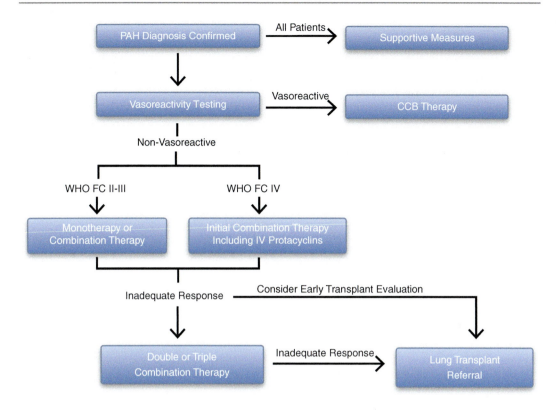

Fig. 5.2 Treatment algorithm for patients with PAH. Published treatment algorithms recommend medical optimization with the use of dual or triple therapy if necessary [2, 20]. Patients should be assessed for acute pulmonary vasoreactivity, and all patients should receive supportive measures, such as pulmonary rehabilitation and supplemental oxygen, if necessary. If a patient has an inadequate response despite maximal medical therapy, lung transplant should be considered. *CCB* calcium channel blocker, *WHO FC* World Health Organization functional class

Table 5.1 FDA-approved treatment options for PAH, listed by pharmacologic class

Prostanoids	ERAs	PDE-5 inhibitors	sGC stimulator
Epoprostenol (IV)	Bosentan	Sildenafil	Riociguat
Treprostinil (IV, SQ, inh, oral)	Ambrisentan	Tadalafil	
Iloprost (inh)	Macitentan		
Selexipag (prostacyclin receptor agonist)			

All medications are available in oral form only unless another route is listed in parentheses
Abbreviations: *IV* intravenous, *SQ* subcutaneous, *inh* inhaled, *ERA* endothelin receptor antagonist, *PDE-5* phosphodiesterase type 5, *sGC* soluble guanylate cyclase

RV while improving left ventricular filling and cardiac output. This can lead to improved tissue perfusion despite a fall in arterial oxygen content [28, 29]. Atrial septostomy, however, is associated with a procedure associated mortality of >10%, and thus its role is limited to palliative or salvage uses at institutions with appropriate expertise [29, 30].

ECMO can be used as a bridge for patients who decompensate while awaiting LT. Successful bridging to transplant has been reported with both conventional veno-arterial ECMO and the use of the pump-free Novalung system with pumpless connection of the pulmonary artery to the left atrium [31–33]. However, the use of such support devices is only recommended in young patients with single organ dysfunction and good potential for rehab [34].

Lung Transplantation for PAH: Overview

Transplant considerations include the need for dual heart/lung transplant (HLT) and the decision to perform single- versus double-lung transplant. The majority of transplants for PAH are double-lung transplants (DLT). LT for PAH makes up only a small percentage of total transplants, and, over time, the percent of transplants being done for PAH has decreased (Fig. 5.3a). From January 1995 to June 2014, only 3.9% of all LT were done for PAH, the majority of these being for patients with IPAH and the rest for patients with congenital heart disease (CHD). Although the total number of HLT done per year has declined to fewer than 100 cases annually, IPAH and CHD represent, respectively, 27.6% and 35.4% of all HLT performed between January 1982 and June 2014 (Fig. 5.3b) [6].

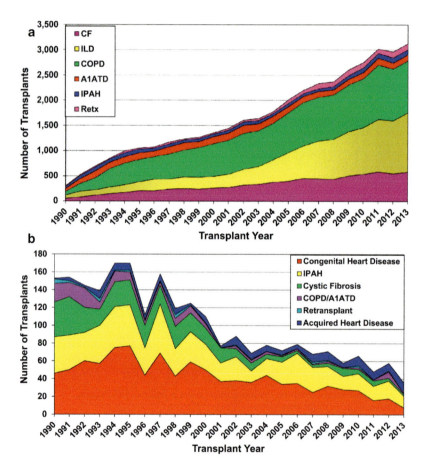

Fig. 5.3 (**a**) Number of lung transplants performed annually broken down by indication. Transplants for IPAH (represented in blue) make up a very small percent of total transplants, and the number of procedures performed annually has failed to increase, despite increases in total number of procedures. (**b**) Number of combined heart/lung transplants performed annually broken down by disease indication. While the number of HLT performed has declined, combined IPAH (represnted by yellow) and con- genital heart disease (represnted by red) account for over half of the transplants (**a**, **b**: Used with permission of Elsevier from Yusen RD, Edwards LB, Kucheryavaya AY, et al. The Registry of the International Society for Heart and Lung Transplantation: Thirty-second Official Adult Lung and Heart-Lung Transplantation Report—2015; Focus Theme: Early Graft Failure. J Heart Lung Transplant 2015;34:1264–77)

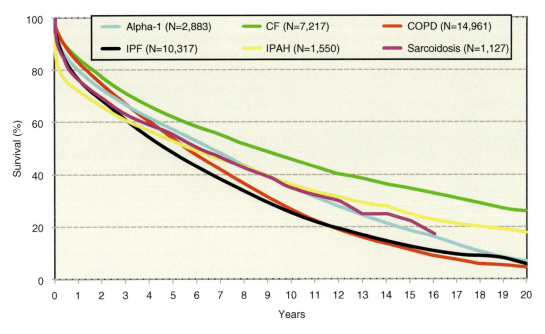

Fig. 5.4 IPAH (yellow line) has the highest mortality at 1 year. However, most of this mortality is related to the initial posttransplant time period, and the 10- and 20-year survival is better than all diseases except for cystic fibrosis (Used with permission of Elsevier from Yusen RD, Edwards LB, Kucheryavaya AY, et al. The Registry of the International Society for Heart and Lung Transplantation: Thirty-second Official Adult Lung and Heart-Lung Transplantation Report—2015; Focus Theme: Early Graft Failure. J Heart Lung Transplant 2015;34:1264–77 (online supplementary material))

LT for IPAH has the highest 1-year mortality of any indication for LT at 23%. For those patients who survive the first posttransplant year, the survival rates are better than that of sarcoidosis, alpha-1 antitrypsin deficiency, COPD, and ILD (Fig. 5.4). The median survival for patients who survive the first year is 10.0 years [6]. Increased experience with LT for PAH combined with advances in management of lung transplant has been associated with improvements in both short- and long-term survival [35, 36].

Listing for Transplant

The decision to list a patient with PAH for lung transplant is complex and fraught with uncertainty. Considered factors include disease severity, prognosis, and expected response to additional treatments. Most experts recommend transplant referral and potential listing when a patient has an inadequate clinical response despite treatment with multiple therapies including intravenous prostacyclin therapy (Fig. 5.2). There is, however, a fair amount of subjectivity in making this determination, although the International Society of Heart and Lung Transplantation (ISHLT) has published recommendations to help guide this decision (Box 5.2) [2, 20, 34].

Markers of disease severity include functional status and hemodynamic measurements. As PAH worsens the right atrial pressure and PVR rise, while the cardiac output falls. In severe disease, the mPAP may actually begin to fall as the RV is no longer able to generate adequate pressure to overcome the increasing vascular resistance. Predictors of mortality include a right atrial pressure >20 mmHg, pericardial effusion, 6MWD <332 m, and New York Heart Association (NYHA) functional class III or IV disease [37–39].

The underlying disease process should play a role in the decision to refer for LT. Compared to patients with IPAH, those with connective tissue disease-associated PAH or familial PAH have worse short- and long-term survival rates, while patients with CHD-related PAH have higher survival rates [27, 37, 38]. As no reliable treatment exists for the treatment of PCH or PVOD, these patients should be referred at the time of diagnosis [2, 40].

Recognizing the above risk factors of mortality, ISHLT recommends using the following criteria in the decision to list: NYHA functional class III or IV despite 3 months of combination therapy including prostanoids, a cardiac index <2 L/min/m^2, mean right atrial pressure >15 mmHg, 6MWD < 350 m or development of hemoptysis, pericardial effusion, or right heart failure [34]. The decision to list should also take into consideration patient preferences, psychosocial support, and comorbid medical conditions.

Wait-List Mortality and the Lung Allocation System

Prior to 2005, wait-list rank was determined by time spent on the list; however, in 2005 the lung allocation score (LAS) system was implemented to attempt to give preference to patients with the highest need and potential benefit from LT [41]. The implementation of the LAS was associated with decreases in number of patients on the wait list, time from listing to transplantation, and, for several diseases, decreased wait-list mortality [42–44]. Despite these improvements, there was concern that the LAS might not accurately reflect disease severity in PAH [44, 45].

In 2009 Chen and colleagues compared rates of transplantation, wait-list mortality, and post-transplant outcomes between patients with IPAH and those with idiopathic pulmonary fibrosis (IPF), COPD, or cystic fibrosis (CF) before and after implementation of the LAS. They found that while patients with IPF, COPD, and CF had decreased wait-list mortality at 12 months, this benefit was not seen in patients with IPAH. Additionally, the relative mortality risk compared to patients with IPF, COPD, and CF increased, and the likelihood of transplant decreased, suggesting that the LAS might not accurately reflect disease severity in PAH [43, 46, 47].

Identified predictors of wait-list mortality in PAH include male gender, worse functional class, 6MWD <300 m, decreased cardiac output, increased right atrial pressure, rise in bilirubin, and the presence of connective tissue disease-associated PAH [36, 44, 46–48]. These findings were incorporated into an updated version of the LAS in February 2015 that now includes cardiac index, central venous pressure, and bilirubin into calculation of the score [49, 50]. Repeat analysis following the implementation of these changes will be necessary to understand their effect. Additionally, physicians may apply for LAS exception points for patients with PAH who are deteriorating on optimal therapy and have a right atrial pressure >15 mmHg and a cardiac index <1.8 L/min/m². If the patient is granted the exception points, he or she receives a LAS equivalent to the 90th percentile nationally [51].

Single- Versus Double-Lung Transplant

The majority of transplants performed for PAH are double-lung transplants (DLT), and this is considered the treatment of choice at most centers. Between January 1995 and June 2014, 90% of transplants done for PAH were DLT [6].

Several centers have reported success using SLT, with improvements in pulmonary vascular hemodynamics as well as mortality rates similar to patients receiving DLT [52–56]. However, there are conflicting results, with other centers reporting trends toward lower mortality and less reperfusion injury in patients who receive DLT [29, 57, 58]. Additionally, there are physiologic reasons why DLT is the procedure of choice for PAH, most notably that in posttransplant there is a large ventilation/perfusion mismatch with ventilation being split evenly between the two lungs but a majority of the perfusion is directed to the transplanted lung. The ventilation/perfusion mismatch may be exacerbated if rejection occurs, as the ventilation will then favor the native lung, which has inadequate perfusion [29, 59].

The ISHLT examined the estimated survival data for over 1500 patients with IPAH over a 12.5-year time period and found a survival benefit for DLT over SLT [60]. This is consistent with an overall survival benefit seen for DLT regardless of the underlying disease [6]. This pooled registry data combined with physiologic rationale makes DLT the preferred treatment over SLT for patients with PAH.

Lung Transplant Versus Heart-Lung Transplant

Originally HLT was the treatment of choice for PAH, and the first HLT performed was actually done in a patient with PAH [6, 61]. However, more recently, fewer HLT are being done for PAH as good outcomes are seen with DLT alone [6].

HLT requires only one airway anastomosis and is associated with fewer vascular complications. [29] Additionally, there were concerns that the RV would not be able to recover following LT only, making HLT a necessity. However, studies demonstrated that the RV has a remarkable ability to recover function following lung-only transplantation [62]. Overall, most comparisons of DLT to HLT for IPAH show similar survival outcomes, with conflicting data about the development of bronchiolitis obliterans syndrome [63–66].

The main challenge in interpreting data comparing DLT to HLT is that all of the studies are retrospective and nonrandomized. In some analyses, the presence of severe RV dilatation or decreased cardiac index was an indication for HLT, making comparison between HLT and DLT challenging as the sickest patients received HLT [65, 66]. Nonetheless, the ISHLT recommends that for most patients with IPAH without RV infarcts or other structural heart disease, BLT is the treatment of choice [34]. Thus, BLT should be used for the majority of patients with IPAH, and the decision to proceed with HLT for an individual patient based on anticipated benefit must be weighed against the risks associated with longer wait-list times [29, 34, 36]. In the event of heart failure posttransplant, there are case reports of ECMO being used successfully as a bridge to recovery [67, 68]. The decision to perform either

DLT or HLT in patients with PAH associated with congenital heart disease is more challenging and will be discussed separately.

Disease-Specific Considerations

Much of the data on PH and transplantation focuses on patients with IPAH. However, PH plays a significant role in transplant decisions for patients with congenital heart disease, and secondary pulmonary hypertension (SPH) can occur in many patients with parenchymal lung disease. Additionally, lung transplant is a treatment option for some patients with non-WHO group 1 PH, particularly those with CTEPH.

Congenital Heart Disease Patients with Need for Heart Transplant

The choice of procedure for patients with CHD is challenging as potential treatment options include DLT, HLT, or heart transplant alone. The presence of PH concurrent with CHD is associated with increased wait-list mortality for patients listed for heart transplant [69]. For some patients, correction of the underlying cardiac defect at the time of LT may be possible and eliminate the need for HLT. This has been done with outcomes similar to that seen with HLT in carefully selected patients [34, 70].

For patients with primary cardiac disease, including acquired heart disease in addition to CHD, pretransplant assessment of associated PH is essential. The presence of pretransplant PH is associated with increased posttransplant mortality [71–73]. The finding of a PVR >5 WU or a transpulmonary gradient > 16–20 mmHg is considered a relative contraindication to heart-only transplant, particularly if the systolic pulmonary artery pressure is >60 mmHg as this is associated with an increased risk of right ventricular failure and early death [34]. A vasodilator challenge can be used to assess for reversibility, although even reversible PH appears to be associated with increased posttransplant mortality, particularly if the use of a vasodilator causes systemic hypotension [34, 71].

Overall, the decision to pursue LT, HLT, or heart-only transplant in a patient with combined heart and lung disease is complex. These decisions should be made in a multidisciplinary fashion with input from both pulmonary and cardiac experts.

Secondary Pulmonary Hypertension

As mentioned previously, many patients who are listed for transplant due to hypoxemic lung disease such as ILD or COPD develop WHO group III PH, often referred to in the transplant literature as secondary pulmonary hypertension (SPH). Overall, the incidence of SPH appears to be higher in patients with COPD than IPF at time of transplant referral, although this may be reflective of shorter disease duration at time of referral in patients with IPF [15]. The presence of concurrent PH is associated with increased wait-list mortality in patients with CF, IPF, and COPD, and the development of pulmonary hypertension in patients with COPD or CF is considered an indication for transplant evaluation according to ISHLT recommendations [13, 14, 34, 74]. As in LT done for PAH, there is debate about the need for DLT in the setting of SPH. Several analyses have found that the presence of SPH was not associated with increased mortality in patients who underwent SLT for underlying lung disease [75, 76]. Nonetheless, as DLT is overall associated with a survival benefit compared to SLT, the procedure choice should be made on an individualized basis.

Chronic Thromboembolic Pulmonary Hypertension

The treatment of choice for patients with CTEPH is pulmonary thromboendarterectomy (PTE) as it is associated with improved mortality (Fig. 5.5) [77]. However, not all patients with CTEPH have surgically accessible disease, and in such patients, LT has been performed successfully [78]. Since the classification of PAH and IPAH in the transplant literature often includes patients who

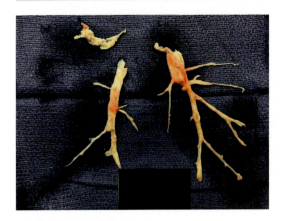

Fig. 5.5 A specimen from a pulmonary thromboendartectomy surgery

underwent transplant for CTEPH, the incidence and outcomes associated with LT for CTEPH are unknown [6, 36]. Over the last several years, treatments for CTEPH in patients with inoperable disease or postoperative PH have expanded to include both FDA approval of the soluble guanylate cyclase stimulator, riociguat, and increased availability of balloon pulmonary angioplasty, a minimally invasive procedure that dilates stenotic pulmonary arteries [79, 80]. Despite these advances, LT will continue to have a role for patients with severe disease that is refractory to available treatments.

Disease Recurrence

The recurrence of IPAH following lung transplant is exceedingly rare, with only a few reported cases in the literature [81, 82]. If PH does recur, the vascular anastomotic site should be evaluated to ensure that stenosis has not developed, as this may be amenable to surgical repair [83]. While fewer transplants are done for PVOD and PCH, there are case reports of both of these diseases recurring posttransplant [84, 85].

Conclusions

Despite significant medical advances in the treatment of PAH over the last 25 years, LT remains an important treatment option for patients with refractory and severe disease.

The decision to list a patient for transplant involves careful review of their comorbidities and risk factors. For most patients with PAH, DLT is the procedure of choice, although both SLT and HLT have been used with success. Additionally, the assessment and recognition of any PH plays an important role in transplant evaluation for all patients undergoing evaluation for any of heart, lung, or combined heart/lung transplant.

References

1. Brown LM, Chen H, Halpern S, et al. Delay in recognition of pulmonary arterial hypertension: factors identified from the REVEAL Registry. Chest. 2011;140:19–26.
2. Galie N, Humbert M, Vachiery JL, et al. 2015 ESC/ERS Guidelines for the diagnosis and treatment of pulmonary hypertension: The Joint Task Force for the Diagnosis and Treatment of Pulmonary Hypertension of the European Society of Cardiology (ESC) and the European Respiratory Society (ERS): Endorsed by: Association for European Paediatric and Congenital Cardiology (AEPC), International Society for Heart and Lung Transplantation (ISHLT). Eur Heart J. 2016;37:67–119.
3. Fisher MR, Forfia PR, Chamera E, et al. Accuracy of Doppler echocardiography in the hemodynamic assessment of pulmonary hypertension. Am J Respir Crit Care Med. 2009;179:615–21.
4. Rich JD, Shah SJ, Swamy RS, Kamp A, Rich S. Inaccuracy of Doppler echocardiographic estimates of pulmonary artery pressures in patients with pulmonary hypertension: implications for clinical practice. Chest. 2011;139:988–93.
5. Hoeper MM, Bogaard HJ, Condliffe R, et al. Definitions and diagnosis of pulmonary hypertension. J Am Coll Cardiol. 2013;62:D42–50.
6. Yusen RD, Edwards LB, Kucheryavaya AY, et al. The Registry of the International Society for Heart and Lung Transplantation: Thirty-second Official Adult Lung and Heart-Lung Transplantation Report—2015; Focus Theme: Early Graft Failure. J Heart Lung Transplant. 2015;34:1264–77.
7. Simonneau G, Gatzoulis MA, Adatia I, et al. Updated clinical classification of pulmonary hypertension. J Am Coll Cardiol. 2013;62:D34–41.
8. Hoeper MM, Simon RGJ. The changing landscape of pulmonary arterial hypertension and implications for patient care. Eur Respiratory Rev. 2014;23: 450–7.
9. Badesch DB, Raskob GE, Elliott CG, et al. Pulmonary arterial hypertension: baseline characteristics from the REVEAL Registry. Chest. 2010;137:376–87.

10. Vachiery JL, Adir Y, Barbera JA, et al. Pulmonary hypertension due to left heart diseases. J Am Coll Cardiol. 2013;62:D100–8.

11. Strange G, Playford D, Stewart S, et al. Pulmonary hypertension: prevalence and mortality in the Armadale echocardiography cohort. Heart. 2012;98:1805–11.

12. Andersen KH, Iversen M, Kjaergaard J, et al. Prevalence, predictors, and survival in pulmonary hypertension related to end-stage chronic obstructive pulmonary disease. J Heart Lung Transplant. 2012;31:373–80.

13. Hayes D Jr, Black SM, Tobias JD, Kirkby S, Mansour HM, Whitson BA. Influence of pulmonary hypertension on patients with idiopathic pulmonary fibrosis awaiting lung transplantation. Ann Thorac Surg. 2016;101:246–52.

14. Hayes D Jr, Black SM, Tobias JD, Mansour HM, Whitson BA. Prevalence of pulmonary hypertension and its influence on survival in patients with advanced chronic obstructive pulmonary disease prior to lung transplantation. COPD. 2016;13:50–6.

15. Solidoro P, Patrucco F, Bonato R, et al. Pulmonary hypertension in chronic obstructive pulmonary disease and pulmonary fibrosis: prevalence and hemodynamic differences in lung transplant recipients at transplant center's referral time. Transplant Proc. 2015;47:2161–5.

16. Seeger W, Adir Y, Barbera JA, et al. Pulmonary hypertension in chronic lung diseases. J Am Coll Cardiol. 2013;62:D109–16.

17. Galiè N, Hoeper MM, Humbert M, et al. Guidelines for the diagnosis and treatment of pulmonary hypertension. Eur Respir J. 2009;34:1219–63.

18. Tunariu N, Gibbs SJ, Win Z, et al. Ventilation-perfusion scintigraphy is more sensitive than multidetector CTPA in detecting chronic thromboembolic pulmonary disease as a treatable cause of pulmonary hypertension: official publication. J Nucl Med. 2007;48:680–4.

19. Auger WR, Fedullo PF, Moser KM, Buchbinder M, Peterson KL. Chronic major-vessel thromboembolic pulmonary artery obstruction: appearance at angiography. Radiology. 1992;182:393–8.

20. Galie N, Corris PA, Frost A, et al. Updated treatment algorithm of pulmonary arterial hypertension. J Am Coll Cardiol. 2013;62:D60–72.

21. Galie N, Barbera JA, Frost AE, et al. Initial use of ambrisentan plus tadalafil in pulmonary arterial hypertension. N Engl J Med. 2015;373:834–44.

22. Sitbon O, Channick R, Chin KM, et al. Selexipag for the treatment of pulmonary arterial hypertension. N Engl J Med. 2015;373:2522–33.

23. Pulido T, Adzerikho I, Channick RN, et al. Macitentan and morbidity and mortality in pulmonary arterial hypertension. N Engl J Med. 2013;369:809–18.

24. Conte JV, Gaine SP, Orens JB, Harris T, Rubin LJ. The influence of continuous intravenous prostacyclin therapy for primary pulmonary hypertension on the timing and outcome of transplantation. J Heart Lung Transplant. 1998;17:679–85.

25. LeVarge BL, Channick RN. The changing paradigm in pulmonary hypertension trials: longer duration, new endpoints. Curr Opin Pulm Med. 2015;21:438–45.

26. Galie N, Manes A, Negro L, Palazzini M, Bacchi-Reggiani ML, Branzi A. A meta-analysis of randomized controlled trials in pulmonary arterial hypertension. Eur Heart J. 2009;30:394–403.

27. Benza RL, Miller DP, Barst RJ, Badesch DB, Frost AE, McGoon MD. An evaluation of long-term survival from time of diagnosis in pulmonary arterial hypertension from the REVEAL Registry. Chest. 2012;142:448–56.

28. Sandoval J, Gaspar J, Pulido T, et al. Graded balloon dilation atrial septostomy in severe primary pulmonary hypertension. A therapeutic alternative for patients nonresponsive to vasodilator treatment. J Am Coll Cardiol. 1998;32:297–304.

29. Doyle RL, McCrory D, Channick RN, Simonneau G, Conte J, American College of Chest Physicians. Surgical treatments/interventions for pulmonary arterial hypertension: ACCP evidence-based clinical practice guidelines. Chest. 2004;126:63S–71S.

30. Kothari SS, Yusuf A, Juneja R, Yadav R, Naik N. Graded balloon atrial septostomy in severe pulmonary hypertension. Indian Heart J. 2002;54:164–9.

31. Rosenzweig EB, Brodie D, Abrams DC, Agerstrand CL, Bacchetta M. Extracorporeal membrane oxygenation as a novel bridging strategy for acute right heart failure in group 1 pulmonary arterial hypertension. ASAIO J. 2014;60:129–33.

32. Mayes J, Niranjan G, Dark J, Clark S. Bridging to lung transplantation for severe pulmonary hypertension using dual central Novalung lung assist devicesdagger. Interact Cardiovasc Thorac Surg. 2016;22(5):677–8.

33. Patil NP, Mohite PN, Reed A, Popov AF, Simon AR. Modified technique using Novalung as bridge to transplant in pulmonary hypertension. Ann Thorac Surg. 2015;99:719–21.

34. Weill D, Benden C, Corris PA, et al. A consensus document for the selection of lung transplant candidates: 2014—an update from the Pulmonary Transplantation Council of the International Society for Heart and Lung Transplantation. J Heart Lung Transplant. 2015;34:1–15.

35. Toyoda Y, Thacker J, Santos R, et al. Long-term outcome of lung and heart-lung transplantation for idiopathic pulmonary arterial hypertension. Ann Thorac Surg. 2008;86:1116–22.

36. de Perrot M, Granton JT, McRae K, et al. Outcome of patients with pulmonary arterial hypertension referred for lung transplantation: a 14-year single-center experience. J Thorac Cardiovasc Surg. 2012;143:910–8.

37. Benza RL, Miller DP, Gomberg-Maitland M, et al. Predicting survival in pulmonary arterial hypertension: insights from the Registry to Evaluate Early and Long-Term Pulmonary Arterial Hypertension Disease Management (REVEAL). Circulation. 2010;122:164–72.

38. Humbert M, Sitbon O, Chaouat A, et al. Survival in patients with idiopathic, familial, and anorexigen-associated pulmonary arterial hypertension in the modern management era. Circulation. 2010;122: 156–63.

39. Miyamoto S, Nagaya N, Satoh T, et al. Clinical correlates and prognostic significance of six-minute walk test in patients with primary pulmonary hypertension. Comparison with cardiopulmonary exercise testing. Am J Respir Crit Care Med. 2000;161:487–92.

40. Mandel J, Mark EJ, Hales CA. Pulmonary veno-occlusive disease. Am J Respir Crit Care Med. 2000;162:1964–73.

41. Egan TM, Murray S, Bustami RT, et al. Development of the new lung allocation system in the United States. Am J Transplant. 2006;6:1212–27.

42. McCurry KR, Shearon TH, Edwards LB, et al. Lung transplantation in the United States, 1998-2007. Am J Transplant. 2009;9:942–58.

43. Chen H, Shiboski SC, Golden JA, et al. Impact of the lung allocation score on lung transplantation for pulmonary arterial hypertension. Am J Respir Crit Care Med. 2009;180:468–74.

44. Chan KM. Idiopathic pulmonary arterial hypertension and equity of donor lung allocation in the era of the lung allocation score: are we there yet? Am J Respir Crit Care Med. 2009;180:385–7.

45. Miller DP, Farber HW. "Who'll be the next in line?" The lung allocation score in patients with pulmonary arterial hypertension. J Heart Lung Transplant. 2013;32:1165–7.

46. Gomberg-Maitland M, Glassner-Kolmin C, Watson S, et al. Survival in pulmonary arterial hypertension patients awaiting lung transplantation. J Heart Lung Transplant. 2013;32:1179–86.

47. Schaffer JM, Singh SK, Joyce DL, et al. Transplantation for idiopathic pulmonary arterial hypertension: improvement in the lung allocation score era. Circulation. 2013;127:2503–13.

48. Benza RL, Miller DP, Frost A, Barst RJ, Krichman AM, McGoon MD. Analysis of the lung allocation score estimation of risk of death in patients with pulmonary arterial hypertension using data from the REVEAL Registry. Transplantation. 2010;90:298–305.

49. Changes to the lung allocation system. 2015. https://optn.transplant.hrsa.gov/news/changes-to-the-lung-allocation-system/.

50. Policies, policy 10: allocation of lungs. 2016. https://optn.transplant.hrsa.gov/media/1200/optn_policies.pdf-nameddest=Policy_10.

51. Submitting LAS exception requests for candidates diagnosed with PH. 2016. https://www.transplantpro.org/news/thoracic/submitting-las-exception-requests-for-candidates-diagnosed-with-ph-2/.

52. Bando K, Armitage JM, Paradis IL, et al. Indications for and results of single, bilateral, and heart-lung transplantation for pulmonary hypertension. J Thorac Cardiovasc Surg. 1994;108:1056–65.

53. Pasque MK, Trulock EP, Cooper JD, et al. Single lung transplantation for pulmonary hypertension. Single institution experience in 34 patients. Circulation. 1995;92(8):2252.

54. Gammie JS, Keenan RJ, Pham SM, et al. Single-versus double-lung transplantation for pulmonary hypertension. J Thorac Cardiovasc Surg. 1998;115:397–402; discussion 402–3.

55. Levine SM, Gibbons WJ, Bryan CL, et al. Single lung transplantation for primary pulmonary hypertension. Chest. 1990;98:1107–15.

56. Ritchie M, Waggoner AD, Davila-Roman VG, Barzilai B, Trulock EP, Eisenberg PR. Echocardiographic characterization of the improvement in right ventricular function in patients with severe pulmonary hypertension after single-lung transplantation. J Am Coll Cardiol. 1993;22(4):1170.

57. Conte JV, Borja MJ, Patel CB, Yang SC, Jhaveri RM, Orens JB. Lung transplantation for primary and secondary pulmonary hypertension. Ann Thorac Surg. 2001;72:1673–9; discussion 1673–80.

58. Boujoukos AJ, Martich GD, Vega JD, Keenan RJ, Griffith BP. Reperfusion injury in single-lung transplant recipients with pulmonary hypertension and emphysema. J Heart Lung Transplant. 1997;16:439–48.

59. Levine SM, Jenkinson SG, Bryan CL, et al. Ventilation-perfusion inequalities during graft rejection in patients undergoing single lung transplantation for primary pulmonary hypertension. Chest. 1992;101:401–5.

60. Yusen RD, Edwards LB, Kucheryavaya AY, et al. The Registry of the International Society for Heart and Lung Transplantation: Thirty-second Official Adult Lung and Heart-Lung Transplantation Report—2015; Focus Theme: Early Graft Failure (Supplementary Online Slides). J Heart Lung Transplant. 2015;34:1264–77.

61. Reitz BA, Wallwork JL, Hunt SA, et al. Heart-lung transplantation: successful therapy for patients with pulmonary vascular disease. N Engl J Med. 1982;306:557–64.

62. Chapelier A, Vouhe P, Macchiarini P, et al. Comparative outcome of heart-lung and lung transplantation for pulmonary hypertension. J Thorac Cardiovasc Surg. 1993;106:299–307.

63. Ueno T, Smith JA, Snell GI, et al. Bilateral sequential single lung transplantation for pulmonary hypertension and Eisenmenger's syndrome. Ann Thorac Surg. 2000;69:381–7.

64. Olland A, Falcoz PE, Canuet M, Massard G. Should we perform bilateral-lung or heart-lung transplantation for patients with pulmonary hypertension? Interact Cardiovasc Thorac Surg. 2013;17:166–70.

65. Fadel E, Mercier O, Mussot S, et al. Long-term outcome of double-lung and heart-lung transplantation for pulmonary hypertension: a comparative retrospective study of 219 patients. Eur J Cardiothorac Surg. 2010;38:277–84.

66. Pielsticker EJ, Martinez FJ, Rubenfire M. Lung and heart-lung transplant practice patterns in pulmo-

nary hypertension centers. J Heart Lung Transplant. 2001;20:1297–304.

67. Pereszlenyi A, Lang G, Steltzer H, et al. Bilateral lung transplantation with intra- and postoperatively prolonged ECMO support in patients with pulmonary hypertension. Eur J Cardiothorac Surg. 2002;21:858–63.

68. Tudorache I, Sommer W, Kuhn C, et al. Lung transplantation for severe pulmonary hypertension—awake extracorporeal membrane oxygenation for postoperative left ventricular remodelling. Transplantation. 2015;99:451–8.

69. Krishnamurthy Y, Cooper LB, Lu D, et al. Trends and outcomes of patients with adult congenital heart disease and pulmonary hypertension listed for orthotopic heart transplantation in the United States. J Heart Lung Transplant. 2016;35(5):619–24.

70. Choong CK, Sweet SC, Guthrie TJ, et al. Repair of congenital heart lesions combined with lung transplantation for the treatment of severe pulmonary hypertension: a 13-year experience. J Thorac Cardiovasc Surg. 2005;129:661–9.

71. Butler J, Stankewicz MA, Wu J, et al. Pre-transplant reversible pulmonary hypertension predicts higher risk for mortality after cardiac transplantation. J Heart Lung Transplant. 2005;24:170–7.

72. Kirklin JK, Naftel DC, Kirklin JW, Blackstone EH, White-Williams C, Bourge RC. Pulmonary vascular resistance and the risk of heart transplantation. J Heart Transplant. 1988;7:331–6.

73. Vakil K, Duval S, Sharma A, et al. Impact of pre-transplant pulmonary hypertension on survival after heart transplantation: a UNOS registry analysis. Int J Cardiol. 2014;176:595–9.

74. Hayes D Jr, Tumin D, Daniels CJ, et al. Pulmonary artery pressure and benefit of lung transplantation in adult cystic fibrosis patients. Ann Thorac Surg. 2016;101:1104–9.

75. Huerd SS, Hodges TN, Grover FL, et al. Secondary pulmonary hypertension does not adversely affect outcome after single lung transplantation. J Thorac Cardiovasc Surg. 2000;119:458–65.

76. Julliard WA, Meyer KC, De Oliveira NC, et al. The presence or severity of pulmonary hypertension does not affect outcomes for single-lung transplantation. Thorax. 2016;71(5):478–80.

77. Condliffe R, Kiely DG, Gibbs JS, et al. Improved outcomes in medically and surgically treated chronic thromboembolic pulmonary hypertension. Am J Respir Crit Care Med. 2008;177:1122–7.

78. D'Armini AM, Cattadori B, Monterosso C, Emmi V, Piovella F, Vigano M. Surgical therapy for chronic thromboembolic pulmonary hypertension: criteria for choosing lung transplant vs thromboendarterectomy. J Heart Lung Transplant. 2001;20:218.

79. Ghofrani HA, D'Armini AM, Grimminger F, et al. Riociguat for the treatment of chronic thromboembolic pulmonary hypertension. N Engl J Med. 2013;369:319–29.

80. Mizoguchi H, Ogawa A, Munemasa M, Mikouchi H, Ito H, Matsubara H. Refined balloon pulmonary angioplasty for inoperable patients with chronic thromboembolic pulmonary hypertension. Circ Cardiovasc Interv. 2012;5:748–55.

81. Massad MG, Powell CR, Kpodonu J, et al. Outcomes of lung transplantation in patients with scleroderma. World J Surg. 2005;29:1510–5.

82. Zhao YD, Peng J, Granton E, et al. Pulmonary vascular changes 22 years after single lung transplantation for pulmonary arterial hypertension: a case report with molecular and pathological analysis. Pulm Circulation. 2015;5:739–43.

83. Soriano CM, Gaine SP, Conte JV, Fairman RP, White C, Rubin LJ. Anastomotic pulmonary hypertension after lung transplantation for primary pulmonary hypertension: report of surgical correction. Chest. 1999;116:564–6.

84. Izbicki G, Shitrit D, Schechtman I, et al. Recurrence of pulmonary veno-occlusive disease after heart-lung transplantation. J Heart Lung Transplant. 2005;24:635–7.

85. Lee C, Suh RD, Krishnam MS, et al. Recurrent pulmonary capillary hemangiomatosis after bilateral lung transplantation. J Thorac Imaging. 2010;25:W89–92.

Psychosocial Evaluation of the Patient Considered for Lung Transplant

6

Thomas M. Soeprono and Ganesh Raghu

Introduction

Lung transplantation can be a very difficult process from many aspects: physically, psychologically, and socially. Although the potential benefits of lung transplantation are significant, there are immense risks that cannot be ignored such as increased pain and suffering, infection, organ rejection, frequent visits and procedures to monitor the status of lung disease, disability, and death. The psychosocial evaluation is an essential component of the lung pre-transplant process and can serve to highlight the potential hazards that may not be illuminated in a medical evaluation. The interview involves appraising a patient's adherence history, care support plan, psychiatric stability, and substance use history (including alcohol and tobacco). Ultimately, there are two primary goals for which we use the information obtained in the assessment: to protect and to advocate for the patient.

When patients are not approved for transplant listing, both patients and the treatment team can think of this as a failure, which can be very demoralizing. An alternative view is that the team is protecting a patient that is not an appropriate candidate for transplant. Lung transplantation, although the only lifesaving measure for many conditions, can cause severe suffering and harm for patients who are not suited for this difficult process. It is the duty of medical practitioners to ensure that they first "do no harm." The psychosocial evaluation enables practitioners to have a better understanding of which patients have the constellation of factors that constitute an appropriate transplant candidate.

Advocacy can take many forms and play a role at various points of treatment, from selection to engagement in the process to care after transplant. It is well established that patients with low socioeconomic status (SES) have poor access to healthcare and are at increased risk for mental illness [1, 2]. Additionally, patients with mental illness tend to receive substandard care [3]. This overlap of low SES, poor access to care, and mental illness could lead the patient to being disregarded in consideration for lung transplant. Appropriate advocacy is necessary to ensure that equivalent care is offered to all individuals in spite of biases. When this cohort of underserved

T. M. Soeprono (✉)
Department of Psychiatry, University of Washington, Seattle, WA, USA
e-mail: thomasms@uw.edu

G. Raghu
Division of Pulmonary, Critical Care, and Sleep Medicine, Department of Medicine University of Washington, Seattle, WA, USA

Center for Interstitial Lung Disease, ILD, Sarcoid and Pulmonary Fibrosis Program, University of Washington Medicine, Seattle, WA, USA

Scleroderma Clinic, University of Washington Medicine, Seattle, WA, USA
e-mail: graghu@uw.edu

© The Author(s) 2018
G. Raghu, R. G. Carbone (eds.), *Lung Transplantation*, https://doi.org/10.1007/978-3-319-91184-7_6

patients does receive care, they are often ill equipped to deal with the stresses and culture of the medical system. This can result in poor outcomes that could have been avoided with appropriate psychosocial treatment. Therefore, advocacy must play a role in the daily process and not just to ensure that patients with chronic mental illness make it onto the transplant list.

The psychosocial evaluation exists to obtain the information necessary to carry out the goals of advocacy and avoid harm. Throughout this chapter, we will discuss the numerous factors that play a role in helping practitioners both advocate for patients and protect them from the potential harms of transplant. This will cover a diverse set of dynamic aspects from a patient's coping style and medical literacy to a patient's history of adherence and substance use. Ultimately, the understanding demonstrated is that medical outcomes improve when psychosocial needs are addressed [4].

Understanding the Patient as a Person

Lung transplantation, although now considered a viable and feasible treatment option for patients with lung diseases in whom all other available treatment interventions have failed, is an intensive treatment that is not without risks and anticipated complications, which are better addressed with detailed and specific knowledge of the patient. Understanding each patient more thoroughly—that is, looking beyond his/her medical illness and at his/her behaviors, coping skills, and social structure—allows providers to be better equipped to anticipate potential difficulties the patient may encounter and can inform the manner in which patients may interact with providers, follow medical advice, and take medications. This is especially important in lung transplantation where patients endure post-lung transplantation complications that require frequent follow-up visits, diagnostic interventions, and close monitoring to promptly identify rejections and infections that require invasive procedures such as ad hoc bronchoscopy, therapeutic interventions, and

associated stresses besides routine postoperative pain during the recovery process and convalescent period.

There are clear behavioral patterns within the individual's life that can give practitioners an insight into their patient's future behaviors. For example, a patient who consistently has had difficulty taking medications will likely continue in this pattern in the posttransplant period. Or a patient's participation in pulmonary rehabilitation helps practitioners anticipate a patient's tenacity and involvement in the recovery process.

While past behavior is the best predictor of future behavior, this is not to say that individuals cannot modify behavior. However, behavior change is an ongoing process that requires insight, conscious effort with clear motivation, and supportive environmental factors [5]. Furthermore, without maintenance, it is easy to return to old habits. Patterns must be recognized and practiced in a different manner before one can assume that the behavior has changed.

Each individual has a unique approach to managing stress and adversity. A further challenge in the rehabilitation process is that patients are often unaware of their coping strategies and that the recovery often takes place in the hospital where patients are isolated from their familiar environment, resources, and supports. By exploring the patient's past, one can uncover difficult times that were overcome with the use of specific strategies and become aware of more adaptive skills and styles that may play or may need to be encouraged in the process of transplantation. On the other hand, evidence and history of inflexible or maladaptive coping skills can guide practitioners in helping patients build resilience and more adaptive strategies that may be employed in the hospital before the transplant process begins. Family and friends can also be encouraged to support and help develop a patient's coping style both before and during the transplantation process.

By understanding a patient's established life routine, a practitioner will be better equipped to anticipate and recommend medical treatment that will be successful. Eliciting information around a typical day—organization/layout, diet, work, and leisure activities, social aspects—sheds light on central components of a person's life. These are all potential avenues for treatment and support as well as potential pitfalls that lead to poor adherence, medical complications, stress, and instability. For example, a military veteran who prides himself on being meticulous and timely throughout his professional and private life is likely to be a very medication-compliant individual. On the other hand, he may have difficulty with the frequent changes in scheduling and having to wait for delayed procedures in the hospital, which could lead to him experiencing anxiety and frustration. A thorough consideration of a patient's thought processes and behaviors is valuable information that supports the process of empathy and effective treatment planning in preparation for lung transplantation.

It is imperative that the patient is fully informed of the foreseen and unforeseen complications and expectations. It is also important that the patient understands the possible consequences of such situations. It is often misunderstood that the mere listing for lung transplantation does not guarantee that the suitable lung will become available during the "waiting" time. As a result, patients benefit from being prepared to cope with continued suffering and endurance of dyspnea, cough, and supplemental oxygen use. At the same time, there is an expectation that patients remain ambulatory despite their disability, maintain their emotional status, and not lose hope. In a disease such as idiopathic pulmonary fibrosis, a relentlessly progressive and fatal disease, every month can be worse than the preceding month, and patients might reach a stage when they cannot get out of bed, become bedridden, and may need to be taken off of the list. If they become too weak and debilitated while waiting for a lung transplant, a transition to palliative and comfort care may be required. Such stressors can understandably be severe and very trying to some patients and caregivers. Because of these high stakes in difficult situations, patients need a tremendous amount of coping skills to manage the overwhelming emotions throughout this process.

Social System

Understanding a patient's social system—care plan, social/family history, finances (including insurance coverage), legal issues—is the expertise of the lung transplant social worker. Social workers play a necessary role throughout the evaluation process by working with patients to optimize these realms of the social system in preparation for transplant.

A patient's care support system is an important indicator of a patient's potential for the success in transplant [6]. Thus, it is necessary to ensure that the patient has adequate support before the transplant process begins. Prior to being approved for listing as an organ recipient, each candidate must provide a care plan that outlines how s/he will receive care throughout the transplant process. The care plan must address issues of transportation, emotional support, postoperative care outside the hospital, and important medical legal documents such as signifying a durable power of attorney (DPOA) in case the patient loses his/her capacity to make medical decisions in the transplant process. An important aspect of creating a care plan is that it allows for patients to get explicit commitments from friends and family. The patient, designated caregivers, and support system must be proactive in working with the social worker to facilitate and accomplish these tasks.

The social support can come in various forms: a dedicated spouse, family members, or a team of friends. The most important aspects are dedication, resilience in the relationship, and appropriate expectations of what will and will not be provided. There are instances in which patients have employed help to assist them through this process. Anecdotally, this type of support system has been found to be less consistent and resilient. Furthermore, financial stressors do not incentivize the continuation of this support after the mandatory period despite often needing ongoing assistance. For these reasons, it is strongly recommended that patients coordinate a solid care plan of invested family and friends.

A patient's family and social history can give practitioners an insight into the patient's social situation, medical literacy, and overall education about the transplant process. Although medical literacy is not pervasive and equivalent within a family, an investigation may highlight potential liaisons within the family who may work as point persons for the medical team or family. This can be especially useful in a patient who has poor health literacy or permanent cognitive deficits. One example would be a patient who is illiterate and English is his non-primary language but has a brother who is a bilingual physical therapist and willing play a major role in the patient's care. Lastly, understanding family dynamics can highlight coping styles, interaction styles, and unique strengths that a particular family might have as noted above in "Understanding the Patient as a Person." It is helpful to enlist the support and motivation of a patient's entire family whenever possible. Understanding how they relate, work through difficulties, and the organization can better equip practitioners to provide patients with support and create individualized care plans for success.

Patients need to be able to come to get to the lung transplant center within 2–3 hours when a suitable lung becomes available. In some situations, patients and caregivers are required to relocate closer to lung transplant centers during the pre- and post-lung transplant period. This can cause additional stress and associated costs. It is not uncommon for patients to be called in for transplant only to find that at the time of harvesting from the donor, the lungs are not suitable for transplant. Preparing a patient for this possibility is imperative. On the other hand, these "practice runs" can be informative and helpful to many candidates in better preparing for the next call. Most lung transplant programs require patients to receive all primary care needs at the lung transplant center for a minimum of 6 months post-lung transplant. During this time, frequent monitoring and surveillance assures satisfactory recovery from lung transplantation and preservation of the lung allograft.

Transplantation has clear financial costs associated with it. The surgery itself has both obvious and unanticipated costs. The most apparent is the limitation on the patient's ability to participate in his/her work both before and after the transplant. Certain types of jobs are not ideal for patients who have undergone transplantation. Jobs that do not allow for appropriate breaks to take medication or that require overly physically demanding work involving heavy lifting may not be ideal. Transplantation may affect one's medical insurance and cost thereof. There are also hidden financial components such as transportation and room and board for friends, family, and the patient while away from home. These factors play a role in helping patients make educated decisions about their course of treatment. Although practitioners try to keep finances from becoming a primary focus in care, it is necessary to address these concerns formally and proactively through the financial services at the transplant center as they can significantly influence the patient's stress level and decision to pursue transplantation.

Legal issues can play a role in a patient's candidacy for transplantation. Immigration status can derail patient's progress through the transplantation process. Current incarceration and the terms of the sentence can also dictate access to care in regard to transplantation. A patient's requirement to be present for court proceedings may influence his or her ability to fully participate in transplantation. Legal issues are not an absolute contraindication to transplantation but rather should be thought of as another psychosocial issue that can lead to increased stress and would best be addressed prior to transplant. Each patient must be addressed on a case-by-case basis due to the inconsistent regional rules that all involved parties have. Inquiring about a patient's legal standing and history is the first step in this process.

Cognitive Status

Cognitive function is a standard component of a medical evaluation. But this realm is also an important part of the psychosocial evaluation due to the additional social supports that must be in place to compensate for any impairment. Patients with rapidly degenerative neurologic diseases are precluded from transplantation because of the scarcity of available organs and the presumed poor prognosis of the patient. Therefore, it is important to ensure that the patient is cognitively stable through testing and interview. Patients who have chronic cognitive impairments or developmental delay, as is the case in a patient with Down syndrome or traumatic brain injury, can successfully transplant as long as there is a clear support system that will enable him/her to adhere to treatment and follow medical recommendations.

At times, cognitive function can impair a patient's ability to make informed medical decisions. Decision-making capacity is no different in transplantation than it is in other medical incidences. In the case in which a patient is unable to make a decision based on an acute etiology such as delirium, non-urgent decisions and procedures should be delayed until the patient's capacity has returned. In urgent cases or acute cases that will not resolve until treatment is rendered, the patient's medical power of attorney becomes the primary decision-maker who attempts to execute what the patient would have wanted. This is another case that demonstrates that establishing a DPOA for each patient as soon as possible is essential. Often times, social work and/or psychiatric services can aid in this complicated and challenging process in order to ensure that the desires of the patient are being met.

Psychiatric Evaluation

Every patient within the pre-transplant lung evaluation process should have psychiatric screening to guarantee that patients who require further evaluation have access to it. Most often, the social work evaluation can screen for possible psychiatric illness that may warrant further evaluation. This can also be done with the use of a questionnaire, which asks about prior psychiatric diagnoses, psychiatric medications, or substance use. Additionally, this screening can take the form of a PHQ-9 and GAD-7, which screen for symptoms associated with depression and anxiety, respectively. Lastly, the medical team, which includes the transplant surgeons, pulmonologists,

anesthesiologists, and others, can and should at any point refer a patient to psychiatry if there are concerns.

Assessment of psychiatric disease should be treated like the assessment of other systems and can be explained as such. In the same way that optimization of cardiac and renal function is ideal in preparation for transplantation in order to improve outcomes and recovery, the optimization of brain function and mental well-being serves an equivalent role in the preparation for transplantation. The transplant process is a severe stressor. Psychiatric illness is precipitated in the environment of stress. Therefore, it stands to reason and has been demonstrated in the literature that there are increased rates of psychiatric illness in the transplantation process [7]. Furthermore, patients with untreated psychiatric illness have increased risk of poor outcomes [8]. It is the goal of the psychiatric evaluation not only to assess for possible psychiatric diagnoses that may hinder a patient's success in transplant but also to treat such processes and enable the patient to become a better transplant candidate. Complicating the picture, psychiatric disorders can be precipitated and/or exaggerated by the use of corticosteroids that are a necessary treatment regimen to prevent rejection.

Primary psychiatric illnesses are categorized into three large groups: mood disorders, anxiety disorders, and psychotic disorders. While there are numerous diagnoses that do not necessarily fit into these major categories, a majority will, and this can provide a good starting point in the evaluation.

Mood disorders and specifically depression are prone to exacerbations under the stress of respiratory illness. The neurovegetative signs of depression (sleep, energy, appetite, concentration, psychomotor) are common symptoms for patients with respiratory illness who do not have depression. Therefore, the psychological symptoms of depression (feeling depressed, anhedonia, guilt, suicidality) are often better indicators of depression in this specific population. Depression is a very treatable illness that should not limit the patient's ability to undergo transplantation in the long term. On the other hand, patients who have active depression should be adequately treated before a transplant takes place. This is because the risks associated with depression—such as poor adherence and suicidal ideation—can put the patient and graft at significant risk of harm and death.

Bipolar disorder, which is characterized by manic episodes, is a fairly rare disease, but, because of the common problems of poor adherence in this population, special screening should take place to ensure that these patients are stable. A patient with bipolar disorder who is well treated and has a history of good adherence can be an appropriate candidate for lung transplant. The common use of steroids in lung disease and transplant is often a concern in patients with bipolar disorder for fear of inducing mania. Although not intuitive, patients with bipolar disorder have no more increased risk of mania under the influence of steroids than the general population [9]. On the other hand, it is important to remember that steroids can also precipitate depressive episodes, especially in patients with a past history of depression.

Anxiety disorders are the most common primary psychiatric disorders in patients with chronic lung disease. There is a clear physiologic explanation for this. A human's natural response to the experience of suffocation and/or drowning is fear and anxiety in order to alert the individual to the risk that he/she is in. The brain tends to generalize these experiences and misinterpret physical symptoms, which results in a cascade of anxious feelings regardless of the stimulus. For example, once a panic attack has occurred, patients will often do everything they can to avoid that experience. As a result, they become hypervigilant and fearful, which may further precipitate anxious feelings. Once this anxiety cycle has begun, it can require extensive treatment, including medication management, cognitive behavioral strategies, or exposure therapy. It is important to validate the medical etiology of these events as well as educate the patient and treat the psychiatric sequelae. It is presumed that the resolution of respiratory function will resolve these anxiety episodes. This is occasionally true, but often times anxiety continues to challenge

patients in the postoperative period while in recovery. For this reason, it is encouraged to aggressively treat anxiety when present in a patient with respiratory failure despite the fact that ultimately not all of the anxiety symptoms will be resolved as long as there is ongoing lung disease progression.

Psychotic disorders are often considered an absolute contraindication to lung transplant. This is most often the case, but there are rare circumstances in which a patient with schizophrenia has demonstrated adequate psychological, social, and environmental stability to warrant transplant. Although the positive symptoms of psychosis (auditory/visual hallucinations, paranoia) are most obvious, it is the negative symptoms (poverty of speech/thought; apathy; loss of motivation; inattention; reduced social drive) that limit a patient's ability to complete transplant. It is important to evaluate each patient on a case-by-case basis when dealing with psychiatric illness given the wide diversity of presentations of the illness and environmental factors that play a role in the diagnosis and treatment of these disorders.

Personality disorders, more specifically cluster B personality disorders (antisocial, borderline, narcissistic, histrionic), are also considered absolute contraindications at many transplant centers because patients with these disorders often have severe nonadherence, difficulty following medical instructions, and poor relationships and interactions with providers and support systems [10]. Other personality disorders within the A and C clusters are not considered contraindications in many instances. Providers are encouraged to consider the functional aspects of these patients rather than focusing on specifically what personality disorder is present. This can best be accomplished by focusing on the patient's coping style and social makeup.

All of the above psychiatric disorders carry with them increased risk of suicide. A recent suicide attempt is a contraindication to transplantation. This is because, as discussed above, past behavior predicts future behavior; thus, the greatest risk factor for suicide is a previous suicide attempt [11]. This does not mean that a patient who had a historical suicide attempt can never receive a lung transplant. Rather, he/she must demonstrate a clear and significant change in the environment and mind-set that led to the previous attempt. Patients who have had repeated incidents of suicide attempts should be excluded from transplant candidacy.

Substance use is a common issue in patients being evaluated for lung transplant. It goes without saying that patients who are currently smoking are not appropriate candidates. But a substance use evaluation extends far beyond this superficial aspect to ensure there are no risk-taking behaviors or substance use that puts the patient or graft at risk due to nonadherence or direct effects of the substance on the lungs. Almost universally, transplant programs have a policy of 6 months of sobriety required prior to approval to be on the organ wait list. There is significant data to suggest that patients who are able to obtain 6 months of sobriety have a diminished risk of relapse [12]. That being said, there is a linear relationship between time from last use and risk of relapse with no specific threshold at the 6-month mark. Sobriety is an incredibly important qualification for transplantation given the extreme risks associated with substance use in the posttransplant period including, but not limited to, infections, rejection, poor adherence, unstable finances, unstable housing, poor social support, and impaired judgment [13]. Patients who have a prior history of substance use may still require chemical dependency evaluation and treatment despite months or years of sobriety depending on the situation. It is important to confirm that patients have developed appropriate alternative coping strategies and social networks to ensure that the stress of transplantation does not provoke a relapse.

A thorough evaluation of a patient's social circles and behaviors that may be associated with past substance use is required. Environmental factors often play the largest role in the relapse process. It is important that patients with substance use disorders find new ways to spend their time, new people to spend their time with, and new places in which to spend their time.

Medical providers can support patients with substance use disorders in maintaining their sobriety by appropriately treating pain, providing monitoring through the use of toxicology screening, providing therapeutic medications that curb cravings and withdrawal symptoms, and counseling that can support motivation to change. Substance use is a treatable illness that necessitates a thorough evaluation and understanding of the patient.

Trauma and abuse can take many forms in the patient's life. These experiences can continue to influence the patient's behavior years later and contribute to the formation of particular coping styles. Post-traumatic stress disorder (PTSD) is the most obvious example of this. Trauma can affect transplantation especially in the setting of the ICU. Because nearly every lung transplant patient goes to the ICU in the postoperative period, it is important that providers understand sensitivities the patient may have. Many patients have experienced re-traumatization as a result of intubation, soft restraints, and other invasive procedures within the ICU [14]. With the knowledge of patient's past trauma, special accommodations and sensitivities can be made to minimize the risk of harm in these patients. Additionally, trauma can drive the formation of maladaptive and immature coping strategies. This can result in unintended interactions with patients that are not therapeutic. Lastly, trauma tends to lead to avoidance behavior. This could lead to poor adherence or other behaviors not conducive to transplantation. Patients should be evaluated for trauma to help practitioners avoid triggers and appropriately support the patient throughout the lung transplant process.

Conclusion

The process involved in a lung transplant is extremely involved and challenging from a physical, psychological, and social perspective. Although this treatment can be lifesaving, it also comes with severe risks that not every patient and his/her caregivers can cope with and/or are prepared to manage. The lung transplantation program and team which include dedicated social workers, psychologists, psychiatrists, primary care providers, and pulmonologists must be prudent to appropriately screen and understand the patients as "individual people." A fully informed patient who understands all the foreseen and unforeseen circumstances associated with the lung transplantation process can be better prepared and is more likely to have a successful outcome. In the case of patients who are not appropriate candidates for transplantation, it is benevolent to protect them from the harm that the transplant process could inflict. But in patients who are appropriate lung transplant candidates, it is prudent for the clinician to advocate and support them through this very difficult process. Advocating and supporting patients are best done with a thorough psychosocial understanding of the patient that involves a discussion about medical adherence, the care support plan, psychiatric stability, and substance use. When done appropriately, these interventions can improve outcomes, prolong life, and lead to a higher quality of life.

References

1. Osborn R, Squires D, Doty M, Sarnak D, Schneider E. In new survey of eleven countries, US adults still struggle with access to and affordability of health care. Health Aff. 2016;35(12):2327–36.
2. Cook B, McGuire T, Miranda J. Measuring trends in mental health care disparities, 2000-2004. Psychiatr Serv. 2007;58(12):1533–40.
3. Thornicroft G, Rose D, Mehta N. Discrimination against people with mental illness: what can psychiatrists do? Adv Psychiatr Treat. 2010;16(1):53–9.
4. Jowsey S, Talor M, Schneekloth T, Clark M. Psychosocial challenges in transplantation. J Psychiatr Pract. 2001;7(6):404–14.
5. Chung T, Noronha A, Carroll K, Potenza M, et al. Brain mechanisms of change in addictions treatment: models, methods, and emerging findings. Curr Addict Rep. 2016;3(3):332–42.
6. Rainer J, Thompson C, Lambros H. Psychological and psychosocial aspects of the solid organ transplant experience—a practice review. Psychotherapy. 2010;47(3):403–12.
7. Dew M, DiMartini A. Psychological disorders and distress after adult cardiothoracic transplantation. J Cardiovasc Nurs. 2005;20(5):S51–66.
8. Ågren S, Sjoberg T, Ekmehag B, Wiborg M, Ivarsson B. Psychosocial aspects before and up to 2 years after heart or lung transplantation: experience of patients and their next of kin. Clin Transplant. 2017;31(3). https://doi.org/10.1111/ctr.12905.
9. Cerullo M. Corticosteroid-induced mania: prepare for the unpredictable. Curr Psychiatry. 2006;5(6):43–50.
10. Yates W, LaBrecque D, Pfab D. Personality disorders as a contraindication for liver transplantation in alcoholic cirrhosis. Psychosomatics. 1998;39(6):501–11.
11. Turecki G, Brent D. Suicide and suicide behavior. Lancet. 2016;387(10024):1227–39.
12. Yates W, Martin M, LaBrecque D, et al. A model to examine the validity of the 6-month abstinence criterion for liver transplantation. Alcohol Clin Exp Res. 1998;22:513–7.
13. Newton S. Recidivism and return to work posttransplant: recipients with substance abuse histories. J Subst Abuse Treat. 1999;17:103–8.
14. Bienvenu O, Gerstenblith T. Posttraumatic stress disorder phenomena after critical illness. Crit Care Clin. 2017;33(3):649–58.

Prognostic Markers and the LAS for Lung Transplantation: Impact of New Revisions for Successful Outcome

M. Patricia George and Matthew R. Pipeling

Introduction

Since the first long-term successful lung transplant in 1983 by Joel Cooper and colleagues [1], the field has evolved and progressed, increasing numbers of patients successfully transplanted and steadily improving outcomes over the years. The growth and improving success in the field stem primarily from technical advancements and medical discoveries; however, one of the interventions that has made one of the most significant impacts on lung transplantation has been the development and adoption of the lung allocation score (LAS). Implemented in 2005, the LAS, a system utilizing prognostic variables in an urgency-based system of organ allocation, instantly changed the prognosis and outlook for many patients with end-stage lung disease, and it continues to evolve today. In this chapter, we will discuss the history of the LAS, its immediate effects on lung transplant outcomes, and how it has shifted the epidemiology of lung transplantation. We will also review the evolution of the LAS and impact of newer prognostic markers recently added to the

LAS. Finally, we will discuss additional prognostic markers of interest and the future of lung allocation.

History of the LAS in Lung Transplantation

To understand the impact of the LAS, one must have an understanding of the history of organ allocation in lung transplantation and the mechanism of how organs are allocated today. When lung transplantation began, organs were initially assigned to patients based on time on the waiting list. The initial Organ Procurement and Transplantation Network (OPTN) issued a 1990 policy that allocated donor lungs based on ABO match and waitlist time. Offers would be made geographically in a donor-centric manner based from the organ procurement organization (OPO) within sequential 300-mile circumferential radii, with the goal of minimizing ischemic time to cadaveric donor lungs [2]. This system was largely unchanged until 1995, when it was decided that 90 days of waiting time would be credited to patients with a diagnosis of idiopathic pulmonary fibrosis (IPF), due to the high rate of mortality on the waiting list.

The effects of this initial first-come, first-served organ allocation policy over the years were that as more patients were listed for lung transplantation, the median time to transplant increased over time. Since patients were awarded donor lungs on the basis of time accrued and since the median waitlist time was more than 2 years, physicians often listed

M. Patricia George (✉)
Department of Medicine, National Jewish Health, Denver, CO, USA
e-mail: georgem@njhealth.org

M. R. Pipeling
Division of Pulmonary, Allergy and Critical Care Medicine, University of Pittsburgh School of Medicine, Pittsburgh, PA, USA
e-mail: pipelingm@upmc.edu

© The Author(s) 2018
G. Raghu, R. G. Carbone (eds.), *Lung Transplantation*, https://doi.org/10.1007/978-3-319-91184-7_7

some patients at the time of diagnosis, well before they were sick enough to require transplant, so that they could accrue time on the waiting list. In other instances, patients who were unlikely to live past 1 year and in whom lung transplant was the only lifesaving option were often not even considered or listed for lung transplant.

In 1998, the Department of Health and Human Services issued the Final Rule, establishing a goal to bring about "allocation policies that make the most effective use of organs, especially by making them available whenever feasible to the most medically urgent patients who are appropriate candidates for transplantation" [3]. Although the Final Rule did not single out lung transplantation, and the follow-up Institute of Medicine Report focused mainly on issues liver transplantation, the OPTN Thoracic Organ Transplantation Committee took action to evaluate and restructure the method of allocating lungs from a time-based system to an urgency-based system through the implementation of a predictive score method (Box 7.1) [2].

234-2005-37011C. The content is the responsibility of the authors alone and does not necessarily reflect the view or policies of the Department of Health and Human Services, nor does mention of trade names, commercial products, or organizations imply endorsement by the US Government.

The OPTN Lung Allocation Subcommittee first divided the main diagnoses into four major groups (Box 7.2) based on the four main indications for lung transplantation: chronic obstructive pulmonary disease, pulmonary arterial hypertension, idiopathic pulmonary fibrosis, and cystic fibrosis. These four diagnoses made up 80% of the indications for transplant. They then created a disease-specific model that examined prognostic factors that predict mortality within 1 year as well as the probability of surviving for the first year after transplant (Table 7.1) [2]. The committee purposefully used the most quantitative variables available in the OPTN database to keep these risk calculations as quantitative as possible. After grouping the remaining 20% diagnostic indications into the four main groups, mostly based on comparable pre- and posttransplant survival, they developed the LAS [2]. However, despite the precision of the calculations using the defined parameter estimates to generate an individual's LAS, it is difficult to generalize a relative "weight" or ranking of any one parameter's impact on an individual's total LAS. One reason for this is the differential use of certain parameters depending on which one of the four major diagnosis groups the patient's disease belongs. For example, a 50% increase in bilirubin or central venous pressure greater than 7 mmHg is only a relevant physiologic parameter in the setting of group B disease. Likewise, the use of the forced vital capacity as a variable depends upon a group D diagnosis as well as also being conditionally dependent on having a forced vital capacity less than 80% predicted. In addition, there are parameters (e.g., 6-min walk test, age, resting oxygen requirement) that are utilized in both the waiting list survival model and the posttransplant survival model.

Box 7.1 Variables Included in Calculation of LAS

- Age
- Assisted ventilation requirement
- Bilirubin (total) and change in bilirubin
- Body mass index
- Cardiac index
- Central venous pressure
- Creatinine and change in creatinine
- Diabetes
- Diagnosis
- Forced vital capacity
- Functional status
- Oxygen requirement at rest
- $PaCO_2$ and change in $PaCO_2$
- Pulmonary artery pressure
- 6-min walk test distance

Data used with permission from Organ Procurement and Transplantation Network (OPTN). Policy 10.1.E. https://optn.transplant. hrsa.gov/media/1200/optn_policies.pdf. This work was supported in part by Health Resources and Services Administration contract

Box 7.2 Transplant Groupings

Group A (obstructive lung disease)

Chronic obstructive pulmonary disease (COPD)/emphysema

Alpha-1-antitrypsin deficiency (A1ATD)

Allergic bronchopulmonary aspergillosis (ABPA)

Bronchopulmonary dysplasia

Constrictive bronchiolitis

Granulomatous lung disease

Kartagener's syndrome

Obstructive lung disease

Primary ciliary dyskinesia

Tuberous sclerosis

Wegener's granulomatosis-bronchiectasis

Ehlers-Danlos syndrome

Inhalation burns/trauma

Sarcoidosis with mean pulmonary artery (PA) pressure ≤30 mmHg

Bronchiectasis

Lymphangioleiomyomatosis (LAM)

Group B (pulmonary vascular disease)

Primary pulmonary hypertension (PPH)

Congenital malformation

Portopulmonary hypertension

Pulmonary thromboembolic disease

Pulmonary venoocclusive disease

Pulmonic stenosis

Right hypoplastic lung

Thromboembolic pulmonary hypertension

CREST-pulmonary hypertension

Pulmonary telangiectasia-pulmonary hypertension

Scleroderma pulmonary hypertension

Eisenmenger's syndrome

Pulmonary vascular disease

Secondary pulmonary hypertension

Group C (cystic fibrosis or immunodeficiency disorders)

Cystic fibrosis (CF)

Common variable immune deficiency (CVID)

Fibrocavitary lung disease

Hypogammaglobulinemia

Shwachman-Diamond syndrome

Group D (restrictive lung disease)

Idiopathic pulmonary fibrosis (IPF)

Wegener's granuloma-restrictive

CREST-restrictive

Pulmonary telangiectasia-restrictive

ANCA positive vasculitis

Scleroderma-restrictive

Alveolar proteinosis

Amyloidosis

Acute respiratory distress syndrome (ARDS)/pneumonia

Bronchiolitis obliterans and organizing pneumonia (BOOP)

Bronchioloalveolar carcinoma (BAC)

Carcinoid tumorlets

Chronic pneumonitis of infancy

Eosinophilic granuloma (EG)

Fibrosing mediastinitis

Graft-vs-host disease (GVHD)

Hermansky-Pudlak syndrome

Hypersensitivity pneumonitis

Idiopathic pulmonary hemosiderosis

Lymphocytic interstitial pneumonia (LIP)

Lupus

Mixed connective tissue disease

Paraneoplastic pemphigus associated Castleman's disease

Polymyositis

Pulmonary hyalinizing granuloma

Sjogren's syndrome

Silicosis

Surfactant protein B deficiency

Teratoma

Lung retransplant/graft failure

Sarcoidosis with mean PA pressure >30 mmHg

Rheumatoid disease

Occupational lung disease other specify cause

Obliterative bronchiolitis (non-retransplant)

Pulmonary fibrosis other specify cause

Used with permission from Organ Procurement and Transplantation Network (OPTN). Policy 10.1.F.i. https://optn.transplant.hrsa.gov/media/1200/optn_policies.pdf. This work was supported in part by Health Resources and Services Administration contract 234-2005-37011C. The content is the responsibility of the authors alone and does not necessarily reflect the view or policies of the Department of Health and Human Services, nor does mention of trade names, commercial products, or organizations imply endorsement by the US Government.

Table 7.1 Predictors in LAS Model

Waiting list survival model		
Characteristic (X)		β and conditions
Age at offer		0.0084*age
Bilirubin (mg/dL)		0.0432*(bilirubin − 1), if bilirubin >1
Bilirubin increase of at least 50%		1.4144, if diagnosis group B
Body mass index (BMI) (kg/m^2)		0.1261*(20 − BMI), if BMI <20 kg/m^2
Cardiac index prior to any exercise (L/min/m^2)		0.5435, if cardiac index <2 L/min/m^2
Central venous pressure (CVP) (mmHg) at rest, prior to any exercise		0.0174*(CVP − 7), if CVP >7 mmHg and diagnosis group B
Continuous mechanical ventilation, if candidate is hospitalized		1.6771
Creatinine (serum) (mg/dL)		0.5034*creatinine, if candidate at least 18 years old at time of offer
Diabetes (regardless of insulin dependency)		0.4680
Diagnosis	Group A	0
	Group B	1.5774
	Group C	1.2314
	Group D	0.6260
Diagnosis detailed	Bronchiectasis (in group A)	0.6681
	Eisenmenger's syndrome (in group B)	−0.6279
	Lymphangioleiomyomatosis (in group A)	−0.3163
	Obliterative bronchiolitis (not retransplant) (in group D)	0.4453
	Pulmonary fibrosis, not idiopathic (in group D)	−0.2091
	Sarcoidosis with PA mean pressure >30 mmHg (in group D)	−0.4578
	Sarcoidosis with PA mean pressure <30 mmHg (in group A)	0.9331
Forced vital capacity (FVC) % predicted		0.1829*(80-FVC)/10, if FVC <80% and diagnosis group D
Functional status		−0.4471, if no assistance needed with activities of daily living
Oxygen need to maintain adequate oxygen saturation (88% or greater) at rest (L/min)		0.0213*O_2, if diagnosis group B 0.1188*O_2, if diagnosis groups A, C, or D
pCO_2		0.1105*pCO_2/10, if pCO_2 > 40
pCO_2 increase of at least 15%		0.2331
Pulmonary artery (PA) systolic pressure at rest, prior to any exercise (mmHg)		0.4155*(PA systolic − 40)/10, if PA systolic >40 mmHg and group A; 0.0462*PA systolic/10, if diagnosis groups B, C, or D
6-min walk distance (feet) obtained while the candidate was receiving supplemental oxygen required to maintain an oxygen saturation of 88% or greater at rest		−0.0845*6-min walk distance/100

Table 7.1 (continued)

Posttransplant survival model		
Characteristic (Y)		α and conditions
Age at transplant (years)		0.0247*(age − 45.9972602), if candidate age >46 years
Cardiac index prior to any exercise (L/min/m²)		0.3499, if cardiac index <2 L/min/m²
Continuous mechanical ventilation, if candidate is hospitalized		0.6094
Creatinine at transplant (mg/dL)		0.0896*creatinine, if candidate age >18 years
Creatinine increase >150%		0.7709
Diagnosis	Group A	0
	Group B	0.6116
	Group C	0.3627
	Group D	0.4641
Diagnosis detailed	Bronchiectasis (in group A)	0.1889
	Eisenmenger's syndrome (in group B)	0.9147
	Lymphangioleiomyomatosis (in group A)	−1.5194
	Obliterative bronchiolitis (not retransplant) (in group D)	−1.2051
	Pulmonary fibrosis, not idiopathic (in group D)	−0.0724
	Sarcoidosis with PA mean pressure >30 mmHg (in group D)	−0.0438
	Sarcoidosis with PA mean pressure <30 mmHg (in group A)	−0.1389
Functional status: if no assistance needed to perform activities of daily living		−0.1900
Oxygen need to maintain adequate oxygen saturation (88% or greater) at rest (L/min)		0.0748*O₂, if diagnosis group A 0.0164*O₂, if diagnosis groups B, C, or D
6-min walk distance (feet) obtained while the candidate was receiving supplemental oxygen required to maintain an oxygen saturation of 88% or greater at rest		0.0005*(1200 − 6-min walk distance)

Used with permission from Organ Procurement and Transplantation Network (OPTN) Policies. Policy 10.1.F. https://optn.transplant.hrsa.gov/media/1200/optn_policies.pdf. This work was supported in part by Health Resources and Services Administration contract 234-2005-37011C. The content is the responsibility of the authors alone and does not necessarily reflect the view or policies of the Department of Health and Human Services, nor does mention of trade names, commercial products, or organizations imply endorsement by the US Government
The predictors in the LAS Model are divided into two categories: Calculating the waiting list model (expected days lived during an additional year on the waiting list) and the posttransplant model (expected days lived during the first year posttransplant). The LAS is a combination of these models to yield the transplant benefit (predicted posttransplant survival minus predicted survival on waiting list), which is then normalized into a score from 0 to 100

Unlike the Model for End-Stage Liver Disease (MELD) score, the predictive model in liver transplant, the LAS not only incorporates waitlist urgency but also purposefully balances the likelihood of posttransplant survival, with the rationale that the rare resource of donor lungs does not go to moribund patients with little chance of survival posttransplant. From this, a calculation known as transplant benefit is devised, which was the difference between predicted posttransplant survival and waitlist survival (Fig. 7.1), and then the LAS was the calculation of transplant benefit minus waitlist urgency. Scores are then normalized on a scale of 0–100, and patients are listed according to that score.

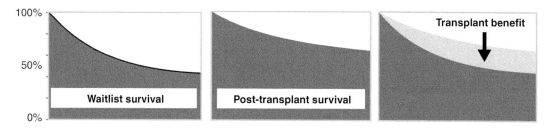

Fig. 7.1 Transplant benefit. The transplant benefit is calculated by subtracting the waitlist survival from posttransplant survival. This is then normalized to fit a scale of 0–100 (Used with permission of Elsevier from Davis SQ, Garrity ER. Organ allocation in lung transplant. Chest 2007;132(5):1646–51)

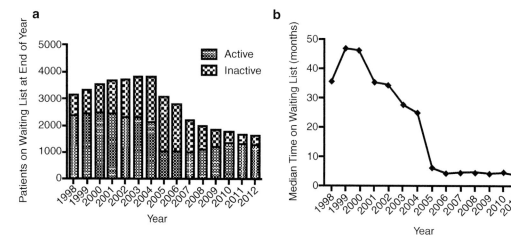

Fig. 7.2 Lung transplant waiting list over time. (**a**) Trends in number of patients on lung transplant waiting list. (**b**) Median time on waiting list by year (**a**, **b**: Data used with permission from Organ Procurement and Transplantation Network (OPTN) and Scientific Registry of Transplant Recipients (SRTR). OPTN/SRTR 2012 Annual Data Report. Rockville, MD: 2014)

Early Impact of the LAS

The LAS had an immediate and significant impact on lung transplantation, with dramatic shifts in waitlist activity. In the 6 years leading up to LAS implementation, there were over 2000 patients active on the transplant waiting list annually, and the median time to transplant was also high, with patients waiting over 2 years to reach transplant [4]. With the implementation of the LAS, the number of patients active on the waiting list plummeted by 54% from 2163 in 2004 to 1005 in 2007, and the median waitlist time dropped from 762 days (95% confidence interval (CI) 666–965 days) in 2004 to 141 days (95% CI 127–157 days) for patients listed in 2007 (Fig. 7.2) [4]. Prior to the LAS, the number

of deaths on the waiting list numbered around 500, and this dropped to 300–400 in the 2 years following the LAS. However, the death rate was not changed, likely due to more urgent patients being listed for transplant post-LAS implementation [4]. Other early studies showed that with the implementation of the LAS, patients were likely sicker at the time of transplant. In an analysis of 176 patients from UNOS region six looking at 2 years before LAS and 1 year after, Gries and colleagues found that the calculated LAS of listed patients was higher after LAS implementation [5]. This shift in LAS was also seen in a study of listed patients in the Veterans Affairs Hospital lung transplantation program, with an increase in calculated LAS from pre-LAS implementation (33.1 ± 1.4) to post-LAS implementation (41.9 ± 9.8; $p < 0.01$) [6]. Despite the increase in urgency of listed patients, none of the early studies showed increase in mortality post-transplant [5–7]. Also, despite sicker patients being transplanted, the hospital lengths of stay post-LAS were shorter in these cohorts [5, 6], although in the five-center study by Kozower and colleagues, an increase in both incidence of primary graft dysfunction and in ICU length of stay was noted [7].

In addition to the impact on waiting times, or perhaps in part due to this very effect, the epidemiology of lung transplantation shifted dramatically after implementation of the LAS (Fig. 7.3). In the study by Gries and colleagues that looked at the impact of LAS implementation, the diagnoses of recipients changed ($p = 0.02$); there were more patients transplanted with pulmonary fibrosis (from 24.4 to 37.8%) and fewer patients with COPD/α_1-antitrypsin deficiency (50 to 26.7%) [5]. This significant shift was also seen in a multicenter study of five transplant centers ($P = 0.002$) [7], and similar change in recipient diagnoses was also seen in the VA cohort ($p < 0.01$) [6]. Aside from underlying diagnoses, the demographics of recipients also changed and persisted. Prior to the LAS era, African-Americans were more likely to die on the waiting list and were less likely to be transplanted than Caucasian recipients, but in the LAS era, these racial disparities were no longer apparent [4, 8]. On the other hand, gender disparities seemed to

have changed as the number of women transplanted decreased in the LAS era compared to pre-LAS era [4], and women were more likely to die after listing or become too sick for transplant in the LAS era ($P < 0.001$) [8].

Continued Impact of LAS on Lung Transplantation

After the implementation of LAS, studies continued to examine whether the changes would be transient or durable, as well as determine the long-term implications of this new system. In their recent analysis, Egan and colleagues analyzed all patients in the OPTN database from 2000 to 2011, encompassing 5 years prior to LAS and 6 years post [9]. Prior to implementation of the LAS, over 500 patients died on the waiting list per year, whereas in the LAS era, this annual death rate on the waiting list decreased by 40% to 300 per year ($P = 0.0062$) (Fig. 7.1) [9]. Similar to the earlier studies, the increase in number of transplants performed for patients with pulmonary fibrosis was significant and sustained, and by 2007 pulmonary fibrosis was the most common indication for lung transplant [9]. There were also significant increases in patients transplanted for other lung diseases (e.g., sarcoidosis; $P = 0.0062$) and retransplanted ($P = 0.0061$) [9, 10]. Although the percentage of patients with COPD who were transplanted did decrease, the

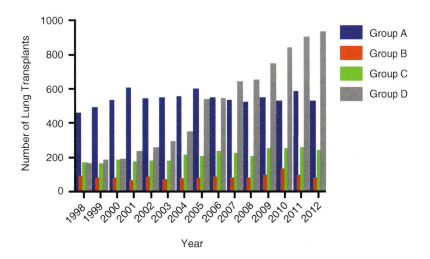

Fig. 7.3 Number of lung transplants per year per each diagnostic group (Data used with permission from Organ Procurement and Transplantation Network (OPTN) and Scientific Registry of Transplant Recipients (SRTR). OPTN/SRTR 2012 Annual Data Report. Rockville, MD: 2014)

absolute numbers of patients with COPD stayed the same [9].

With the shift in lung transplant patients' diagnoses in the LAS era, the early trend of transplanting older and sicker patients continued. Although the number of patients over the age of 65 was already on the rise pre-LAS, there was a more rapid increase in the number of patients transplanted who were older than 65, likely reflecting the greater number of transplants in pulmonary fibrosis patients [9]. Additionally, there was a trend toward transplanting sicker patients, as the median LAS at transplant has consistently continued to rise post-LAS implementation [9]. Despite these factors, 1-year survival has increased significantly post-LAS [9, 11]. These trends likely reflect that improvements in expertise and technological advances have paralleled the willingness to take on challenging cases.

Impact of LAS on Long-Term Survival and Resource Utilization

Since its inception, the LAS has helped to alter the transplant landscape, with preserved 1-year posttransplant survival, yielding an overall positive net transplant benefit in patients transplanted. Many researchers have further investigated the mid- and long-term implications and trends that have developed since its implementation.

Liu and colleagues used an LAS of 46 at the time of lung transplant as a starting point to conduct a retrospective cohort study on patients in the OPTN database from 2005 to 2009, and after adjusting for age, center volume, diagnosis, waiting list times, they found that patients with an LAS of 60 or greater had an increased risk of death than those at 46 or below despite shorter waitlist times (LAS 60–79: hazard ratio [HR], 1.52; 95% CI 1.21–1.90; LAS $\geq$ 80: HR 2.03; 95% CI 1.61–2.55; $p < 0.001$) [12]. When they looked at subgroups, this increased mortality risk was seen in IPF patients with LAS $\geq$ 60 and in COPD patients with LAS $\geq$ 80 [12]. They reconciled their findings with the prior study by Merlo by stating that the previous study did not break down the groups above an LAS of 46; hence, the

increased risk seen by Merlo in that cohort was likely driven by the LAS $\geq$ 60 group [12, 13]. While some may see these data as an argument for an LAS cutoff, Liu and colleagues stopped short of that in their discussion.

While overall there has not been a decrease in 1-year survival post-LAS, when comparing patients in the highest LAS quintile (LAS > 46) to the rest, Merlo and colleagues found that the risk of death was significantly greater in the highest quintile. These patients were also sicker at the date of transplant, as they were more likely to have IPF and diabetes and be on a mechanical ventilator at the time of transplant [13]. In a study looking at the impact of the LAS on IPF patient outcomes alone, it was found that patients with an LAS > 50 had a 10% lower cumulative survival at 1 year than patients in the lowest quartile and had a higher mortality risk [14]. These patients were more likely to have higher baseline oxygen requirements, require mechanical ventilation, have diabetes, and have worse pulmonary function testing [14]. The authors made an important observation: because LAS is designed to predict posttransplant benefit, defined as posttransplant survival subtracted from waitlist urgency, even patients with a high LAS (70–79) and predicted posttransplant mortality of 39.5% have a positive posttransplant benefit, meaning their survival is better than expected without lung transplant [14].

In a subsequent study, Russo and colleagues looked at 3836 patients entered into the OPTN database between April 5, 2006, and December 31, 2007, and analyzed survival and outcomes of the index hospitalization [15]. They found that patients with LAS of 75 or greater had a decreased survival and a significantly increased incidence of posttransplant complications, such as the need for dialysis, and increased hospital length of stay. They argued in their discussion for continued review of LAS methodology, stating that although the patients had a transplant survival benefit by LAS, that given those with higher LAS had a median survival of only 1.56 years (LAS 90–100) or 2.28 years (LAS 80–89), the additional survival gained may not be in the best interest of long-term survival of scarce donor lungs [15].

As researchers tried to hone in on the optimal LAS for transplant, Russo and colleagues studied transplant survival benefit in smaller subsets of the OPTN dataset to try to find the most optimal range for LAS yielding the greatest net transplant benefit with a likelihood of surviving consistent with actuarial survival. They discovered that the lowest priority (LAS < 40 and LAS 40–49) and highest priority (LAS 80–90 and LAS 90+) groups had the lowest net survival benefit. In fact, candidates with a LAS < 40 had better survival without a lung transplant. From their work, they suggested that further work is done to optimize organ allocation to the patient who would receive the greatest benefit [16].

Maxwell and colleagues examined the impact of the LAS on survival beyond 1 year and found that although 1-year survival has remained similar post-LAS consistent with the pre-LAS era, survival conditional on 1 year in the post-LAS cohort was worse, especially at months 13 and 14 where the hazard of death was significantly increased in the post-LAS cohort [17]. The authors postulated that this is the effect of a shift from patient-centered outcomes to focusing on the metric of 1-year survival in challenging cases and then withdrawing care after that point [17]. Hayanga and colleagues corroborated these studies in their analysis of the OPTN dataset from 2005 to 2012, reporting that higher LAS is associated with worse survival and noted that at their center, up to 45% of listed candidates cross the threshold of LAS > 50 between time of listing and transplant [18]. Single-center studies have come to similar conclusions that higher LAS is associated with increased posttransplant mortality [19, 20]. Looking at the impact of high LAS on survival in a large, single-center retrospective study of 527 consecutive patients, survival was significantly lower in patients with LAS ≥ 50 compared with those with LAS < 50 (92.6% vs. 96.9% at 30 days, 71.5% vs. 83.2% at 1 year, 52% vs. 73.9% at 3 years) [19].

Higher LAS has been associated with increased resource use in several studies. In the study by Horai and colleagues, patients who had an LAS of 50 of greater had an increased need for tracheostomy, prolonged mechanical ventilation,

and longer intensive care unit (ICU) length of stay (LOS) [19]. Arnaoutakis and colleagues looked at 84 patients who underwent lung transplantation at the Johns Hopkins Hospital between May 2004 and December 2009 [21]. They divided up recipients by LAS into quartiles to analyze resource utilization compared to LAS. Those patients who were in the highest quartile of LAS (LAS ≥ 49.9) had shorter waitlist times and were sicker with higher oxygen requirements, and a greater likelihood of needing pretransplant ICU care, and also had higher median index admission charges than the other quartiles combined [21]. They also had longer median length of stay and ICU LOS, longer duration of mechanical ventilation, a higher rate of reintubation, and greater need for tracheostomy [21]. Expanding on earlier reports of increased resource use, Maxwell and colleagues used the National Inpatient Sample data from 2000 to 2011 and found an association between LAS implementation and increased healthcare resource use. At the time of the LAS implementation, there was a decrease in mortality but a 40% growth in hospital charges at the time of index hospitalization not seen in other organ transplants, with increases in hospital length of stay, use of ECMO, tracheostomy, and other daily charges as well as increase in disposition to rehabilitation or a facility other than home [22].

Impact of Worsening LAS on Posttransplant Outcomes

Aside from the direct association of increased risk of 1-year mortality with LAS, clinicians often worry about patients on the waiting list who are on an acute decline in their lung disease. In a post-LAS study from the OPTN database, an acute increase in LAS of five or greater comparing the time of transplant to 30 days prior was associated with significantly worse posttransplant survival (HR 1.31, 95% CI 1.11–1.54, $P = 0.001$) [23]. This effect of the change in LAS was independent of the LAS at time of transplant, center volume, underlying diagnosis, or donor characteristics [23]. Fortunately, a patient's LAS can be updated at any time and as frequently as is necessary such that the score most accurately represents the degree of urgency and transplant benefit that is attempted to be predicted by the equation. In fact, centers are required to update the data on actively listed patients at least every 6 months (with the exception of data from cardiac catheterization which can be less frequent due to the invasive nature of data acquisition), and most centers update these data every 3 months. Any variables for the LAS equation that are missing or have expired from previously entered data are given substitute values to represent "normal" or that are least beneficial in the final LAS calculation (Table 7.2).

Table 7.2 Values substituted for missing or expired actual values in calculating the LAS

If this covariate's value	Is	Then the LAS calculation will use this substituted value
Bilirubin	Missing, expired, or less than 0.7 mg/dL	0.7 mg/dL
Body mass index (BMI)	Missing or expired	100 kg/m^2
Cardiac index	Missing	3.0 L/min/m^2
Central venous pressure (CVP)	Missing or less than 5 mmHg	5 mmHg
Continuous mechanical ventilation	Missing or expired	No mechanical ventilation in the waiting list model Continuous mechanical ventilation while hospitalized in the posttransplant survival measure
Creatinine: serum	Missing or expired	0.1 mg/dL in the waiting list model 40 mg/dL in the posttransplant survival measure for candidates at least 18 years old 0 mg/dL in the posttransplant survival measure for candidates less than 18 years old
Diabetes	Missing or expired	No diabetes
Forced vital capacity (FVC)	Missing or expired	150% for diagnosis group D
Functional status	Missing or expired	No assistance needed in the waiting list model Some or total assistance needed in the posttransplant survival measure
Oxygen needed at rest	Missing or expired	No supplemental oxygen needed in the waiting list model 26.33 L/min in the posttransplant survival measure
pCO$_2$	Missing, expired, or less than 40 mmHg	40 mmHg
Pulmonary artery (PA) systolic pressure	Missing or less than 20 mmHg	20 mmHg
6-min walk distance	Missing or expired	4000 ft in the waiting list urgency measure 0 ft in the posttransplant survival measure

Used with permission from Organ Procurement and Transplantation Network (OPTN) Policies. Policy 10.1.E. https://optn.transplant.hrsa.gov/media/1200/optn_policies.pdf. This work was supported in part by Health Resources and Services Administration contract 234-2005-37011C. The content is the responsibility of the authors alone and does not necessarily reflect the view or policies of the Department of Health and Human Services, nor does mention of trade names, commercial products, or organizations imply endorsement by the US Government

Impact of LAS on Certain Subgroups: Special Consideration of Pulmonary Arterial Hypertension

The LAS has shifted the epidemiology of lung transplant, with its biggest impact on shortening the waiting list time for sicker IPF patients, improving their net transplant survival, and changing the demographics of transplant recipient with more patients with IPF undergoing transplant. However, the benefits seen in the IPF patient cohort have not completely transcended the diagnostic group, and the most important area of discrepancy has been in patients with IPAH (Fig. 7.3).

There have been two studies that on the surface seem to give different results with concerning the impact of LAS on transplant outcomes in IPAH patients. In one of the largest to date, Schaffer and colleagues studied all IPAH patients ($n = 1403$) in the OPTN database from 1998 to 2011 and reported that in the LAS era, both patient survival on the waiting list and posttransplant survival improved [24]. In an earlier study by Chen and colleagues examining the UNOS database between 2002 and 2008, they reported that implementation of the LAS enhanced the likelihood of transplantation for patients with IPAH; however, waitlist mortality was unchanged, and there was also no change in posttransplant mortality [25]. The most notable difference between these two studies was the length of time (approximately 80 months) pre- and post-LAS used in Schaffer's study, making it a report more about different transplant eras, which encompass many more changes (e.g., candidate selection and optimization, medical and surgical advances, etc.) than about the impact of LAS per se.

Perhaps more controversial, several studies have reported that waiting list mortality decreased for all diagnoses except IPAH, which has remained unchanged [5, 7, 25, 26]. While the likelihood of transplantation *among* patients in the IPAH patient group increased after LAS

implementation when comparing this group to other diagnostic groups, this is not the case. Patients with IPAH are less likely to receive a lung transplant than patients with IPF or CF, and they are more likely to die on the waiting list than patients with COPD or CF [25, 26]. Therefore, although more IPAH patients who were listed underwent lung transplant, the proportion of IPAH patients transplanted remained small compared to other diagnostic categories after implementation of the LAS. This relative disadvantage of having a group B (pulmonary hypertension) diagnosis among lung transplant candidates was acknowledged early by UNOS policy 10.2.B, and it was established that requests for an exception for candidates with pulmonary hypertension could qualify for an increase in LAS granted by the Lung Review Board if the patient is deteriorating on optimal therapy *and* the patient has a right atrial pressure greater than 15 mmHg or a cardiac index less than 1.8 L/min/m^2.

Why the discrepancy in the LAS effect on IPAH vs. other diseases? Benza and colleagues proposed in their impactful 2010 study that it likely was because while LAS was a good predictor of waiting list urgency in IPF and COPD, it was a poorer predictor of this in IPAH, putting PAH patients at a disadvantage. The most significant predictors of mortality in patients with PAH have been shown to be cardiac index (CI), mean right atrial pressure (mRAP), New York Heart Association Functional Class, and 6-min walk distance (6MWD) [27]. When the LAS was first developed, CI and mRAP were not included, and 6MWD was used as a threshold value at 150 ft (45.7 m) rather than as a continuous variable. Furthermore, pulmonary function tests, which are part of the LAS calculator, are more predictive of clinical worsening in patients with COPD or pulmonary fibrosis than IPAH. Therefore, Benza and colleagues looked at the Registry to Evaluate Early and Long-Term PAH Disease Management (REVEAL) to compare actual mortality in the large cohort to the predicted mortality based on LAS. They then performed an analysis to identify additional variables to include in the LAS that could improve its predictive function in IPAH patients and identified two subsets of patients who had a greater 1-year mortality than predicted by LAS: those with an mRAP of 14 mmHg or more and those with a 6MWD less than 300 m [27].

Building on these important findings, Gomberg-Maitland and colleagues identified and developed predictive equations for 1-year survival in a waitlisted cohort [28]. They used the OPTN database and analyzed all 827 patients listed with a primary diagnosis of PAH after 1991 and followed them until March 1, 2012. Through their study, they derived a new predictive equation that incorporated cardiac output, 6MWD, and baseline oxygen level at rest. They reported that the predicted 1-year survival curves were very similar between the LAS and the new model, but the new model performed better in terms of sensitivity and specificity than the LAS, especially in the post-2006 era [28]. Their work laid the groundwork for the LAS revisions that went into effect on February 19, 2015.

In addition to these model changes, simultaneously there has been discussion of total bilirubin as another prognostic marker highly predictive of mortality in PAH patients. This was based on data from a large study demonstrating that total bilirubin was the strongest predictor of poor prognosis in congestive heart failure patients[29] and borne out in studies of PAH patients in a single-center and lung transplant patients as a whole from the OPTN cohort [30, 31].

Given the potentially detrimental effects of LAS on transplantation of patients with pulmonary vascular disease (group B patients), it was decided that the LAS should be modified to include the following revisions: total bilirubin, cardiac output, CVP, and 6-min walk data as a continuous variable, and on February 19, 2015, new changes were put into place for the lung allocation score. Although no published data are yet available to know the impact on waitlist or transplant outcomes, the UNOS Thoracic Organ Transplantation Committee met in early 2016 and discussed the early impact of the LAS revisions [32]. The committee noted that the waiting list mortality did trend toward a decrease in all diagnostic groups except for group C. All groups showed an increased posttransplant survival measure. The LAS for group B patients (pulmonary hypertension) did show an absolute increase as well as relative increase compared with other diagnostic groups. There has been a decrease in requests for modification of LAS, as well as a reduction in difference in the calculated and requested exceptions as well [32]. The committee concluded that it will remain to be seen whether these changes persist over time and what their implications on longer-term outcomes are.

Future Directions in Lung Allocation

It is difficult to argue the profound impact of the LAS has had on lung transplantation on patients with end-stage lung disease in the United States. In a relatively short time, it has led to more equitable distribution of organs to those who are predicted to have the greatest transplant benefit and greatly reduced deaths on the waiting list in a consistent and sustained fashion. And this has happened in 10 years, with open access to OPTN datasets allowing investigators to evaluate the performance of the LAS and the need for continued development of prognostic markers. In the next section, we discuss specific prognostic markers on the horizon in lung transplant.

Prognostic Factors on the Horizon in Lung Transplant

As the field continues to evolve, prognostic markers—whether existing in the LAS or new—will continue to shift in terms of their impact on lung transplant outcomes. In this section, we discuss several prognostic factors that have been areas of attention in the field of lung transplantation. At many transplant centers, these factors already play a role in transplant evaluation and organ allocation, and, as we accumulate more experience and evidence, these or other variables may become part of our formalized LAS in future updates.

The Impact of Pulmonary Hypertension on Underlying Lung Disease

One prognostic factor recently under study in lung transplant candidates is that of pulmonary hypertension associated with lung disease, namely, the impact of WHO Group 3 pulmonary hypertension on patient outcomes. In a single-center study from Denmark, postcapillary (mean pulmonary artery pressure (mPAP) ≥ 25 and pulmonary capillary wedge pressure (PCWP) >15) and precapillary pulmonary hypertension (mPAP > 25, PCWP $\leq$ 15) were both associated with significantly worse 90-day survival [33]. PGD was the major cause of death in the first 90 days, and, in subgroup analyses, postcapillary and precapillary pulmonary hypertensions were associated with worse outcomes in COPD patients [33]. These findings that pulmonary hypertension was associated with increased risk of 1-year mortality in COPD patients were corroborated by a post-LAS study from the OPTN database, in which COPD patients with precapillary PH had a 1.74 times higher risk of 1-year posttransplant mortality than COPD patients without PH [34]. This increased risk associated with postcapillary PH has not been demonstrated in patients with idiopathic pulmonary fibrosis or cystic fibrosis [34–36]. Time will tell if we see this reflected in the new LAS given that hemodynamics are now in the calculation.

Severity of Illness Not Accounted for by LAS: Mechanical Ventilation and Extracorporeal Life Support

Studies looking at the impact of mechanical ventilation on posttransplant survival have shown that the need for continuous mechanical ventilation is a significant risk factor for increased mortality on the waiting list as well as posttransplant mortality [37–39]. In an analysis of OPTN data in the LAS era, Singer and colleagues noted that the greatest posttransplant mortality risk in those who were mechanically ventilated pretransplant is within the first 6 months; however, and, after

that time, it is no different with nonmechanically ventilated patients [37]. They also found that pretransplant mechanical ventilation in non-cystic fibrosis obstructive lung disease was not associated with increased posttransplant mortality [37]. Mechanical ventilation is already accounted for in the LAS calculator and is heavily weighted in the calculation of transplant urgency (Table 7.1). However, the use of extracorporeal life support (ECLS), another predictor of urgency as well as death posttransplant, is not included.

In recent years, technology has improved to be able to help even sicker patients pretransplant with the use and continued improvement in ECLS technology. While early studies showed variable outcomes posttransplant, more recent reports continue to provide equipoise for the use of ECLS as a bridge to transplant to give patients a net transplant benefit. However, despite the level of critical illness of a patient on ECLS, it is still not included in the LAS. Pretransplant ECLS has been associated with decreased posttransplant survival in studies pre-LAS era and the LAS era [31, 38, 39]. However, as centers have gained experience and comfort with the procedure, we have begun to see improvement in posttransplant outcomes after pretransplant ECLS. In one of the centers with the most ECLS experience, Lang and colleagues reported that although posttransplant survival in patients who had received ECLS was significantly lower than those who had not, mortality conditional on 3-month survival was no different between these groups [40]. They argued that pretransplant mortality in these patients without ECLS was certainly 100%, supporting the net transplant benefit in this group as a justification for the use of the technology [40]. Outcomes with ECLS have seemed to improve in the LAS era. Toyoda and colleagues reported on single-center experience using ECLS in 24 patients pretransplant, and, despite the increased incidence of primary graft dysfunction and longer LOS posttransplant, they reported no significant difference in actuarial survival compared to non-ECLS patients [41]. In another report from two centers on their experience using ECLS as a bridge to transplant, Hoopes and colleagues shared their clinical algorithm to use the technology to work to get patients to an ambulatory state prior to transplant and reported good outcomes at the 1–3- and 5-year time points with 93%, 80%, and 66% survival, respectively, though still decreased survival in their center's patients compared to those not requiring ECLS [42]. They stated that their experience challenged the notion that ECLS is expensive and futile and suggested future multicenter trials to examine how best to use this technology as a bridge to transplant [42].

Hayanga and colleagues looked at the OPTN database to compare trends in survival over time in patients in whom ECLS was used as a bridge to transplant and demonstrated that, while ECLS was associated with decreased 1-year survival compared to non-ECLS transplanted patients, 1-year survival has progressively improved over time and, as of 2009–2011 period, it was 74.4% in ECLS-bridged patients vs. 85.7% in non-ECLS bridged patients ($P = 0.004$) [43]. In an analysis of the OPTN database from 2010 to 2015 looking at posttransplant outcomes of patients on ECLS and including center volume in the comparison, Hayes and colleagues showed that in historically low-volume centers (those in lower 50% in terms of annual lung transplants performed), ECLS was associated with increased posttransplant mortality (HR 1.968, 95% CI 1.083–3.577, $P = 0.026$); however, this increased risk was not seen in historically high-volume centers (those in the top 25% of annual transplants performed) meaning they have performed at least 170 transplants in the first 5 years in the post-LAS era (HR 0.853, 95% CI 0.596–1.222, $P = 0.386$) [44]. The authors suggested that these data be used as evidence that the LAS system should be revised to account for use of ECLS support and that perhaps center expertise should be accounted for too. They also called for ongoing studies of ECLS outcomes to try to determine in which candidates it yielded the greatest benefit and also to monitor poor results that may be due to centers with less expertise [44].

In summary, the advancement of transplant and supportive technologies in critically ill patients has led to ECLS being used as a bridge to transplant. Ongoing studies are needed to continue to review outcomes and perhaps prospectively study treatment algorithms and, most of all, work toward incorporating ECLS usage into the LAS calculation.

Age, Body Composition, Functional Status, and Frailty

As mentioned earlier, as the general population has aged and with the demographic shift of lung transplantation that came with the LAS era (more patients with ILD being transplanted, thus being an older population), several studies have looked at the implications of advancing age on posttransplant outcomes. In recipients who underwent lung transplant from 2007 to 2009, survival was lowest in those whose age ≥65 years old [45]. Looking more specifically at the impact of age and performing a multivariate regression analysis, although age over 70 years old was a risk factor for 1-year posttransplant mortality prior to the LAS, in the LAS era, 1-year survival in patients aged 70 or higher is comparable to outcomes in those of age 60–69 [46]. Although age is incorporated already as a continuous variable in the LAS, in reality many centers use threshold or cutoff values in the evaluation of transplant candidates. Given variable practices among centers as well as success in older candidates [46], there has been a push to look beyond chronologic age at other risk factors that could impact one's physiologic age, such as body composition and functional status or frailty.

Body mass index is already incorporated in the LAS calculation; however, as we push our limits of transplantation and as the obesity epidemic continues to grow, many investigators have renewed their interest in looking at BMI as a prognostic factor in lung transplantation. In a study from the OPTN database of 9073 adults transplanted in the LAS era, Singer and colleagues found that being underweight (BMI ≤ 18.5) and in class II–III obesity (BMI ≥ 35) was associated with a twofold increase in 1-year mortality [47]. Hypoalbuminemia, a marker of malnutrition, at the time of listing is an independent risk factor for posttransplant mortality [48]. Obesity has also been associated with a twofold risk of primary graft dysfunction, a major risk factor of early death after transplant [49]. Fortunately, it appears that obesity may be a modifiable risk factor as weight loss in patients with BMI $\geq$ 25 prior to transplantation had improved survival (HR 0.85, 95% CI 0.77–0.95, P = 0.004) with decreased median ventilator days and a trend toward decreased ICU LOS [50].

In recent years, physicians have been interested in the impact of functional status and frailty on surgical and posttransplant outcomes. The frail phenotype was initially defined by Fried as "a clinical syndrome in which three or more of the following criteria [are] present: unintentional weight loss ($\geq$10 pounds in the past year), self-reported exhaustion, weakness (grip strength), slow walking speed, and low physical activity" [51]. In a multicenter prospective study in lung transplant candidates, frailty has been associated with increased risk of delisting or death before transplant [52]. These findings were corroborated by a single-center retrospective cohort analysis that showed preoperative frailty was associated with increased risk of death, though no increase in mechanical ventilator days or LOS [53]. In a study looking at pretransplant muscle mass measured on CT scan in 117 transplant recipients, it was found that those within the lowest 25th percentile of muscle index had decreased survival (HR 3.83, 95% CI 1.42–10.3, P = 0.007) and a significantly longer hospital LOS [54]. In a study of a related field of performance status in the OPTN dataset, there was a significant difference in mortality rates between patients who preoperatively needed assistance and those who did not (P < 0.001), and preoperative functional independence as measured by Karnofsky scale $\geq$50 was protective in terms of 1-year mortality [55]. In patients undergoing redo lung transplantation, poor functional status based on Karnofsky scale has been identified as a risk factor for increased 1-year mortality [56]. Given the potential impact of frailty on lung transplant outcomes, as we accumulate more data, we may see more of these data measures in preoperative assessment and counseling of lung transplant candidates, and the hope is that these risk factors of frailty are potentially modifiable through rehabilitation and nutritional measures to reduce risk of poor outcomes posttransplant.

Conclusions

The implementation of the lung allocation score greatly shifted the landscape of lung transplantation, making it possible to allocate organs on a need-based rather than a time-based system. The LAS helped enable the scarce resource of organs to go to the sickest of patients with the greatest potential benefit and also allowed more patients to survive to lung transplant. By allowing transplant centers to update patient data pretransplant at any time (and on average every 3 months), the LAS helps centers make sure that the patients who need organs most urgently are the ones given highest priority. Concomitantly, our technical and medical abilities have improved to enable improved outcomes, further pushing the envelope and potentially helping more patients survive their end-stage lung disease. As our abilities and successes change and as new prognostic markers are identified, continued evaluation of the LAS by the OPTN Thoracic Committee will help assure that the limited supply of organs goes to patients with the greatest potential benefit and may also lead to universal adoption of this system of organ allocation.

References

1. Cooper JD, Pearson FG, Patterson GA, et al. Technique of successful lung transplantation in humans. J Thorac Cardiovasc Surg. 1987;93(2):173–81.
2. Egan TM, Murray S, Bustami RT, et al. Development of the new lung allocation system in the United States. Am J Transplant. 2006;6(5 Pt 2):1212–27.
3. Health Resources and Services Administration, HHS. Organ procurement and transplantation network. Final rule. Fed Regist. 2007;72(46):10616–9.
4. McCurry KR, Shearon TH, Edwards LB, et al. Lung transplantation in the United States, 1998-2007. Am J Transplant. 2009;9(4 Pt 2):942–58.
5. Gries CJ, Mulligan MS, Edelman JD, Raghu G, Curtis JR, Goss CH. Lung allocation score for lung transplantation: impact on disease severity and survival. Chest. 2007;132(6):1954–61.
6. Osaki S, Maloney JD, Meyer KC, Cornwell RD, Edwards NM, De Oliveira NC. The impact of the lung allocation scoring system at the single national Veterans Affairs Hospital lung transplantation program. Eur J Cardiothorac Surg. 2009;36(3):497–501.

7. Kozower BD, Meyers BF, Smith MA, et al. The impact of the lung allocation score on short-term transplantation outcomes: a multicenter study. J Thorac Cardiovasc Surg. 2008;135(1):166–71.

8. Wille KM, Harrington KF, deAndrade JA, Vishin S, Oster RA, Kaslow RA. Disparities in lung transplantation before and after introduction of the lung allocation score. J Heart Lung Transplant. 2013;32(7):684–92.

9. Egan TM, Edwards LB. Effect of the lung allocation score on lung transplantation in the United States. J Heart Lung Transplant. 2016;35(4):433–9.

10. Osho AA, Castleberry AW, Snyder LD, et al. Differential outcomes with early and late repeat transplantation in the era of the lung allocation score. Ann Thorac Surg. 2014;98(6):1914–20, discussion1920–1.

11. Iribarne A, Russo MJ, Davies RR, et al. Despite decreased wait-list times for lung transplantation, lung allocation scores continue to increase. Chest. 2009;135(4):923–8.

12. Liu V, Zamora MR, Dhillon GS, Weill D. Increasing lung allocation scores predict worsened survival among lung transplant recipients. Am J Transplant. 2010;10(4):915–20.

13. Merlo CA, Weiss ES, Orens JB, et al. Impact of U.S. Lung Allocation Score on survival after lung transplantation. J Heart Lung Transplant. 2009;28(8):769–75.

14. Weiss ES, Allen JG, Merlo CA, Conte JV, Shah AS. Lung allocation score predicts survival in lung transplantation patients with pulmonary fibrosis. Ann Thorac Surg. 2009;88(6):1757–64.

15. Russo MJ, Iribarne A, Hong KN, et al. High lung allocation score is associated with increased morbidity and mortality following transplantation. Chest. 2010;137(3):651–7.

16. Russo MJ, Worku B, Iribarne A, et al. Does lung allocation score maximize survival benefit from lung transplantation? J Thorac Cardiovasc Surg. 2011;141(5):1270–7.

17. Maxwell BG, Levitt JE, Goldstein BA, et al. Impact of the lung allocation score on survival beyond 1 year. Am J Transplant. 2014;14(10):2288–94.

18. Hayanga JWA, Lira A, Aboagye JK, Hayanga HK, D'Cunha J. Extracorporeal membrane oxygenation as a bridge to lung transplantation: what lessons might we learn from volume and expertise? Interact Cardiovasc Thorac Surg. 2016;22(4):406–10.

19. Horai T, Shigemura N, Gries C, et al. Lung transplantation for patients with high lung allocation score: single-center experience. Ann Thorac Surg. 2012;93(5):1592–7–discussion1597.

20. Shafii AE, Mason DP, Brown CR, et al. Too high for transplantation? Single-center analysis of the lung allocation score. Ann Thorac Surg. 2014;98(5):1730–6.

21. Arnaoutakis GJ, Allen JG, Merlo CA, et al. Impact of the lung allocation score on resource utilization after lung transplantation in the United States. J Heart Lung Transplant. 2011;30(1):14–21.

22. Maxwell BG, Mooney JJ, Lee P. Increased resource use in lung transplant admissions in the lung allocation score era. Am J Respir Crit Care Med. 2015 Feb 1;191(3):302–8.

23. Tsuang WM, Vock DM, Copeland C. An acute change in lung allocation score and survival after lung transplantation: a cohort study. Ann Intern Med. 2013;158(9):650–7.

24. Schaffer JM, Singh SK, Joyce DL, Reitz BA. Transplantation for idiopathic pulmonary arterial hypertension: improvement in the lung allocation score era. Circulation. 2013;127(25):2503–13.

25. Chen H, Shiboski SC, Golden JA, et al. Impact of the lung allocation score on lung transplantation for pulmonary arterial hypertension. Am J Respir Crit Care Med. 2009;180(5):468–74.

26. Chan KM. Idiopathic pulmonary arterial hypertension and equity of donor lung allocation in the era of the lung allocation score: are we there yet? Am J Respir Crit Care Med. 2009;180(5):385–7.

27. Benza RL, Miller DP, Frost A, Barst RJ, Krichman AM, Mcgoon MD. Analysis of the lung allocation score estimation of risk of death in patients with pulmonary arterial hypertension using data from the REVEAL Registry. Transplantation. 2010;90(3):298–305.

28. Gomberg-Maitland M, Glassner-Kolmin C, Watson S, et al. Survival in pulmonary arterial hypertension patients awaiting lung transplantation. J Heart Lung Transplant. 2013;32(12):1179–86.

29. Allen LA, Felker GM, Pocock S, et al. Liver function abnormalities and outcome in patients with chronic heart failure: data from the Candesartan in Heart Failure: Assessment of Reduction in Mortality and Morbidity (CHARM) program. Eur J Heart Fail. 2009;11(2):170–7.

30. Takeda Y, Takeda Y, Tomimoto S, Tani T, Narita H, Kimura G. Bilirubin as a prognostic marker in patients with pulmonary arterial hypertension. BMC Pulm Med. 2010;10:22.

31. Russo MJ, Davies RR, Hong KN, et al. Who is the high-risk recipient? Predicting mortality after lung transplantation using pretransplant risk factors. J Thorac Cardiovasc Surg. 2009;138(5):1234–1238.e1.

32. Committee OUT. Thoracic Organ Transplatation Committee Meeting Summary [Internet]. 2016;1–3. Available from: http://optn.transplant.hrsa.gov.

33. Andersen KH, Schultz HHL, Nyholm B, Iversen MP, Gustafsson F, Carlsen J. Pulmonary hypertension as a risk factor for survival after lung transplantation. Clin Transplant. 2016;30(4):357–64.

34. Singh VK, Patricia George M, Gries CJ. Pulmonary hypertension is associated with increased post-lung transplant mortality risk in patients with chronic obstructive pulmonary disease. J Heart Lung Transplant. 2015;34(3):424–9.

35. Hayes D, Higgins RS, Black SM, et al. Effect of pulmonary hypertension on survival in patients with idiopathic pulmonary fibrosis after lung transplantation: an analysis of the United Network of Organ Sharing registry. J Heart Lung Transplant. 2015;34(3):430–7.

36. Hayes D, Higgins RS, Kirkby S, et al. Impact of pulmonary hypertension on survival in patients

with cystic fibrosis undergoing lung transplantation: an analysis of the UNOS registry. J Cyst Fibros. 2014;13(4):416–23.

37. Singer JP, Blanc PD, Hoopes C, et al. The impact of pretransplant mechanical ventilation on short- and long-term survival after lung transplantation. Am J Transplant. 2011;11(10):2197–204.

38. Mason DP, Thuita L, Nowicki ER, Murthy SC, Pettersson GB, Blackstone EH. Should lung transplantation be performed for patients on mechanical respiratory support? The US experience. J Thorac Cardiovasc Surg. 2010;139(3):765–773.e1.

39. Gottlieb J, Warnecke G, Hadem J, et al. Outcome of critically ill lung transplant candidates on invasive respiratory support. Intensive Care Med. 2012;38(6):968–75.

40. Lang G, Taghavi S, Aigner C, et al. Primary lung transplantation after bridge with extracorporeal membrane oxygenation: a plea for a shift in our paradigms for indications. Transplantation. 2012;93(7):729–36.

41. Toyoda Y, Bhama JK, Shigemura N, et al. Efficacy of extracorporeal membrane oxygenation as a bridge to lung transplantation. J Thorac Cardiovasc Surg. 2013;145(4):1065–70, discussion1070–1.

42. Hoopes CW, Kukreja J, Golden J, Davenport DL, Diaz-Guzman E, Zwischenberger JB. Extracorporeal membrane oxygenation as a bridge to pulmonary transplantation. J Thorac Cardiovasc Surg. 2013;145(3):862–7, discussion 867–8.

43. Hayanga AJ, Aboagye J, Esper S, et al. Extracorporeal membrane oxygenation as a bridge to lung transplantation in the United States: an evolving strategy in the management of rapidly advancing pulmonary disease. J Thorac Cardiovasc Surg. 2015;149(1):291–6.

44. Hayes D, Tobias JD, Tumin D. Center volume and extracorporeal membrane oxygenation support at lung transplantation in the Lung Allocation Score Era. Am J Respir Crit Care Med. 2016;194(3):317–26.

45. Valapour M, Skeans MA, Smith JM, et al. OPTN/SRTR annual data report 2014: lung. Am J Transplant. 2016;16:141–68.

46. Kilic A, Merlo CA, Conte JV, Shah AS. Lung transplantation in patients 70 years old or older: have outcomes changed after implementation of the lung allocation score? J Thorac Cardiovasc Surg. 2012;144(5):1133–8.

47. Singer JP, Peterson ER, Snyder ME, et al. Body composition and mortality after adult lung transplantation in the United States. Am J Respir Crit Care Med. 2014;190(9):1012–21.

48. Baldwin MR, Arcasoy SM, Shah A, et al. Hypoalbuminemia and early mortality after lung transplantation: a cohort study. Am J Transplant. 2012;12(5):1256–67.

49. Lederer DJ, Kawut SM, Wickersham N, et al. Obesity and primary graft dysfunction after lung transplantation: the Lung Transplant Outcomes Group Obesity Study. Am J Respir Crit Care Med. 2011;184(9):1055–61.

50. Chandrashekaran S, Keller CA, Kremers WK, Peters SG, Hathcock MA, Kennedy CC. Weight loss prior to lung transplantation is associated with improved survival. J Heart Lung Transplant. 2015;34(5):651–7.

51. Fried LP, Tangen CM, Walston J, et al. Frailty in older adults: evidence for a phenotype. J Gerontol A Biol Sci Med Sci. 2001;56(3):M146–56.

52. Singer JP, Diamond JM, Gries CJ, et al. Frailty phenotypes, disability, and outcomes in adult candidates for lung transplantation. Am J Respir Crit Care Med. 2015;192(11):1325–34.

53. Wilson ME, Vakil AP, Kandel P, Undavalli C. Pretransplant frailty is associated with decreased survival after lung transplantation. J Heart Lung Transplant. 2015;35(2):173–8.

54. Kelm DJ, Bonnes SL, Jensen MD. Pretransplant wasting (as measured by muscle index) is a novel prognostic indicator in lung transplantation. Clin Transplant. 2016 Mar;30(3):247–55.

55. Grimm JC, Valero V, Kilic A, et al. Preoperative performance status impacts perioperative morbidity and mortality after lung transplantation. Ann Thorac Surg. 2015;99(2):482–9.

56. Kilic A, Beaty CA, Merlo CA, Conte JV, Shah AS. Functional status is highly predictive of outcomes after redo lung transplantation: an analysis of 390 cases in the modern era. Ann Thorac Surg. 2013;96(5):1804–11, discussion1811.

Part II

The Donor Lung and the Lung Transplant Recipient

Management of the Donor and Recipient: Surgical Management

8

Andrea Mariscal and Shaf Keshavjee

Introduction

Lung transplantation is a standard lifesaving therapy for patients suffering from end-stage lung disease. Over the past three to four decades, we have witnessed major advancements in lung preservation, surgical technique, immunosuppression, and posttransplantation management that have led to markedly improved outcomes and to an increasing number of lung transplants performed each year. The number of patients being listed, however, continues to increase in greater proportion than the number of available donor lungs, which translates to more patients dying on wait list.

Worldwide, still only 15–20% of the offered lungs are being used for transplantation. The lung is susceptible to a series of injuries during the donation process (such as brain death, ventilator-acquired pneumonia, neurogenic and hydrostatic pulmonary edema, barotraumas, etc.), which translates into very low utilization rates.

A. Mariscal · S. Keshavjee (✉)
Division of Thoracic Surgery, Toronto General Hospital, University Health Network, Toronto, ON, Canada

Toronto Lung Transplant Program,
Toronto General Hospital, University Health Network,
University of Toronto, Toronto, ON, Canada
e-mail: andrea.mariscal@uhn.ca;
Shaf.keshavjee@uhn.ca

Meticulous management of potential lung donors and appropriate preservation and treatment of potentially transplantable lungs is critical to expand the donor pool. Careful donor management and lung preservation refer to the steps taken after determination of death to preserve lung quality in the multiorgan donor to optimize function after transplantation.

Donor Lung

Donor Selection Criteria

The current lung donor criteria were empirically established in the early years of lung transplantation. These criteria initially included a donor age below 55 years old, an arterial partial pressure of oxygen (PaO_2/FiO_2) ratio greater than 300 mmHg, no or a moderate smoking history, a clear chest X-ray, clear bronchoscopy, gram stain negative, intubation time less than 5 days, and a minimal ischemic time [1] (Box 8.1).

Most centers today agree that these criteria are likely too conservative and often use extended criteria donors (ECD) that do not completely meet the traditional empiric criteria [1]. Although results have varied outcomes of transplantation, using extended criteria donor lungs has generally become acceptable, in weighing the risk balance

Table 8.1 Donation after cardiac death: Maastricht categories

Maastricht category	Description	Condition
I	Dead on arrival at hospital	Uncontrolled
II	Unsuccessful resuscitation	Uncontrolled
III	Anticipated circulatory arrest	Controlled
IV	Circulatory arrest in patient previously declared brain death	Controlled
V	Circulatory arrest in hospital	Uncontrolled

1-year survival. These results are comparable to contemporary cohort of DBD lung transplants. A better understanding of how the DCD process affects donor lungs will continue to have a major impact in expanding the utilization of DCD organs.

Donor Management During the Pre-retrieval Phase

The main goals during the pre-retrieval phase are related to maintaining the stability of the donor and to maintaining as many organs as possible suitable for transplant. In a review by Munshi and colleagues on donor management and lung preservation [10], the recommendations to achieve a suitable donor lung are described (Table 8.2). These recommendations include ventilation with ideal tidal volume (6–8 mL/kg); fraction of inspired oxygen of 50%; positive end-expiratory pressure of 5–10 cmH_2O; euvolemia with a target central venous pressure of 6–8 mmHg; vasopressin as the initial vasopressor of choice; norepinephrine, epinephrine, or phenylephrine as second-line treatment for hemodynamic instability; and the use of methylprednisolone and other hormone therapy replacements. Previously published studies have shown that standardization of donor management protocols including: setting goals for mean arterial pressure, pH, oxygenation, sodium, glucose, vasopressor use, urine output, and central venous pressure can increase

to death on the waiting list. Thus, many centers advocate use of ECD to effectively increase the donor pool with acceptable similar transplant outcomes [2–4].

The use of donors after cardiac death (DCD) has been explored and is a valuable source of lungs. In the last decade, the DCD donor pool has become by far the largest source for the increase in multiorgan donors. From 2006 to 2008, there was an increase of 24% in the DCD category compared with a 2% decrease in the number of consented dead brain donors (DBD) [4]. There are four types of DCD donors [5]: uncontrolled donors include Categories I (dead on arrival) and II (unsuccessful resuscitation) and controlled donors include Categories III (cardiac arrest after withdrawal of life support) and IV (cardiac arrest in brain-dead donors). In this setting, (Category III) several series have been reported with acceptable results and have described an increase in use [6–9] (Table 8.1). Although the initial series with small numbers of patients showed conflicting results, more recent studies with a larger numbers of patients have demonstrated excellent results including the multicenter study by Cypel and colleagues. [6–9] In that study, in which the experience from 10 centers (300 DCD transplants) was reviewed, they reported a 97% 30-day and 89%

Table 8.2 Recommendations for donor management

	Goal	Management
Ventilation	Protective ventilation	Low tidal volume FiO_2 50% PEEP 8–10 Recruitment maneuvers
Hemodynamics	Hemodynamic stability	Euvolemia (CVP ≤ 6–8 mmHg) Vasopressin (first-line vasopressor) Alpha-1 agonist (second-line vasopressor)
Hormone therapy	Lung protection Diabetes insipidus Hypothyroidism	Glucocorticoids (metilprednisolone 15 mg/kg) Vasopressin (100–200 mL/h) Thyroid replacement (thyroid hormone T4)
Donor management protocols	Achievement of previous set goals	Adhesion to established goals

Adapted with permission of Elsevier from Munshi L, Keshavjee S, Cypel M. Donor management and lung preservation for lung transplantation. Lancet Respir Med. 2013;1(4):318–28
FiO_2 fraction of inspired oxygen, *PEEP* positive end-expiratory pressure

the rate of successful organ donation, particularly in lung transplantation [11].

Donor Lung Retrieval Surgery

Before starting the retrieval, the trend of arterial blood gases and airway pressure should be examined. The retrieval team should perform a bronchoscopy to inspect for signs of aspiration, infection, anatomical abnormalities, endobronchial lesions, or compression. Bronchoscopy is also essential to clear any retained secretions to facilitate complete recruitment and expansion of the lung, which in turn will ensure uniform flushing of the lung bed during flush preservation. During the whole donor operating room phase of the retrieval procedure, the lungs are ventilated with FiO_2 50%, PEEP 5 cmH$_2$O, and V_T 8 mL/kg.

Access is gained through a standard median sternotomy incision. Both pleural spaces are entered and examined. Recruitment of all atelectatic lung segments is carried out in situ by gentle massage of both lungs as the anesthesiologist inflates them to a sustained pressure of up to 30 cmH$_2$O. Palpation of both lungs and visual evaluation of deflation capacity (recruitment with 20 cmH$_2$O or 30 cmH$_2$O for 30 s followed by opening of the airway to room air) is performed. While relatively subjective, this observation is a good indication of the absence of significant obstructive airways disease. The results of this examination, as well as the latest results of the arterial blood gas, chest radiograph, and bronchoscopic examination, are immediately communicated to the lung recipient implant surgeon for final decision-making. The anticipated cross-clamp time and estimated arrival time to the recipient operating room is also updated for logistical planning purposes. Individual pulmonary vein gas sampling can be useful in evaluating unilateral or lobar dysfunction. This is particularly useful in rescuing one well-functioning lung for a single-lung transplant when the donor systemic (two lung) blood gases are suboptimal due to one severely damaged lung.

After opening the pericardium, the superior vena cava is dissected free of all circumferential mediastinal attachments up to its bifurcation into the innominate veins and is encircled using a 0 silk tie; the ascending aorta is encircled with an umbilical tape making sure it is completely separated from pulmonary artery (PA). A purse string suture of 4-0 polypropylene suture (Prolene®; Ethicon, Inc, Somerville, NJ, USA) is then placed in the main pulmonary artery (midway between PA valve and the bifurcation) to later secure the PA flush cannula.

Once the abdominal teams have completed their pre-dissection, the donor is heparinized 3–5 min before cannulation (300 IU/kg). The lung flush solution (low potassium dextran, Perfadex®, [XVIVO Perfusion, Göteborg, Sweden]) should be ready kept cold on ice; the flush solution bag is hung *not more than 30 cm above the level of the heart.* A minimum of 3 min after heparin administration, the cannula is inserted into the PA and connected to the infusion tube. The tip of the PA cannula must be positioned before the pulmonary arterial bifurcation in order to avoid the preferential perfusion of one lung over the other. The organ preservation procedure is initiated by the bolus administration of prostaglandin E_1 (500 µg in 10 mL normal saline) into the main pulmonary artery immediately adjacent to the PA cannula. Once the blood pressure drops indicating PGE_1 circulation and effect, the aorta is then cross-clamped. The superior vena cava is ligated with the previously placed supra-azygos silk ligature. The inferior vena cava is then vented by complete transection just above the diaphragm. The left atrium is vented by transecting the tip of the left atrial appendage to create a drainage hole at least 2 cm in diameter. The cardioplegia for cardiac preservation is then initiated. (Note that, if desired, the aorta can also be cross-clamped after ligating the superior vena cava, venting of the left atrium, and venting of the inferior vena cava to optimize the decompression of the left ventricle.) The pulmonary preservation flush is then initiated. It is administered into the pulmonary arteries through the high-flow perfusion cannula (diameter 22 French) at 30 cm height gravity pressure only. The LPD flush solution emanating from the atrial appendage is allowed to drain into the pleural space to provide additional topical cooling of the lungs. Note that ventilation of the lung on the ventilator must be continued throughout this phase. The color of the flush solution draining is usually clear at the end of the antegrade flushing procedure (60 mL/kg—usually 4 L), but it is not absolutely necessary. The tip of the PA cannula must be monitored to confirm it remains in the main PA and proximal to the bifurcation during the whole procedure. Both lungs should appear equally blanched after the administration of the pulmonary flush. After the completion of thoracic organ preservation infusions, the heart is excised first. The lungs remain cooled, and gently ventilating in the chest for the few minutes is required to excise the heart.

Excision of the Donor Heart

The pulmonary artery is transected at its midpoint, halfway between the pulmonary valve and the arterial bifurcation (at the site of the PA cannulation suture). The aorta is transected, taking whatever length is desired by the cardiac team. The IVC transection is completed if not already done, and the SVC is transected just below the previously tied suture. This leaves the heart connected only by the pulmonary veins.

The apex of the heart is elevated to expose the posterior left atrium and pulmonary veins. The left atrial incision is started halfway between the now visible left inferior pulmonary vein and the coronary sinus (atrioventricular groove). Then, under direct vision inside the LA, further extension of the initial left atrial incision is then carried out parallel to the atrioventricular groove toward the base of the left atrial appendage on the left and toward inferior pulmonary vein orifice on the right. At all times, the pulmonary vein orifices should be kept in sight to make sure that an adequate cuff is maintained both on the left atrium on the heart and on the left atrium on the lung side. It is not necessary to take an excessive cuff on the donor heart for implantation, and a reasonably experienced surgeon should be able to do this without compromising the pulmonary vein orifices on the lung graft. It is almost always possible in the adult donor to stay 5–10 mm out of the pulmonary vein orifices. The excision of the heart is now complete and it is removed from the field.

The retrograde pulmonary flush is then initiated by infusing 1 L of Perfadex® through an inflated Foley catheter (18 or 20 French) with its tip sequentially positioned in each individual pulmonary vein orifice (250 mL for each vein). The return of retrograde flush solution into the pulmonary artery often reveals some debris or pulmonary emboli (if present).

After the retrograde flush is completed, the mediastinum is dissected. Both inferior pulmonary ligaments are carefully mobilized and divided by reaching behind the lung and gently retracting each lower lobe anteriorly and laterally. The dissection continues following the anterior wall of the esophagus until reaching the azygos vein on the right side and aorta on the left side, which are transected. All mediastinal tissue is divided down to the level of the upper trachea which is then encircled. Note that the lungs are still being ventilated on the ventilator to this point. Prior to stapling the trachea, the lungs are recruited with a sustained airway pressure of 15–20 cmH$_2$O and a FiO$_2$ of 50%; the lungs should be about 75% inflated. The proximal trachea is stapled twice with a TA-30 stapling device (Covidien, Minneapolis, MN, USA) and transected between the staple lines. This is to prevent contamination of the operative field with any respiratory tract organisms. The knife or scissors used to transect the airway is considered "contaminated" and handed back to the nurse separately so that it is not used again by other surgical teams in the donor operation. The trachea should be transected as close to the larynx as possible; this is particularly important for donor lungs that might be treated with ex vivo lung perfusion (EVLP) as intubation of the double lung block requires enough length of trachea to accommodate and secure an endotracheal tube for ventilation. The lung block is removed. The lungs are examined for unexpected pathologic conditions, reviewing each lobe, especially the posterior and dependent areas that might not have been adequately observed while in the chest. The lungs are place in a triple plastic bag containing 3 L of Perfadex®, sitting on ice, which has been prepared on the back table. Do *not* place any ice in the bag in direct contact with the lungs as this could cause freezing injury to the tissue. The preservation bags are tied, and the lungs are placed into a cooler surrounded by ice for transport. The principal steps of the brain death donor surgery are described in Box 8.2.

Donation After Cardiac Death (DCD) Lung Retrieval

For donation after cardiac death (DCD) lung retrievals, the team usually waits in the operating room for the donor to arrive. Two members of the lung recovery team should be present. Arrive in the donor OR at least 30 min prior to withdrawal of life-support therapies to ensure all equipment is ready for use and the ventilator is set on the

---

Box 8.2 Brain-Dead Donor Surgery: Principal Steps

1. Arterial blood gases
2. Bronchoscopy
3. Ventilation setting: FiO$_2$ 50%, PEEP 5 cmH$_2$O, and V$_T$ 8 mL/kg
4. Sternotomy
5. Recruitment maneuvers: Transient sustained breath hold to 30 cmH$_2$O
6. Palpation of both lungs and evaluation of deflation capacity
7. Pericardium opening
8. Dissection and encircling of superior vena cava, inferior vena cava, and aorta
9. Purse string suture 4-0 polypropylene suture in midpoint of main pulmonary artery
10. Heparin 300 IU/kg
11. Insertion of PA cannula
12. Inject prostaglandin E$_1$ (500 µg in 10 cm^3 of normal saline) into the main pulmonary artery
13. Aorta cross-clamp
14. Ligation of superior vena cava, transection of inferior vena cava
15. Transection of the tip of the left atrial appendage (create a 2 cm diameter orifice)
16. Perfusion start. Allow flush solution to drain into pleural spaces for topical cooling
17. Cardiectomy
18. Retrograde flush into each pulmonary vein in situ with inflated Foley catheter
19. Pulmonary ligament mobilization
20. Mediastinal dissection, transection of azygous vein and aorta
21. Dissection of peritracheal tissue—high subglottic
22. Lung recruitment and tracheal stapling (double stapling with TA-30)
23. Excision of the lung block. Final examination of the lungs
24. Place lungs in 2 L of LPD solution in sterile bags and place in cooler (do *not* put ice in the bag with the lung)

FiO$_2$ fraction of inspired oxygen, *PEEP* positive end-expiratory pressure, *T$_v$* tidal volume

---

appropriate parameters (similar to brain death donor procedures). Although different hospitals may have different protocols, ideally the donor should receive heparin (500–1000 U/kg) 5 min before withdrawal. The head of the bed should be slightly elevated, and a nasogastric tube should be placed to decompress the stomach and avoid aspiration after extubation.

Upon arrival in the OR, the donor is re-intubated by one member of the lung donor team, and the donor is placed on standard ventilation (V_T of 8–10 mL/kg, FiO$_2$ of 50% PEEP of 5 cmH$_2$O).

The intubating surgeon then performs a bronchoscopy to examine and clear the airways, making sure there are no signs of aspiration. The second surgeon meanwhile expeditiously preps and drapes the donor and performs the sternotomy. The pericardium is opened, the PA is cannulated, and the lungs are recruited. PGE$_1$ (500 µg) is injected into the PA, and 3–5 cardiac manual compressions are performed. Cold Perfadex® flush is then infused in the standard fashion. Subsequent steps are similar to brain death donors. Frequently, the final decision for lung utilization is made after explantation and detailed examination of the lungs. The principal steps of DCD donor surgery are described in Box 8.3.

Box 8.3 Donor After Cardiac Death Surgery: Principal Steps

1. Heparin (500–1000 U/kg) 5 min before withdrawal
2. Donor arrival to the OR
3. Donor reintubation. Ventilation setting: FiO$_2$ 50%, PEEP 5 cmH$_2$O, and V_T 8 cm L/kg
4. Simultaneous bronchoscopy and sternotomy
5. Pericardium opening
6. Cannulation of the pulmonary artery
7. Recruitment maneuvers: Sustain pressure of 30 cmH$_2$O for 30–60 s as needed
8. Dissection and encircling of superior vena cava and aorta
9. Purse string stitch 4-0 polypropylene suture in the main pulmonary artery
10. Insertion of the cannula
11. Prostaglandin E$_1$ (500 µg in 10 cc of normal saline) into the main pulmonary artery
12. 3–5 cardiac compressions
13. Transection of inferior vena cava and SVC
14. Transection of the tip of the left atrial appendage (2 cm drainage orifice)

---

15. Start pulmonary flush. (LPD 60 mL/kg. Ice saline slush into both pleural spaces
16. Cardiectomy
17. Retrograde flush with inflated Foley catheter inserted into each pulmonary vein (250 mL each)
18. Pulmonary ligament mobilization
19. Mediastinal dissection, transection of azygous vein and aorta
20. Dissection of peritracheal tissue
21. Lung recruitment and tracheal stapling (high in the subglottic area, double staple with TA-30 stapler)
22. Excision of the lung block. Final examination of the lungs
23. Decision for ex vivo perfusion assessment

FiO$_2$ fraction of inspired oxygen, *PEEP* positive end-expiratory pressure, *T$_v$* tidal volume

---

Donor Lung Dissection on the Back Table in the Recipient Operating Room

The outer bag of the triple-bagged donor lungs is removed by the OR nurse as the surgeon lifts the sterile now double-bagged lungs and places them in a bucket on the back table that is prefilled with crushed ice. The double bags are cut open, and the lungs thus remain in the same Perfadex solution they arrived in, on ice for the back table preservation and dissection phase. Two towels are wet with the Perfadex® from the lung bag and then used to wrap the lungs to keep them cool while exposing the hilum and middle mediastinal structures for the dissection. The separation of the two lungs is initiated by identifying and dividing the pulmonary arteries at the bifurcation. The left atrium is visualized and then divided in the midline with direct visualization of all four pulmonary veins. The rest of the mediastinal tissue (posterior pericardium) is also divided in the midline, leaving the airway isolated. The airway is divided with little to no disruption of the peribronchial tissue which carries the blood supply to the bronchi. The division of the lungs is completed by firing a GIA 60 blue stapler (Covidien, Minneapolis, MN, USA) across the longer left bronchus at the carina.

Preparation of the hilar structures (PA, pulmonary vein cuff and main bronchus) of the first lung to be implanted is then performed. This starts by dissecting the proximal PA from the surrounding tissue until the first branch. The proximal PA then can be trimmed to the appropriate length. The left atrial cuff is released from the surrounding tissue; usually not much dissection is required.

The bronchus is then opened by cutting off the staple line. By visualizing *on the inside*, the surgeon can see approximately where the transection of the donor bronchus will be, approximately one ring proximal to the lobar bifurcation. Then, the dissection of the peribronchial tissue *on the outside* of the bronchus is carried out guided by this, being very careful to *not* dissect beyond where the final transection will be. This is very important as the nutritive blood supply to the donor bronchus comes from collaterals from the donor lung pulmonary circulation and is carried through the microcirculation in this peribronchial tissue. If this tissue is excessively "cleaned off," then sewing the anastomosis may be technically easier, but the risk of bronchial ischemia will be greater. A flap of peribronchial tissue is preserved anteriorly as it is dissected, to be used to buttress the bronchial anastomosis.

Potential Complications During the Donor Surgery

Donor Instability

The main goal at the time of organ harvesting is to maintain hemodynamic stability using fluid resuscitation to maintain normovolemia and vasoactive drugs as required to maintain blood pressure. In case of severe hemodynamic instability, a decision should be made to proceed with the PA cannulation, clamp the aorta, and start flushing the lung with the perfusion solution. If there is severe intraoperative bleeding which compromises the stability of the donor, the lung harvest can be handled in the same manner as a DCD donor.

Previous Surgery

A relative donor exclusion criterion is the history of previous cardiac surgery. Several thoracic trans-plant centers have been using donors with previous cardiac surgeries successfully [12, 13]. During donor harvesting, careful technique is necessary to avoid injury of the lung and heart during dissection. As in any redo sternotomy, it is desirable to use the oscillating saw to reopen the sternum: first the anterior and then the posterior plates, making sure the lungs are not ventilating in the meantime. The dissection under the sternum should be enough to insert the chest retractor. Lungs are assessed as usual, opening the pleural spaces. If the lungs have adhesions, they should be dissected as close as possible to the chest wall and just enough to assess the lungs; the rest of the adhesions can be removed after perfusion. The dissection of the heart starts at the diaphragmatic surface, finding a good and safe plane toward the inferior and superior vena cava and right atrium. The aorta is dissected and separated from the pulmonary artery. SVC is encircled as usual with a silk tie. The posterior surface of the heart can be dissected after cross-clamp. The rest of the procedure is performed in the same manner as a regular donor.

Congenital Abnormalities

Some congenital abnormalities are acceptable for the lungs to be safely used for transplant.

Tracheal Bronchus

Tracheal bronchus is an aberrant bronchus most commonly arising from the right lateral wall of the trachea. The population incidence varies between 0.1 and 5% [14]. There are several options to do the airway anastomosis depending on the recipient and donor characteristics. The simplest technique is to implant a patch of the donor tracheal bronchus and bronchus intermedius at the right tracheobronchial anastomosis [15]. Anatomical resections (segmentectomy or lobectomy) can be performed depending on the donor-recipient size mismatch [16]. Reconstruction techniques can also be performed.

Anomalous Pulmonary Venous Return

Anomalous pulmonary venous return (APVR) is a rare congenital malformation where the aberrant vein returns to the superior vena cava or right atrium instead of returning to the left atrium.

Its incidence ranges from 0.4 to 0.7% [17]. APVR in a donor requires reconstruction to avoid venous infarction or massive bleeding after the implantation. The most common variant is flow from the right superior pulmonary vein to the superior vena cava. In that case, the donor aberrant pulmonary vein can be anastomosed to the recipient left atrial cuff with a conduit of autologous pericardium [14]. Other reconstruction techniques have been described using iliac vein conduits [14], as well as direct anastomosis of the aberrant vessels to atrial appendages [18]. Anatomic resection (lobectomy) can be performed to avoid the aberrant vein [19]. If any congenital abnormality of the heart or great vessels is noted in the donor assessment, it is advisable to check pulmonary artery pressures to make sure there is no element of secondary pulmonary hypertension. If the donor does not have a Swan-Ganz catheter, this can be done with direct intraoperative measurement of PA pressure with a needle inserted into the PA at sternotomy.

Donor Lung Preservation

Conventional Lung Preservation

Improvements in the technique for lung preservation and the use of preservation solutions specifically designed for the lungs have been key to achieving improved results in lung transplantation. Static cold preservation, which has been the cornerstone of organ preservation, aims to slow cell metabolism and thus reduce consumption oxygen and other substrates in an attempt to prevent organ deterioration. This strategy reduces cellular activity in a nonselective way, including processes that lead to edema and cell damage [20, 21].

Preservation solutions can be divided in two groups: intracellular solutions with high potassium and low sodium such as University of Wisconsin solution and Euro-Collins and extracellular solutions with low potassium and high sodium such as low-potassium dextran (Perfadex®) and Celsior® (IGL, Waters Medical Solutions, Rochester, MN, USA) [22]. The concept of an extracellular solution for lung preservation was introduced in the early 1980s by Fujimura and colleagues [23]. Keshavjee and colleagues

demonstrated improvement of lung function by adding dextran 40 to the low-potassium solution as a rheologic and oncotic agent that minimizes edema. Dextran improves erythrocyte deformability and prevents erythrocyte aggregation. It also has an antithrombotic effect [24]. Date and colleagues proposed the addition of 1% glucose to the low-potassium dextran solution to allow the sustained aerobic metabolism and maintain the cellular integrity [25]. The benefits of low-potassium dextran solutions over the intracellular solutions in lung preservation have been demonstrated in multiple studies [26–28]. Currently, most transplant centers in the world use low-potassium, dextran and glucose solutions.

The optimal temperature of the perfusion solution has been subject of various studies. Some groups have shown beneficial effects when the solution was used at higher temperatures (15–20 °C). Nevertheless, the majority of these studies have been done in small animals [29–31]. Because the potential deleterious effect of the cold flushing is minimal in comparison to the damage induced by warm ischemia, flushing the lungs with hypothermic solutions is still a recommended practice.

The retrograde flush (administration of the flush solution through each pulmonary vein with drainage through the pulmonary artery) has been proven to improve lung preservation. It is thought that this is because of improved distribution of the flush to vascular beds in the lung that may not have been flushed through the antegrade route as well as for its capacity to remove clots from the pulmonary circulation [32].

The benefits of keeping the lungs inflated with oxygen during the cold ischemic period have been shown in many studies [33, 34]. There are three principal mechanisms of protection: maintenance of aerobic metabolism, preservation of epithelial fluid transport, and preservation of the integrity of pulmonary surfactant [22]. Atelectasis is associated with higher pulmonary vascular resistance, but it is known that hyperinflation of the lung is also detrimental. Over-inflation during cold ischemia can lead to barotrauma and increased pulmonary capillary filtration coefficient that translates into edema [35]. Hyperinflation can occur inadvertently when the lungs are transported in airplanes. It is important not to fully inflate the lungs when the trachea is stapled so that there is room for some expansion at increased altitude. In our clinical practice, we perform a gentle recruitment maneuver to ensure that the lung is fully expanded before flush perfusion and ventilate the lungs with peak pressure of 20 cm and a PEEP of 5 cmH$_2$O and FiO$_2$ of 50% during the perfusion period.

Some experiments have shown a possible beneficial effect of maintaining slightly higher temperatures in the lung during cold storage (10 °C), but other groups have not confirmed this [30, 36, 37]. This is also not easily or practically achievable, and it decreases the margin of safety. Thus, aiming for a preservation temperature in the range of to 8 °C is easily and safely achievable.

Prostaglandin E$_1$ is used during lung donor retrieval to induce pulmonary vasodilatation and for its anti-inflammatory properties [38]. Prostaglandin E$_1$ is also helpful in improving pulmonary dynamic compliance after reperfusion [39]. The Toronto Lung Transplant Program strategy for static lung preservation is described in Table 8.3.

Table 8.3 Toronto Lung Transplant Program technique for lung preservation

Preservation solution	Low-potassium dextran solution (Perfadex®)
Pharmacological additives	Prostaglandin E1, heparin, methylprednisolone
Anterograde flush (volume)	60 mL/kg
Retrograde flush (volume)	250 mL/ pulmonary vein
Pressure during flush	30 cm H$_2$0 (gravity drain by height above OR table)
Lung ventilation during flush	PEEP 5 cmH$_2$O and V$_T$ 8 mL/kg
Temperature of perfusion solution	4–8 °C
Oxygenation	FiO$_2$ 50%
Airway pressure	15–20 cmH$_2$O (visualize nearly complete expansion of lungs but not overexpansion)
Storage temperature	4–8 °C

Modified with permission of Elsevier from de Perrot M, Keshavjee S. Lung preservation. Semin Thorac Cardiovasc Surg 2004;16;300–8
FiO$_2$ fraction of inspired oxygen, *PEEP* positive end-expiratory pressure, *T$_v$* tidal volume

Ex Vivo Lung Perfusion

Despite the advances in lung transplantation, this therapy continues to be limited by the shortage of available donors. A common strategy used to increase utilization of donor lungs has been to transplant extended criteria organs.

Primary graft dysfunction (PGD) is a serious early complication after lung transplantation. Severe PGD is associated with a 20–30% mortality rate, and PGD also predisposes lung transplant recipients for development of chronic lung allograft dysfunction (CLAD), the leading cause of late death in lung transplant recipients. The pathogenesis of PGD is multifactorial. Ischemia-reperfusion injury is a major contributing component in the development of PGD. Ischemia-reperfusion injury affects the transplanted lung by stimulating mechanisms of inflammation and generation of reactive oxygen species (ROS) [40]. At some point, the use of extended criteria donors can increase the incidence of PGD.

Ex vivo lung perfusion (EVLP) represents an opportunity to further assess the function of the lung and, more importantly, to even treat them before transplantation into the recipient. This strategy provides a non-injurious maintenance strategy to ventilate and perfuse the lungs at normothermia outside the body.

In an attempt to evaluate the lungs after retrieval, Steen and colleagues developed a short-term ex vivo perfusion system [41]. They developed a buffered, extracellular solution with an optimal colloid osmotic pressure to act as the lung perfusate (Steen Solution™, XVIVO Perfusion, Göteborg, Sweden) [42]. This strategy was used for short-term assessment of lungs after DCD. Erasmus and colleagues first attempted to extend the EVLP duration to 6 h; however, that circuit induced injury and became problematic with increased PVR and airway pressures at 6 h [43].

The Toronto group developed an EVLP system capable of reliably achieving long-term (12 h) ex vivo lung perfusion and making detailed evaluation and even treatment of the lung outside the body a reality [44] (Fig. 8.1).

In the Toronto technique, an acellular perfusate is used. Maximal flow is limited to 40% of calculated cardiac output, reducing the hydrostatic edema caused by perfusion pressure. A positive

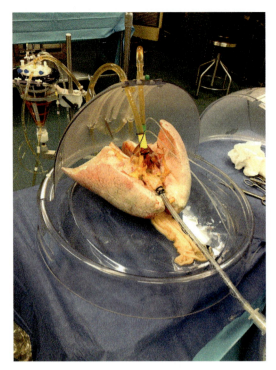

Fig. 8.1 Ex vivo lung perfusion

Table 8.4 Ex vivo perfusion protocol: Toronto Lung Transplant Program

Perfusion	Ventilation
Target: 40% cardiac output	Volume control mode
Start: 150 mL/min	V_T: 7 mL/kg
PA pressure: <15 mmHg	Respiratory rate: 7/min
Left atrial pressure: 3–5 mmHg	PEEP: 5 cmH$_2$O
Centrifugal pump	FiO$_2$ 21%
2L Steen solution	

PA pulmonary artery, *T$_v$* tidal volume, *FiO$_2$* fraction of inspired oxygen, *PEEP* positive end-expiratory pressure

Portable Ex Vivo Lung Perfusion

A portable ex vivo lung perfusion allows for earlier connection of the donor lung to a normothermic EVLP system instead of using conventional cold preservation for transport. Warnecke and colleagues published the first report of a portable EVLP system in a study in which they investigated the effect of normothermic preservation and transportation of standard criteria human donor lungs on a portable device. Lungs were preserved by normothermic perfusion and ventilation on the transportable Organ Care System™ (OCS) Lung (TransMedics, Inc., Andover, MA, USA) [47]. The results showed that the device could be used safely [48]. It is important to note that, while initially marketed to provide preservation with "no cold ischemia," it became evident to the investigators that this led to potential increased risk of lung injury, and it was recognized that a period of pre-EVLP and post-EVLP cold preservation is still required.

The OCS protocol used in the pilot study was a combination of some factors from the Lund and the Toronto EVLP protocols. A cellular perfusate based on Steen Solution™ supplemented with erythrocytes and an open LA was combined with a perfusate flow of 2.5 L/min, resembling the protective approach developed by the Toronto group. The Steen Solution™ was later replaced by a low-potassium dextran solution with glucose.

The OCS protocol is currently being evaluated on a larger scale in a prospective randomized multicenter trial (OCS™ Lung INSPIRE Trial)

left atrial pressure of 3–5 mmHg is maintained in order to maintain the intrapulmonary alveolar vessels open and prevent collapse during inspiration. Oxygen is removed, and carbon dioxide is supplied via a membrane oxygenator to create a venous admixture of the PA inflow. Removal of oxygen allows for the measure of lung function by taking the difference between post-lung and pre-lung PaO_2, and addition of carbon dioxide helps maintain the pH of the perfusate [4]. The Toronto EVLP technique is summarized in Table 8.4. Using this EVLP strategy, a clinical trial was performed for assessment of high-risk donor lungs, which otherwise would not be used. Lungs that demonstrated stable or improved compliance and pulmonary vascular resistance and had a pO_2/FiO_2 of more than 350 mmHg were transplanted and resulted in posttransplant outcomes comparable to control standard donor lungs [4, 45]. The potential for repair of injured donor lungs is greatly increased with the development of this safe prolonged normothermic perfusion of lungs [46].

comparing transplant outcomes of standard criteria lungs preserved and transported by either normothermic EVLP or standard cold preservation alone. The International EXPAND Lung Pivotal Trial was started as a clinical pilot to evaluate the OCS Lung portable system as a device to assess lungs that otherwise were unusable for transplantation [47]. Several other companies are in the process of developing automated ex vivo lung perfusion devices as interest in this field continues to expand. A note of caution to the reader is that all devices do not have the same technical characteristics and this will need to be evaluated over time as to what is the optimal technique to perform EVLP.

Recipient

Lung Transplant Procedure

Prior to intubation, an intravenous and a radial arterial line are placed. The patient is intubated with a double-lumen endotracheal tube, and position of the tube is confirmed with bronchoscopy. Central venous access is established in the neck. Placement of a Swan-Ganz pulmonary artery (PA) catheter is performed.

In bilateral sequential lung transplants, the decision on which side should be transplanted first is usually made preoperatively depending on the function testing in which the side with the least perfusion (worst side) is transplanted first. There may be other donor and recipient characteristics that influence the decision.

The patient is positioned supine with arms abducted, to expose the whole chest. The chest, abdomen, and bilateral groins are prepped in the sterile field to allow for access to the femoral vessels in case of need for additional lines or extracorporeal support. The traditional incision used for bilateral lung transplantation is the clamshell incision (Fig. 8.2). The procedure may also be performed using separate bilateral anterior thoracotomies. Single-lung transplants can be also performed through posterolateral thoracotomies,

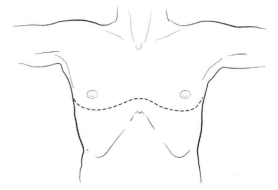

Fig. 8.2 Clamshell incision

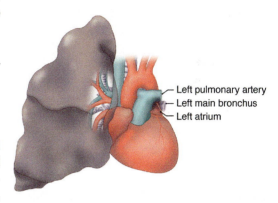

Left pulmonary artery
Left main bronchus
Left atrium

Fig. 8.3 Pneumonectomy

but the anterior approach has the advantage of having a faster and easier access to central cannulation in case of urgent need.

The incision is usually performed in the fourth intercostal space. The mammary vessels are legated and transected. Sternum is divided transversely using a sternal saw which is held obliquely to create a bevel that improves stability after secure closure with sternal wires. Two chest retractors are placed. Adhesions if found are taken down with cautery. The hilar dissection is started, carefully protecting the phrenic nerve. Extra caution is used near the recurrent laryngeal nerve while dissecting the left hilum. The pneumonectomy (Fig. 8.3) is started by dissecting the PA, superior pulmonary vein, releasing the inferior pulmonary ligament until the inferior pulmonary vein and the bronchus. The PA is encircled making sure the PA catheter is not in that side.

Temporary manual occlusion of the PA may be performed for a few minutes to assess hemodynamic stability. The pericardium may be opened at any time if central cannulation is anticipated or to assist with the hilar dissection. The pulmonary veins are encircled separately. The first branch of the PA is divided between silk ties.

The PA and the pulmonary veins are divided with vascular staplers as distally as possible. The bronchus is liberated from the surrounding tissues. The cartilage of the bronchus is divided with cautery. Once the lung is excised, a fresh edge of the bronchus is created with a scalpel, and two anchoring sutures at the membrano-cartilaginous junction (3-0 PDS suture) are placed before cutting the back wall of the bronchus using a valve scissor. The length of the bronchus is adjusted to be quite short, approximately two rings from the carina, to "mediastinalize" the anastomotic site. All secretions are suctioned, and bleeding from the bronchial vessels is controlled, avoiding denudation of the bronchus to prevent damage to its blood supply and subsequent ischemic complications. The hilum is then prepared by opening the pericardium circumferentially, allowing mobilization of the pulmonary vein stumps.

The donor bronchus is opened and trimmed to within approximately one ring from the lobar takeoffs. It is very important to *not* trim off the peribronchial fatty tissue. This tissue carries the critical blood supply coming through pulmonary arterial to bronchial artery collaterals that the bronchial anastomosis is critically dependent on for healing. As a rule of thumb, do not trim more than 1–2 mm from the cut edge of the bronchus. A cooling jacket is placed in the recipient thoracic cavity to keep the graft cool during implantation. The implantation is then conducted sequentially beginning with the bronchial anastomosis. Using the previously placed stiches, the donor bronchial membrano-cartilaginous edge is attached. The donor airway tissue is handled as minimally as possible and gently when necessary. The membranous portion of the airway is sutured with a 4-0 polypropylene running suture, and the anterior cartilaginous airway is anastomosed with interrupted 4-0 Prolene sutures about

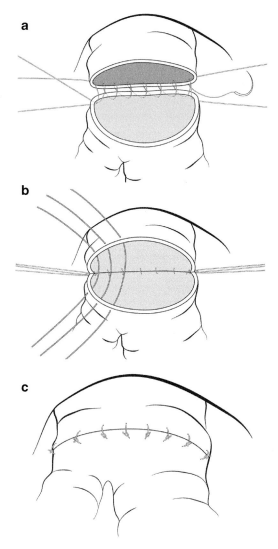

Fig. 8.4 Bronchial anastomosis

2–3 mm apart (Fig. 8.4). The bronchial anastomosis is then buttressed using the peribronchial donor bronchus tissue that is sutured to the recipient peribronchial tissue. The anastomosis is immediately inspected using a bronchoscope, and intra-airway secretions are cleared.

A curved vascular clamp is placed proximally on the PA, and the staple line is excised. The donor PA is trimmed, avoiding leaving the donor PA too long to avoid kinking of the artery. Stay sutures are placed at both ends starting from the donor PA, using the position of the first branch of the PA to orient the anastomosis and avoid

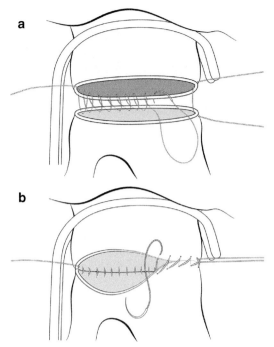

Fig. 8.5 Arterial anastomosis

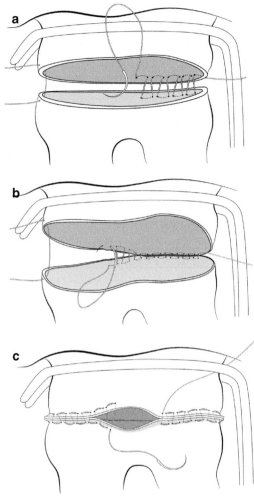

Fig. 8.6 Venous anastomosis

torsion. The anastomosis is performed in a continuous manner using a running 5-0 polypropylene suture interrupted in two places to prevent stenosis. After completing the front wall, 10–15 mL of saline is instilled into the PA lumen with 14 G angiocatheter to de-air. The PA sutures are then tied (Fig. 8.5).

The venous stumps are grasped with Judd-Allice clamps, and a left atrial clamp designed for use in this position (Scanlan Instruments, St. Paul, MN, USA) is placed proximally on the left atrium. The staple lines on the pulmonary veins are excised, and the orifices are joined to form a single atrial orifice for the atrial anastomosis. Corner stitches are placed. An "everting mattress" technique with clearly visualized endothelial to endothelial apposition is then performed using a running 4-0 polypropylene suture [49]. The suture is left untied at the anterior midpoint of the anastomosis for antegrade de-airing (Fig. 8.6).

The cooling jacket is removed, and the implanted lung allograft is gently inflated to a sustained airway pressure of 20 cmH$_2$O before reperfusion and then ventilated with an FiO$_2$ of less than 50%, PEEP of 5 cmH$_2$O, and pressure control ventilation limiting the peak airway pressure usually to 15–20 mmHg. When re-expansion of the graft is achieved, the PA clamp is partially opened to gradually reperfuse the lung, and, after de-airing, the atrial anastomosis suture is secured. The PA is kept partially clamped for 10 min to provide protective low-pressure, low shear stress initial reperfusion of the lung [50]. The patient is ventilated under pressure control or with tidal volumes approximately 5–7 mL/kg. Positive end-expiratory pressure (PEEP) is set at 5 cmH$_2$O. Hemostasis is carefully checked. The second lung is implanted in the same fashion. Two chest tubes are placed in each pleural space.

A straight one is placed toward the apex in the chest, and a curve chest tube is placed along the diaphragm on each side.

The transverse thoracosternotomy (clamshell) incision is closed using four figure of eight intercostal sutures on each side, and the sternum is approximated using three sternal wires. It is important to tie the pericostal sutures before securing the wires to avoid undue stress on the important wire closure.

Intraoperative Management of the Allograft

Cardiopulmonary Bypass/ECLS

The more commonly used device for intraoperative cardiopulmonary support during lung transplantation historically was standard cardiopulmonary bypass (CPB). Today, extracorporeal lung support (ECLS or ECMO) is being increasingly used. Approximately 60% of patients can undergo SLT or sequential BLT without the need for CPB support. The use of cardiorespiratory support is usually limited to patients with pulmonary hypertension or patients who cannot tolerate unilateral ventilation or perfusion. There are some centers that routinely use cardiopulmonary bypass for lung transplantation with positive outcomes [51]. One potentially beneficial effect is the ability to reperfuse the graft with controlled pulmonary artery pressures over a prolonged period of time. This benefit of providing controlled low-pressure reperfusion is counterbalanced by the pump-related inflammatory response leading to coagulopathy, neutrophil, and complement activation that can lead to organ injury [52, 53].

The use of extracorporeal membrane oxygenation (ECMO) as a bridge to transplant has been increasing. An increasing number of programs have expanded their use for the intraoperative period of lung transplantation. Some of the advantages of (ECMO) are the need for less anticoagulation (ACT 160–180 s is sufficient), a minimized circuit that requires lower priming volumes, and the lack of air-blood contact and

> **Box 8.4 Modifications of the ECMO Circuit: Toronto Lung Transplant Program**
>
> 1. For the right atrial cannulation, two purse strings are used with an umbilical tape snared around the cannula
> 2. Centrifugal pump with a lock mechanism in case of air entrainment
> 3. Maquet Quadrox oxygenator with de-airing ports
> 4. CPB circuit as a backup always available in operating room in the eventuality of any problem with the ECMO circuit
>
> Data from Machuga TN, Collaud S, Mercier O, Cheung M., Cunningham V, Kim SJ, et al.. Outcomes of intraoperative extracorporeal membrane oxygenation versus cardiopulmonary bypass for lung transplantation. J Thorac Cardiovasc Surg. 2015;149(4):1152–7

cardiotomy suction. All these translate into less coagulopathy and less systemic inflammatory response [54]. The Toronto Lung Transplant Program recently published their experience in which they demonstrated the advantages of using ECMO instead of CPB for intraoperative support in lung transplantation. The Toronto Lung Transplant Program Modifications of the ECMO circuit are described in Box 8.4. Patients who were supported intraoperatively with ECMO instead of CPB demonstrated a shorter duration of mechanical ventilation, had shorter ICU and hospital length of stay, and required less blood products during the perioperative period when compared with matched recipients who were supported with conventional CPB [54].

These findings suggest that ECLS/ECMO may be considered to be the preferred choice for intraoperative cardiopulmonary support for lung transplantation. Conventional CPB of course is required for patients undergoing lung transplantation and concomitant cardiac repair procedures, or in cases of complex atrial anastomosis requiring heart arrest, and in emergency situations such as massive intraoperative bleeding [54]. If one is on ECMO and the operative situation dictates the need for CPB, the circuits can be switched from ECMO to a full CPB circuit readily.

Protective Measures at the Time of Reperfusion

Mechanical ventilation can potentially add additional injury to already injured lungs. A number of studies have demonstrated that mechanical ventilation can worsen preexisting lung injury [22]. The exact effect of different modes of ventilation has not been addressed yet. Animal studies have shown better lung function if protective ventilation is implemented. The lung graft should be re-inflated first with a sustained airway pressure of 20 cmH_2O to gently recruit alveolar units before reperfusion and then ventilated with a low FiO_2, PEEP of 5 cmH_2O, and pressure control with a peak airway pressure of less than 25 cmH_2O [55].

The pulmonary artery pressure is crucial during the initial period of reperfusion. The endothelial permeability is increased during this phase. Pulmonary edema and further lung damage can be the consequence of a rapid reperfusion [22]. Studies have shown an improved lung function in transplanted lungs reperfused gradually in a controlled fashion over a 10-min period [50].

Surgical Complications in the Recipient

Early Postoperative Complications

Ischemia-Reperfusion-Induced Injury: Primary Graft Dysfunction

Ischemia-reperfusion (IR)-induced lung injury is an acute syndrome that occurs within the first 72 h of the posttransplant period [56, 57]. It is characterized by alveolar damage (pulmonary infiltrates in chest X-ray), lung edema, and hypoxemia [40]. The severe form of IR injury leads to primary graft dysfunction (PGD), and it represents one of the most serious complications during the early postoperative period. PGD is the end result of a series of aggressions starting in the donor and until the lung reperfusion after transplantation. Ischemia-reperfusion injury has been identified as the main cause of primary graft failure, but there are other insults that happen to the

donor before retrieving the lungs (mechanical ventilation, brain death, aspiration, contusion, infection, edema, hypotension, atelectasis, etc.) that also exacerbate the inflammatory response of ischemia and reperfusion [40].

The incidence reported of severe PGD varies between 11 and 25% [56, 58]. When it comes to the clinical presentation, this syndrome behaves similar to the acute respiratory distress syndrome (ARDS) [59]. PGD is also associated with a 20–30% mortality rate in the first month after lung transplant, and studies have demonstrated worse long-term survival [58, 60, 61]. The International Society for Heart and Lung Transplantation (ISHLT) established a classification in 2005 giving the clinical syndrome a grading system from 1 to 3 based on PaO_2/FiO_2 (P/F) and pulmonary edema represented by radiographic infiltrates in the transplanted lung [56, 60]. The specific pathophysiologic mechanisms leading to IR lung injury and PGD are multifactorial and represent an active field of investigation.

At the present time, there is no recognized effective therapy for the prevention or treatment of PGD. The treatment remains mainly supportive using lung-protective ventilation strategies. Inhaled nitric oxide may be useful in patients with refractory hypoxemia secondary to PGD [62]. Patients with severe graft failure may need extracorporeal membrane oxygenation (ECMO) for ventilatory support.

Therapies delivered in vivo and ex vivo to treat or avoid PGD are currently being tested in different settings. Ex vivo lung perfusion (EVLP) is a normothermic preservation method initially described by Steen and colleagues to assess organs from donors after cardiac death [63]. This method has been further developed by Cypel and colleagues to potentially improve lung quality and repair injured donor lungs aiming to avoid the development of PGD after transplantation [64]. During EVLP, drugs can be delivered for different possible targets including treatment of infections with antibiotics, antiviral, and antifungal agents; disintegration of microthrombi with fibrinolytic agents; and removal of interstitial edema with high osmotic agents among others. These drugs can also be administered at higher than usual doses directly to the lungs without the fear of collateral drug toxicity to other organs. Drugs can be added to the perfusate or injected into the afferent tubing running to the vasculature of the lung. They can also be delivered endotracheally [65].

Mesenchymal stem cells (MSCs) intrapulmonary and intravascular are being studied for their potential anti-inflammatory and antibacterial properties [66, 67]. IL-10 gene therapy delivered intrabronchial during EVLP has proven in preclinical studies to attenuate posttransplant injury [46, 68–74]. Other therapies include complement inhibition with a soluble complement receptor-1 [75] and bronchoscopic administration of exogenous surfactant [76], before reperfusion pioglitazone treatment [77], among others [78].

Atrial Arrhythmias

Atrial arrhythmias presented as atrial fibrillation (AF) and atrial tachycardia (AT) represent a common complication after any cardiothoracic surgery. The exact mechanisms that conducts to atrial arrhythmias are unknown and include electrophysiological abnormalities that may be worsened by inflammation in the early postoperative period [79].

The incidence reported varies between 10 and 50% and is more frequent during the immediate postoperative period and during the first month after transplant, usually before hospital discharge [80].

Pulmonary fibrosis, advance age, coronary disease diagnosed pretransplant, enlarged LA, and postoperative vasopressors are factors known to increase the risk for developing AF [81].

It is known that the pulmonary veins play a major role in the development and maintenance of several kinds of atrial arrhythmias. Atrial fibrillation (AF) can be initiated by ectopic beats from pulmonary veins [82, 83]. During the lung transplant surgery, the recipient superior and inferior pulmonary veins are manipulated, divided, and anastomosed as a single venous cuff to the donor left atrium. This left atrial anastomosis may produce blockages or slow the conduction that can lead to electroanatomic substrate for reentry [80].

The presence of posttransplant atrial arrhythmias has been associated in several studies with prolonged hospital stay and increased mortality [81, 84, 85].

Pleural Complications

A significant population of lung transplant patients present with a pleural complication during the postoperative period. The incidence in series reported is between 22 [86] and 35% [87]. This is not surprising since the pleural space is exposed and gets manipulated during the surgery. Many of the patients have had previous procedures involving the pleural space such as lung resections, biopsies, or pleurodesis. The underlying disease can play a major role in the incidence of pleural complications, such as patients with pulmonary infection (cystic fibrosis) or previous pneumothoraces. The transbronchial biopsies performed as part of transplant surveillance protocols can also be the cause of chronic pleural complications. Immunosuppression can lead to infection of the pleural space [86].

Pleural Effusion

Most lung transplant recipients develop effusions in the immediate postoperative period. This early postoperative effusion is generally ipsilateral to the transplanted lung. The pleural fluid in the immediate postoperative period is a combination of blood and lymphatic drainage, rich in neutrophils and lactate dehydrogenase, that decreases progressively in the following 7 days [88, 89].

There are several explanations for the accumulation of pleural fluid in the early postoperative period after lung transplantation. It is well known that alveolar capillaries have increased permeability for the first several days. That is because of allograft ischemia, denervation, or disruption and remodeling of the capillaries, which occurs between the second and fourth week after transplantation [87]. The pleural effusion often resolves by itself. Pleural drainage should stay in place until the output is less than 200 mL/24 h [87, 89]. Other causes of pleural effusion after lung transplant include a significant positive fluid balance in the postoperative state and acute graft rejection [87].

Hemothorax

Hemothorax is one of the most common surgical complications immediately after lung transplant and the primary reason for reoperation. The persistence of bleeding can lead to hemodynamic problems increasing the fluid and blood product transfusion requirements. Hemothorax can present at any time after transplant either early on or even weeks after the procedure. The blood rarely comes from the vascular anastomosis since that is addressed during the surgery. The main cause is bleeding from the mediastinal dissection or divided pleural adhesions [90]. Factors that contribute to bleeding from adhesions include fibrotic and vascular pleuropulmonary adhesions (bronchiectasis, tuberculosis, silicosis, previous thoracic surgery). Cardiopulmonary bypass or ECMO during transplant, ECMO after transplant, and patients requiring anticoagulants or antiplatelet agents are more at risk to bleed after transplant. This complication is associated with increased postoperative morbidity and mortality [91]. Treatment of hemothorax includes correction of the coagulation abnormalities, fluid management, and early surgical intervention to evacuate clot and optimize hemostasis.

Chylothorax

Chylothorax has a low incidence after transplant. It is usually the result of thoracic duct injuries. An appropriate diet combined with chest drains is usually enough to achieve chylothorax resolution. Lymphangioleiomyomatosis can be a cause of refractory bilateral chylothorax. Postoperative refractory chylothorax may cause nutritional deficiencies, respiratory dysfunction, and dehydration [92]. Refractory chylothorax has been effectively controlled in some cases with somatostatin administration, pleuroperitoneal shunt, and chemical pleurodesis with sclerosing agents including talc. The combination of the immunosuppressed patient and significant lymph loss (protein, fluid, lymphocytes) can be life-threatening. If chyle drainage is excessive and persistent, lymphatic embolization by an inter-ventional radiologist or reoperation to ligate the duct and/or seal the leak may be required.

Pneumothorax

Pneumothorax can occur any time after chest drains removal. It is most likely to happen when the lung does not fill the cavity because of a size discrepancy between donor's graft and recipient. This may occur in patients with emphysema who have significant pretransplant lung hyperinflation. Pneumothorax can also occur in the non-transplanted lung in patients receiving single-lung transplantation. Patients receiving a single-lung for emphysema can experience hyperinflation of the native lung with mediastinal compression. It is important to prevent this event with early extubation. Most pneumothoraces are related to pleural issues such as small tears in the donor lung or related to surgery. If a new pneumothorax appears 7–10 days after transplant, a bronchoscopy should be performed to make sure that it is not due to a rare, but possible, bronchial dehiscence.

Vascular Anastomotic Complications

Vascular complications should be and are rare. They occur in 1–3% of lung transplants [90, 93]. These complications have very high mortality and morbidity. Vascular complications can be kinking of the anastomosis developing obstruction because of excessive length of the artery or anastomotic misalignment. Other problems include stricture of the suture anastomosis due to technique or technical issues. Other complications described include intraluminal obstruction to flow (thrombosis or dissection). It has been proposed that lower pulmonary veins and particularly the left lower vein are more predisposed to stenosis and thrombosis because of their anatomical disposition [90]. Women with restrictive pathology have increased incidence of anastomotic complications. This may be related to smaller thoracic cavities, making the anastomoses more challenging and a relatively restricted space for the larger implanted lung. Pulmonary vein obstruction is an early complication presenting the first hours after transplant. The risk of infarction is greater immediately after transplant because the new lung does not have alternative blood flow from the bronchial circulation [94]. It should be clinically suspected when a patient presents with severe hypoxia and pulmonary edema. This must be differentiated from primary graft dysfunction (sometimes difficult to do), infection, and rejection.

Transthoracic or transesophageal echocardiogram should be performed by an experienced operator due to the challenging visualization and interpretation after recent surgery. CT angiography with reconstructions assesses the pulmonary arterial anastomosis and distal vascularization. A CT angiogram can also clearly visualize the venous anastomoses. Arterial vascular complications are less common, and they present later after transplant. Patients develop pulmonary hypertension with hypoxia. Some degree of relative stenosis seen on CT angiography is common due to donor-recipient size differences. Significant stenosis is due to kinking or thrombosis at the suture.

The treatment depends on the degree of the vascular complication. Conservative management is sufficient for mild obstruction, especially if the stenosis is in one lung in a bilateral lung transplant recipient. Some stenoses can be treated with balloon angioplasty dilatation. Patients with thrombosis should receive anticoagulant therapy. If the thrombosis is severe enough to cause infarction of the lung, surgical intervention should be considered even knowing the poor prognosis. Significant stenosis in the arterial or venous anastomosis with clinical compromise requires urgent intervention either with a catheter (angioplasty, dilatation with or without stenting) or surgery. The type of intervention depends on the time that has elapsed after transplant; endovascular procedures are used more often for alterations found weeks after transplant. Urgent surgery should be considered in patients diagnosed at an earlier stage presenting with severe respiratory and hemodynamic compromise, especially if the alteration is due to a misorientation. Infarction of the graft because of prolonged ischemia may need anatomic resection of the lung or even re-transplantation. Re-intervention in these types of patients has a high morbidity and mortality rate even in expert hands. Prognosis of the vascular complications depends on the early diagnosis and the selection of the most appropriate therapy.

Late Postoperative Complications

Pleural Complications

Empyema
Empyema is an uncommon complication; however, it is associated with increased morbidity and mortality. Empyema usually occurs within the first 6 months following transplant surgery and generally not during the immediate postoperative period. The development of empyema is likely related to the usual issues: major surgery, "clean-contaminated" surgery where the airway was open, persistent spaces in the pleural cavity where the new lungs may incompletely fill or fit the recipient chest, and an immunosuppressed patient. In general, significant pleural collections should be sampled and rained in the lung transplant patient, as immunosuppression may mask the usual signs of sepsis.

Airway Complications
The reported incidence of airway complications is very variable and could be explained by the absence of standardized definitions. The incidence varies from 1.6 to 33% [95]. According to a number of studies, 9–13% of all bronchial anastomoses at some point may develop complications severe enough to require intervention [96, 97]. The incidence today, however, is much lower than in the early experience of lung transplantation [98].

Airway complications are primarily attributed to ischemia of the bronchus during the immediate posttransplant period. This can be largely prevented by meticulous attention to lung preservation and to surgical technique. Donor lungs lose the bronchial flow component of the dual blood supply that normal lungs have at the level of the main bronchus. The implanted donor lung bronchus depends completely on the collateral perfusion (pulmonary artery to bronchial collateral circulation) until revascularization by the recipient's bronchial arteries is achieved (2–4 weeks) [96].

Postoperative factors such as low cardiac output, sepsis, hypotension, severe vasoconstriction, or dehydration may decrease the blood flow in this fragile microcirculation, increasing the risk of airway ischemia. The length of donor bronchus is vital in order to decrease the ischemia. Shortening the donor bronchus as close as possible to the secondary carina has been demonstrated to reduce anastomotic ischemia [99–101]. During the surgery (donor and recipient), surgical dissection is performed with minimal manipulation using a "no touch" technique to leave the peribronchial tissue as intact as possible, preserving the collateral microvasculature. Reinforcing the anastomosis with peribronchial vascularized tissue helps protect the bronchial anastomosis. Preoperative and postoperative pulmonary infections are known as an important risk factor for airway complications [102, 103]. Posttransplant anastomotic infections predispose to the development of dehiscence, stenosis, malacia, fistulas, and granulation tissue [95]. Sirolimus in posttransplant should be avoided since it has shown to increase the rate of severe airway complications including dehiscence. Reperfusion injury increases interstitial edema and compromises pulmonary microcirculatory blood flow [97, 102].

Bronchial Dehiscence

Dehiscence is thankfully a rare complication nowadays and presents usually in the early postoperative period as a result of poor airway healing. The clinical presentation depends on the severity of the dehiscence (partial or complete). Most frequently, air leakage through chest drains is noted, or a pneumothorax and subcutaneous emphysema is noted when drains have already been removed. Patients with more extensive dehiscence present with sepsis. Other common presentations include dyspnea, inability to wean from mechanical ventilation, pneumomediastinum, lung collapse, or persistent air leak. Diagnosis is based on bronchoscopy and CT scan. On CT, dehiscence can be identified as bronchial wall defects, bronchial narrowing, bronchial wall irregularities, and air around the

anastomosis [104]. CT has 100% sensitivity and 94% specificity for dehiscence detection compared with bronchoscopy [105]. However, the CT does not show mucosal necrosis which is the earliest sign and a useful predictor of dehiscence. Flexible bronchoscopy is required for the definitive diagnosis [105]. Management of dehiscence depends on the severity of the dehiscence and on the clinical presentation. Severe cases require open surgical repair for reanastomosis, flap bronchoplasty, or even re-transplantation. These procedures have a very high risk, and the results are generally poor. Some groups have reported good outcomes with temporary placement of self-expanding metallic stents in life-threatening dehiscences [95]. Small defects (4 mm or less) often have excellent clinical outcomes with conservative management. The chest drains must remain in place. Regular aspiration and monitoring bronchoscopies should be performed to follow the healing process. Proper antibiotic and antifungal therapy should be given if needed. Any fluid collections in the mediastinum should be drained.

Bronchial Stenosis

Bronchial stenosis is a more commonly seen airway complication. It is usually not an immediate posttransplant complication: most of them present after 2–3 months posttransplant. They are the result of an abnormal healing process. There are two types of bronchial stenosis: one that appears at the surgical anastomosis and the other at the segmental non-anastomotic bronchus. Segmental non-anastomotic bronchial stenosis is less frequent. The more frequent among them is involving the bronchus intermedius (BI) [106, 107]. The so-called vanishing bronchus intermedius syndrome is a severe form of bronchial stenosis of the BI associated with high morbidity and mortality. Bronchial stenosis is thought to be the consequence of airway inflammation and immunologic cytolytic airway damage and possibly complicated by vasospasm, ischemia, or microvascular injury. Perivascular mononuclear cells injure the endothelium, decreasing the blood flow to the proximal airways and exacerbating the already reduced flow from the loss of the bronchial circulation [108]. Diagnosis requires flexible bronchoscopy. Computed tomography should be performed in order to assess the stenosis length and plan a possible treatment if the stenosis is greater than 50% of the bronchus diameter. Multisection CT with 2D and 3D reconstructions is very useful, allowing measurements required to address the possible treatments. Spirometry can show a decline in the forced expiratory flow (FEF 25–75) and the peak expiratory flow (PEF). Standard management includes endoscopic therapies including balloon dilatation, dilatation with rigid bronchoscopy, and stent placement. Other therapies such as electrocautery, cryotherapy, laser, and brachytherapy have also been described, but evidence for efficacy in this setting is scant. Mild stenosis without granulation tissue can be managed with periodic fiberoptic bronchoscopy-guided balloon dilatations or rigid bronchoscopic dilatations. It is a relatively safe procedure with very low morbidity and can provide immediate relief and improvement of the flows. Dilatation induces less granulation tissue, but in some patients a fibrotic scar may form in the area of previous dilatations. It is important to relieve the obstruction from a stricture not only for airway flows but also to decrease the entrapment of secretions that perpetuates an inflammation-swelling-stenosis-infection cycle. If repeated dilatations are not sufficient to maintain airway patency, then one resorts to stent placement. There are many types of stents constructed of various different materials: silicone, metal, fixed or self-expanding, etc. Whenever possible, it is desirable to use a removable silicone stent, which is capable of stenting the airway for 2–3 months, while it heals and remodels; it can then be removed. If all interventions fail, there are surgical procedures that can be performed including reconstruction, sleeve resections of the strictured area, lobar resections, or re-transplantation.

Granulation Tissue

Exophytic benign granulating tissue can sometimes present weeks to months after surgery. It is likely the result of the ischemia, healing, and remodeling process that involves overstimulation and inflammation. *Aspergillus* at the anastomosis can produce more granulation and inflammation, worsening the problem. Some of these granulations are small and resolve spontaneously. However, sometimes they present clinically with symptoms of obstruction: cough, dyspnea, hypoxia, or obstructive pneumonia. Spirometry shows a decrease in pulmonary function, and bronchoscopy confirms the diagnosis. The treatment is the debridement of the tissue, usually with forceps in either fiber-optic or rigid bronchoscopy, as required. Cryotherapy, YAG laser vaporization, argon plasma, or electrocautery has also been used in this setting [109], but care must be taken not to induce further injury to the airway with these energy and ablative modalities. Topical mitomycin C has also been applied to granulation tissue with the theoretical intent to reduce the proliferation of fibroblasts and so to halt the development of granulation tissue and stenosis.

Bronchomalacia

Bronchomalacia is sometimes seen in a transplanted lung. It is defined as a narrowing of 50% or more of the airway lumen on expiration. Bronchomalacia is most commonly seen more than 3–4 months after lung transplantation. It behaves as a dynamic stenosis. Patients present with cough, dyspnea, difficulty to expectorate, stridor, recurrent infections, and changes in spirometry behaving as an obstructive disease (decrease in the forced expiratory flow of 25–75%, low peak expiratory rate, and reduction of the FEV_1). Diagnosis requires bronchoscopy and CT reconstructions or dynamic inspiratory-expiratory CT. The treatment depends on the severity of the airway narrowing and airway collapse. Asymptomatic patients do not require any treatment. Symptomatic patients may need nocturnal noninvasive positive-pressure ventilation or airway stenting. The etiology of this is often related to leaving too long a recipient or donor airway, although sometimes it is idiopathic. This issue can be avoided by keeping both the recipient and the donor bronchi short at the time of anastomosis as described above.

Summary

More than 30 years after the first successful clinical lung transplant, this procedure is now being applied more and more commonly around the world. With advances in donor management and the ability to salvage more donor organs, the application of lung transplantation as effective therapy for patients with end-stage lung disease will continue to increase.

A lung transplant operation remains a complex procedure with multiple steps and significant technical challenges. Optimal results depend on the meticulous attention to detail in donor lung management and preservation, the conduct of the implant operation, and the management of the recipient intraoperatively and postoperatively by an experienced lung transplant team. As in any major surgery, the best results are achieved with attention to detail and preventative steps to avoid complications but also with astute and early recognition and management of complications when they occur.

References

1. Orens JB, Boehler A, de Perrot M, Estenne M, Glanville AR, Keshavjee S, et al. A review of lung transplant donor acceptability criteria. J Heart Lung Transplant. 2003;22(11):1183–200.
2. Pierre AF, Keshavjee S. Lung transplantation: donor and recipient critical care aspects. Curr Opin Crit Care. 2005;11(4):339–44.
3. Botha P. Extended donor criteria in lung transplantation. Curr Opin Organ Transplant. 2009;14(2):206–10.
4. Cypel M, Keshavjee S. Strategies for safe donor expansion: donor management, donations after cardiac death, ex-vivo lung perfusion. Curr Opin Organ Transplant. 2013;18(5):513–7.
5. Daemen JW, Kootstra G, Wijnen RM, Yin M, Heineman E. Nonheart-beating donors: the Maastricht experience. Clin Transpl. 1994:303–16.
6. Levvey BJ, Harkess M, Hopkins P, Chambers D, Merry C, Glanville AR, et al. Excellent clinical outcomes from a national donation-after-determination-of-cardiac-death lung transplant collaborative. Am J Transplant. 2012;12(9):2406–13.
7. Cypel M, Sato M, Yildirim E, Karolak W, Chen F, Yeung J, et al. Initial experience with lung dona-tion after cardiocirculatory death in Canada. J Heart Lung Transplant. 2009;28(8):753–8.
8. De Oliveira NC, Osaki S, Maloney JD, Meyer KC, Kohmoto T, D'Alessandro AM, et al. Lung transplantation with donation after cardiac death donors: long-term follow-up in a single center. J Thorac Cardiovasc Surg. 2010;139(5):1306–15.
9. Love RB. Perspectives on lung transplantation and donation-after-determination-of-cardiac-death donors. Am J Transplant. 2012;12(9):2271–2.
10. Munshi L, Keshavjee S, Cypel M. Donor management and lung preservation for lung transplantation. Lancet Respir Med. 2013;1(4):318–28.
11. Franklin GA, Santos AP, Smith JW, Galbraith S, Harbrecht BG, Garrison RN. Optimization of donor management goals yields increased organ use. Am Surg. 2010;76(6):587–94.
12. Toyoda Y, McCurry KR. Prior cardiac surgery is not a contraindication for lung donor. Ann Thorac Surg. 2007;84(1):314–6.
13. Das De S, Nenekidis I, Itrakjy A, Mascaro J. Bilateral lung transplantation from a donor with previous aortic valve surgery. Asian Cardiovasc Thorac Ann. 2016;24(4):375–7.
14. Schmidt F, McGiffin DC, Zorn G, Young KR, Weill D, Kirklin JK. Management of congenital abnormalities of the donor lung. Ann Thorac Surg. 2001;72(3):935–7.
15. Sekine Y, Fischer S, de Perrot M, Pierre AF, Keshavjee S. Bilateral lung transplantation using a donor with a tracheal right upper lobe bronchus. Ann Thorac Surg. 2002;73(1):308–10.
16. Brichon PY, Blin D, Perez I, Pison C, Blanc-Jouvan F, Pin I, et al. Double-lung transplantation using donor lungs with a right tracheal bronchus. Ann Thorac Surg. 1992;54(4):777–8.
17. Olland A, Reeb J, Falcoz PE, Garnon J, Germain P, Santelmo N, et al. Anomalous pulmonary venous return of the left upper lobe in a donor lung. Ann Thorac Surg. 2015;99(6):2199–202.
18. Khasati NH, MacHaal A, Thekkudan J, Kumar S, Yonan N. An aberrant donor pulmonary vein during lung transplant: a surgical challenge. Ann Thorac Surg. 2005;79(1):330–1.
19. Melvan JN, Force SD, Sancheti MS. Anatomic resection to manage donor partial anomalous pulmonary venous return during lung transplantation: a case report and review. Transplant Proc. 2015;47(3):846–8.
20. Machuca TN, Cypel M, Keshavjee S. Advances in lung preservation. Surg Clin North Am. 2013;93(6):1373–94.
21. Hall SM, Komai H, Reader J, Haworth SG. Donor lung preservation: effect of cold preservation fluids on cultured pulmonary endothelial cells. Am J Physiol. 1994;267(5 Pt 1):L508–17.
22. de Perrot M, Keshavjee S. Lung preservation. Semin Thorac Cardiovasc Surg. 2004;16(4):300–8.

23. Fujimura S, Handa M, Kondo T, Ichinose T, Shiraishi Y, Nakada T. Successful 48-hour simple hypothermic preservation of canine lung transplants. Transplant Proc. 1987;19(1 Pt 2):1334–6.

24. Keshavjee SH, Yamazaki F, Cardoso PF, McRitchie DI, Patterson GA, Cooper JD. A method for safe twelve-hour pulmonary preservation. J Thorac Cardiovasc Surg. 1989;98(4):529–34.

25. Date H, Matsumura A, Manchester JK, Obo H, Lima O, Cooper JM, et al. Evaluation of lung metabolism during successful twenty-four-hour canine lung preservation. J Thorac Cardiovasc Surg. 1993;105(3):480–91.

26. Thabut G, Vinatier I, Brugiere O, Leseche G, Loirat P, Bisson A, et al. Influence of preservation solution on early graft failure in clinical lung transplantation. Am J Respir Crit Care Med. 2001;164(7):1204–8.

27. Fischer S, Matte-Martyn A, De Perrot M, Waddell TK, Sekine Y, Hutcheon M, et al. Low-potassium dextran preservation solution improves lung function after human lung transplantation. J Thorac Cardiovasc Surg. 2001;121(3):594–6.

28. Arnaoutakis GJ, Allen JG, Merlo CA, Baumgartner WA, Conte JV, Shah AS. Low potassium dextran is superior to University of Wisconsin solution in high-risk lung transplant recipients. J Heart Lung Transplant. 2010;29(12):1380–7.

29. Wang LS, Nakamoto K, Hsieh CM, Miyoshi S, Cooper JD. Influence of temperature of flushing solution on lung preservation. Ann Thorac Surg. 1993;55(3):711–5.

30. Date H, Lima O, Matsumura A, Tsuji H, d'Avignon DA, Cooper JD. In a canine model, lung preservation at 10 degrees C is superior to that at 4 degrees C. A comparison of two preservation temperatures on lung function and on adenosine triphosphate level measured by phosphorus 31-nuclear magnetic resonance. J Thorac Cardiovasc Surg. 1992;103(4):773–80.

31. Albes JM, Fischer F, Bando T, Heinemann MK, Scheule A, Wahlers T. Influence of the perfusate temperature on lung preservation: is there an optimum? Eur Surg Res. 1997;29(1):5–11.

32. Struber M, Hohlfeld JM, Kofidis T, Warnecke G, Niedermeyer J, Sommer SP, et al. Surfactant function in lung transplantation after 24 hours of ischemia: advantage of retrograde flush perfusion for preservation. J Thorac Cardiovasc Surg. 2002;123(1):98–103.

33. Baretti R, Bitu-Moreno J, Beyersdorf F, Matheis G, Francischetti I, Kreitmayr B. Distribution of lung preservation solutions in parenchyma and airways: influence of atelectasis and route of delivery. J Heart Lung Transplant. 1995;14(1 Pt 1):80–91.

34. Sakuma T, Tsukano C, Ishigaki M, Nambu Y, Osanai K, Toga H, et al. Lung deflation impairs alveolar epithelial fluid transport in ischemic rabbit and rat lungs. Transplantation. 2000;69(9):1785–93.

35. Haniuda M, Hasegawa S, Shiraishi T, Dresler CM, Cooper JD, Patterson GA. Effects of inflation volume during lung preservation on pulmonary capillary permeability. J Thorac Cardiovasc Surg. 1996;112(1):85–93.

36. Kirk AJ, Colquhoun IW, Dark JH. Lung preservation: a review of current practice and future directions. Ann Thorac Surg. 1993;56(4):990–100.

37. Kayano K, Toda K, Naka Y, Pinsky DJ. Identification of optimal conditions for lung graft storage with Euro-Collins solution by use of a rat orthotopic lung transplant model. Circulation. 1999;100(19 Suppl):II257–61.

38. de Perrot M, Fischer S, Liu M, Jin R, Bai XH, Waddell TK, et al. Prostaglandin E1 protects lung transplants from ischemia-reperfusion injury: a shift from pro- to anti-inflammatory cytokines. Transplantation. 2001;72(9):1505–12.

39. Chen CZ, Gallagher RC, Ardery P, Dyckman W, Donabue S, Low HB. Retrograde flush and cold storage for twenty-two to twenty-five hours lung preservation with and without prostaglandin E1. J Heart Lung Transplant. 1997;16(6):658–66.

40. de Perrot M, Liu M, Waddell TK, Keshavjee S. Ischemia-reperfusion-induced lung injury. Am J Respir Crit Care Med. 2003;167(4):490–511.

41. Steen S, Liao Q, Wierup PN, Bolys R, Pierre L, Sjoberg T. Transplantation of lungs from non-heart-beating donors after functional assessment ex vivo. Ann Thorac Surg. 2003;76(1):244–52, discussion 252

42. Steen S, Ingemansson R, Eriksson L, Pierre L, Algotsson L, Wierup P, et al. First human transplantation of a nonacceptable donor lung after reconditioning ex vivo. Ann Thorac Surg. 2007;83(6):2191–4.

43. Erasmus ME, Fernhout MH, Elstrodt JM, Rakhorst G. Normothermic ex vivo lung perfusion of non-heart-beating donor lungs in pigs: from pretransplant function analysis towards a 6-h machine preservation. Transpl Int. 2006;19(7):589–93.

44. Cypel M, Yeung JC, Hirayama S, Rubacha M, Fischer S, Anraku M, et al. Technique for prolonged normothermic ex vivo lung perfusion. J Heart Lung Transplant. 2008;27(12):1319–25.

45. Cypel M, Yeung JC, Machuca T, Chen M, Singer LG, Yasufuku K, et al. Experience with the first 50 ex vivo lung perfusions in clinical transplantation. J Thorac Cardiovasc Surg. 2012;144(5):1200–6.

46. Cypel M, Liu M, Rubacha M, Yeung JC, Hirayama S, Anraku M, et al. Functional repair of human donor lungs by IL-10 gene therapy. Sci Transl Med. 2009;1(4):4ra9.

47. Andreasson AS, Dark JH, Fisher AJ. Ex vivo lung perfusion in clinical lung transplantation–state of the art. Eur J Cardiothorac Surg. 2014;46(5):779–88.

48. Warnecke G, Moradiellos J, Tudorache I, Kuhn C, Avsar M, Wiegmann B, et al. Normothermic perfusion of donor lungs for preservation and assessment with the Organ Care System Lung before bilateral transplantation: a pilot study of 12 patients. Lancet. 2012;380(9856):1851–8.

49. de Perrot M, Keshavjee S. Everting mattress running suture: an improved technique of atrial anastomosis

in human lung transplantation. Ann Thorac Surg. 2002;73(5):1663–4.

50. Pierre AF, DeCampos KN, Liu M, Edwards V, Cutz E, Slutsky AS, et al. Rapid reperfusion causes stress failure in ischemic rat lungs. J Thorac Cardiovasc Surg. 1998;116(6):932–42.

51. Marczin N, Royston D, Yacoub M. Pro: lung transplantation should be routinely performed with cardiopulmonary bypass. J Cardiothorac Vasc Anesth. 2000;14(6):739–45.

52. McRae K. Con: lung transplantation should not be routinely performed with cardiopulmonary bypass. J Cardiothorac Vasc Anesth. 2000;14(6):746–50.

53. Zangrillo A, Garozzo FA, Biondi-Zoccai G, Pappalardo F, Monaco F, Crivellari M, et al. Miniaturized cardiopulmonary bypass improves short-term outcome in cardiac surgery: a meta-analysis of randomized controlled studies. J Thorac Cardiovasc Surg. 2010;139(5):1162–9.

54. Machuca TN, Collaud S, Mercier O, Cheung M, Cunningham V, Kim SJ, et al. Outcomes of intraoperative extracorporeal membrane oxygenation versus cardiopulmonary bypass for lung transplantation. J Thorac Cardiovasc Surg. 2015;149(4):1152–7.

55. de Perrot M, Imai Y, Volgyesi GA, Waddell TK, Liu M, Mullen JB, et al. Effect of ventilator-induced lung injury on the development of reperfusion injury in a rat lung transplant model. J Thorac Cardiovasc Surg. 2002;124(6):1137–44.

56. Christie JD, Carby M, Bag R, Corris P, Hertz M, Weill D, et al. Report of the ISHLT Working Group on Primary Lung Graft Dysfunction part II: definition. A consensus statement of the International Society for Heart and Lung Transplantation. J Heart Lung Transplant. 2005;24(10):1454–9.

57. Christie JD, Bavaria JE, Palevsky HI, Litzky L, Blumenthal NP, Kaiser LR, et al. Primary graft failure following lung transplantation. Chest. 1998;114(1):51–60.

58. Yusen RD, Edwards LB, Kucheryavaya AY, Benden C, Dipchand AI, Goldfarb SB, et al. The Registry of the International Society for Heart and Lung Transplantation: thirty-second official adult lung and heart-lung transplantation report–2015; focus theme: early graft failure. J Heart Lung Transplant. 2015;34(10):1264–77.

59. Christie JD, Bellamy S, Ware LB, Lederer D, Hadjiliadis D, Lee J, et al. Construct validity of the definition of primary graft dysfunction after lung transplantation. J Heart Lung Transplant. 2010;29(11):1231–9.

60. Porteous MK, Diamond JM, Christie JD. Primary graft dysfunction: lessons learned about the first 72 h after lung transplantation. Curr Opin Organ Transplant. 2015;20(5):506–14.

61. Lee JC, Christie JD, Keshavjee S. Primary graft dysfunction: definition, risk factors, short- and long-term outcomes. Semin Respir Crit Care Med. 2010;31(2):161–71.

62. Meade MO, Granton JT, Matte-Martyn A, McRae K, Weaver B, Cripps P, et al. A randomized trial of inhaled nitric oxide to prevent ischemia-reperfusion injury after lung transplantation. Am J Respir Crit Care Med. 2003;167(11):1483–9.

63. Steen S, Sjoberg T, Pierre L, Liao Q, Eriksson L, Algotsson L. Transplantation of lungs from a non-heart-beating donor. Lancet. 2001;357(9259):825–9.

64. Cypel M, Yeung JC, Liu M, Anraku M, Chen F, Karolak W, et al. Normothermic ex vivo lung perfusion in clinical lung transplantation. N Engl J Med. 2011;364(15):1431–40.

65. Van Raemdonck D, Neyrinck A, Cypel M, Keshavjee S. Ex-vivo lung perfusion. Transpl Int. 2015;28(6):643–56.

66. Lee JW, Fang X, Gupta N, Serikov V, Matthay MA. Allogeneic human mesenchymal stem cells for treatment of E. coli endotoxin-induced acute lung injury in the ex vivo perfused human lung. Proc Natl Acad Sci U S A. 2009;106(38):16357–62.

67. Lee JW, Krasnodembskaya A, McKenna DH, Song Y, Abbott J, Matthay MA. Therapeutic effects of human mesenchymal stem cells in ex vivo human lungs injured with live bacteria. Am J Respir Crit Care Med. 2013;187(7):751–60.

68. Cassivi SD, Liu M, Boehler A, Tanswell AK, Slutsky AS, Keshavjee S, et al. Transgene expression after adenovirus-mediated retransfection of rat lungs is increased and prolonged by transplant immunosuppression. J Thorac Cardiovasc Surg. 1999;117(1):1–7.

69. de Perrot M, Fischer S, Liu M, Imai Y, Martins S, Sakiyama S, et al. Impact of human interleukin-10 on vector-induced inflammation and early graft function in rat lung transplantation. Am J Respir Cell Mol Biol. 2003;28(5):616–25.

70. de Waal Malefyt R, Abrams J, Bennett B, Figdor CG, de Vries JE. Interleukin 10(IL-10) inhibits cytokine synthesis by human monocytes: an autoregulatory role of IL-10 produced by monocytes. J Exp Med. 1991;174(5):1209–20.

71. Fischer S, De Perrot M, Liu M, MacLean AA, Cardella JA, Imai Y, et al. Interleukin 10 gene transfection of donor lungs ameliorates posttransplant cell death by a switch from cellular necrosis to apoptosis. J Thorac Cardiovasc Surg. 2003;126(4):1174–80.

72. Fischer S, Liu M, MacLean AA, de Perrot M, Ho M, Cardella JA, et al. In vivo transtracheal adenovirus-mediated transfer of human interleukin-10 gene to donor lungs ameliorates ischemia-reperfusion injury and improves early posttransplant graft function in the rat. Hum Gene Ther. 2001;12(12):1513–26.

73. Martins S, de Perrot M, Imai Y, Yamane M, Quadri SM, Segall L, et al. Transbronchial administration of adenoviral-mediated interleukin-10 gene to the donor improves function in a pig lung transplant model. Gene Ther. 2004;11(24):1786–96.

74. Yeung JC, Wagnetz D, Cypel M, Rubacha M, Koike T, Chun YM, et al. Ex vivo adenoviral vector gene delivery results in decreased vector-associated inflammation pre- and post-lung transplantation in the pig. Mol Ther. 2012;20(6):1204–11.

75. Keshavjee S, Davis RD, Zamora MR, de Perrot M, Patterson GA. A randomized, placebo-controlled trial of complement inhibition in ischemia-reperfusion injury after lung transplantation in human beings. J Thorac Cardiovasc Surg. 2005;129(2):423–8.

76. Kermeen FD, McNeil KD, Fraser JF, McCarthy J, Ziegenfuss MD, Mullany D, et al. Resolution of severe ischemia-reperfusion injury post-lung transplantation after administration of endobronchial surfactant. J Heart Lung Transplant. 2007;26(8):850–6.

77. Ito K, Shimada J, Kato D, Toda S, Takagi T, Naito Y, et al. Protective effects of preischemic treatment with pioglitazone, a peroxisome proliferator-activated receptor-gamma ligand, on lung ischemia-reperfusion injury in rats. Eur J Cardiothorac Surg. 2004;25(4):530–6.

78. den Hengst WA, Gielis JF, Lin JY, Van Schil PE, De Windt LJ, Moens AL. Lung ischemia-reperfusion injury: a molecular and clinical view on a complex pathophysiological process. Am J Physiol Heart Circ Physiol. 2010;299(5):H1283–99.

79. Echahidi N, Pibarot P, O'Hara G, Mathieu P. Mechanisms, prevention, and treatment of atrial fibrillation after cardiac surgery. J Am Coll Cardiol. 2008;51(8):793–801.

80. See VY, Roberts-Thomson KC, Stevenson WG, Camp PC, Koplan BA. Atrial arrhythmias after lung transplantation: epidemiology, mechanisms at electrophysiology study, and outcomes. Circ Arrhythm Electrophysiol. 2009;2(5):504–10.

81. Nielsen TD, Bahnson T, Davis RD, Palmer SM. Atrial fibrillation after pulmonary transplant. Chest. 2004;126(2):496–500.

82. Chen SA, Hsieh MH, Tai CT, Tsai CF, Prakash VS, Yu WC, et al. Initiation of atrial fibrillation by ectopic beats originating from the pulmonary veins: electrophysiological characteristics, pharmacological responses, and effects of radiofrequency ablation. Circulation. 1999;100(18):1879–86.

83. Haissaguerre M, Jais P, Shah DC, Takahashi A, Hocini M, Quiniou G, et al. Spontaneous initiation of atrial fibrillation by ectopic beats originating in the pulmonary veins. N Engl J Med. 1998;339(10):659–66.

84. D'Angelo AM, Chan EG, Hayanga JW, Odell DD, Pilewski J, Crespo M, et al. Atrial arrhythmias after lung transplantation: Incidence and risk factors in 652 lung transplant recipients. J Thorac Cardiovasc Surg. 2016;152(3):901–9.

85. Sacher F, Vest J, Raymond JM, Stevenson WG. Incessant donor-to-recipient atrial tachycardia after bilateral lung transplantation. Heart Rhythm. 2008;5(1):149–51.

86. Herridge MS, de Hoyos AL, Chaparro C, Winton TL, Kesten S, Maurer JR. Pleural complications in lung transplant recipients. J Thorac Cardiovasc Surg. 1995;110(1):22–6.

87. Ferrer J, Roldan J, Roman A, Bravo C, Monforte V, Pallissa E, et al. Acute and chronic pleural complications in lung transplantation. J Heart Lung Transplant. 2003;22(11):1217–25.

88. Judson MA, Handy JR, Sahn SA. Pleural effusions following lung transplantation. Time course, characteristics, and clinical implications. Chest. 1996;109(5):1190–4.

89. Nunley DR, Grgurich WF, Keenan RJ, Dauber JH. Empyema complicating successful lung transplantation. Chest. 1999;115(5):1312–5.

90. de la Torre M, Fernandez R, Fieira E, Gonzalez D, Delgado M, Mendez L, et al. Postoperative surgical complications after lung transplantation. Rev Port Pneumol (2006). 2015;21(1):36–40.

91. Gammie JS, Cheul Lee J, Pham SM, Keenan RJ, Weyant RJ, Hattler BG, et al. Cardiopulmonary bypass is associated with early allograft dysfunction but not death after double-lung transplantation. J Thorac Cardiovasc Surg. 1998;115(5):990–7.

92. Hussein M, Aljehani YM, Nizami I, Saleh W. Successful management of bilateral refractory chylothorax after double lung transplantation for lymphangioleiomyomatosis. Ann Thorac Med. 2014;9(2):124–6.

93. Clark SC, Levine AJ, Hasan A, Hilton CJ, Forty J, Dark JH. Vascular complications of lung transplantation. Ann Thorac Surg. 1996;61(4):1079–82.

94. Siddique A, Bose AK, Ozalp F, Butt TA, Muse H, Morley KE, et al. Vascular anastomotic complications in lung transplantation: a single institution's experience. Interact Cardiovasc Thorac Surg. 2013;17(4):625–31.

95. Santacruz JF, Mehta AC. Airway complications and management after lung transplantation: ischemia, dehiscence, and stenosis. Proc Am Thorac Soc. 2009;6(1):79–93.

96. Hyytinen TA, Heikkila LJ, Verkkala KA, Sipponen JT, Vainikka TL, Halme M, et al. Bronchial artery revascularization improves tracheal anastomotic healing after lung transplantation. Scand Cardiovasc J. 2000;34(2):213–8.

97. Date H, Trulock EP, Arcidi JM, Sundaresan S, Cooper JD, Patterson GA. Improved airway healing after lung transplantation. An analysis of 348 bronchial anastomoses. J Thorac Cardiovasc Surg. 1995;110(5):1424–32, discussion 1432–3

98. Awori Hayanga JW, Aboagye JK, Shigemura N, Hayanga HK, Murphy E, Khaghani A, et al. Airway complications after lung transplantation: contemporary survival and outcomes. J Heart Lung Transplant. 2016;35(10):1206–11.

99. Shennib H, Massard G. Airway complications in lung transplantation. Ann Thorac Surg. 1994;57(2):506–11.

100. Garfein ES, Ginsberg ME, Gorenstein L, McGregor CC, Schulman LL. Superiority of end-to-end versus telescoped bronchial anastomosis in single lung transplantation for pulmonary emphysema. J Thorac Cardiovasc Surg. 2001;121(1):149–54.

101. Van De Wauwer C, Van Raemdonck D, Verleden GM, Dupont L, De Leyn P, Coosemans W, et al. Risk

factors for airway complications within the first year after lung transplantation. Eur J Cardiothorac Surg. 2007;31(4):703–10.

102. Mulligan MS. Endoscopic management of airway complications after lung transplantation. Chest Surg Clin N Am. 2001;11(4):907–15.

103. Herrera JM, McNeil KD, Higgins RS, Coulden RA, Flower CD, Nashef SA, et al. Airway complications after lung transplantation: treatment and long-term outcome. Ann Thorac Surg. 2001;71(3):989–93, discussion 993–4

104. Krishnam MS, Suh RD, Tomasian A, Goldin JG, Lai C, Brown K, et al. Postoperative complications of lung transplantation: radiologic findings along a time continuum. Radiographics. 2007;27(4):957–74.

105. Mughal MM, Gildea TR, Murthy S, Pettersson G, DeCamp M, Mehta AC. Short-term deployment of self-expanding metallic stents facilitates healing of bronchial dehiscence. Am J Respir Crit Care Med. 2005;172(6):768–71.

106. De Gracia J, Culebras M, Alvarez A, Catalan E, De la Rosa D, Maestre J, et al. Bronchoscopic balloon dilatation in the management of bronchial stenosis following lung transplantation. Respir Med. 2007;101(1):27–33.

107. Marulli G, Loy M, Rizzardi G, Calabrese F, Feltracco P, Sartori F, et al. Surgical treatment of posttransplant bronchial stenoses: case reports. Transplant Proc. 2007;39(6):1973–5.

108. Hasegawa T, Iacono AT, Orons PD, Yousem SA. Segmental nonanastomotic bronchial stenosis after lung transplantation. Ann Thorac Surg. 2000;69(4):1020–4.

109. Madden BP, Kumar P, Sayer R, Murday A. Successful resection of obstructing airway granulation tissue following lung transplantation using endobronchial laser (Nd:YAG) therapy. Eur J Cardiothorac Surg. 1997;12(3):480–5.

Immunology in Lung Transplantation

9

Idoia Gimferrer and Karen A. Nelson

Immunology of the Native Lung

One of the most important characteristics of the lung is that it is an "open" organ in constant contact with the environment. Every day 8000–9000 L of air are filtered by the lungs allowing the inhalation of particles, allergens, and microbes. The anatomical structure of the lung, the physical barrier formed by the epithelial cells with mucus secretions, and the presence of many types of immune cells contribute to keep the lung free of pathogens, infections, and inflammation.

Epithelial Cells and Secretions

The conducting airways of the lungs, from the trachea to terminal bronchioles, are lined by a ciliated pseudostratified epithelium with few secretory cells. The submucosal glands surround the airways and secrete fluids, mucins, and host-defense proteins that form the mucus gel. The mucus traps foreign particles, cell debris, and pathogens. The motile cilia on the epithelial cells allow the clearance of the mucus. These two factors work together

I. Gimferrer (✉) · K. A. Nelson
Department of Immunogenetics/HLA, Bloodworks Northwest, Seattle, WA, USA
e-mail: igimferrer@bloodworksnw.org;
knelson@bloodworksnw.org

to keep the lung free of pathogens and maintain homeostasis, with, of course, the collaboration of resident immune cells [1].

Macrophages and Dendritic Cells (DC)

The lung is populated with several native immune cell types—such as eosinophils, granulocytes, DC, and macrophages—which play an important role in protecting the lung from external insults. DC and macrophages are the main players due to their capacity to directly interact with lymphocytes. The main function of the DC is to sample antigens in the lumen of the alveoli and the conducting air way. When found, infectious pathogens initiate the appropriate immune response. Three different types of DC have been identified in the lung, conventional (cDC), monocyte-derived (moDC), and plasmacytoid (pDC). Their origin is not yet clear, but at least for cDC, it appears they arise in the lung from a bone marrow DC precursor. pDC are considered potent antiviral cells due to their high production of type I interferons, although in steady state their main function is to maintain tolerance to harmless antigens. cDC are very important for cytotoxic CD8-T-cell activation and to promote long-term protection. The role of moDC has not yet been well studied [2].

Macrophages located in the alveoli have been implicated in the defense against bacterial, viral,

G. Raghu, R. G. Carbone (eds.), *Lung Transplantation*, https://doi.org/10.1007/978-3-319-91184-7_9

and fungal infections due to their potent phago- cytic function. As shown in Fig. 9.1a–c, alveolar macrophages (AM) express inhibitory and acti- vating receptors and can deliver pro-inflammatory or anti-inflammatory signals depending on the environment. For instance, recognition of patho- gens through their Toll-like receptors (TLR) acti- vates the production of inflammatory cytokines. On the other hand, binding to ligands on epithe- lial cells promotes tolerance and has anti-

inflammatory effects (Fig. 9.1a–c) [3]. In summary, it is the cross talk among the AM, DC, and epithelium airway that is responsible for the final immune response.

T and B Lymphocytes

T lymphocytes (T cells) play a critical role in the immune system: CD4+T cells "help" B cells to

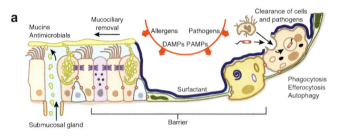

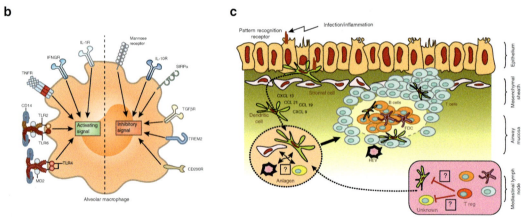

Fig. 9.1 (**a–c**) Native lung immunology. (**a**) Epithelium lung structure: ciliated cells clear mucus with foreign par- ticles trapped. PAMPs, DAMPs, and other pathogens acti- vate epithelial cells, which increase the production of protective cytokines, mucin recruits, and other immune cells. PAMPs, pathogen-associated molecular patterns; DAMPs, damage-associated molecular patterns (Reprinted with permission of Springer Nature from Whitsett JA, Alenghat T. Respiratory epithelial cells orchestrate pulmonary innate immunity. Nature immunol- ogy. 2015;16(1):27-35.). (**b**) Balancing act of macrophage activation: alveolar macrophage (AM) activation is tightly controlled through direct cell-cell contact and soluble mediator interactions. AM express activating and inhibitor receptors and the net sum of their signals determine the final outcome. Per example, during inflammatory pro- cesses, epithelial cell may loss expression of inhibitory ligands, which in consequence will promote alveolar

macrophage activation. IFNGR, interferon-γ receptor; IL 1R, IL 1 receptor; TGFβR, TGFβ receptor; TNFR, TNF receptor (Used with permission of Springer Nature from Hussell T, Bell TJ. Alveolar macrophages: plasticity in a tissue-specific context. Nature reviews Immunology. 2014;14(2):81-93). (**c**) iBALT formation. iBALT is an organized immunological structure with T and B areas that is induced through the release of chemokines and cytokines and the expression of a unique combination of adhesion molecules. Follicular DCs are located in the B-cell region and present antigen and costimulatory sig- nals to the B cells. Tregs located in mediastinal LNs are able to attenuate iBALT formation through a still unknown mechanism (Used with permission of Springer Nature from Foo SY, Phipps S. Regulation of inducible BALT formation and contribution to immunity and pathology. Mucosal immunology. 2010;3(6):537-44) mount antibody responses and also influence CD8+ T-cell function; T cells interact with DC and macrophages driving the production of cytokines and phagocytosis; CD8+ T cells have a direct antiviral function; γδ T cells, NKT, and innate lymphoid cells (ILC) are very important on early responses to many lung infections; and T cells can mature to memory cells for long-term protection. These memory T cells are located in lymphoid tissues or circulating in blood, but more recently a subset of "tissue-resident" memory T cells has been described in the lung which might provide early innate-like cell-mediated protection [4].

The main function of B lymphocytes (B cells) is to produce antibodies, which have an important protective effect against infections. However, since the lung is susceptible to airborne pathogens, serum IgG does not correlate with protection; instead this role is played by mucosal antibodies, mainly dimeric IgA [5].

Both T and B cells are commonly primed by activated DC carrying antigens. Naïve CD8+ T cell will acquire cytolytic activity and will migrate to the inflamed sites. CD4+ T cells differentiate to different subsets depending on the environment, although in the presence of a viral infection, the immune response is biased to Th1 with high INFγ production. B cell differentiation is classically T cell dependent. Hence, B lymphocytes carrying antigens present these peptides to T cells through HLA class II, which leads to class switch from IgM to IgG or IgA and memory B-cell production [5].

Induced Bronchus-Associated Lymphoid Tissue (iBALT)

iBALT is an organized ectopic lymphoid tissue that forms in the human lungs during diseases involving chronic inflammation, infection, or autoimmunity and seems to be dependent on the present of IL-17. iBALT is composed of separate T- and B-cell areas, follicular and resident DCs, high endothelial venules (HEVs) in the T-cell zone, and an overlying lympho-epithelium containing cells similar to microfold cells of Peyer's patches (PPs). iBALT functions as a lymphatic tissue, collecting antigens and activated DCs, supporting B-cell differentiation and generating effector and memory T cells and long-lived plasma cells. Whether iBALT is beneficial or detrimental appears to be context dependent. A correlation has been described between iBALT formation and severity in chronic obstructive pulmonary disease and tissue damage in rheumatoid arthritis patients [6]. However, iBALT have been able to protect against airborne microbes in lymph node-deficient mice [7]. In conclusion, iBALT promotes rapid and efficient local immune responses to pulmonary pathogens [8].

Immune Response Against the Lung Allograft

Despite important advances in the field of lung transplantation, rejection remains the most important problem for long-term survival of the graft. In the first year posttransplant, over 50% of lung transplant recipients are treated for acute allograft rejection, and, at 5 years, about 50% of them have developed chronic lung allograft dysfunction (CLAD) or bronchiolitis obliterans syndrome (BOS) [9].

Both arms of the immune system—innate and adaptive—are implicated in recognition of the allograft as foreign. In addition, activation of the innate immune system by ischemia-reperfusion injury during organ retrieval and implantation can promote the initiation and amplification of an adaptive immune response. In the absent of immunosuppressive agents, naïve T cells will be primed by DCs carrying donor antigens and can differentiate into effector cells with different phenotypes and functions [10]. B cells will be also activated by T cells to produce antibodies against the graft. The main targets of these antibodies are human leukocyte antigens (HLA), although other proteins could be the target too. Antibodies can cause both complement depending cell cytotoxicity and, after binding to target antigens, interact with Fc receptors on immune cells and mediate antibody-dependent cellular cytotoxicity (ADCC) [11].

Cellular Immunity

When naïve T cells are activated depending on the environment and other factors, the naïve T cells differentiate to various subsets, each one secreting characteristic cytokines that shape the immune repose against the graft.

Mechanism of T-Alloimmunity

The physiologic function of T lymphocytes is to scan the body looking for infected or damaged cells that should be eliminated in order maintain homeostasis. The T-cell receptor (TCR) has been selected during thymic development to recognize the unique combination of a self-HLA protein loaded with a specific self-peptide. Therefore, when a TCR encounters a different HLA-peptide combination, it triggers T-cell activation and induces an immune response. The general rule is that HLA class I proteins present peptides derived from the degradation of intracellular proteins to

CD8+ T-cells and HLA class II proteins present peptides originating from extracellular proteins to CD4+ T cells. As the HLA system is the most polymorphic human system, donors and recipients are highly likely to have inherited different genetic variants and are said to be mismatched. Although HLA antigens are the main target of allorecognition, other less polymorphic proteins could also promote immune responses, acting as minor histocompatibility antigens [12].

After organ transplant, recipient T cells are exposed to donor cells and proteins and potentially initiate an allorecognition process that, if not controlled, will end up with the destruction of the transplanted organ [11]. During this allorecognition process, autologous T cells may be primed by three different pathways (Fig. 9.2). The indirect pathway consists of T-cell recognition of peptides derived from donor's HLA antigens and presented by self-HLA on self-antigen-presenting cells (APC). This is the physiological pathway that the

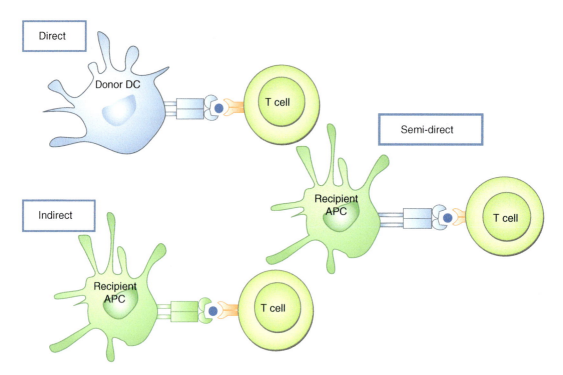

Fig. 9.2 Mechanism of T-alloimmunity. T cells recognize alloantigens through the interaction of their TCR with APC in three different ways. Direct: TCR directly recognize the foreign HLA on donor's APC. Indirect: TCR recognizes a foreign peptide presented by a self-HLA on self-APC. Semi-indirect: the foreign HLA is presented by self-APC to the TCR (Used with permission of Wolters Kluwer Health Inc from Wood KJ, Goto R. Mechanisms of rejection: current perspectives. Transplantation. 2012;93(1):1-10)

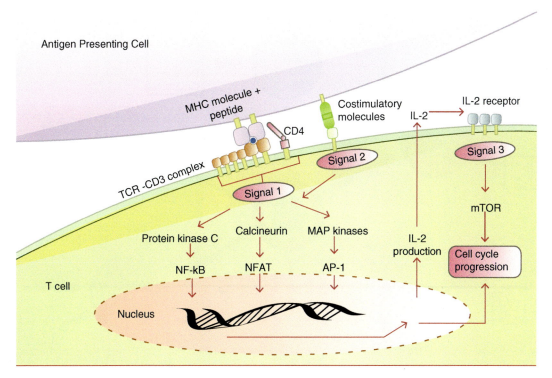

Fig. 9.3 Full T-cell activation requires three signals. Signal 1 is delivered by the interaction of the TCR with its ligand, the HLA-peptide complex on the APC. The binding of other costimulatory receptors on the T cell triggers signal 2. Finally cytokines produced by the T cell or other immune cells provides the last signal. The final fate of the T cell will be the net result of all three signals (Used with permission of Wolters Kluwer Health Inc from Wood KJ, Goto R. Mechanisms of rejection: current perspectives. Transplantation. 2012;93(1):1-10)

immune system uses to defend against virus and other pathogens. The direct pathway involves the direct recognition of the donor HLA antigens on donor cells. Finally, due to the capability of the cells to interchange membrane fragments, recipient's APCs could incorporate donor HLA antigens and present it to autologous T cells. This pathway is the semi-direct pathway [11] (Fig. 9.2). All three pathways could be implicated during a rejection episode, but it is believed that the direct mechanism is primarily implicated soon after transplant, and later on the indirect presentation is the prevalent one [13].

Although the interaction of the TCR with a HLA-peptide complex is necessary to initiate the activation of naïve T cell, a full activation requires also ligation of costimulatory receptors. The final fate of the naïve T cell is the net result of the avidity of the TCR-HLA-peptide recognition, the balance of signals from positive and negative costimulatory receptors, and also the environmental cytokines secreted by the APC and other participant immune cells (Fig. 9.3). CD4+ T cells usually acquire helper function and differentiate into CD4+ T phenotypes, including induced Treg (iTreg), and all have unique transcription factors and cytokine signatures (Fig. 9.4) [14].

Naïve CD8+ T cells usually transform into cytotoxic cells, killing the target cells by exocytosis of toxic granules or ligation of death receptors. CD8+ T cells can also be differentiated in subsets (Tc1, Tc2, Tc17) [15], although their characteristics have been less well studied [11].

Cytokines and Chemokines

The within graft protective regulatory T cells and graft destructive effector T cells largely depends on the balance of pro-inflammatory and anti-inflammatory cytokines. In this way, the presence of TGFβ without pro-inflammatory cytokines

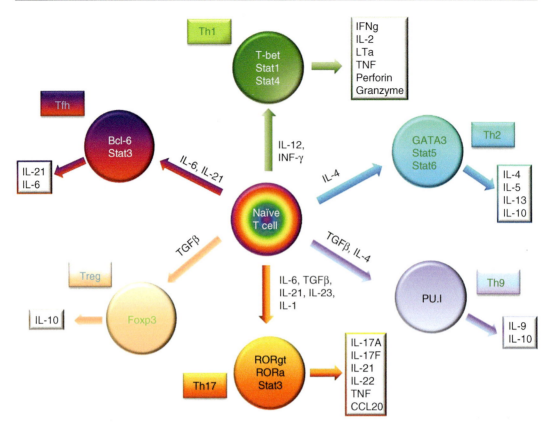

Fig. 9.4 CD4 T-cell phenotypes. Once a naïve CD4 T cell has received signals through its TCR and co-receptors, it starts its differentiation to helper T cell (Th). The local cytokine milieu will determine the final Th phenotype and each phenotype secretes a distinct cytokines profile

directs commitment to induce T regulatory (iTreg) phenotype. On the contrary, the presence of TGFβ together with the pro-inflammatory cytokines IL-6/IL-21/IL-23 turns the development to T helper (Th) 17, and, in the presence of IL-4, T cells become Th9. Other cytokines, like IL-12 and IL-4, will induce naïve T-cell commitment to Th1 and Th2, respectively [16] (Fig. 9.4). Each subset of T cells secretes characteristic cytokines that will influence the clinical outcome. For example, a Th1 response correlates with a more acute rejection episode, due to the production of INFγ, IL-2, IL-12, TNFα, and GM-CSF. This cytokine profile will attract other immune cells to the graft, some with cytotoxic activity (CD8+T, NK) increasing the graft damage. A Th2 response can also cause rejection of the graft with secretion of IL-4 and recruitment of eosinophils. Th17 is a very pro-inflammatory cell subset that has been involved in chronic rejection and autoimmunity. Th17 secretes cytokines, such as IL-17, IL-21, and IL-22. iTreg suppress other Th cell functions and promote tolerance through the secretion of IL-10. These cells are developed when there is a lack of pro-inflammatory cytokines, but, importantly, their differentiation is reversible, and they can acquire a pro-inflammatory phenotype under pro-inflammatory conditions [17].

In lung transplantation, elevated level of pro-inflammatory cytokines early posttransplant has been correlated with an increased risk of chronic rejection [18]. In particular, several studies correlate the increase of IL-17 with the development of chronic rejection or BOS [19], and a more recent study using a murine model pointed out that IL-17-secreting CD4+T cells, and not Th17 cells, are the ones required for the development of BOS [20].

Chemokines are a subset of cytokines whose function is to control the migration of leukocytes under both basal and inflammatory conditions. Not surprisingly, they are also involved during the alloimmune response from initial ischemic damage to acute inflammation, rejection process, or eventual resolution [21]. In lung transplantation, it has been described that higher values of the chemokine CXCL10 (IP-10) in BAL fluids are associated with acute cellular rejection (ACR) [22]. Similarly, the persistence of CXCL9 and CXCL10 suggest worsening of lung allograft function [23]. In a recent study, 34 different cytokines, chemokines, and growth factors were measured in the BAL fluid from 77 patients either stable or with different types of CLAD (non-neutrophilic BOS, neutrophilic BOS, and restrictive allograft syndrome (RAS)). Major differences in cytokine and chemokine expression were found between CLAD and stable patients. In particular IL-6, CXCL10, and VEGF were identified as potential important mediators in the development of RAS [24].

Testing Cellular Immunity

Although T-cell-mediated alloreactivity is the driving force during the alloimmune response, monitoring of immune responses to transplants has mainly focused on detecting B-cell immune responses by measuring antibodies against the graft. Here we summarize potential T-cell immunity tests that could be used in lung transplantation.

Mixed Lymphocyte Culture (MLC)

This was the first assay developed to measure T-cell reactivity to allergenic cells. It was used by histocompatibility laboratories for long time until more modern techniques were developed [25]. This is a very labor-intensive assay requiring several days of incubation time and significant variability that made this test not practical in clinical settings.

ELISPOT

The ELISPOT technique combines MLC and ELISA assays. It is very useful for monitoring cell-mediated immunity and detection of rare antigen-specific T cells (or B cells).

Briefly, cells are cultured in plates and stimulated with the antigen of interest. Activated T cells secrete cytokines that are trapped by antibodies coating the bottom of the culture well. Using antibodies specific for different cytokines allows for customization of the assay and the ability to phenotype the T-cell reactivity. As previously indicated for MLC, this method also requires long incubation times, has moderate reproducibility, and is very labor-intensive [26]. There are few commercially available kits used mainly in research.

Measurement of ATP Production by CD4+ T Cell (ImmuKnow®, Cylex, Columbia, MD, USA)

ImmuKnow® is a commercial available assay to measure the overall capability of peripheral CD4+ T cells to be activated. This assay was originally developed to monitor CD4+ T-cell function in HIV patients and later on adapted to the transplant field [27]. Briefly, whole blood is incubated overnight with phytohemagglutinin (PHA), a non-specific T-cell activator, and ATP production by CD4+ cells is measured the next day.

Several studies have used ImmuKnow to monitor patients' immune activity after transplantation with disparate results. Some have indicated that low T-cell function results correlate with an increased risk for infection, but high T-cell activity did not correlate with rejection [28]. Other studies have not found this association [29, 30]. Therefore, although ImmuKnow assay may identify an immunocompromised patient and be used to monitor immunosuppression treatment, the clinical utility of this assay in transplantation field still needs to be proven.

Bronchoalveolar Lavage (BAL)

BAL is a procedure that recovers cellular and noncellular components of the alveolar and bronchial space. In lung transplantation, BAL may be used to diagnose inflammatory processes like acute and chronic rejection and infections [31]. Reduction of BAL fluid recovery and an increase in neutrophils were associated with rejection or infection in comparison with stable patients. Analysis of BAL product in chronic rejection

(BOS) patients demonstrated a higher proportion of macrophages; in contrast, patients with infection had the highest increase in lymphocytes. IL-8 was elevated in both groups [19]. Other studies found that an increase in neutrophils in BAL from stable lung transplant recipients had a negative predictive value for transplant survival [32].

Humoral Immunity

B cells have a bivalent role in the alloresponse against the graft. On the one hand, they can be activated by T cells to produce antibodies against proteins in the graft (humoral alloimmunity) [11]. On the other hand, B cells can act as APC, due to their high expression of HLA class I and II and costimulatory molecules. B cells can also produce cytokines to support T-cell activation, differentiation, and development to memory T cells. B cells can be subtyped in B1, B2, and B regulatory (Breg) (Fig. 9.5). B1 cells are mainly located in pleural and peritoneal cavity but also in small numbers in the spleen and secrete low affinity natural antibodies without T-cell collaboration. B2 cells are the classical B cells. They mature in the bone marrow and once activated in a germinal center can produce high affinity antibodies. This antibody production is T cell dependent. After activation, some of the B cells can differentiate into memory or plasma cells. The third subset, Breg, has regulatory capabilities and may secrete IL-10 or TGF-β or even inhibit T-cell responses by direct contact [33].

The target of the alloantibodies produced by the B cells could be any protein expressed in the graft. Since HLA molecules are the most polymorphic protein in humans and usually mismatched between donor and recipient, they are the main immune target. Other less polymorphic donor proteins or even monomorphic proteins that are upregulated in the graft could also trigger an antibody response.

The mechanisms by which antibodies promote lung allograft injury remain poorly understood and are the focus of intense research. Antibody binding to donor HLA or other targets on endothelial or epithelial cells could lead to activation of the complement (C′) cascade with C′ deposits leading to cell injury, production of pro-inflammatory molecules, and recruitment of inflammatory cells. Also, antibodies can produce organ damage independently of C′, by marking cells for destruction through ADCC or by

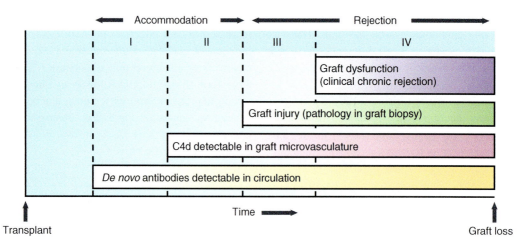

Fig. 9.5 Antibody-mediated rejection. Any time post-transplant, a patient can develop antibodies against graft antigens, being HLA proteins the most common target. In some cases, not shown, patient has these antibodies present before transplant. These antibodies can cause organ damage, which initially could be asymptomatic (accommodation) but eventually will cause graft loss (AMR). Depending on the timing, inflammation, and symptom, the AMR could be acute or chronic (Used with permission of Springer Nature from Colvin RB, Smith RN. Antibody-mediated organ-allograft rejection. Nature reviews Immunology. 2005;5(10):807-17)

inducing endothelial or epithelial cell activation with increased gene expression and subsequent proliferation [34].

Mechanisms of Antibody-Mediated Rejection (AMR)

An antibody has two functional parts: the constant fraction (Fc) which can bind C′ or be recognized by Fc receptors (FcR) carried by immune cells and the variable region (Fab) which binds to the specific target potentially triggering C′ activation. C1 is the first component of the C′ cascade, and the C1q subunit changes conformation when bound to immunoglobulin molecules. The cascade continues through C1r cleavage and then C1s, activation of C2 and C4 which activate C3 and C5, and finally the lytic complex, C5–9. HLA antibodies by activating C′ produce a direct lysis of the target cell. Both the concentration of the antibody and the nature of the immunoglobulin play a role. C1q has five arms and needs to cross-link to be activated; since IgM is pentameric, a single molecule is sufficient. On the contrary, IgG molecules must be closely clustered, and, recently, it has been described that six IgG units are required [35] for optimal C′ activation. Also, the different IgG subclasses have different C1q binding properties: from higher to lower binding capabilities IgG3, IgG1, IgG2, and IgG4 [36, 37]. The activation of the C′ cascade ends up with the formation of membrane attack complexes (MAC), which essentially are pores in the membrane, and the lysis of the cell. Importantly, other components of the C′ cascade, like C3a and C5a, are potent chemotactic molecules that activated endothelial cells and attract immune cells to the graft promoting inflammation [36, 38].

When antibodies bind via Fab to antigens, it activates their Fc region which allows binding to Fc receptors (FcR) present on the surface of some cells. This interaction signals the FcR-carrying cell, which releases cytokines and attracts other immune cells to the graft causing local inflammation. If the FcR is on a cell with cytotoxic capability, like NK or CD8, it could induce ADCC [36].

Another mechanism through which antibodies may damage the graft depends on the target of the antibodies and its ability for signal transduction, as well as on the nature of the signal pathway activated, and the type and location of the cell carrying the targeted antigen [39–41].

Antibodies Against HLA

It has been described that antibodies against HLA class I antigens upregulate fibrogenic growth factors promoting fibrinogenesis and apoptosis [42]. In laboratory models, low levels of antibodies against HLA class I induce survival signals through mTOR2, but contrarily high antibody levels activate mTOR1 signaling inducing cell proliferation and fibrosis [43–45]. The role of anti-HLA class II antibodies has been less investigated, mainly due to its restricted expression pattern. However, B cells and fibroblasts stimulated with anti-HLA class II antibodies demonstrated release of pro-inflammatory factors (IL-6, RANTES) and became activated or underwent apoptosis [46].

Although antibodies to HLA expressed in the allograft have been implicated in both acute and chronic rejection in solid organ transplants, their role in lung transplantation setting was controversial. A recent study [47] following 441 first-time lung recipients over a 10-year period describes that approximately one-third of lung transplant recipients have detectable HLA antibodies posttransplant and one-third of these patients have donor-specific antibodies (DSA). Also, it correlates the presence of HLA antibodies with BOS and the presence of DSA with worse survival. Other studies confirmed the correlation of the presence of de novo DSA and BOS [48–50]. The association of pre-formed DSA with worse survival was much more evident in the C′ binding DSA group and when DSA was against class I HLA [51]. Acute AMR was also described in lung recipients who developed DSA posttransplant. The acute episode was survived by 70% of the patients, but 93% of the survivors developed CLAD or BOS during the 4 years of follow-up [52]. Table 9.1 shows a selection of clinical studies describing the role of antibodies against HLA in human lung transplantation.

Table 9.1 Clinical studies evaluating the role of anti-HLA antibodies in lung transplantation

Citations	Design[a]	# subjects	Antibody[b]	Clinical outcomes	Hazard ratio	p value	Assay
Palmer et al. [53]	R	90	DSA	BOS	4.08	0.002	Flow-PRA
Girnita et al. [54]	P	51	HLA	BOS	ND	0.005	ELISA
Snyder et al. [47]	P	441	HLA	BOS, mortality	2.42	0.001	Flow
Ius et al. [55]	R	546	dn DSA	mortality	1.9	0.04	Luminex
Morrel et al. [48]	P	445	dn DSA	BOS, mortality	4.91–19.78	0.001	Luminex
Safavi et al. [49]	P	148	dn DSA	BOS, mortality	5.74	0.001	Luminex
Smith et al. [51]	R	425	DSA	Survival	3.57	0.004	Luminex
Tikkanen et al. [56]	P	340	dn DSA	CLAD	2.04	0.01	Luminex
Roux et al. [57]	R	209	DSA/AMR	CLAD Survival	7.28, 3.06	0.0026, <0.0001	Luminex

[a]*P* prospective, *R* retrospective
[b]*dn DSA* de novo DSA

Antibodies Against Non-HLA Antigens

The role of antibodies to non-HLA antigens in solid organ transplantation is a hot topic in the histocompatibility and transplant community, since there are several reports describing their association with rejection and worse survival outcomes. Non-HLA antibodies form a heterogeneous group that includes antibodies against monomorphic proteins (autoantibodies) and antibodies against polymorphic proteins (alloantibodies) expressed on the graft.

Since the endothelium is in direct contact with the blood stream, where these potential detrimental antibodies are located, it is not surprising that it is the first target for these non-HLA antibodies (and also HLA antibodies). Antibodies that bind to any unknown protein expressed on endothelial cells are referred as anti-endothelial cell antibodies (AECA). The target proteins could potentially be any protein expressed by the endothelial cells. These AECA have been traditionally detected using assays with human umbilical vein endothelial cells (HUVEC). However, a commercial flow crossmatch kit using donor-derived pre-endothelial cells as target is available. The role of AECA in rejection and correlation with worse outcomes is supported by several publications [58–60].

MHC class I polypeptide-related sequence A (MICA), a polymorphic protein often mismatched between donor and recipient, is expressed on endothelial cells under inflammatory conditions. There are studies that indicate that antibodies against polymorphisms on this protein could play a role in solid organ rejection including the lung [61–63].

Angiotensin II type 1 receptor (AT1R), a protein with a role in blood pressure, seems to be the target of autoantibodies implicated in kidney and heart rejection with decreased graft survival [64–66]. Only two studies have been reported so far on the role of anti-AT1R antibodies in lung transplant. One study concluded that the presence of these antibodies was not correlated with reduced short-term survival at 1 year [67]. The other study described a reduction of freedom from cell-mediated rejection in patient with AT1R antibodies [68].

Besides the abovementioned non-HLA antibodies, other ones have been associated with decreased graft survival. These non-HLA antibodies usually target monomorphic proteins present in recipient and donor cells and are therefore considered autoantibodies, and some of them seem to be organ specific. In this way, antibodies against myosin and vimentin have been described in patients with chronic allograft vasculopathy (CAV) after heart transplant [69, 70]; collagen IV, fibronectin, and agrin seem to be the target for autoantibodies implicated in transplant glomerulopathy [71, 72]; antibodies against K-α1-tubulin and collagen V have been correlated with BOS in lung transplantation [73, 74] and CAV in heart allograft [75].

The list of potential targets of autoantibodies implicated in solid organ transplant outcomes is

Table 9.2 Clinical studies evaluating the role of non-HLA antibodies in lung transplantation

Citations	# subjects	Protein(s) target of antibodies[a]	Antibody associations[b]	Sample timing
Jaramillo [76]	27	AEC	Associated with BOS	Post
Burlingham [77]	54	Collagen l V	Associated with BOS	Post
Goers [78]	36	K alpha tubulin	Associated with BOS	Post
Iwata [79]	10	Collagen V	Associated with PGD	Post
Hagedorn [80]	48	28 identified on multiarray	Positive and negative association with BOS	Post
Angaswamy [61]	80	MICA	Associated with BOS	Post
Bharat [81]	142	Collagen I/V, K alpha tubulin	Associated with PGD	Pre
Paantjens [82]	49	MICA	No association seen with BOS	Pre and post
Arnaoutakis [67]	89	AT1R	No association with early outcomes	Pre
Hachem [74]	108	Collagen V, K alpha tubulin	Associated with BOS, chronic rejection	Post
Tiriveedhi [73]	317	Collagen V, K alpha tubulin	Associated with increased risk of PGD, BOS	Pre

[a]*AEC* endothelial cell, *MICA*, MHC class I polypeptide-related sequence A
[b]*BOS* bronchiolitis obliterative syndrome, *PGD* primary graft dysfunction

accumulating. Table 9.2 show a selection of the reports describing the role of non-HLA antibodies in lung transplantation.

AMR Controversy and Treatment

In contrast to other solid organs, there is a lack of a standardized definition for AMR in lung transplantation; each transplant center has a unique AMR characterization. This makes it a challenge to develop treatment or to establish prognostics and risk factors, complicating interpretation of the literature. A consensus conference proposed to defining ARM as "definite," "probable," or "possible" based on the presence of all, two, or one of the following items (respectively): lung histology compatible with AMR, C4d staining, and the presence of DSA. Importantly, this classification allows the diagnoses of AMR in the absence of HLA-DSA [83]. Figure 9.5 depicts a proposed sequence of the humoral rejection process, where de novo antibodies against the graft are present and may or may not damage the organ early on. If the clinical and histological presentation shows a lot of inflammatory features accompanied by a rapid decrease in graft function, this is considered acute rejection. More often, rejection mediated by antibodies is more indolent and only diagnosed by biopsy (subclinical rejection)

or by a slow loss of graft function, considered chronic rejection [36].

Antibody Detection Techniques

Sensitization against HLA (and also non-HLA proteins) may occur with exposure during pregnancy, transfusion with blood products, transplantation, and even infections. Monitoring for the presence of these antibodies pre- and post-lung transplantation has become standard of care for many transplant programs. The technologies for HLA and non-HLA antibody detection include cell- and solid-phase-based assays, each one with different pros and cons [26].

Cell-Based Assays

These assays use live cells, mainly lymphocyte obtained either from blood or lymph nodes. T lymphocytes are used to detect antibodies against HLA class I and B lymphocytes for detection of antibodies against HLA class I and II. Importantly, both T and B cell express multiple other proteins that could be the target of non-HLA antibodies or autoantibodies, causing positive reactions. Briefly, lymphocytes are incubated with patient's sera. And, after washes, rabbit C′ and vital dyes (cytotoxicity assay) or fluorochrome-labeled antibodies (flow cytometric assay) are added.

Cytotoxicity PRA and Crossmatch

This technique, also named complement-dependent cytotoxicity (CDC) (Fig. 9.6), relies on the ability of antibodies (IgG and IgM) to activate the classical pathway of the C′ cascade. Hence, donor lymphocytes carrying HLA antigens to which patient has antibodies will die. This technique could be used for antibody specificity testing or as a crossmatch, depending on whether a panel of cell carrying known HLA antigens or cells from a specific potential organ donor (crossmatch) are used.

The main limitations of cytotoxicity assays are they are labor-intensive, there are positive reactions in the presence of IgG or IgM autoantibodies or antibodies to non-HLA targets [84], and a threshold amount of immunoglobulins of a specific subclass is required to activate the C′ cascade potentially resulting in a false-negative assay [35]. The main advantage is that the clinical relevance of a cytotoxic positive assay is well established [85]. In this way, transplanting a patient against HLA antibody specificities detected by CDC assay has demonstrated the reduced survival of the graft [85]. For this reason, in the lung transplantation setting, many programs do not transplant if there is a positive CDC crossmatch due to HLA antibodies, but exceptions are made based on patient's clinical situation.

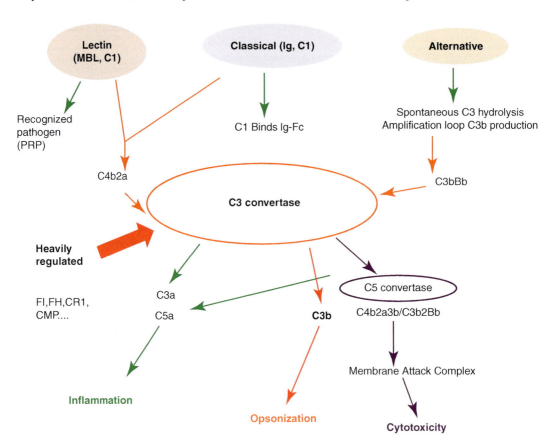

Fig. 9.6 Complement cascade. There are three C′ activation pathways: lectin, classical, and alternative. The classical pathway involves Ig recognition of its target and consequent C1 binding. The lectin pathway is activated when the mannose-binding lectin (MBL) or ficolins recognize mannose or fucose residues, common on pathogens, which allows C1 binding. The alternative pathway is a physiological spontaneous C3 hydrolysis that can also occur after lectin or classical pathway activation. All they converse to a key point with the creation of C3 convertase enzyme. This process is heavily regulated. Downstream of the C3 convertase, there is the production of C3a and C5a, which are the split products of C3 and C5, respectively, and are pro-inflammatory. C3b is the other split product of C3, and it is a potent opsonizating factor. C5 convertase is the first step to the formation of MAC, which will cause cell death

Flow Cytometric Crossmatch

A flow cytometer and fluorochrome-labeled antibodies are used to identify both the cell populations of interest and the presence of antibodies binding to cells (Fig. 9.7). This assay has higher sensitivity than the above described CDC crossmatch. Therefore, positive crossmatches due to anti-HLA antibodies are considered an increased risk for transplantation, and the risk correlates with the intensity of the reaction. Importantly, some non-HLA or autoantibodies can cause positive crossmatch, too, and the transplant risk for these cases should be individually considered.

Flow crossmatch is the main technique used by all solid organ transplants center in USA for the evaluation of a donor-recipient pair transplant risk. For kidney and pancreas transplantations, these flow crossmatches are performed pretransplant. For the other solid organs, including the lung, the cold ischemia time allowed for organ viability is shorter decreasing the opportunity to perform a prospective flow crossmatch. In these cases, flow crossmatches are done peri- or posttransplant, and results are used to stratify the risk for rejection and adjust immunosuppression.

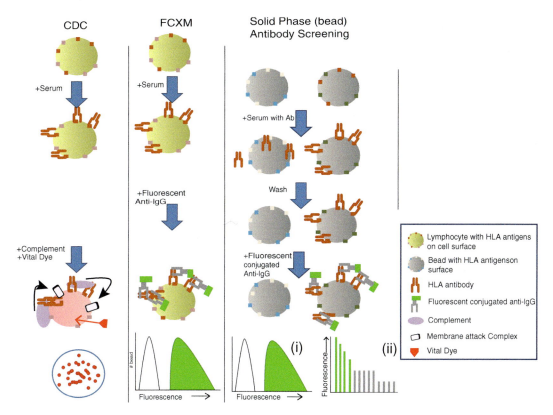

Fig. 9.7 Antibody detection techniques. Schematic representation of three different assays used to detect antibodies against donor antigens. All three assays have a first step where patient's serum is incubated with either cells or beads carrying proteins, and then they differentiate in the way this reaction is detected. CDC: it takes advantage of antibodies capability of activating the C′ cascade, which ends with the formation of the membrane attack complex (MAC) and the death of the cell. The MAC forms pores on the cell surface allowing the vital dye to pass in. Dead and alive cells are easily identified by the change in color and morphology. Flow cytometric crossmatch (FCXM): cell bound antibodies are marked by fluorochrome and light detected by cytometric instruments. Solid phase: plastic beads covered with HLA proteins are used as antibodies target, instead of cells. Again, bound antibodies are marked by fluorochrome and analyzed by Luminex instrument. In both FCXM and solid phase assay, measured fluorescence is relative to a negative control (Used with permission of Elsevier from Tinckam K. Histocompatibility methods. Transplantation reviews (Orlando, Fla). 2009;23(2):80-93)

Solid Phase Assays for HLA Antibody Detection and Specificity

These methods use purified soluble or recombinant HLA proteins attached to a solid surface, which could be a plastic tray (ELISA) or microbeads (Luminex, Austin, TX, USA) to detect antibodies against HLA. By using pure HLA proteins, the interference of non-HLA antigens and autoimmunity is circumvented, although nonspecific positive reactions against artifacts introduced during manipulation of the HLA proteins have been described [86].

There are also commercial kits available to detect some non-HLA antibodies: AT1R or MICA.

ELISA

This was the first solid-phase assay for clinical use and was introduced in 1993 [87]. Briefly, plastic trays with adhered HLA proteins are incubated with patient's sera. Enzyme-conjugated antibody to human IgG (or IgM) is added to detect bound antibodies. This method is more sensitive than a CDC antibody assay but less commonly used in transplantation than bead-based assays.

Luminex Bead Arrays

Luminex technology is based on an array of fluorochrome-labeled plastic microbeads to which proteins have been bound. There are several commercially available assays for the detection of antibodies against HLA antigens. These assays differ in the display of HLA antigens. Assays where each bead carries several HLA antigens (mixed antigen beads) are used for the qualitative detection of antibodies, and assays where each bead carries a single HLA antigen (single antigen beads, SAB) facilitate the identification of the HLA antigen target of an antibody (Fig. 9.6). The higher sensitivity of the SAB assay allowed detection of antibodies to HLA-DQA1 and HLA-DP, which were not detected in CDC or ELISA assays. Antibody reactivity in bead assays is measured in fluorescent units, mean fluorescent intensity (MFI), which provides an estimation of the antibody levels.

False-negative or weak-positive reactions in bead assays have been also described and may be due to the prozone effect. Modification of the serum sample—by using heat inactivation, dithiothreitol (DTT), or ethylenediaminetetra acid (EDTA)—overcomes this problem, which is usually due to a blocking effect caused by C1 or IgM [88]. In addition, false-positive reactions also exist. They are attributed to the reaction of "natural" IgG antibodies against plastic beads itself or "cryptic" epitopes on denaturalized HLA proteins introduced during bead manufacturing. These antibodies tend to be more prevalent in patients with autoimmune diseases [86, 89]; however, they do not appear to be correlated with transplant outcomes. Due to artifacts in these assays, it is strongly advised that interpretation of bead assay results involves the expertise and knowledge of an immunohistocompatibility expert.

Variations of the HLA bead assays to detect the more clinically relevant C' binding HLA antibodies (named C1q and C3d assays) have been developed [90, 91].

Luminex microarray bead technology is the most sensitive assay available to detect and identify HLA antibodies. However, the clinical relevance of the low levels of HLA antibodies only detectable in these assays has been questioned [92–95]. Consensus is building that persistent low levels of donor-specific HLA antibodies are potentially detrimental for the transplanted organ and required close monitoring [96–98].

Unacceptable Antigens and Calculated PRA (cPRA)

Targets of HLA antibodies detected by a solid phase technology that are above an arbitrary cutoff are considered unacceptable antigens (UA). That means that, if a patient's serum with identified antibodies to UA is crossmatched with a donor carrying any of these UA, the flow crossmatch is expected to be positive, and therefore the risk for this transplant is increased.

UNOS, United Network for Organ Sharing, introduced the concept of cPRA in 2007, in an effort to prevent some of the inherent variabilities of traditional PRA. The cPRA accounts for the frequency of the antigen detected as UA in the donor population; thus, a person with one UA which is highly represented in the population (like HLA-A2) will have a higher cPRA than another patient with several antibodies targeting less frequent antigens. In summary, cPRA reflexes better the chance for a patient to find a compatible donor. Importantly, high cPRA do not always correlate with high levels/titer of antibodies. Therefore, some patients with high cPRA but low to moderate titers could benefit from desensitization protocols, with the goal to reduce the antibodies to levels acceptable for transplantation. On the contrary, patients with high cPRA and high titer will be difficult to transplant and usually have longer waiting time and may have to be transplanted in the context of positive crossmatches.

Virtual Crossmatch

Thanks to the introduction of SAB assays for HLA antibody identification, a patient's antibody profiles may now be characterized more accurately. A virtual crossmatch is when the information obtained from this technology is used to predict a crossmatch result (without physically doing the crossmatch) based on a given donor HLA type. Since the predictions are not 100% accurate, a physical crossmatch should still be performed to ensure patient's safety.

In lung transplantation and the other solid organs with short cold ischemia time, a virtual crossmatch is usually performed to evaluate a recipient-donor transplant risk. Transplant centers are highly encouraged to seek expertise advice from their histocompatibility consultant when considering accepting an organ offer for a sensitized patient.

Complement

Both allo- and autoantibodies can bind complement (C′), which can lead to direct cell damage or cell activation with the production of cytokines and inflammation.

The C′ system is an important component of the innate immunity that functions primarily as a

first-line of host defense against pathogens. Additionally, C′ has been implicated in other functions such as regulation of the adaptive response, promotion of tissue regeneration, angiogenesis, development of the central nervous system, and control embryo implantation [99]. Activation of the C′ system (Fig. 9.6) generates three mayor types of effectors: anaphylatoxins (C3a and C5a), opsonins (C3b, iC3b and C3d), and the membrane attack complex (MAC).

Due to the potentially dangerous effect of over activation of the C′ cascade, it must be tightly regulated. Several soluble and membrane-attached proteins act as C′ regulator and are part of the C′ system (Fig. 9.8). In fact, upregulation of regulatory C′ proteins (CD55 and CD59) on endothelial cells after incompatible ABO antibody stimulation has been described in an in vitro model and proposed as the basis for tolerogenicity in ABO incompatible transplants. Unfortunately, this upregulation seems to be missing when stimulation is mediated by anti-HLA antibodies [100]. The import role-play by the C′ in the homeostasis of our body is supported by the association of mutation on some C′ genes with different diseases, like hereditary angioedema or paroxysmal nocturnal hemoglobinuria [101]. Furthermore, T-cell regulation and antibody production are also influenced by elements of the C′ system. In this way, it has been described that the deficit of C1q, C2, C4, or CR1/2 leads to impaired antibody responses [102], and anaphylatoxins may influence CD4+ and CD8+ T-cell function [103–105]. Of course, other elements of the innate immune system, such as TLRs, may also influence T- and B-cell responses.

In lung-related disease, the downregulation of CD55/DAF during asthma episodes has been described [106], and murine models demonstrated the implication of C3aR in the physiopathology of allergic asthma [107, 108]. BOS, the most common chronic complication after lung transplantation, seems also to be partially caused by C′ system dysregulation. Hence, C′ regulators (CRP, CD55/DAF, and CD46) expression was downregulated; meanwhile C3a and IL-17 were

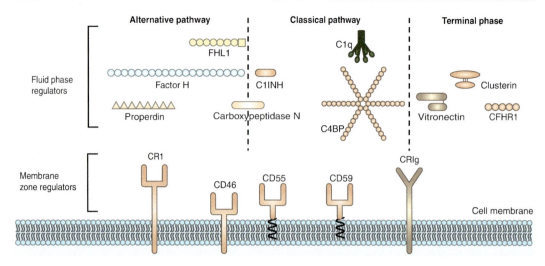

Fig. 9.8 Complement regulator (CR). There are C′ regulators that are membrane-bound and others found soluble. CRs are specific for a pathway, are expressed by different cells, and have different mechanism of action. In this way C1INH blocks C1r and C1s affecting the initiation of the classical and lectin pathways; CR1, expressed on B cells, binds to C3b instructing the B cell to produce Abs to the foreign antigen (Used with permission of Springer Nature from Zipfel PF, Skerka C. Complement regulators and inhibitory proteins. Nature reviews Immunology. 2009;9(10):729-40)

upregulated. This study demonstrated that C3a induces IL-17, which promotes auto- and alloimmunity, and that IL-17 downregulates the expression of epithelial cell-derived C′ regulators. Altogether, it suggested a feedforward loop between IL-17 and C′ activation [109].

The role of C′ in other organ transplants has been also demonstrated [103]. Kidneys from C3-deficient donors survived longer than normal kidneys, suggesting that local C′ protein production is relevant during the rejection process [110]. Also, mouse hearts from DAF$^{-/-}$ knockouts survived longer than wild type [111]. It has also been implicated in the role of C3 during hematopoietic stem cell (HSC) engraftment [112].

Innate Immunity

Activation of the innate immune system in the early phase posttransplant is largely a non-specific response to tissue damage and will occur irrespective of whether there is a genetic difference between the donor and recipient. Although innate immune system contributes to graft rejection, it is not sufficient to do so on its own and requires the participation of the adaptive immune system. One can say that the transplant act itself initiates events that contribute to its own destruction.

The inflammatory cells (dendritic cells, monocytes, macrophages, neutrophils, and other cells) from the innate immune system express germ line-encoded pattern recognition receptors (PRR) have limited clonal expansion and do not usually generate memory cells. This system is the first element implicated in the self-/non-self-recognition events that ultimately lead to productive T- and B-cell immunity. There are several families of PRRs, including transmembrane, intracellular, and secreted proteins.

PRRs recognize microbes carrying pathogen-associated molecular patterns (PAMPs) and markers of cell stress or death (danger-associated molecular patterns (DAMPs) or "alarmins"). During graft ischemia-reperfusion injury, the upregulation of some DAMP members [113] and the activation of PRRs, like Toll-like receptors (TLR) (membrane-bound PRR), have been reported [114, 115]. Although DAMs seems to participate in graft rejection [116, 117], no single DAMP or group of related DAMP has emerged as necessary and sufficient [118]. To the contrary, the absence of TLR signaling has been shown to facilitate tolerance [119].

Neutrophils and monocytes are the first recipient cells to appear in the allograft after transplant. It has been visualized that monocytes infiltrate lung allografts before neutrophils do and that neutrophil migration is indeed monocyte-dependent [120]. Monocyte migration is dependent on the chemokine receptor CCR2, and, once inside the graft, these monocytes differentiate into DC [121]. Some have observed the accumulation of patient-derived DC in the graft and lymph node early posttransplant, raising the hypothesis that monocytes could link innate and adaptive immunity after transplantation [118], as it has been already described during infections [122].

NK cells were originally considered part of the innate immune system, but they share the same lymphoid progenitor as T and B cells. NK cell receptors recognize self-HLA class I: this interaction triggers inhibitory signals preventing activation and cell death. In a solid organ transplant setting, it is highly likely that donor and recipient are mismatched for HLA class I, therefore lacking the NK inhibitory signals ("missing-self" theory). Despite this, it has been demonstrated that NK are not necessary for acute rejection in solid organ graft [123], although they still participate in the process [124]. In contrast, activated NK cells can reject a hematopoietic stem cell (HSC) graft [125]. Therefore, missing-self recognition by NK cells contributes to allograft rejection and to the regulation of the alloimmune response but does not appear to be critical [118].

In summary, the main role of innate immunity is to defend us from pathogenic microorganisms, and, although it may start and promote allorecognition after transplantation, it seems to be neither sufficient nor totally necessary for that. Inflammatory mediators released as a response to ischemia-reperfusion injury promote an inflammatory process that sets up the adaptive system to respond against the graft, but do not explain how alloimmunity can still be triggered long after transplantation. It is possible that innate "allorecognition" mechanisms exist, as it has been described for ancestral species [126, 127], and elucidating those will bring a better understanding of the pathogenesis of acute and chronic rejection.

Applications to Transplant

Patients waiting for a lung transplant are listed with the OPTN database or UNET. From an immunological standpoint, ABO type and an anti-HLA antibody profile are the two main considerations for matching with a potential donor. OPTN policy allows for donor to be ABO identical or compatible with the recipient. Anti-ABO antibodies develop after infancy, and, since ABO determinants are expressed in tissues, transplantation crossing major ABO barriers is considered high risk. Exceptions to allow incompatible ABO lung transplants in patients younger than 2 years have been approved [128]. In adult lung transplantation, few cases of incompatible ABO transplant have been described, and the longest graft survival was 9 years [129].

In this chapter, it is apparent that allosensitization with production of antibodies to donor HLA adds risk to a lung transplant. The highest level of risk appears to be conferred by high levels of DSA at transplant or by a history of multiple instances of allosensitization: pregnancy, transfusion, or prior transplantation. Desensitization protocols are designed to lower the levels of antibody primarily through plasma exchange and interruption of antibody production mainly with agents targeting B cells or plasma cells [130]. Plasma exchange benefit is twofold: it reduces antibody levels in the graft and increases the activity of plasma cells raising their sensitivity to agents like bortezomib. These protocols do not work for everyone, and the challenge is to keep antibody levels low until a suitable organ is allocated. The risk involved in transplanting across a history of allosensitization can be mitigated by closely monitoring for the appearance of DSA after transplant, with prompt intervention using the same tools identified for desensitization protocols.

Lung transplantation is a lifesaving event. In 2015, 2072 lung transplants were performed in the USA. The median patient survival is 5 years with CLAD being the major cause of death [128]. Efforts are needed to better understand the immunological events implicated in the rejection process, which will allow for the development of new immunotherapies.

References

1. Whitsett JA, Alenghat T. Respiratory epithelial cells orchestrate pulmonary innate immunity. Nat Immunol. 2015;16(1):27–35.
2. Kopf M, Schneider C, Nobs SP. The development and function of lung-resident macrophages and dendritic cells. Nat Immunol. 2015;16(1):36–44.
3. Hussell T, Bell TJ. Alveolar macrophages: plasticity in a tissue-specific context. Nat Rev Immunol. 2014;14(2):81–93.
4. Cauley LS, Lefrancois L. Guarding the perimeter: protection of the mucosa by tissue-resident memory T cells. Mucosal Immunol. 2013;6(1):14–23.
5. Chiu C, Openshaw PJ. Antiviral B cell and T cell immunity in the lungs. Nat Immunol. 2015;16(1):18–26.
6. Rangel-Moreno J, Hartson L, Navarro C, Gaxiola M, Selman M, Randall TD. Inducible bronchus-associated lymphoid tissue (iBALT) in patients with pulmonary complications of rheumatoid arthritis. J Clin Invest. 2006;116(12):3183–94.
7. Moyron-Quiroz JE, Rangel-Moreno J, Kusser K, Hartson L, Sprague F, Goodrich S, et al. Role of inducible bronchus associated lymphoid tissue (iBALT) in respiratory immunity. Nat Med. 2004;10(9):927–34.
8. Foo SY, Phipps S. Regulation of inducible BALT formation and contribution to immunity and pathology. Mucosal Immunol. 2010;3(6):537–44.
9. Aurora P, Boucek MM, Christie J, Dobbels F, Edwards LB, Keck BM, et al. Registry of the International Society for Heart and Lung Transplantation: tenth official pediatric lung and heart/lung transplantation report--2007. J Heart Lung Transplant. 2007;26(12):1223–8.
10. Kim IK, Bedi DS, Denecke C, Ge X, Tullius SG. Impact of innate and adaptive immunity on rejection and tolerance. Transplantation. 2008;86(7):889–94.
11. Wood KJ, Goto R. Mechanisms of rejection: current perspectives. Transplantation. 2012;93(1):1–10.
12. Neefjes J, Jongsma ML, Paul P, Bakke O. Towards a systems understanding of MHC class I and MHC class II antigen presentation. Nat Rev Immunol. 2011;11(12):823–36.
13. Afzali B, Lombardi G, Lechler RI. Pathways of major histocompatibility complex allorecognition. Curr Opin Organ Transplant. 2008;13(4):438–44.
14. Palmer MT, Weaver CT. Autoimmunity: increasing suspects in the CD4+ T cell lineup. Nat Immunol. 2010;11(1):36–40.
15. Vukmanovic-Stejic M, Vyas B, Gorak-Stolinska P, Noble A, Kemeny DM. Human Tc1 and Tc2/Tc0 CD8 T-cell clones display distinct cell surface and functional phenotypes. Blood. 2000;95(1):231–40.
16. Strom TB, Koulmanda M. Recently discovered T cell subsets cannot keep their commitments. J Am Soc Nephrol. 2009;20(8):1677–80.
17. Hanidziar D, Koulmanda M. Inflammation and the balance of Treg and Th17 cells in transplant rejection and tolerance. Curr Opin Organ Transplant. 2010;15(4):411–5.
18. Hall DJ, Baz M, Daniels MJ, Staples ED, Klodell CT, Moldawer LL, et al. Immediate postoperative inflammatory response predicts long-term outcome in lung-transplant recipients. Interact Cardiovasc Thorac Surg. 2012;15(4):603–7.
19. Vanaudenaerde BM, Wuyts WA, Geudens N, Nawrot TS, Vos R, Dupont LJ, et al. Broncho-alveolar lavage fluid recovery correlates with airway neutrophilia in lung transplant patients. Respir Med. 2008;102(3):339–47.
20. Wu Q, Gupta PK, Suzuki H, Wagner SR, Zhang C, Cummings OW, et al. CD4 T Cells but Not Th17 Cells Are Required for Mouse Lung Transplant Obliterative Bronchiolitis. Am J Transplant. 2015;15(7):1793–804.
21. O'Boyle G, Ali S, Kirby JA. Chemokines in transplantation: what can atypical receptors teach us about anti-inflammatory therapy? Transplant Rev. 2011;25(4):136–44.
22. Husain S, Resende MR, Rajwans N, Zamel R, Pilewski JM, Crespo MM, et al. Elevated CXCL10 (IP-10) in bronchoalveolar lavage fluid is associated with acute cellular rejection after human lung transplantation. Transplantation. 2014;97(1):90–7.
23. Neujahr DC, Perez SD, Mohammed A, Ulukpo O, Lawrence EC, Fernandez F, et al. Cumulative exposure to gamma interferon-dependent chemokines CXCL9 and CXCL10 correlates with worse outcome after lung transplant. Am J Transplant. 2012;12(2):438–46.
24. Verleden SE, Ruttens D, Vos R, Vandermeulen E, Moelants E, Mortier A, et al. Differential cytokine, chemokine and growth factor expression in phenotypes of chronic lung allograft dysfunction. Transplantation. 2015;99(1):86–93.
25. Bach F, Hirschhorn K. Lymphocyte interaction: a potential histocompatibility test in vitro. Science. 1964;143(3608):813–4.
26. Tinckam K. Histocompatibility methods. Transplant Rev. 2009;23(2):80–93.
27. Holl V, Schmidt S, Aubertin AM, Moog C. The major population of PHA-stimulated PBMC infected by

R5 or X4 HIV variants after a single cycle of infection is predominantly composed of CD45RO+CD4+ T lymphocytes. Arch Virol. 2007;152(3):507–18.

28. Rodrigo E, Lopez-Hoyos M, Corral M, Fabrega E, Fernandez-Fresnedo G, San Segundo D, et al. ImmuKnow as a diagnostic tool for predicting infection and acute rejection in adult liver transplant recipients: a systematic review and meta-analysis. Liver Transpl. 2012;18(10):1245–53.

29. Torio A, Fernandez EJ, Montes-Ares O, Guerra RM, Perez MA, Checa MD. Lack of association of immune cell function test with rejection in kidney transplantation. Transplant Proc. 2011;43(6):2168–70.

30. Ling X, Xiong J, Liang W, Schroder PM, Wu L, Ju W, et al. Can immune cell function assay identify patients at risk of infection or rejection? A meta-analysis. Transplantation. 2012;93(7):737–43.

31. Reynaud-Gaubert M, Thomas P, Gregoire R, Badier M, Cau P, Sampol J, et al. Clinical utility of bronchoalveolar lavage cell phenotype analyses in the postoperative monitoring of lung transplant recipients. Eur J Cardiothorac Surg. 2002;21(1):60–6.

32. Neurohr C, Huppmann P, Samweber B, Leuschner S, Zimmermann G, Leuchte H, et al. Prognostic value of bronchoalveolar lavage neutrophilia in stable lung transplant recipients. J Heart Lung Transplant. 2009;28(5):468–74.

33. Clatworthy MR. Targeting B cells and antibody in transplantation. Am J Transplant. 2011;11(7):1359–67.

34. Martinu T, Howell DN, Palmer SM. Acute cellular rejection and humoral sensitization in lung transplant recipients. Semin Respir Crit Care Med. 2010;31(2):179–88.

35. Diebolder CA, Beurskens FJ, de Jong RN, Koning RI, Strumane K, Lindorfer MA, et al. Complement is activated by IgG hexamers assembled at the cell surface. Science. 2014;343(6176):1260–3.

36. Colvin RB, Smith RN. Antibody-mediated organ-allograft rejection. Nat Rev Immunol. 2005;5(10):807–17.

37. Vidarsson G, Dekkers G, Rispens T. IgG subclasses and allotypes: from structure to effector functions. Front Immunol. 2014;5:520.

38. Albrecht EA, Chinnaiyan AM, Varambally S, Kumar-Sinha C, Barrette TR, Sarma JV, et al. C5a-induced gene expression in human umbilical vein endothelial cells. Am J Pathol. 2004;164(3):849–59.

39. Al-Daccak R, Mooney N, Charron D. MHC class II signaling in antigen-presenting cells. Curr Opin Immunol. 2004;16(1):108–13.

40. Li F, Atz ME, Reed EF. Human leukocyte antigen antibodies in chronic transplant vasculopathy-mechanisms and pathways. Curr Opin Immunol. 2009;21(5):557–62.

41. Zhang X, Reed EF. HLA class I: an unexpected role in integrin beta4 signaling in endothelial cells. Hum Immunol. 2012;73(12):1239–44.

42. Jaramillo A, Smith CR, Maruyama T, Zhang L, Patterson GA, Mohanakumar T. Anti-HLA class I

antibody binding to airway epithelial cells induces production of fibrogenic growth factors and apoptotic cell death: a possible mechanism for bronchiolitis obliterans syndrome. Hum Immunol. 2003;64(5):521–9.

43. Jindra PT, Zhang X, Mulder A, Claas F, Veale J, Jin YP, et al. Anti-HLA antibodies can induce endothelial cell survival or proliferation depending on their concentration. Transplantation. 2006;82(1 Suppl):S33–5.

44. Jindra PT, Jin YP, Rozengurt E, Reed EFHLA, class I. antibody-mediated endothelial cell proliferation via the mTOR pathway. J Immunol. 2008;180(4):2357–66.

45. Zhang X, Reed EF. Effect of antibodies on endothelium. Am J Transplant. 2009;9(11):2459–65.

46. Valenzuela NM, Reed EF. Antibodies in transplantation: the effects of HLA and non-HLA antibody binding and mechanisms of injury. Methods Mol Biol. 2013;1034:41–70.

47. Snyder LD, Wang Z, Chen DF, Reinsmoen NL, Finlen-Copeland CA, Davis WA, et al. Implications for human leukocyte antigen antibodies after lung transplantation: a 10-year experience in 441 patients. Chest. 2013;144(1):226–33.

48. Morrell MR, Pilewski JM, Gries CJ, Pipeling MR, Crespo MM, Ensor CR, et al. De novo donor-specific HLA antibodies are associated with early and high-grade bronchiolitis obliterans syndrome and death after lung transplantation. J Heart Lung Transplant. 2014;33(12):1288–94.

49. Safavi S, Robinson DR, Soresi S, Carby M, Smith JD. De novo donor HLA-specific antibodies predict development of bronchiolitis obliterans syndrome after lung transplantation. J Heart Lung Transplant. 2014;33(12):1273–81.

50. Brugiere O, Suberbielle C, Thabut G, Lhuillier E, Dauriat G, Metivier AC, et al. Lung transplantation in patients with pretransplantation donor-specific antibodies detected by Luminex assay. Transplantation. 2013;95(5):761–5.

51. Smith JD, Ibrahim MW, Newell H, Danskine AJ, Soresi S, Burke MM, et al. Pre-transplant donor HLA-specific antibodies: characteristics causing detrimental effects on survival after lung transplantation. J Heart Lung Transplant. 2014;33(10):1074–82.

52. Witt CA, Gaut JP, Yusen RD, Byers DE, Iuppa JA, Bennett Bain K, et al. Acute antibody-mediated rejection after lung transplantation. J Heart Lung Transplant. 2013;32(10):1034–40.

53. Palmer SM, Davis RD, Hadjiliadis D, Hertz MI, Howell DN, Ward FE, et al. Development of an antibody specific to major histocompatibility antigens detectable by flow cytometry after lung transplant is associated with bronchiolitis obliterans syndrome. Transplantation. 2002;74(6):799–804.

54. Girnita AL, Duquesnoy R, Yousem SA, Iacono AT, Corcoran TE, Buzoianu M, et al. HLA-specific antibodies are risk factors for lymphocytic bronchiolitis and

chronic lung allograft dysfunction. Am J Transplant. 2005;5(1):131–8.

55. Ius F, Sommer W, Tudorache I, Kuhn C, Avsar M, Siemeni T, et al. Early donor-specific antibodies in lung transplantation: risk factors and impact on survival. J Heart Lung Transplant. 2014;33(12):1255–63.

56. Tikkanen JM, Singer LG, Kim SJ, Li Y, Binnie M, Chaparro C, et al. De Novo DQ donor-specific antibodies are associated with chronic lung allograft dysfunction after lung transplantation. Am J Respir Crit Care Med. 2016;194(5):596–606.

57. Roux A, Bendib Le Lan I, Holifanjaniaina S, Thomas KA, Hamid AM, Picard C, et al. Antibody-mediated rejection in lung transplantation: clinical outcomes and donor-specific antibody characteristics. Am J Transplant. 2016;16(4):1216–28.

58. Ferry BL, Welsh KI, Dunn MJ, Law D, Proctor J, Chapel H, et al. Anti-cell surface endothelial antibodies in sera from cardiac and kidney transplant recipients: association with chronic rejection. Transpl Immunol. 1997;5(1):17–24.

59. Sun Q, Liu Z, Chen J, Chen H, Wen J, Cheng D, et al. Circulating anti-endothelial cell antibodies are associated with poor outcome in renal allograft recipients with acute rejection. Clin J Am Soc Nephrol. 2008;3(5):1479–86.

60. Sun Q, Cheng Z, Cheng D, Chen J, Ji S, Wen J, et al. De novo development of circulating anti-endothelial cell antibodies rather than pre-existing antibodies is associated with post-transplant allograft rejection. Kidney Int. 2011;79(6):655–62.

61. Angaswamy N, Saini D, Ramachandran S, Nath DS, Phelan D, Hachem R, et al. Development of antibodies to human leukocyte antigen precedes development of antibodies to major histocompatibility class I-related chain A and are significantly associated with development of chronic rejection after human lung transplantation. Hum Immunol. 2010;71(6):560–5.

62. Zhang Q, Cecka JM, Gjertson DW, Ge P, Rose ML, Patel JK, et al. HLA and MICA: targets of antibody-mediated rejection in heart transplantation. Transplantation. 2011;91(10):1153–8.

63. Luo L, Li Z, Wu W, Luo G, Mei H, Sun Z, et al. The effect of MICA antigens on kidney transplantation outcomes. Immunol Lett. 2013;156(1-2):54–8.

64. Dragun D, Muller DN, Brasen JH, Fritsche L, Nieminen-Kelha M, Dechend R, et al. Angiotensin II type 1-receptor activating antibodies in renal-allograft rejection. N Engl J Med. 2005;352(6):558–69.

65. Giral M, Foucher Y, Dufay A, Van Huyen JP, Renaudin K, Moreau A, et al. Pretransplant sensitization against angiotensin II type 1 receptor is a risk factor for acute rejection and graft loss. Am J Transplant. 2013;13(10):2567–76.

66. Reinsmoen NL, Lai CH, Mirocha J, Cao K, Ong G, Naim M, et al. Increased negative impact of donor HLA-specific together with non-HLA-specific antibodies on graft outcome. Transplantation. 2014;97(5):595–601.

67. Arnaoutakis GJ, Eng HS, George TJ, Beaty CA, Merlo CA, Shah AS, et al. The impact of angiotensin II type 1 receptor auto-antibodies and early lung transplant outcomes. Am J Transplant. 2012;12(S3):170.

68. Reinsmoen NL, Mirocha J, Ensor C, Marrari M, Chaux GE, Lai C, Levine D, Zeevi A. A three center study reveals new insights into the impact of non-HLA antibodies on the acute rejection process in lung transplantation. J Heart Lung Transplant. 2015;34(4):S119–S20.

69. Kalache S, Dinavahi R, Pinney S, Mehrotra A, Cunningham MW, Heeger PS. Anticardiac myosin immunity and chronic allograft vasculopathy in heart transplant recipients. J Immunol. 2011;187(2):1023–30.

70. Nath DS, Illias Basha H, Saini D, Ramachandran S, Ewald GA, Moazami N, Mohanakumar T. The important role of immune responses to self-antigen in pathogenesis of coronary artery vasculopathy following human cardiac transplantation. J Heart Lung Transplant. 2010;29(2):S84–S5.

71. Angaswamy N, Klein C, Tiriveedhi V, Gaut J, Anwar S, Rossi A, et al. Immune responses to collagen-IV and fibronectin in renal transplant recipients with transplant glomerulopathy. Am J Transplant. 2014;14(3):685–93.

72. Joosten SA, Sijpkens YW, van Ham V, Trouw LA, van der Vlag J, van den Heuvel B, et al. Antibody response against the glomerular basement membrane protein agrin in patients with transplant glomerulopathy. Am J Transplant. 2005;5(2):383–93.

73. Tiriveedhi V, Gautam B, Sarma NJ, Askar M, Budev M, Aloush A, et al. Pre-transplant antibodies to Kalpha1 tubulin and collagen-V in lung transplantation: clinical correlations. J Heart Lung Transplant. 2013;32(8):807–14.

74. Hachem RR, Tiriveedhi V, Patterson GA, Aloush A, Trulock EP, Mohanakumar T. Antibodies to K-alpha 1 tubulin and collagen V are associated with chronic rejection after lung transplantation. Am J Transplant. 2012;12(8):2164–71.

75. Nath DS, Tiriveedhi V, Basha HI, Phelan D, Moazami N, Ewald GA, et al. A role for antibodies to human leukocyte antigens, collagen-V, and K-alpha1-Tubulin in antibody-mediated rejection and cardiac allograft vasculopathy. Transplantation. 2011;91(9):1036–43.

76. Jaramillo A, Naziruddin B, Zhang L, Reznik SI, Smith MA, Aloush AA, et al. Activation of human airway epithelial cells by non-HLA antibodies developed after lung transplantation: a potential etiological factor for bronchiolitis obliterans syndrome. Transplantation. 2001;71(7):966–76.

77. Burlingham WJ, Love RB, Jankowska-Gan E, Haynes LD, Xu Q, Bobadilla JL, et al. IL-17-dependent cellular immunity to collagen type V pre-

disposes to obliterative bronchiolitis in human lung transplants. J Clin Invest. 2007;117(11):3498–506.

78. Goers TA, Ramachandran S, Aloush A, Trulock E, Patterson GA, Mohanakumar T. De novo production of K-alpha1 tubulin-specific antibodies: role in chronic lung allograft rejection. J Immunol. 2008;180(7):4487–94.

79. Iwata T, Philipovskiy A, Fisher AJ, Presson RG Jr, Chiyo M, Lee J, et al. Anti-type V collagen humoral immunity in lung transplant primary graft dysfunction. J Immunol. 2008;181(8):5738–47.

80. Hagedorn PH, Burton CM, Carlsen J, Steinbruchel D, Andersen CB, Sahar E, et al. Chronic rejection of a lung transplant is characterized by a profile of specific autoantibodies. Immunology. 2010;130(3):427–35.

81. Bharat A, Saini D, Steward N, Hachem R, Trulock EP, Patterson GA, et al. Antibodies to self-antigens predispose to primary lung allograft dysfunction and chronic rejection. Ann Thorac Surg. 2010;90(4):1094–101.

82. Paantjens AW, van de Graaf EA, Kwakkel-van Erp JM, Hoefnagel T, van Ginkel WG, Fakhry F, et al. The induction of IgM and IgG antibodies against HLA or MICA after lung transplantation. Pulm Med. 2011;2011:432169.

83. Levine DJ, Glanville AR, Aboyoun C, Belperio J, Benden C, Berry GJ, et al. Antibody-mediated rejection of the lung: a consensus report of the International Society for Heart and Lung Transplantation. J Heart Lung Transplant. 2016;35(4):397–406.

84. Book BK, Agarwal A, Milgrom AB, Bearden CM, Sidner RA, Higgins NG, et al. New crossmatch technique eliminates interference by humanized and chimeric monoclonal antibodies. Transplant Proc. 2005;37(2):640–2.

85. Patel R, Terasaki PI. Significance of the positive crossmatch test in kidney transplantation. N Engl J Med. 1969;280(14):735–9.

86. Grenzi PC, de Marco R, Silva RZ, Campos EF, Gerbase-DeLima M. Antibodies against denatured HLA class II molecules detected in luminex-single antigen assay. Hum Immunol. 2013;74(10):1300–3.

87. Kao KJ, Scornik JC, Small SJ. Enzyme-linked immunoassay for anti-HLA antibodies--an alternative to panel studies by lymphocytotoxicity. Transplantation. 1993;55(1):192–6.

88. Weinstock C, Schnaidt M. The complement-mediated prozone effect in the Luminex single-antigen bead assay and its impact on HLA antibody determination in patient sera. Int J Immunogenet. 2013;40(3):171–7.

89. Poli F, Benazzi E, Innocente A, Nocco A, Cagni N, Gianatti A, et al. Heart transplantation with donor-specific antibodies directed toward denatured HLA-A*02:01: a case report. Hum Immunol. 2011;72(11):1045–8.

90. Yabu JM, Higgins JP, Chen G, Sequeira F, Busque S, Tyan DB. C1q-fixing human leukocyte antigen antibodies are specific for predicting transplant glomerulopathy and late graft failure after kidney transplantation. Transplantation. 2011;91(3):342–7.

91. Zeevi A, Lunz J, Feingold B, Shullo M, Bermudez C, Teuteberg J, et al. Persistent strong anti-HLA antibody at high titer is complement binding and associated with increased risk of antibody-mediated rejection in heart transplant recipients. J Heart Lung Transplant. 2013;32(1):98–105.

92. Gebel HM, Bray RA, Nickerson P. Pre-transplant assessment of donor-reactive, HLA-specific antibodies in renal transplantation: contraindication vs. risk. Am J Transplant. 2003;3(12):1488–500.

93. Aubert V, Venetz JP, Pantaleo G, Pascual M. Low levels of human leukocyte antigen donor-specific antibodies detected by solid phase assay before transplantation are frequently clinically irrelevant. Hum Immunol. 2009;70(8):580–3.

94. Susal C, Dohler B, Sadeghi M, Ovens J, Opelz G. HLA antibodies and the occurrence of early adverse events in the modern era of transplantation: a collaborative transplant study report. Transplantation. 2009;87(9):1367–71.

95. Singh N, Djamali A, Lorentzen D, Pirsch JD, Leverson G, Neidlinger N, et al. Pretransplant donor-specific antibodies detected by single-antigen bead flow cytometry are associated with inferior kidney transplant outcomes. Transplantation. 2010;90(10):1079–84.

96. Everly MJ. Summarizing the use of donor specific anti-HLA antibody monitoring in transplant patients. Clin Transpl. 2011:333–6.

97. Sicard A, Amrouche L, Suberbielle C, Carmagnat M, Candon S, Thervet E, et al. Outcome of kidney transplantations performed with preformed donor-specific antibodies of unknown etiology. Am J Transplant. 2014;14(1):193–201.

98. Morath C, Opelz G, Zeier M, Susal C. Clinical relevance of HLA antibody monitoring after kidney transplantation. J Immunol Res. 2014;2014:845040.

99. Ricklin D, Hajishengallis G, Yang K, Lambris JD. Complement: a key system for immune surveillance and homeostasis. Nat Immunol. 2010;11(9):785–97.

100. Iwasaki K, Miwa Y, Ogawa H, Yazaki S, Iwamoto M, Furusawa T, et al. Comparative study on signal transduction in endothelial cells after anti-a/b and human leukocyte antigen antibody reaction: implication of accommodation. Transplantation. 2012;93(4):390–7.

101. Zipfel PF, Skerka C. Complement regulators and inhibitory proteins. Nat Rev Immunol. 2009;9(10):729–40.

102. Sorman A, Zhang L, Ding Z, Heyman B. How antibodies use complement to regulate antibody responses. Mol Immunol. 2014;61(2):79–88.

103. Dunkelberger JR, Song WC. Role and mechanism of action of complement in regulating T cell immunity. Mol Immunol. 2010;47(13):2176–86.

104. Abe M, Shibata K, Akatsu H, Shimizu N, Sakata N, Katsuragi T, et al. Contribution of anaphylatoxin C5a

to late airway responses after repeated exposure of antigen to allergic rats. J Immunol. 2001;167(8):4651–60.

105. Baelder R, Fuchs B, Bautsch W, Zwirner J, Kohl J, Hoymann HG, et al. Pharmacological targeting of anaphylatoxin receptors during the effector phase of allergic asthma suppresses airway hyperresponsiveness and airway inflammation. J Immunol. 2005;174(2):783–9.

106. Agrawal A, Sinha A, Ahmad T, Aich J, Singh P, Sharma A, et al. Maladaptation of critical cellular functions in asthma: bioinformatic analysis. Physiol Genomics. 2009;40(1):1–7.

107. Drouin SM, Corry DB, Hollman TJ, Kildsgaard J, Wetsel RA. Absence of the complement anaphylatoxin C3a receptor suppresses Th2 effector functions in a murine model of pulmonary allergy. J Immunol. 2002;169(10):5926–33.

108. Wills-Karp M. Complement activation pathways: a bridge between innate and adaptive immune responses in asthma. Proc Am Thorac Soc. 2007;4(3):247–51.

109. Suzuki H, Lasbury ME, Fan L, Vittal R, Mickler EA, Benson HL, et al. Role of complement activation in obliterative bronchiolitis post-lung transplantation. J Immunol. 2013;191(8):4431–9.

110. Pratt JR, Basheer SA, Sacks SH. Local synthesis of complement component C3 regulates acute renal transplant rejection. Nat Med. 2002;8(6):582–7.

111. Pavlov V, Raedler H, Yuan S, Leisman S, Kwan WH, Lalli PN, et al. Donor deficiency of decay-accelerating factor accelerates murine T cell-mediated cardiac allograft rejection. J Immunol. 2008;181(7):4580–9.

112. Ratajczak MZ, Reca R, Wysoczynski M, Kucia M, Baran JT, Allendorf DJ, et al. Transplantation studies in C3-deficient animals reveal a novel role of the third complement component (C3) in engraftment of bone marrow cells. Leukemia. 2004;18(9):1482–90.

113. Rao DA, Pober JS. Endothelial injury, alarmins, and allograft rejection. Crit Rev Immunol. 2008;28(3):229–48.

114. Goldstein I, Ben-Horin S, Li J, Bank I, Jiang H, Chess L. Expression of the alpha1beta1 integrin, VLA-1, marks a distinct subset of human CD4+ memory T cells. J Clin Invest. 2003;112(9):1444–54.

115. Shimamoto A, Pohlman TH, Shomura S, Tarukawa T, Takao M, Shimpo H. Toll-like receptor 4 mediates lung ischemia-reperfusion injury. Ann Thorac Surg. 2006;82(6):2017–23.

116. Kaczorowski DJ, Tsung A, Billiar TR. Innate immune mechanisms in ischemia/reperfusion. Front Biosci (Elite Ed). 2009;1:91–8.

117. Tsung A, Sahai R, Tanaka H, Nakao A, Fink MP, Lotze MT, et al. The nuclear factor HMGB1 mediates hepatic injury after murine liver ischemia-reperfusion. J Exp Med. 2005;201(7):1135–43.

118. Oberbarnscheidt MH, Zecher D, Lakkis FG. The innate immune system in transplantation. Semin Immunol. 2011;23(4):264–72.

119. Kim JI, Lee MK IV, Moore DJ, Sonawane SB, Duff PE, O'Connor MR, et al. Regulatory T-cell counter-regulation by innate immunity is a barrier to transplantation tolerance. Am J Transplant. 2009;9(12):2736–44.

120. Kreisel D, Nava RG, Li W, Zinselmeyer BH, Wang B, Lai J, et al. In vivo two-photon imaging reveals monocyte-dependent neutrophil extravasation during pulmonary inflammation. Proc Natl Acad Sci U S A. 2010;107(42):18073–8.

121. Gelman AE, Okazaki M, Sugimoto S, Li W, Kornfeld CG, Lai J, et al. CCR2 regulates monocyte recruitment as well as CD4 T1 allorecognition after lung transplantation. Am J Transplant. 2010;10(5):1189–99.

122. Dominguez PM, Ardavin C. Differentiation and function of mouse monocyte-derived dendritic cells in steady state and inflammation. Immunol Rev. 2010;234(1):90–104.

123. Heidecke CD, Araujo JL, Kupiec-Weglinski JW, Abbud-Filho M, Araneda D, Stadler J, et al. Lack of evidence for an active role for natural killer cells in acute rejection of organ allografts. Transplantation. 1985;40(4):441–4.

124. Maier S, Tertilt C, Chambron N, Gerauer K, Huser N, Heidecke CD, et al. Inhibition of natural killer cells results in acceptance of cardiac allografts in CD28-/- mice. Nat Med. 2001;7(5):557–62.

125. Murphy WJ, Kumar V, Bennett M. Acute rejection of murine bone marrow allografts by natural killer cells and T cells. Differences in kinetics and target antigens recognized. J Exp Med. 1987;166(5):1499–509.

126. Nicotra ML, Powell AE, Rosengarten RD, Moreno M, Grimwood J, Lakkis FG, et al. A hypervariable invertebrate allodeterminant. Curr Biol. 2009;19(7):583–9.

127. Rosengarten RD, Nicotra ML. Model systems of invertebrate allorecognition. Curr Biol. 2011;21(2):R82–92.

128. Valapour M, Skeans MA, Smith JM, Edwards LB, Cherikh WS, Uccellini K, et al. OPTN/SRTR 2015 Annual Data Report: Lung. Am J Transplant. 2017;17(Suppl 1):357–424.

129. Snell GI, Holmes M, Levvey BJ, Shipp A, Robertson C, Westall GP, et al. Lessons and insights from ABO-incompatible lung transplantation. Am J Transplant. 2013;13(5):1350–3.

130. Pouliquen E, Koenig A, Chen CC, Sicard A, Rabeyrin M, Morelon E, et al. Recent advances in renal transplantation: antibody-mediated rejection takes center stage. F1000Prime Rep. 2015;7:51.

Physiologic and Epigenetic Changes with Pulmonary Vascular Injury After Lung Transplantation

10

Steven Kenneth Huang, Roberto G. Carbone, and Giovanni Bottino

Abbreviations

ARDS	Acute respiratory distress syndrome
BOS	Bronchiolitis obliterans syndrome
COPD	Chronic obstructive pulmonary disease
DNMT	DNA methyltransferase
ECMO	Extracorporeal membrane oxygenation
EVLP	Ex vivo lung perfusion
HIF	Hypoxia-inducible factor
IFN	Interferon
IL	Interleukin
miRNA	MicroRNA
NET	Neutrophil extracellular trap
NO	Nitric oxide
PAF	Platelet-activating factor
PGD	Primary graft dysfunction
ROS	Reactive oxygen species
TET	Ten-eleven translocation
TLR	Toll-like receptor
TNF	Tumor necrosis factor

S. K. Huang (✉)
Department of Pulmonary and Critical Care Medicine, University of Michigan,
Ann Arbor, MI, USA
e-mail: stehuang@umich.edu

R. G. Carbone
Department of Internal Medicine, University of Genoa, Genoa, Italy

G. Bottino
Department of Medicine, University of Genoa—DIMI, Genoa, Italy

Introduction

Primary graft dysfunction (PGD) is one of the most important complications limiting the success of lung transplantation and continues to exact significant morbidity and mortality [1, 2]. PGD is a term used to describe the severe end of a spectrum of clinical responses that occur as a consequence of vascular injury immediately after transplantation. Many terms—including ischemia-reperfusion injury, reimplantation response, reimplantation edema, reperfusion edema, early graft dysfunction, primary graft failure, and posttransplant acute respiratory distress syndrome (ARDS) [3]—are often used synonymously with PGD. This syndrome occurs, by definition, within the first 72 h of transplantation and is pathologically characterized by pulmonary edema and diffuse alveolar damage in a pattern consistent with acute lung injury. Despite improvements in surgical technique, PGD still affects an estimated 10–25% of lung transplant recipients and carries an eightfold higher risk of mortality in the first 30 days with an overall mortality of 20–30% in the first month after lung transplant [1, 2, 4]. Long-term PGD is a major risk factor for the development of bronchiolitis obliterans syndrome (BOS) [5]. In this chapter, we will discuss the physiologic and pathophysiologic changes that occur in this condition and the potential mechanisms that account for this form of lung injury. For most of the chapter, the

© The Author(s) 2018

G. Raghu, R. G. Carbone (eds.), *Lung Transplantation*, https://doi.org/10.1007/978-3-319-91184-7_10

Fig. 10.1 (**a**, **b**) Normal pulmonary arterial vasculature. Reconstructed images from an MRI of a healthy patient demonstrate the ability to comprehensively map the vasculature of pulmonary arteries. (**a**) axial view; (**b**) posterior view

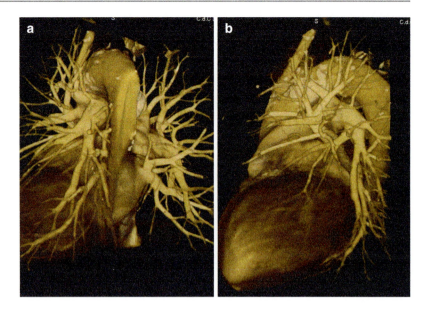

terms ischemia-reperfusion injury or pulmonary vascular injury will be used to emphasize the underlying etiology and pathophysiology of this form of injury, and we exclude from discussion PGD that may occur from infection or acute antibody-mediated reactions such as hyperacute rejection. An image of normal human vasculature is shown in Fig. 10.1a, b, and the vasculature is the site of much of the initial injury during ischemia and reperfusion. This chapter will begin by discussing the risk factors for vascular injury before moving onto a discussion of the current knowledge of its pathophysiology. We will then discuss whether epigenetic mechanisms may be important, before ending with a discussion of the clinical strategies to diagnose and limit or treat ischemia-reperfusion injury.

Risk Factors for Ischemia-Reperfusion and Vascular Injury

Factors related to the donor, the procurement of the donor organ, the recipient, and the care of patients after transplant contribute to the risk of ischemia-reperfusion injury [2]. Identification of these risk factors has impacted the process of organ procurement, the surgical techniques, and care of patients perioperatively (Box 10.1).

Box 10.1 Risk Factors for Ischemia-Reperfusion Injury

Donor-related risk factors
   Donor age
   >10 pack-year smoking history
   History of obesity in donor
   Elevated pulmonary pressures
   Diagnosis of sarcoidosis
   Presence of venous thromboembolism
   Hypotension
Organ retrieval and storage
   Alveolar overdistension
   Duration of cold ischemia time
   Target temperature
   Type of lung perfusate
Recipient
   Pulmonary arterial hypertension
   Idiopathic pulmonary fibrosis
Posttransplant factors
   Ventilator-induced overdistension
   Aspiration
   Pneumonia
   Fluid overload

Donor Risk Factors

Several studies have identified that demographics and baseline characteristics of the donor are independent risk factors for the development of ischemia-reperfusion injury [6]. Donor age and donors with greater than a 10-pack-year smoking history were identified by multilevel regression analysis as risk factors for PGD [7]. Another study of 255 lung transplants identified female gender and donors of African-American origin as also important independent risk factors for ischemia-reperfusion injury, although the reasons for this are less clear [8]. The condition of the donor organ prior to harvest certainly contributes to the success of the organ after transplantation, as the presence of donor thromboembolism [9], donor smoking history, donor diagnosis of sarcoidosis, presence of elevated pulmonary arterial pressures, and donor obesity have also been shown to be risk factors for PGD [10].

Risk Factors Related to Donor Organ Retrieval

In addition to the baseline characteristics of the donor, the condition of the donor upon retrieval and storage of the organ also significantly impact the development of ischemia-reperfusion injury. Brain death is associated with the release of many inflammatory cytokines including interleukin (IL)-8 and IL-6, which correlate with the development of PGD [11]. Donor hypotension and alveolar overdistension resulting in ventilator-induced lung injury also contribute to the development of ischemia-reperfusion injury and have influenced the management of donors in the intensive care unit prior to procurement.

The process of organ procurement plays a major role in the rate of ischemia-reperfusion injury, which has impacted how surgery is performed [12]. This is discussed in further detail in Chap. 8. The duration of cold ischemia storage may be particularly important; however, the maximal duration for cold storage is unclear. Early studies suggest that ischemia times up to 8 h did not significantly increase the risk for short- or long-term complications [13, 14], whereas later studies of larger cohorts identify cold ischemia times of greater than 6 h to pose a significant risk [15]. As will be discussed later in the chapter, the use of ex vivo lung perfusion (EVLP) strategies may preserve function of the graft beyond 12 h

without affecting patient survival or incidence of PGD [16]. Although hypothermia, which decreases metabolic rate, is necessary for cold storage, it has the potential to contribute to ischemia-reperfusion injury as hypothermia is associated with increased oxidative stress [17], inactivation of the Na^+/K^+-ATPase pump [18], increasing intracellular calcium [19], and increasing apoptotic cell death [20].

Recipient

Interestingly, the underlying diagnosis of the recipient also influences the risk for developing PGD, even if the recipient receives a double lung transplant. Recipients with pulmonary arterial hypertension possess the greatest risk for ischemia-reperfusion injury [8], followed by recipients with pulmonary fibrosis [21]. Recipients with chronic obstructive pulmonary disease possess the lowest risk, with reported incidence as low as 3% [22]. The reason for the differences in risk is unknown but may be related to comorbidities associated with these diagnoses or systemic changes in biology associated with either pulmonary hypertension or fibrosis. Pulmonary hypertension is often associated with cardiac dysfunction, and the changes in shear stress of a hypertrophied right ventricle may contribute to reperfusion injury [23]. Recipient age and other comorbidities such as obesity, diabetes, renal impairment, and left-ventricular dysfunction have not correlated with an increased risk of ischemia-reperfusion injury [22].

Posttransplant Factors

A number of posttransplant factors can contribute to the risk of developing reperfusion injury. Single lung transplant, as opposed to double lung transplant, has the advantage of providing more organs to a larger group of recipients, but differences in vascular perfusion and physiology between the donor organ and native lung after transplantation may increase the risk of reperfusion injury to the single transplanted lung. Single lung transplant itself has been demonstrated to be a risk factor for PGD, and the odds are further increased in recipients with preoperative evidence of pulmonary arterial hypertension [10]. It is believed that the presence of a nonperfused, native pulmonary arterial hypertensive lung causes hyperperfusion and, thus, injury to the transplanted lung, and pathologic studies of pulmonary arterial hypertensive patients undergoing single lung transplant demonstrate the presence of vascular remodeling and upregulation of apoptotic markers in the donor lung [24]. Most transplant centers recommend double lung transplantation in patients with pulmonary arterial hypertension as several studies demonstrate that these patients have improved survival compared to those that obtain a single lung [25, 26]. This practice, however, continues to remain controversial as other studies demonstrate no difference in mortality between single and double lung transplant recipients of pulmonary arterial hypertension [27, 28]. Aspiration, pneumonia, fluid overload, and overdistension resulting in ventilator-induced lung injury are additional postsurgical risk factors for PGD [22]. Complications from the surgical procedure and transfusions may also lead to lung injury. There remains significant debate as to whether cardiopulmonary bypass surgery itself is a risk factor for ischemia-reperfusion injury [8, 22, 29, 30].

Pathophysiology of Ischemia-Reperfusion Injury

Identification of the risk factors that contribute to PGD has significantly enhanced the understanding of the pathophysiology. Pathologically, it is characterized by diffuse alveolar damage, and thus, the mechanisms that contribute to PGD are likely similar to that observed in non-transplant-related acute lung injury. However, the physiologic changes that occur during procurement (including cold ischemia) and implantation (including reperfusion) also provide unique circumstances that trigger different pathways and further the risk of injury.

Although still an area of intense study, the following summarizes the broad category of cells, molecules, and pathways that encompass the current state of knowledge of how injury from ischemia-reperfusion is felt to occur (Box 10.2). An illustration of their interactions is shown in Fig. 10.2.

Injury Due to Dysregulated Energy Metabolism Associated with Ischemia

During organ procurement, circulation to the lung is lost, anoxia develops locally in the tissue, and aerobic metabolism is halted. ATP is rapidly depleted, leading to loss of mitochondrial membrane potential. Loss of mitochondrial membrane potential leads to release of calcium, as well as

Box 10.2 Mechanisms of Ischemia-Reperfusion Injury

Dysregulated energy metabolism
  Loss of mitochondrial membrane potential
  Cellular apoptosis
Oxidative stress and generation of ROS
  Mitochondrial release
  Activation of xanthine oxidase
  NADPH-dependent superoxide generation
  Nitric oxide synthetase
  Neutrophil granules
Endothelial disruption
  Increase integrin expression
  Increased hypoxia-inducible factor
  Increased transient receptor potential vanilloid 4
  Increased intercellular adhesion molecule 1
Release of pro-inflammatory mediators
  Pro-thrombotic state
  Activation of complement cascade
  Release of pro-inflammatory cytokines
  Endothelin activation
  Increase in platelet-activating factor
  Increase in phospholipase A_2 and its metabolites
Leukocyte activation
  Macrophages
  Neutrophils
  T cells

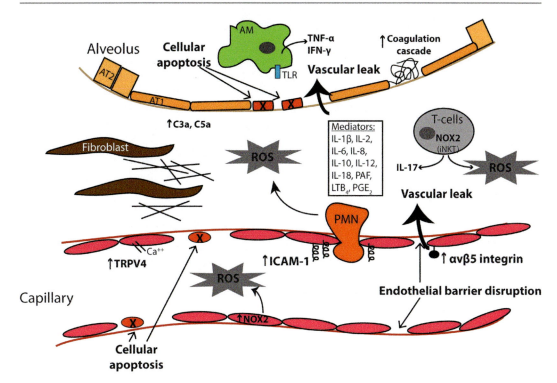

Fig. 10.2 Multiple mechanisms that contribute to lung ischemia-reperfusion injury. Ischemia-reperfusion injury is a consequence of multiple events in the vascular, interstitium, and alveolar space. The vascular space is characterized by oxidant injury, leakiness of the endothelial barrier, and adhesion and migration of neutrophils and T cells, which, together with macrophages, lead to damage of the alveolar epithelium, triggering of the coagulation cascade, activation of complement, and production of pro-inflammatory cytokines and lipid mediators. These then lead to further damage and amplification of lung injury. *NOX2* NADPH oxidase 2, *ROS* reactive oxygen species, *TRPV* transient receptor potential vanilloid, *ICAM-1* intercellular adhesion molecule-1, *PMN* polymorphonuclear cells, *iNKT* invariant natural killer T cells, *AM* alveolar macrophage, *AT1* alveolar epithelial cell type 1, *TLR* toll-like receptor, *TNF-α* tumor necrosis factor (TNF), *IFN-γ* interferon-γ, *IL* interleukin, *PAF* platelet-activating factor, *LTB4* leukotriene B$_4$, *PGE2* prostaglandin E$_2$

pro-apoptotic proteins such as members of the Bcl-2 family and cytochrome-*c*, which activates caspase 9 and the apoptotic pathway. The presence of apoptotic cells is a hallmark of ischemia-reperfusion injury [31]. Longer ischemia times are associated with greater evidence of apoptosis and eventual necrosis in lung tissue [20]. Cold temperatures preserve lung function by decreasing cellular metabolism and limiting ATP depletion [32].

Oxidative Stress and Generation of Reactive Oxygen Species (ROS)

At least some degree of organ ischemia is unavoidable during procurement, and rapid reperfusion of the organ helps to limit the damage from ischemia (and is ultimately necessary for organ function in the recipient). However, as critical as ischemia time is to organ injury, many studies have demonstrated that the process of reperfusion itself is just as important, if not more so, to tissue injury. The damage induced by reperfusion is generally considered a result of reactive oxygen species, resulting in oxidative stress. Animal models have shown that reperfusion of lungs results in a burst of free radicals within 1 h of reperfusion [33]. ROS intermediates can even be measured in the systemic circulation after reperfusion [33]. ROS can be derived from the mitochondria during energy depletion, from the activation of xanthine oxidase, from NADPH-dependent superoxide generation, from nitric oxide synthases, or from neutrophils themselves. The relative contribution from each of these sources of ROS is uncertain, but damage or shear stress to the endothelium may lead to upregulation of many of these pathways. It has been shown that a lack of perfusion may be "sensed" by mechanotransduction signals that lead to endothelial membrane depolarization and activation of NADPH oxidase 2, which contributes to ROS generation [34].

Endothelial Injury and Barrier Disruption

Not only are endothelial cells a potential source of ROS but also the targets of ROS damage. Endothelial injury and disruption of the endothelial barrier are often considered sentinel events in the development of ischemia-reperfusion injury and are often characterized by apoptosis [35]. Endothelial injury may occur as a consequence of ischemia or as a result of reperfusion which results in a burst of oxidative stress. The injury, whether due to hypoxia-induced apoptosis, shear stress due to alterations in blood flow, or a direct result of ROS, results in barrier disruption, leading to increased vascular permeability [34]. Integrins on the endothelial cell surface mediate vascular leak, and a recent study demonstrated that inhibition of the integrin $\alpha v \beta 5$ with blocking antibody decreased vascular leak in a mouse model of lung transplant [36]. Agonists to the sphingosine-1-phosphate receptors on endothelial cells have also been shown in animal models to decrease vascular leak after ischemia-reperfusion injury [37], indicating that these molecules are also important in regulating endothelial barrier dysfunction. Many cells including the endothelium express hypoxia-inducible factors (HIF) as they sense hypoxic or ischemic injury and that stabilization of HIF-1α [38] and HIF-2α [39] can assist in angiogenesis and resolution of ischemia-reperfusion injury. Stress to the endothelium, as sensed by transient receptor potential vanilloid 4, can result in increased opening of

calcium channels which can also contribute to lung injury [40]. Finally, ischemia-reperfusion injury may trigger endothelial dysfunction that leads to the upregulation of intercellular adhesion molecule 1 which contributes to leukocyte recruitment and extravasation [34].

Release of Pro-inflammatory Mediators

As with other forms of acute lung injury, ischemia-reperfusion injury is associated with increased production and release of a host of soluble enzymes, pro-inflammatory cytokines, and bioactive lipid mediators.

Complement and Procoagulation Cascade

Members of the complement cascade, including C3 and C5a, become activated during ischemia-reperfusion injury and amplify inflammation through neutrophil chemoattraction [41], increased vascular permeability, and increased smooth muscle contraction [17]. Complement activation antagonists improve vascular repair and limit vascular injury and chronic rejection. Injury is also associated with a pro-thrombotic state and is accompanied by an increase in tissue factor [42] and plasminogen inhibitor-1 [43] and a decrease in urokinase-type plasminogen activator and thrombomodulin [44]. This pro-thrombotic state contributes to microvascular thrombosis.

Cytokines

Ischemia-reperfusion injury is associated with a release of a number of pro-inflammatory cytokines, including tumor necrosis factor (TNF)-α, interferon-γ, IL-1β, IL-2, IL-6, IL-8, IL-10, IL-12, and IL-18 [45, 46]. Many of these cytokines have been shown to be elevated in other forms of acute lung injury. IL-8, in particular, negatively correlates with PaO_2/FiO_2 ratio and is associated with higher rates of PGD [47]. These cytokines, mostly derived from macrophages and lymphocytes, often amplify or potentiate the inflammatory process by upregulating adhesion molecules, increasing the sensitivity and contraction of vascular smooth muscle cells, and recruiting leukocytes to areas of inflammation. Notably, some of these cytokines may be derived from the donor organ as a consequence of brain death [11]. Many of these cytokines signal through activation of transcription factors NF-κB and AP-1 [48, 49].

Lipid Mediators

A number of bioactive lipids are also released to contribute to lung injury. These lipids are generated and released from the membrane predominantly by phospholipase A_2, which is activated in various forms of lung injury [50]. Platelet-activating factor (PAF) is one of the most potent lipid mediators that is critical to lung injury [51], and antagonists to PAF have been shown to reduce ischemia-reperfusion injury in animal models of lung transplant [52]. The incidence of posttransplant ischemia-reperfusion injury may be further reduced when PAF antagonists are combined with antagonists to endothelin-1 [53], a mediator elevated in ischemia-reperfusion injury that contributes to increased vascular endothelial growth factor and vascular permeability [54, 55]. Phospholipase A_2 also results in the generation of arachidonic acid-derived metabolites including leukotrienes B_4, C_4, D_4, and E_4 and the prostaglandins E_2, I_2, and F_{2a}, all of which recruit immune cells and contribute to inflammation.

Leukocyte Activation

Ischemia-reperfusion injury has been described as occurring in a biphasic pattern where donor characteristics influence injury in the first 24 h and recipient factors influence delayed phase of injury that occurs in the ensuing 24 h [56]. The activation of leukocytes is felt to play a critical role in the inflammatory response of both phases where donor-derived alveolar macrophages participate in the initial injury [57] and recipient neutrophils [58, 59] and T lymphocytes infiltrate the lung in the later phase of inflammation.

Alveolar macrophages may become activated from danger-associated molecular pattern molecules that trigger signaling through toll-like receptors (TLR) leading to the increased production of cytokines such as TNF-α and IFN-γ [45, 46, 60]. TLR4 plays an important role in ischemia-reperfusion injury, and knockdown of TLR4 attenuates injury after hypoxia-reoxygenation [61, 62]. Depletion of macrophages through the use of clodronate has also been suggested to attenuate ischemia-reperfusion injury [63].

Neutrophils are recruited by eicosanoids and chemokines such as CXCL2 and IL-8 produced by macrophages and adhesion molecules such as intercellular adhesion molecule 1 and P-selectin expressed by the endothelium [34, 64]. Neutrophils are felt to contribute to the "delayed" phase of injury [56, 58] through the release of other pro-inflammatory cytokines, proteases, and further generation of ROS. More recently, neutrophils have also been shown to generate neutrophil extracellular traps (NETs), and one study showed that NETs are induced after ischemia-reperfusion injury and are more abundant in patients with PGD [65].

Both donor-derived and recipient-recruited T lymphocytes also play a role in ischemia-reperfusion injury. Important donor-derived T cells include natural killer T cells which produce IL-17A through NADPH oxidase 2, leading to further inflammation and neutrophil infiltration [66]. CD4+ T lymphocytes also accumulate in lung tissue after reperfusion and contribute to the delayed phase of reperfusion injury by releasing IFN-γ [67].

Epigenetic Changes After Vascular Injury

In light of the acute damage that occurs during primary graft dysfunction, ischemia-reperfusion injury is also a major risk for chronic rejection and bronchiolitis obliterans syndrome (BOS) [5]. Despite being an acute event that occurs within the first 72 h after transplant, PGD carries a

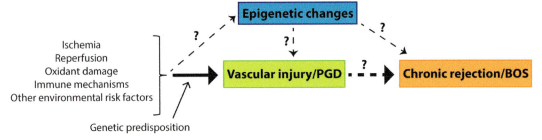

Fig. 10.3 Gene-environment interactions in the development of vascular injury factors that contribute to vascular injury and primary graft dysfunction (PGD) have the potential to also cause epigenetic changes which may be a mechanism by which late stage transplant complications occur

two- to threefold risk of developing chronic BOS that is independent of acute rejection, infection, and lymphocytic bronchitis [5]. One might thus conclude that ischemia-reperfusion injury and PGD result in changes at the molecular and cellular level that persist, even after clinical signs of injury have resolved. The pathophysiology of ischemia-reperfusion injury is reviewed above, but how seemingly short-term changes contribute to chronic rejection that is observed months to years later is unknown. Epigenetic alterations are often used to explain how early life environmental exposures contribute to chronic disease later in life and may be one mechanism by which PGD contributes to BOS (Fig. 10.3). Studies of epigenetic changes in the context of lung transplantation and ischemia-reperfusion injury are limited; however, other models and conditions of lung injury, repair, and fibrosis provide examples of how epigenetic alterations arise in the lung and lead to disease.

Overview of Epigenetic Mechanisms

Epigenetics refers to the heritable regulation of genes and their regulation that is not part of the DNA code itself (Fig. 10.4a–e). Originally coined by C.H. Waddington in 1942, the term epigenetics was used to describe how cells interact with their environment to differentiate and maintain phenotype as part of development. Today, it is recognized that methylation of DNA, covalent modifications of histones, and the actions of noncoding RNA all regulate and make up part of the "epigenetic code." This code influences which genes are transcribed and thus play an important role in cell fate and cell identity. Epigenetic mechanisms are evolutionarily conserved across species and are crucial for normal development. Aberrations in epigenetic patterns are also critical to the development of many diseases.

DNA Methylation

DNA methylation refers to the addition of methyl groups to DNA base pairs and occurs predominantly on the 5′ position of cytosine. DNA methylation typically occurs within the context of cytosine-guanine (CG) dinucleotide sequences, sometimes also termed CpG where the "p" represents the phosphate group between the nucleotides. Methylation has also been recognized to occur in non-CG contexts (designated CH where H is A, C, or T) as well [68]. CG sequences are unequally distributed throughout the genome but concentrate in high proportion designated as "CpG islands." These islands are often found in gene promoters, and, traditionally, methylation of these islands results in gene chromatin condensation and gene silencing [69]. Recent data, however, suggest that DNA methylation of CG sites distant from these islands, often termed "shores," may be just as important if not more so than CpG islands in gene regulation [70] and that methylation within gene bodies may increase expression [71]. Methylated cytosine can undergo further modification to form hydroxymethylcytosine which can lead to base excision, repair, and eventually an unmethylated state.

Methylation of DNA is carried out by the actions of DNA methyltransferases (DNMTs), where the DNMT1 isoform plays a role in the maintenance of methylation during replication, and DNMT3a and DNMT3b are enzymes

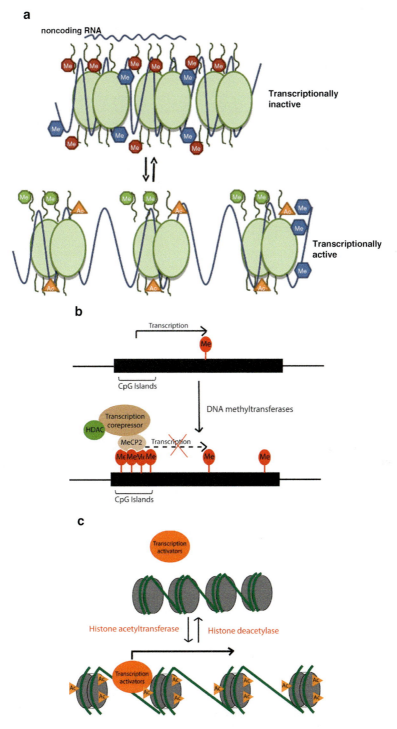

Fig. 10.4 (a–e) Epigenetic mechanisms. (a) Various epigenetic mechanisms, including DNA methylation, histone modifications, and actions of noncoding RNA work in concert to modulate chromatin rendering sections of the genome transcriptionally poised and/or active versus inactive. Histone modifications include acetylation and methylation (mono-, di-, and tri-), among others, at different amino acid residues often on the tails of various histone proteins. (b) DNA methylation at certain sites within genes can lead to recruitment of methyl-binding proteins (such as MeCP2) and transcription repression. (c, d) Acetylation or deacetylation of histones can alter the chromatin from an open or closed conformation, respectively, and affect accessibility of transcription factors. (e) Various histone marks at different amino acid residues are often associated with transcriptionally active or inactive chromatin

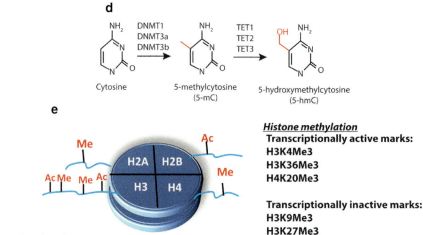

Fig. 10.4 (continued)

generally associated with de novo DNA methylation. Ten-eleven translocation (TET) enzymes were discovered to participate in hydroxymethylation [72]. DNA methylation is important for normal development and is a major mechanism for X-chromosome inactivation. However, it is also dynamic and tunable by the environment [73], and alterations in DNA methylation patterns play a role in aging and disease.

Histone Modifications

DNA is wound around histones in a coordinated and energy-dependent manner, and the structure of DNA-protein interactions contribute to the transcriptional activity of genes. Histones assemble into octamers consisting of two of each H3, H4, H2A, and H2B subunits. Each of the four core histone subunits contain a "tail" that sticks out from the octamer and contain amino acid residues by covalent modifications such as acetylation and methylation. The type, position, and degree of modification on each histone form a "histone code" [74] that affects whether genes are open as euchromatin and transcriptionally active or condensed and inactive. Certain histone marks, such as trimethylation of histone 3 at lysine 4 position, are found at transcriptional start sites and correlate with active transcription, whereas trimethylation of histone 3 at lysine 9 and 27 are associated with transcriptional repression. Many different enzymes form complexes that establish these marks, erase modifications, or remodel histone positioning. Many cancers are associated with mutations in these enzymes, and inhibitors to these enzymes are in development to treat many potential diseases. Histone marks and modifying complexes are also known to associate and affect DNA methylation patterns.

Noncoding RNA

Large sections of the genome are transcribed into RNA that do not code for protein and are collectively termed noncoding RNA. These include microRNA (miRNA), piwi-interacting RNA, short interfering RNA, and long noncoding RNA (lncRNA). These RNAs affect not just stability and protein translation of other mRNAs but also chromatin structure and the establishment of other epigenetic marks, including DNA methylation and histone modifications. Small RNAs (20–30 bp) are often expressed in a cell-type-specific manner, and miRNAs in particular have been shown to regulate over 60% of the human genome [75].

Epigenetic Changes in the Context of Other Lung Diseases

To date, there have been limited studies that have interrogated whether epigenetic changes occur after vascular injury in the context of lung transplantation, per se. However, epigenetic changes have been identified in other forms of lung injury

Box 10.3 Epigenetic Changes in Other Lung Diseases

Pulmonary fibrosis
DNA methylation
Thy-1
EP2 receptor
P14^{ARF}
Histone modifications
COX-2
IP-10
Fas receptor
miRNA
miR-17~92
miR-29
miR-145
miR-155
miR-199a-5p
miR-200
Pulmonary hypertension
DNA methylation
Superoxide dismutase 2
Histone modifications
Nitric oxide synthase
miRNA
Let-7b
Let-7d
miR-21
miR-204
Chronic obstructive pulmonary disease
Asthma

are enriched in repair and extracellular matrix generation. Although the etiology of IPF is unknown, repeated epithelial injury and dysregulated repair by fibroblasts and other mesenchymal cells are felt to be cardinal features of its pathophysiology. Lung fibroblasts from IPF patients, in particular, have been shown to exhibit increased DNA methylation that contribute to the decreased expression of the Thy-1 receptor [78], the E prostanoid 2 receptor [79], and p14^{ARF} [80]. The decreased expression of these proteins has been shown to contribute to the pro-fibrotic and anti-apoptotic features of these cells. Global DNA methylation analyses of fibroblasts have revealed that both hyper- and hypomethylated changes are present throughout the genome in IPF cells compared to nonfibrotic lung fibroblasts and have identified potentially hundreds of novel genes that are epigenetically dysregulated and important in IPF [81]. Modifications in histone marks have also been shown to contribute to decreased expression of cyclooxygenase-2 [82], IP-10 [83], and Fas receptor [84] in IPF fibroblasts, which may account for their resistance to apoptosis. Abnormal expression of a host of miRNAs including miR-17~92 [85], miR-29 [86], miR-145 [87], miR-155 [88], miR-199a-5p [89], and miR-200 [90] are dysregulated in IPF and contribute to IPF pathogenesis. Finally, differential expression of several lncRNAs have also been shown to be associated with fibrosis, though the functions of these lncRNAs are still being investigated [91].

Epigenetic Changes in Pulmonary Hypertension

Primary arterial pulmonary hypertension is characterized by remodeling of the vasculature and, in many regards, exhibits many pathophysiologic features similar to transplant-related BOS and vascular injury. Indeed, hypoxia and ischemia are important environmental stressors that play a key role in the pathogenesis of pulmonary hypertension, and induction of hypoxia is often employed to model pulmonary hypertension in animals. Epigenetic modifications of several pro-inflammatory cytokines have been shown to develop in arterial fibroblasts and are reversed

and repair and provide insight into the importance and possible mechanisms of how epigenetic changes may occur in the setting of transplantation (Box 10.3).

Epigenetic Changes in Diseases of Parenchymal Lung Injury and Pulmonary Fibrosis

Idiopathic pulmonary fibrosis (IPF) is the most common fibrotic disease among the diffuse parenchymal lung diseases, and numerous studies have demonstrated that epigenetic changes are present and widespread throughout the IPF lung. At least two independent studies of IPF lung tissue have demonstrated genome-wide level changes in DNA methylation [76, 77]. These changes occur in genes whose ontologies with histone deacetylase inhibitors [92]. Increased H3 and H4 acetylation at the promoter of endothelial nitric oxide synthase has been demonstrated in rat models of pulmonary hypertension [93]. DNA hypermethylation of superoxide dismutase 2 in pulmonary arterial smooth muscle has been demonstrated in strains of rats with spontaneous pulmonary arterial hypertension [94]. Finally, multiple studies have demonstrated that a multitude of miRNAs—including Let-7b [95], Let-7d [96], miR-21 [97], miR-204 [98] to name a few—are decreased in vascular endothelial cells and contribute to pulmonary hypertension in both patients and animal models. A recent study demonstrated that miR-21 was downregulated, leading to increased toll-like receptor signaling in PGD [99].

Epigenetic Changes in Airway Diseases

In no other lung disorder is the importance of epigenetic changes more evident than in obstructive airway diseases. A comprehensive list of all of the epigenetic abnormalities associated with asthma and chronic obstructive pulmonary disease (COPD) is beyond the scope of this chapter. However, a few illustrated examples demonstrate how epigenetic changes that occur in the airway and that lead to airway remodeling may inform us of potential epigenetic changes that may develop in the airways and parenchyma of lung transplant recipients that can lead to airway remodeling and bronchiolitis obliterans. One of the earliest studies in COPD that demonstrated the importance of histone modifications showed that decreased histone deacetylase activity was associated with increased severity of disease [100], and this was due in part to decreased steroid responsiveness [101]. Epigenetic modifications have also been shown to be important in the development of asthma, where DNA methylation changes have been identified in studies of individual genes [102] and in whole-genome analyses [103]. Importantly, many of these epigenetic changes arise in utero, which may explain how maternal diet and exposure to tobacco smoke and air pollution contribute to the development of asthma in children later in life. Pollution and tobacco smoke trigger many of the same inflammatory and oxidative pathways shared by vascular injury during transplantation, and epigenetic modifications may thus occur through similar mechanisms. Indeed, cigarette smoke has been shown to decrease levels of DNMT3b [104].

Evidence for Epigenetic Changes After Transplantation of Other Solid Organs

Outside of lung transplantation, important epigenetic modifications have been identified in the context of other solid organ transplants. These are often associated with ischemia-reperfusion injury as well. For example, demethylation of the *C3* gene has been associated with chronic nephropathy after kidney transplantation [105]. Detection of *CALCA* gene hypermethylation in urine has been proposed as a potential biomarker of acute kidney injury after kidney transplantation [106].

Mechanisms by Which Epigenetic Modifications May Arise After Lung Transplantation

Ischemia and Oxidative Stress

As alluded to earlier, epigenetic changes have been identified in various lung diseases, and ischemia and/or oxidative stress are mechanisms by which these changes may occur. Hypoxia is associated with changes in expression of DNMT and TET enzymes [107, 108]. Oxidative stress induces damage to DNA that can affect binding of epigenetic modifying enzymes [109]. Oxidative stress, often as a consequence of cigarette smoking and particulate matter, can also affect the expression of DNMT and TET enzymes that regulate DNA methylation. These data all support the notion that oxidative stress can influence epigenetic patterns after lung transplantation.

Epigenetic Changes Associated with Immune Responses

Since epigenetic modifications play a key role in cell identity and cellular phenotype, it is no surprise that epigenetic changes are crucial to leukocyte differentiation and the development of particular immune responses. Specific DNA methylation profiles play a direct role in the segregation of Th1 and Th2 cells [110], and DNA methylation is recognized to regulate expression of Foxp3 [111], a key transcription factor that induces Treg development. Epigenetic factors also affect the differentiation of myeloid cells and polarization of macrophages that are important in innate immunity [112]. Factors that influence the epigenetic patterns of all of these cell types may thus play an important role in the modulation of immune responses that critically affect rates of acute and chronic allograft rejection.

Epigenetic Considerations for Future Therapy and Biomarker of Injury in Lung Transplantation

Many of the features that dictate the success of lung transplantation—age of the donor organ, modulation of immune responses, duration of ischemia and degree of reperfusion, and development of fibrotic repair—are all factors that have been demonstrated in varying degrees to affect epigenetic patterns. As a consequence, acquired epigenetic changes play an important role in long-term gene expression patterns and, in the case of transplantation, can influence immediate and longer-lasting effects on organ survival and organ failure. Because different diseases often provide a distinct epigenetic profile, assaying epigenetic profiles in different compartments can serve as a potential biomarker for the presence of disease. Finally, many drugs have been designed to target epigenetic modifying enzymes such as DNA methylation inhibitors, histone deacetylase inhibitors, and bromodomain inhibitors, and these drugs offer the opportunity to treat diseases dependent on epigenetic changes.

Clinical Assessment of Vascular Injury and Graft Dysfunction

Diagnosis and Differential Diagnosis

The International Society for Heart and Lung Transplantation has standardized the definition of PGD as occurring within the first 72 h after transplant [3], but other conditions associated with hypoxemia and diffuse pulmonary infiltrates must be excluded. The differential diagnosis of PGD includes cardiogenic pulmonary edema, pneumonia, transfusion-related lung injury, antibody-mediated acute rejection, and thromboembolism.

Pulmonary Edema

Transplantation is often accompanied by significant fluid shifts perioperatively, and one should rule out pulmonary edema in the differential. Depending on the pretransplant diagnosis, some patients may also have cardiac dysfunction as a result of pulmonary hypertension. An echocardiogram and some measure of fluid status, through either invasive or noninvasive means, should be performed. In some cases, a pulmonary artery catheter may help guide fluid management.

Pneumonia

Although elevated white count, fever, and radiographic infiltrates are often useful in making a clinical diagnosis of pneumonia, these features are also often found in patients posttransplant without evidence of infection, making pneumonia difficult to distinguish from cases of PGD. Bronchoscopy or cultures from endotracheal aspirates can be useful in this setting, as well as blood cultures from the recipient and cultures from the donor lung. Bacterial pneumonia continues to be a cause of morbidity and mortality posttransplant despite prophylactic antibiotics.

Antibody-Mediated Rejection

Hyperacute rejection is a rare cause of organ dysfunction that occurs within the first 24 h and is due preformed antibodies against the donor organ. If hyperacute rejection is suspected, the pretransplant panel reactive antibody test could be reviewed, and increased cross-reactivity, especially greater than 10%, is more suggestive of hyperacute rejection [113]. Acute rejection due to newly derived antibodies from the host typically occurs after 24 h and is often suppressed by the significant immunosuppression given immediately after transplant. Bronchoscopy with transbronchial biopsies can help diagnose this.

Grading System

The International Society of Heart and Lung Transplantation has proposed criteria used to grade the severity of PGD based on the ratio of the partial pressure of oxygen in the artery to the fraction of inspired oxygen (PaO_2/FiO_2) (Table 10.1) [3]. These criteria are akin to criteria often used to define or grade ARDS. Consensus criteria for diagnosing and grading PGD are important in order to standardize terminology, capture the spectrum of severity, and establish criteria that assist in clinical studies and future scientific inquiry.

It is recommended that grading and diagnostic criteria be assessed serially at 24, 48, and 72 h. Some clinicians recommend the use of additional time points such as 6 and 12 h which may help identify patients early for more aggressive treatment.

Table 10.1 Grading severity of ischemia-reperfusion injury

Grade 0	$PaO_2/FiO_2 > 300$ and normal chest radiograph
Grade 1	$PaO_2/FiO_2 > 300$ and diffuse allograft infiltrates on chest radiograph
Grade 2	PaO_2/FiO_2 between 200 and 300
Grade 3	$PaO_2/FiO_2 < 200$

Adapted with permission of Elsevier from Christie JD, Carby M, Bag R, Corris P, Hertz M, Weill D, ISHLT Working Group on Primary Lung Graft Dysfunction. Report of the ISHLT Working Group on Primary Lung Graft Dysfunction part II: definition. A consensus statement of the International Society for Heart and Lung Transplantation. J Heart Lung Transplant 2005;24: 1454-1459

Prevention and Treatment Strategies to Limit Vascular Injury and PGD

Since many factors are involved in the pathophysiology of vascular injury and PGD, prevention strategies target multiple steps along the transplant process, including retrieval, preservation, implantation, reperfusion, and posttransplant care that might mitigate these risks (Box 10.4).

Lung Preservation Techniques

Historically, different preservative solutions—including the Euro-Collins, the University of Wisconsin, the low potassium dextran, and the Celsior—have all been used and vary by electrolyte and metabolite composition. There is no clear solution of choice, with various studies often supporting one solution over another and randomized controlled trials showing only

---

Box 10.4 Preventive and Treatment Strategies for PGD

Lung preservation techniques
- Preservation solution
- Addition of prostaglandin E1 in preservation
- Cold temperature 4–8 °C
- Minimize ischemia time
- Low-pressure, slow reperfusion
- Ex vivo lung perfusion strategies

Postoperative management
- Low tidal volume, lung protective strategies
- Consideration of inhaled nitric oxide
- Consideration of inhaled prostacyclin
- Extracorporeal membrane oxygenation

Experimental therapies
- Ex vivo lung perfusion (EVLP)
- Bronchial artery revascularization
- Antagonist to platelet-activating factor
- Antagonist to soluble complement receptor 1
- Antioxidants such as *N*-acetylcysteine
- DNA methylation inhibitors
- Inhibitors to histone modifying enzymes

modest impact. The volume, pressure, and temperature of the flush solution are also variables that need to be taken into account. These decisions are discussed in greater detail in Chap. 8.

Most organs are stored between 4 and 8 °C, though optimal temperatures and storage times are unknown. Cold ischemia times of up to 8 h are generally considered acceptable, and it is debated as to whether longer ischemia times contribute to PGD [6]. Donor risk factors (such as age and smoking history) and recipient risk factors (such as the underlying diagnosis) may be more important than duration of cold ischemia and may allow for transplantation of organs up to 12 h of cold ischemia time [6]. Recent advancements in EVLP have prolonged the viability of the donor lung at normothermic conditions, improved the suitability of higher-risk donor organs, and have the potential to dramatically change how organs are preserved and allocated. Although it is unclear if EVLP by itself decreases the incidence of PGD, the use of EVLP allows for a longer preservation times (>12 h) without increasing the risk for PGD [16].

Since mechanical stress and oxidative damage are major factors that contribute to vascular injury, approaches that minimize damage during reperfusion may be even more critical than ischemia time in limiting PGD. It is recommended that a gradual reintroduction of blood flow over a 10-min period be performed which has been shown to reduce the incidence of lung injury in animal models [114, 115]. Lower pressure during reperfusion, such as between 20 and 30 mmHg, is also recommended to reduce the incidence of reperfusion injury [116]. With its vasodilatory properties, inhaled nitric oxide has been proposed as a possible strategy to prevent injury during reperfusion, but small prospective randomized trials have not shown this to be beneficial [117]. The addition of prostaglandin E_1 to the preservation solution [118] or to the patient directly during reperfusion has also been suggested as means of limiting injury given the vasodilatory and anti-inflammatory properties of prostaglandins.

Current Treatment of PGD

The treatment of patients with ischemia-reperfusion injury is mainly supportive and parallels strategies for patients with ARDS. Low tidal volume protective ventilation strategies should be employed. Although inhaled nitric oxide has not been shown to be beneficial in preventing PGD, case series suggest that it may be beneficial in treating patients with established ischemia-reperfusion injury [119, 120]. Inhaled prostacyclin is another vasodilator that has been used and may be beneficial as well. Finally, although extracorporeal membrane oxygenation (ECMO) is often considered a salvage therapy reserved in cases of severe, life-threatening hypoxemia, early initiation of ECMO may be beneficial and associated with a 40–80% survival [119, 121].

Future Considerations in Prevention and Treatment

With improved knowledge of the pathophysiology of ischemia-reperfusion injury, many targets can be considered for future treatment and prevention. Improvements in surgical techniques and perioperative management are discussed in Chap. 8. This includes strategies for EVLP and consideration of bronchial artery revascularization. Although predominantly thought to decrease rates of anastomosis dehiscence and stenosis, bronchial artery revascularization may also improve tissue perfusion and protect epithelium and endothelium from damage. Prostaglandins, as discussed earlier, require clinical trials to support its efficacy. Exogenous surfactant therapy may help improve the structure and function of the lung [122].

Among the many mediators that contribute to injury, targeting PAF with the antagonist BN52021 is one of the more promising and has been shown in clinical trials to improve oxygenation [123]. Since leukocytes play a key role in mediating damage associated with ischemia-reperfusion, inhibition of complement, such as with soluble complement receptor-1, has also been shown in small randomized controlled trials to be beneficial [124]. All of these studies require further follow-up with larger-scale randomized controlled trials.

Given that oxidant injury plays a critical role in the pathogenesis, antioxidants such as N-acetylcysteine may be beneficial [125]. Inhibition of xanthine oxidase or NADPH oxidase may also be beneficial in limiting oxidative injury, as has been shown in animal models [126]. Since macrophages and neutrophils play a key role in the inflammatory cascade, selective depletion of these cells and/or the cytokines they produce may be beneficial. In contrast, infusion of cell-based therapies, such as mesenchymal stem cells that participate in regeneration and repair, may attenuate the severity of injury [127, 128]. Given the potential for epigenetic modifications to arise in the lung after injury, methylation inhibitors and bromodomain inhibitors that target epigenetic modifying enzymes may also have a role.

Conclusion

PGD lies at the severe end of the broader spectrum of ischemia-reperfusion injury. Despite advances in transplant surgery, PGD remains a frequent cause of morbidity and mortality after transplantation. Factors related to the donor, organ procurement, organ preservation, recipient condition, and postoperative care all contribute to the risk of ischemia-reperfusion injury. The pathophysiology of ischemia-reperfusion injury is complex and involves (1) damage due to ischemia including apoptosis, (2) oxidative injury caused by ROS, (3) damage to the endothelial barrier, (4) an influx of inflammatory leukocytes including neutrophils, and (5) release of a myriad of pro-inflammatory cytokines, lipids, and other mediators. Because of the injurious environment, ischemia-reperfusion injury may be associated with epigenetic changes, which may be a source of persistent abnormalities that contribute to organ dysfunction, such as bronchiolitis obliterans syndrome, later in the posttransplant course. The diagnosis of ischemia-reperfusion injury should be considered in any posttransplant patient with hypoxia and pulmonary infiltrates, and appropriate diagnostic, preventive, and treatment measures should be taken. Future treatment strategies require vigorous testing at the clinical level but provide optimism in the prevention and treatment of this highly morbid condition.

References

1. Christie JD, Sager JS, Kimmel SE, Ahya VN, Gaughan C, Blumenthal NP, Kotloff RM. Impact of primary graft failure on outcomes following lung transplantation. Chest. 2005;127:161–5.
2. Arcasoy SM, Fisher A, Hachem RR, Scavuzzo M, Ware LB, ISHLT Working Group on Primary Lung Graft Dysfunction. Report of the ISHLT Working Group on Primary Lung Graft Dysfunction part V: predictors and outcomes. J Heart Lung Transplant. 2005;24:1483–8.
3. Christie JD, Carby M, Bag R, Corris P, Hertz M, Weill D, ISHLT Working Group on Primary Lung Graft Dysfunction. Report of the ISHLT Working Group on Primary Lung Graft Dysfunction part II: definition. A consensus statement of the International Society for Heart and Lung Transplantation. J Heart Lung Transplant. 2005;24:1454–9.
4. Lee JC, Christie JD. Primary graft dysfunction. Proc Am Thorac Soc. 2009;6:39–46.
5. Daud SA, Yusen RD, Meyers BF, Chakinala MM, Walter MJ, Aloush AA, Patterson GA, Trulock EP, Hachem RR. Impact of immediate primary lung allograft dysfunction on bronchiolitis obliterans syndrome. Am J Respir Crit Care Med. 2007;75:507–13.
6. de Perrot M, Bonser RS, Dark J, Kelly RF, McGiffin D, Menza R, Pajaro O, Schueler S, Verleden GM, ISHLT Working Group on Primary Lung Graft Dysfunction. Report of the ISHLT Working Group on Primary Lung Graft Dysfunction part III: donor-related risk factors and markers. J Heart Lung Transplant. 2005;24:1460–7.
7. Whitson BA, Nath DS, Johnson AC, Walker AR, Prekker ME, Radosevich DM, Herrington CS, Dahlberg PS. Risk factors for primary graft dysfunction after lung transplantation. J Thorac Cardiovasc Surg. 2006;131:73–80.
8. Christie JD, Kotloff RM, Pochettino A, Arcasoy SM, Rosengard BR, Landis JR, Kimmel SE. Clinical risk factors for primary graft failure following lung transplantation. Chest. 2003;124:1232–41.
9. Oto T, Excell L, Griffiths AP, Levvey BJ, Snell GI. The implications of pulmonary embolism in a multiorgan donor for subsequent pulmonary, renal, and cardiac transplantation. J Heart Lung Transplant. 2008;27:78–85.

10. Diamond JM, Lee JC, Kawut SM, Shah RJ, Localio AR, Bellamy SL, Lederer DJ, Cantu E, Kohl BA, Lama VN, Bhorade SM, Crespo M, Demissie E, Sonett J, Wille K, Orens J, Shah AS, Weinacker A, Arcasoy S, Shah PD, Wilkes DS, Ware LB, Palmer SM, Christie JD, Lung Transplant Outcomes Group. Clinical risk factors for primary graft dysfunction after lung transplantation. Am J Respir Crit Care Med. 2013;187:527–34.

11. Kaneda H, Waddell TK, de Perrot M, Bai XH, Gutierrez C, Arenovich T, Chaparro C, Liu M, Keshavjee S. Pre-implantation multiple cytokine mRNA expression analysis of donor lung grafts predicts survival after lung transplantation in humans. Am J Transplant. 2006;6:544–51.

12. Pasque MK. Standardizing thoracic organ procurement for transplantation. J Thorac Cardiovasc Surg. 2010;139:13–7.

13. Fiser SM, Kron IL, Long SM, Kaza AK, Kern JA, Cassada DC, Jones DR, Robbins MC, Tribble CG. Influence of graft ischemic time on outcomes following lung transplantation. J Heart Lung Transplant. 2001;20:1291–6.

14. Novick RJ, Bennett LE, Meyer DM, Hosenpud JD. Influence of graft ischemic time and donor age on survival after lung transplantation. J Heart Lung Transplant. 1999;18:425–31.

15. Thabut G, Mal H, Cerrina J, Dartevelle P, Dromer C, Velly JF, Stern M, Loirat P, Leseche G, Bertocchi M, Mornex JF, Haloun A, Despins P, Pison C, Blin D, Reynaud-Gaubert M. Graft ischemic time and outcome of lung transplantation: a multicenter analysis. Am J Respir Crit Care Med. 2005;171:786–91.

16. Yeung JC, Krueger T, Yasufuku K, de Perrot M, Pierre AF, Waddell TK, Singer LG, Keshavjee S, Cypel M. Outcomes after transplantation of lungs preserved for more than 12 h: a retrospective study. Lancet Respir Med. 2017;5:119–24.

17. de Perrot M, Liu M, Waddell TK, Keshavjee S. Ischemia-reperfusion-induced lung injury. Am J Respir Crit Care Med. 2003;167:490–511.

18. Ware LB, Golden JA, Finkbeiner WE, Matthay MA. Alveolar epithelial fluid transport capacity in reperfusion lung injury after lung transplantation. Am J Respir Crit Care Med. 1999;159:980–8.

19. Clavien PA, Harvey PR, Strasberg SM. Preservation and reperfusion injuries in liver allografts. An overview and synthesis of current studies. Transplantation. 1992;53:957–78.

20. Fischer S, Maclean AA, Liu M, Cardella JA, Slutsky AS, Suga M, Moreira JF, Keshavjee S. Dynamic changes in apoptotic and necrotic cell death correlate with severity of ischemia-reperfusion injury in lung transplantation. Am J Respir Crit Care Med. 2000;162:1932–9.

21. Fang A, Studer S, Kawut SM, Ahya VN, Lee J, Wille K, Lama V, Ware L, Orens J, Weinacker A, Palmer SM, Crespo M, Lederer DJ, Deutschman CS, Kohl BA, Bellamy S, Demissie E, Christie JD, Lung Transplant Outcomes Group. Elevated pulmonary artery pressure is a risk factor for primary graft dysfunction following lung transplantation for idiopathic pulmonary fibrosis. Chest. 2011;139:782–7.

22. Barr ML, Kawut SM, Whelan TP, Girgis R, Bottcher H, Sonett J, Vigneswaran W, Follette DM, Corris PA, ISHLT Working Group on Primary Lung Graft Dysfunction. Report of the ISHLT Working Group on Primary Lung Graft Dysfunction part IV: recipient-related risk factors and markers. J Heart Lung Transplant. 2005;24:1468–82.

23. Dudek SM, Garcia JG. Cytoskeletal regulation of pulmonary vascular permeability. J Appl Physiol (1985). 2001;91:1487–500.

24. Zhao YD, Peng J, Granton E, Lin K, Lu C, Wu L, Machuca T, Waddell TK, Keshavjee S, de Perrot M. Pulmonary vascular changes 22 years after single lung transplantation for pulmonary arterial hypertension: a case report with molecular and pathological analysis. Pulm Circ. 2015;5:739–43.

25. Bando K, Keenan RJ, Paradis IL, Konishi H, Komatsu K, Hardesty RL, Griffith BP. Impact of pulmonary hypertension on outcome after single-lung transplantation. Ann Thorac Surg. 1994;58:1336–42.

26. Conte JV, Borja MJ, Patel CB, Yang SC, Jhaveri RM, Orens JB. Lung transplantation for primary and secondary pulmonary hypertension. Ann Thorac Surg. 2001;72:1673–9, discussion 1679–80

27. Huerd SS, Hodges TN, Grover FL, Mault JR, Mitchell MB, Campbell DN, Aziz S, Chetham P, Torres F, Zamora MR. Secondary pulmonary hypertension does not adversely affect outcome after single lung transplantation. J Thorac Cardiovasc Surg. 2000;119:458–65.

28. Julliard WA, Meyer KC, De Oliveira NC, Osaki S, Cornwell RC, Sonetti DA, Maloney JD. The presence or severity of pulmonary hypertension does not affect outcomes for single-lung transplantation. Thorax. 2016;71:478–80.

29. Aeba R, Griffith BP, Kormos RL, Armitage JM, Gasior TA, Fuhrman CR, Yousem SA, Hardesty RL. Effect of cardiopulmonary bypass on early graft dysfunction in clinical lung transplantation. Ann Thorac Surg. 1994;57:715–22.

30. Triantafillou AN, Pasque MK, Huddleston CB, Pond CG, Cerza RF, Forstot RM, Cooper JD, Patterson GA, Lappas DG. Predictors, frequency, and indications for cardiopulmonary bypass during lung transplantation in adults. Ann Thorac Surg. 1994;57:1248–51.

31. Stammberger U, Gaspert A, Hillinger S, Vogt P, Odermatt B, Weder W, Schmid RA. Apoptosis induced by ischemia and reperfusion in experimental lung transplantation. Ann Thorac Surg. 2000;69:1532–6.

32. Shoji T, Omasa M, Nakamura T, Yoshimura T, Yoshida H, Ikeyama K, Fukuse T, Wada H. Mild hypothermia ameliorates lung ischemia reperfusion injury in an ex vivo rat lung model. Eur Surg Res. 2005;37:348–53.

33. Gielis JF, Boulet GA, Briede JJ, Horemans T, Debergh T, Kusse M, Cos P, Van Schil PE. Longitudinal quantification of radical bursts during pulmonary ischaemia and reperfusion. Eur J Cardiothorac Surg. 2015;48:622–9.

34. Chatterjee S, Nieman GF, Christie JD, Fisher AB. Shear stress-related mechanosignaling with lung ischemia: lessons from basic research can inform lung transplantation. Am J Physiol Lung Cell Mol Physiol. 2014;307:L668–80.

35. Gilmont RR, Dardano A, Engle JS, Adamson BS, Welsh MJ, Li T, Remick DG, Smith DJ Jr, Rees RS. TNF-alpha potentiates oxidant and reperfusion-induced endothelial cell injury. J Surg Res. 1996;61:175–82.

36. Mallavia B, Liu F, Sheppard D, Looney MR. Inhibiting integrin alphavbeta5 reduces ischemia-reperfusion injury in an orthotopic lung transplant model in mice. Am J Transplant. 2016;16:1306–11.

37. Stone ML, Sharma AK, Zhao Y, Charles EJ, Huerter ME, Johnston WF, Kron IL, Lynch KR, Laubach VE. Sphingosine-1-phosphate receptor 1 agonism attenuates lung ischemia-reperfusion injury. Am J Physiol Lung Cell Mol Physiol. 2015;308:L1245–52.

38. Zhao X, Jin Y, Li H, Wang Z, Zhang W, Feng C. Hypoxia-inducible factor 1 alpha contributes to pulmonary vascular dysfunction in lung ischemia-reperfusion injury. Int J Clin Exp Pathol. 2014;7:3081–8.

39. Ge H, Zhu H, Xu N, Zhang D, Ou J, Wang G, Fang X, Zhou J, Song Y, Bai C. Increased lung ischemia-reperfusion injury in aquaporin 1-null mice is mediated via decreased hypoxia-inducible factor 2alpha stability. Am J Respir Cell Mol Biol. 2016;54:882–91.

40. Balakrishna S, Song W, Achanta S, Doran SF, Liu B, Kaelberer MM, Yu Z, Sui A, Cheung M, Leishman E, Eidam HS, Ye G, Willette RN, Thorneloe KS, Bradshaw HB, Matalon S, Jordt SE. TRPV4 inhibition counteracts edema and inflammation and improves pulmonary function and oxygen saturation in chemically induced acute lung injury. Am J Physiol Lung Cell Mol Physiol. 2014;307:L158–72.

41. Ivey CL, Williams FM, Collins PD, Jose PJ, Williams TJ. Neutrophil chemoattractants generated in two phases during reperfusion of ischemic myocardium in the rabbit. Evidence for a role for C5a and interleukin-8. J Clin Invest. 1995;95:2720–8.

42. Compeau CG, Ma J, DeCampos KN, Waddell TK, Brisseau GF, Slutsky AS, Rotstein OD. In situ ischemia and hypoxia enhance alveolar macrophage tissue factor expression. Am J Respir Cell Mol Biol. 1994;11:446–55.

43. Pinsky DJ, Liao H, Lawson CA, Yan SF, Chen J, Carmeliet P, Loskutoff DJ, Stern DM. Coordinated induction of plasminogen activator inhibitor-1 (PAI-1) and inhibition of plasminogen activator gene expression by hypoxia promotes pulmonary vascular fibrin deposition. J Clin Invest. 1998;102:919–28.

44. Ogawa S, Gerlach H, Esposito C, Pasagian-Macaulay A, Brett J, Stern D. Hypoxia modulates the barrier and coagulant function of cultured bovine endothelium. Increased monolayer permeability and induction of procoagulant properties. J Clin Invest. 1990;85:1090–8.

45. Krishnadasan B, Naidu BV, Byrne K, Fraga C, Verrier ED, Mulligan MS. The role of proinflammatory cytokines in lung ischemia-reperfusion injury. J Thorac Cardiovasc Surg. 2003;125:261–72.

46. Ng CS, Wan S, Arifi AA, Yim AP. Inflammatory response to pulmonary ischemia-reperfusion injury. Surg Today. 2006;36:205–14.

47. De Perrot M, Sekine Y, Fischer S, Waddell TK, McRae K, Liu M, Wigle DA, Keshavjee S. Interleukin-8 release during early reperfusion predicts graft function in human lung transplantation. Am J Respir Crit Care Med. 2002;165:211–5.

48. Lan Q, Mercurius KO, Davies PF. Stimulation of transcription factors NF kappa B and AP1 in endothelial cells subjected to shear stress. Biochem Biophys Res Commun. 1994;201:950–6.

49. den Hengst WA, Gielis JF, Lin JY, Van Schil PE, De Windt LJ, Moens AL. Lung ischemia-reperfusion injury: a molecular and clinical view on a complex pathophysiological process. Am J Physiol Heart Circ Physiol. 2010;299:H1283–99.

50. Arbibe L, Koumanov K, Vial D, Rougeot C, Faure G, Havet N, Longacre S, Vargaftig BB, Bereziat G, Voelker DR, Wolf C, Touqui L. Generation of lysophospholipids from surfactant in acute lung injury is mediated by type-II phospholipase A2 and inhibited by a direct surfactant protein A-phospholipase A2 protein interaction. J Clin Invest. 1998;102:1152–60.

51. Nagase T, Ishii S, Kume K, Uozumi N, Izumi T, Ouchi Y, Shimizu T. Platelet-activating factor mediates acid-induced lung injury in genetically engineered mice. J Clin Invest. 1999;104:1071–6.

52. Kawahara K, Tagawa T, Takahashi T, Akamine S, Nakamura A, Yamamoto S, Muraoka S, Tomita M. The effect of the platelet-activating factor inhibitor TCV-309 on reperfusion injury in a canine model of ischemic lung. Transplantation. 1993;55:1438–9.

53. Stammberger U, Carboni GL, Hillinger S, Schneiter D, Weder W, Schmid RA. Combined treatment with endothelin- and PAF-antagonists reduces posttransplant lung ischemia/reperfusion injury. J Heart Lung Transplant. 1999;18:862–8.

54. Shennib H, Serrick C, Saleh D, Adoumie R, Stewart DJ, Giaid A. Alterations in bronchoalveolar lavage and plasma endothelin-1 levels early after lung transplantation. Transplantation. 1995;59:994–8.

55. Taghavi S, Abraham D, Riml P, Paulus P, Schafer R, Klepetko W, Aharinejad S. Co-expression of endothelin-1 and vascular endothelial growth factor mediates increased vascular permeability in lung grafts before reperfusion. J Heart Lung Transplant. 2002;21:600–3.

56. Fiser SM, Tribble CG, Long SM, Kaza AK, Cope JT, Laubach VE, Kern JA, Kron IL. Lung transplant

reperfusion injury involves pulmonary macrophages and circulating leukocytes in a biphasic response. J Thorac Cardiovasc Surg. 2001;121:1069–75.

57. Naidu BV, Krishnadasan B, Farivar AS, Woolley SM, Thomas R, Van Rooijen N, Verrier ED, Mulligan MS. Early activation of the alveolar macrophage is critical to the development of lung ischemia-reperfusion injury. J Thorac Cardiovasc Surg. 2003;126:200–7.

58. Welbourn CR, Goldman G, Paterson IS, Valeri CR, Shepro D, Hechtman HB. Pathophysiology of isch-aemia reperfusion injury: central role of the neutro-phil. Br J Surg. 1991;78:651–5.

59. Adoumie R, Serrick C, Giaid A, Shennib H. Early cellular events in the lung allograft. Ann Thorac Surg. 1992;54:1071–6, discussion 1076–7.

60. Chen GY, Nunez G. Sterile inflammation: sens-ing and reacting to damage. Nat Rev Immunol. 2010;10:826–37.

61. Merry HE, Phelan P, Doak MR, Zhao M, Hwang B, Mulligan MS. Role of toll-like receptor-4 in lung ischemia-reperfusion injury. Ann Thorac Surg. 2015;99:1193–9.

62. Zanotti G, Casiraghi M, Abano JB, Tatreau JR, Sevala M, Berlin H, Smyth S, Funkhouser WK, Burridge K, Randell SH, Egan TM. Novel criti-cal role of Toll-like receptor 4 in lung ischemia-reperfusion injury and edema. Am J Physiol Lung Cell Mol Physiol. 2009;297:L52–63.

63. Zhao M, Fernandez LG, Doctor A, Sharma AK, Zarbock A, Tribble CG, Kron IL, Laubach VE. Alveolar macrophage activation is a key ini-tiation signal for acute lung ischemia-reperfusion injury. Am J Physiol Lung Cell Mol Physiol. 2006;291:L1018–26.

64. Moore TM, Khimenko P, Adkins WK, Miyasaka M, Taylor AE. Adhesion molecules contribute to isch-emia and reperfusion-induced injury in the isolated rat lung. J Appl Physiol (1985). 1995;78:2245–52.

65. Sayah DM, Mallavia B, Liu F, Ortiz-Munoz G, Caudrillier A, DerHovanessian A, Ross DJ, Lynch JP III, Saggar R, Ardehali A, Lung Transplant Outcomes Group, Ware LB, Christie JD, Belperio JA, Looney MR. Neutrophil extracellular traps are pathogenic in primary graft dysfunction after lung transplantation. Am J Respir Crit Care Med 2015;191:455–63.

66. Sharma AK, LaPar DJ, Stone ML, Zhao Y, Mehta CK, Kron IL, Laubach VE. NOX2 activation of natu-ral killer T cells is blocked by the adenosine A2A receptor to inhibit lung ischemia-reperfusion injury. Am J Respir Crit Care Med. 2016;193:988–99.

67. de Perrot M, Young K, Imai Y, Liu M, Waddell TK, Fischer S, Zhang L, Keshavjee S. Recipient T cells mediate reperfusion injury after lung transplantation in the rat. J Immunol. 2003;171:4995–5002.

68. Lister R, Pelizzola M, Dowen RH, Hawkins RD, Hon G, Tonti-Filippini J, Nery JR, Lee L, Ye Z, Ngo QM, Edsall L, Antosiewicz-Bourget J, Stewart R, Ruotti V, Millar AH, Thomson JA, Ren B, Ecker

JR. Human DNA methylomes at base resolution show widespread epigenomic differences. Nature. 2009;462:315–22.

69. Suzuki MM, Bird A. DNA methylation landscapes: provocative insights from epigenomics. Nat Rev Genet. 2008;9:465–76.

70. Irizarry RA, Ladd-Acosta C, Wen B, Wu Z, Montano C, Onyango P, Cui H, Gabo K, Rongione M, Webster M, Ji H, Potash JB, Sabunciyan S, Feinberg AP. The human colon cancer methylome shows similar hypo- and hypermethylation at conserved tissue-specific CpG island shores. Nat Genet. 2009;41:178–86.

71. Hellman A, Chess A. Gene body-specific meth-ylation on the active X chromosome. Science. 2007;315:1141–3.

72. Tahiliani M, Koh KP, Shen Y, Pastor WA, Bandukwala H, Brudno Y, Agarwal S, Iyer LM, Liu DR, Aravind L, Rao A. Conversion of 5-methylcytosine to 5-hydroxymethylcytosine in mammalian DNA by MLL partner TET1. Science. 2009;324:930–5.

73. Feil R, Fraga MF. Epigenetics and the environment: emerging patterns and implications. Nat Rev Genet. 2012;13:97–109.

74. Jenuwein T, Allis CD. Translating the histone code. Science. 2001;293:1074–80.

75. Lewis BP, Burge CB, Bartel DP. Conserved seed pairing, often flanked by adenosines, indicates that thousands of human genes are microRNA targets. Cell. 2005;120:15–20.

76. Rabinovich EI, Kapetanaki MG, Steinfeld I, Gibson KF, Pandit KV, Yu G, Yakhini Z, Kaminski N. Global methylation patterns in idiopathic pulmonary fibro-sis. PLoS One. 2012;7:e33770.

77. Sanders YY, Ambalavanan N, Halloran B, Zhang X, Liu H, Crossman DK, Bray M, Zhang K, Thannickal VJ, Hagood JS. Altered DNA methylation profile in idiopathic pulmonary fibrosis. Am J Respir Crit Care Med. 2012;186:525–35.

78. Sanders YY, Pardo A, Selman M, Nuovo GJ, Tollefsbol TO, Siegal GP, Hagood JS. Thy-1 pro-moter hypermethylation: a novel epigenetic patho-genic mechanism in pulmonary fibrosis. Am J Respir Cell Mol Biol. 2008;39:610–8.

79. Huang SK, Fisher AS, Scruggs AM, White ES, Hogaboam CM, Richardson BC, Peters-Golden M. Hypermethylation of PTGER2 confers pros-taglandin E2 resistance in fibrotic fibroblasts from humans and mice. Am J Pathol. 2010;177:2245–55.

80. Cisneros J, Hagood J, Checa M, Ortiz-Quintero B, Negreros M, Herrera I, Ramos C, Pardo A, Selman M. Hypermethylation-mediated silencing of p14(ARF) in fibroblasts from idiopathic pulmo-nary fibrosis. Am J Physiol Lung Cell Mol Physiol. 2012;303:L295–303.

81. Huang SK, Scruggs AM, McEachin RC, White ES, Peters-Golden M. Lung fibroblasts from patients with idiopathic pulmonary fibrosis exhibit genome-wide differences in DNA methylation compared to fibroblasts from nonfibrotic lung. PLoS One. 2014;9:e107055.

82. Coward WR, Watts K, Feghali-Bostwick CA, Knox A, Pang L. Defective histone acetylation is responsible for the diminished expression of cyclooxygenase 2 in idiopathic pulmonary fibrosis. Mol Cell Biol. 2009;29:4325–39.

83. Coward WR, Watts K, Feghali-Bostwick CA, Jenkin G, Pang L. Repression of IP-10 by interactions between histone deacetylation and hypermethylation in idiopathic pulmonary fibrosis. Mol Cell Biol. 2010;30:2874–86.

84. Huang SK, Scruggs AM, Donaghy J, Horowitz JC, Zaslona Z, Przybranowski S, White ES, Peters-Golden M. Histone modifications are responsible for decreased Fas expression and apoptosis resistance in fibrotic lung fibroblasts. Cell Death Dis. 2013;4:e621.

85. Dakhlallah D, Batte K, Wang Y, Cantemir-Stone CZ, Yan P, Nuovo G, Mikhail A, Hitchcock CL, Wright VP, Nana-Sinkam SP, Piper MG, Marsh CB. Epigenetic regulation of miR-17~92 contributes to the pathogenesis of pulmonary fibrosis. Am J Respir Crit Care Med. 2013;187:397–405.

86. Cushing L, Kuang PP, Qian J, Shao F, Wu J, Little F, Thannickal VJ, Cardoso WV, Lu J. miR-29 is a major regulator of genes associated with pulmonary fibrosis. Am J Respir Cell Mol Biol. 2011;45:287–94.

87. Yang S, Cui H, Xie N, Icyuz M, Banerjee S, Antony VB, Abraham E, Thannickal VJ, Liu G. miR-145 regulates myofibroblast differentiation and lung fibrosis. FASEB J. 2013;27:2382–91.

88. Pottier N, Maurin T, Chevalier B, Puissegur MP, Lebrigand K, Robbe-Sermesant K, Bertero T, Lino Cardenas CL, Courcot E, Rios G, Fourre S, Lo-Guidice JM, Marcet B, Cardinaud B, Barbry P, Mari B. Identification of keratinocyte growth factor as a target of microRNA-155 in lung fibroblasts: implication in epithelial-mesenchymal interactions. PLoS One. 2009;4:e6718.

89. Lino Cardenas CL, Henaoui IS, Courcot E, Roderburg C, Cauffiez C, Aubert S, Copin MC, Wallaert B, Glowacki F, Dewaeles E, Milosevic J, Maurizio J, Tedrow J, Marcet B, Lo-Guidice JM, Kaminski N, Barbry P, Luedde T, Perrais M, Mari B, Pottier N. miR-199a-5p Is upregulated during fibrogenic response to tissue injury and mediates TGFbeta-induced lung fibroblast activation by targeting caveolin-1. PLoS Genet. 2013;9:e1003291.

90. Yang S, Banerjee S, de Freitas A, Sanders YY, Ding Q, Matalon S, Thannickal VJ, Abraham E, Liu G. Participation of miR-200 in pulmonary fibrosis. Am J Pathol. 2012;180:484–93.

91. Sun H, Chen J, Qian W, Kang J, Wang J, Jiang L, Qiao L, Chen W, Zhang J. Integrated long noncoding RNA analyses identify novel regulators of epithelial-mesenchymal transition in the mouse model of pulmonary fibrosis. J Cell Mol Med. 2016;20:1234–46.

92. Li M, Riddle SR, Frid MG, El Kasmi KC, McKinsey TA, Sokol RJ, Strassheim D, Meyrick B, Yeager ME, Flockton AR, McKeon BA, Lemon DD, Horn TR, Anwar A, Barajas C, Stenmark KR. Emergence of fibroblasts with a proinflammatory epigenetically altered phenotype in severe hypoxic pulmonary hypertension. J Immunol. 2011;187:2711–22.

93. Xu XF, Ma XL, Shen Z, Wu XL, Cheng F, Du LZ. Epigenetic regulation of the endothelial nitric oxide synthase gene in persistent pulmonary hypertension of the newborn rat. J Hypertens. 2010;28:2227–35.

94. Archer SL, Marsboom G, Kim GH, Zhang HJ, Toth PT, Svensson EC, Dyck JR, Gomberg-Maitland M, Thebaud B, Husain AN, Cipriani N, Rehman J. Epigenetic attenuation of mitochondrial superoxide dismutase 2 in pulmonary arterial hypertension: a basis for excessive cell proliferation and a new therapeutic target. Circulation. 2010;121:2661–71.

95. Guo L, Yang Y, Liu J, Wang L, Li J, Wang Y, Liu Y, Gu S, Gan H, Cai J, Yuan JX, Wang J, Wang C. Differentially expressed plasma microRNAs and the potential regulatory function of Let-7b in chronic thromboembolic pulmonary hypertension. PLoS One. 2014;9:e101055.

96. Wang L, Guo LJ, Liu J, Wang W, Yuan JX, Zhao L, Wang J, Wang C. MicroRNA expression profile of pulmonary artery smooth muscle cells and the effect of let-7d in chronic thromboembolic pulmonary hypertension. Pulm Circ. 2013;3:654–64.

97. Caruso P, MacLean MR, Khanin R, McClure J, Soon E, Southgate M, MacDonald RA, Greig JA, Robertson KE, Masson R, Denby L, Dempsie Y, Long L, Morrell NW, Baker AH. Dynamic changes in lung microRNA profiles during the development of pulmonary hypertension due to chronic hypoxia and monocrotaline. Arterioscler Thromb Vasc Biol. 2010;30:716–23.

98. Courboulin A, Paulin R, Giguere NJ, Saksouk N, Perreault T, Meloche J, Paquet ER, Biardel S, Provencher S, Cote J, Simard MJ, Bonnet S. Role for miR-204 in human pulmonary arterial hypertension. J Exp Med. 2011;208:535–48.

99. Xu Z, Sharma M, Gelman A, Hachem R, Mohanakumar T. Significant role for microRNA-21 affecting toll-like receptor pathway in primary graft dysfunction after human lung transplantation. J Heart Lung Transplant. 2017;36(3):331–9.

100. Ito K, Ito M, Elliott WM, Cosio B, Caramori G, Kon OM, Barczyk A, Hayashi S, Adcock IM, Hogg JC, Barnes PJ. Decreased histone deacetylase activity in chronic obstructive pulmonary disease. N Engl J Med. 2005;352:1967–76.

101. Ito K, Yamamura S, Essilfie-Quaye S, Cosio B, Ito M, Barnes PJ, Adcock IM. Histone deacetylase 2-mediated deacetylation of the glucocorticoid receptor enables NF-kappaB suppression. J Exp Med. 2006;203:7–13.

102. Karmaus W, Ziyab AH, Everson T, Holloway JW. Epigenetic mechanisms and models in the ori-

gins of asthma. Curr Opin Allergy Clin Immunol. 2013;13:63–9.

103. Yang IV, Pedersen BS, Liu A, O'Connor GT, Teach SJ, Kattan M, Misiak RT, Gruchalla R, Steinbach SF, Szefler SJ, Gill MA, Calatroni A, David G, Hennessy CE, Davidson EJ, Zhang W, Gergen P, Togias A, Busse WW, Schwartz DA. DNA methylation and childhood asthma in the inner city. J Allergy Clin Immunol. 2015;136:69–80.

104. Liu H, Zhou Y, Boggs SE, Belinsky SA, Liu J. Cigarette smoke induces demethylation of prometastatic oncogene synuclein-gamma in lung cancer cells by downregulation of DNMT3B. Oncogene. 2007;26:5900–10.

105. Parker MD, Chambers PA, Lodge JP, Pratt JR. Ischemia- reperfusion injury and its influence on the epigenetic modification of the donor kidney genome. Transplantation. 2008;86:1818–23.

106. Mehta TK, Hoque MO, Ugarte R, Rahman MH, Kraus E, Montgomery R, Melancon K, Sidransky D, Rabb H. Quantitative detection of promoter hypermethylation as a biomarker of acute kidney injury during transplantation. Transplant Proc. 2006;38:3420–6.

107. Huang N, Tan L, Xue Z, Cang J, Wang H. Reduction of DNA hydroxymethylation in the mouse kidney insulted by ischemia reperfusion. Biochem Biophys Res Commun. 2012;422:697–702.

108. Watson CJ, Collier P, Tea I, Neary R, Watson JA, Robinson C, Phelan D, Ledwidge MT, McDonald KM, McCann A, Sharaf O, Baugh JA. Hypoxia-induced epigenetic modifications are associated with cardiac tissue fibrosis and the development of a myofibroblast-like phenotype. Hum Mol Genet. 2014;23:2176–88.

109. Franco R, Schoneveld O, Georgakilas AG, Panayiotidis MI. Oxidative stress, DNA methylation and carcinogenesis. Cancer Lett. 2008;266:6–11.

110. Wilson CB, Rowell E, Sekimata M. Epigenetic control of T-helper-cell differentiation. Nat Rev Immunol. 2009;9:91–105.

111. Lal G, Zhang N, van der Touw W, Ding Y, Ju W, Bottinger EP, Reid SP, Levy DE, Bromberg JS. Epigenetic regulation of Foxp3 expression in regulatory T cells by DNA methylation. J Immunol. 2009;182:259–73.

112. Zaslona Z, Scruggs AM, Peters-Golden M, Huang SK. Protein kinase A inhibition of macrophage maturation is accompanied by an increase in DNA methylation of the colony-stimulating factor 1 receptor gene. Immunology. 2016;149:225–37.

113. Masson E, Stern M, Chabod J, Thevenin C, Gonin F, Rebibou JM, Tiberghien P. Hyperacute rejection after lung transplantation caused by undetected low-titer anti-HLA antibodies. J Heart Lung Transplant. 2007;26:642–5.

114. Pierre AF, DeCampos KN, Liu M, Edwards V, Cutz E, Slutsky AS, Keshavjee SH. Rapid reperfusion causes stress failure in ischemic rat lungs. J Thorac Cardiovasc Surg. 1998;116:932–42.

115. Clark SC, Sudarshan C, Khanna R, Roughan J, Flecknell PA, Dark JH. Controlled reperfusion and pentoxifylline modulate reperfusion injury after single lung transplantation. J Thorac Cardiovasc Surg. 1998;115:1335–41.

116. Halldorsson AO, Kronon MT, Allen BS, Rahman S, Wang T. Lowering reperfusion pressure reduces the injury after pulmonary ischemia. Ann Thorac Surg. 2000;69:198–203, discussion 204.

117. Botha P, Jeyakanthan M, Rao JN, Fisher AJ, Prabhu M, Dark JH, Clark SC. Inhaled nitric oxide for modulation of ischemia-reperfusion injury in lung transplantation. J Heart Lung Transplant. 2007;26:1199–205.

118. Chiang CH, Wu K, Yu CP, Yan HC, Perng WC, Wu CP. Hypothermia and prostaglandin E(1) produce synergistic attenuation of ischemia-reperfusion lung injury. Am J Respir Crit Care Med. 1999;160:1319–23.

119. Shargall Y, Guenther G, Ahya VN, Ardehali A, Singhal A, Keshavjee S, ISHLT Working Group on Primary Lung Graft Dysfunction. Report of the ISHLT Working Group on Primary Lung Graft Dysfunction part VI: treatment. J Heart Lung Transplant. 2005;24:1489–500.

120. Kemming GI, Merkel MJ, Schallerer A, Habler OP, Kleen MS, Haller M, Briegel J, Vogelmeier C, Furst H, Reichart B, Zwissler B. Inhaled nitric oxide (NO) for the treatment of early allograft failure after lung transplantation. Munich Lung Transplant Group. Intensive Care Med. 1998;24:1173–80.

121. Fischer S, Bohn D, Rycus P, Pierre AF, de Perrot M, Waddell TK, Keshavjee S. Extracorporeal membrane oxygenation for primary graft dysfunction after lung transplantation: analysis of the Extracorporeal Life Support Organization (ELSO) registry. J Heart Lung Transplant. 2007;26:472–7.

122. Kermeen FD, McNeil KD, Fraser JF, McCarthy J, Ziegenfuss MD, Mullany D, Dunning J, Hopkins PM. Resolution of severe ischemia-reperfusion injury post-lung transplantation after administration of endobronchial surfactant. J Heart Lung Transplant. 2007;26:850–6.

123. Wittwer T, Grote M, Oppelt P, Franke U, Schaefers HJ, Wahlers T. Impact of PAF antagonist BN 52021 (Ginkolide B) on post-ischemic graft function in clinical lung transplantation. J Heart Lung Transplant. 2001;20:358–63.

124. Keshavjee S, Davis RD, Zamora MR, de Perrot M, Patterson GA. A randomized, placebo-controlled trial of complement inhibition in ischemia-reperfusion injury after lung transplantation in human beings. J Thorac Cardiovasc Surg. 2005;129:423–8.

125. Forgiarini LF, Forgiarini LA Jr, da Rosa DP, Silva MB, Mariano R, Paludo Ade O, Andrade CF. N-acetylcysteine administration confers lung protection in different phases of lung ischaemia-reperfusion injury. Interact Cardiovasc Thorac Surg. 2014;19:894–9.

126. Zhu C, Bilali A, Georgieva GS, Kurata S, Mitaka C, Imai T. Salvage of nonischemic control lung from injury by unilateral ischemic lung with apocynin, a nicotinamide adenine dinucleotide phosphate (NADPH) oxidase inhibitor, in isolated perfused rat lung. Transl Res. 2008;152:273–82.

127. Lu W, Si YI, Ding J, Chen X, Zhang X, Dong Z, Fu W. Mesenchymal stem cells attenuate acute ischemia-reperfusion injury in a rat model. Exp Ther Med. 2015;10:2131–7.

128. Tian W, Liu Y, Zhang B, Dai X, Li G, Li X, Zhang Z, Du C, Wang H. Infusion of mesenchymal stem cells protects lung transplants from cold ischemia-reperfusion injury in mice. Lung. 2015;193:85–95.

Part III

The Lung Transplant Recipient: Medical Management

Medical Management of the Lung Transplant Recipient: Extrapulmonary Issues

11

Erika D. Lease and Ganesh Raghu

Abbreviations

BCC	Basal cell carcinoma
BMP	Basic metabolic panel
BOS	Bronchiolitis obliterans syndrome
Ca	Calcium
CBC	Complete blood count
CF	Cystic fibrosis
CLAD	Chronic lung allograft dysfunction
CMV	Cytomegalovirus
COPD	Chronic obstructive pulmonary disease
CXR	Chest radiograph (X-ray)
EBV	Epstein-Barr virus
FEV1	Forced expiratory volume in 1 s
GERD	Gastroesophageal reflux disease
GFR	Glomerular filtration rate
HUS	Hemolytic uremic syndrome
IPF	Idiopathic pulmonary fibrosis
ISHLT	International Society for Heart and Lung Transplantation
IU/mL	International units per milliliter
LFT	Liver function testing
MDS	Myelodysplastic syndrome
Mg	Magnesium
MRI	Magnetic resonance imaging
PCR	Polymerase chain reaction
PFT	Pulmonary function testing
PLS	Passenger leukocyte syndrome
PO_4	Phosphorus
PRBCs	Packed red blood cells
PRES	Posterior reversible encephalopathy syndrome
PTLD	Posttransplant lymphoproliferative disorder
RBCs	Red blood cells
SCC	Squamous cell carcinoma
SIR	Standardized incidence ration
TTP	Thrombotic thrombocytopenic purpura

E. D. Lease (✉)
Division of Pulmonary, Critical Care, and Sleep
Medicine, University of Washington, Seattle,
WA, USA
e-mail: edlease@uw.edu

G. Raghu
Division of Pulmonary, Critical Care, and Sleep Medicine,
Department of Medicine University of Washington,
Seattle, WA, USA

Center for Interstitial Lung Disease, ILD, Sarcoid
and Pulmonary Fibrosis Program, University
of Washington Medicine, Seattle, WA, USA

Scleroderma Clinic, University of Washington
Medicine, Seattle, WA, USA
e-mail: graghu@uw.edu

Introduction

Following transplantation, medical management of the lung transplant recipient is vital for maintaining the health of the allograft and to promote an overall successful outcome after a lung transplant surgery. This includes vigilant and meticulous monitoring for all lung transplant-related

© The Author(s) 2018
G. Raghu, R. G. Carbone (eds.), *Lung Transplantation*, https://doi.org/10.1007/978-3-319-91184-7_11

issues including administering appropriate immunosuppression with antirejection medications while monitoring for associated toxicities and drug interactions as well as prompt detection of infection and lung allograft rejection. A large number of non-pulmonary complications that may arise following lung transplantation are related to immunosuppressant effects and/or toxicities; therefore, the transplant pulmonologist must balance the management of these effects and/or toxicities in the setting of the patient's other comorbidities without compromising the functional status of the lung allograft. Non-pulmonary complications include but are not limited to renal dysfunction, hematologic abnormalities, gastrointestinal complications, neurologic sequelae, oncologic manifestations, and metabolic derangements. While monitoring lung allograft function following transplantation is critical to overall survival, monitoring for the subsequent non-pulmonary complications is also important to avoid increased morbidity and mortality in lung transplant recipients. See Table 11.1 for a sample of post-lung transplant routine monitoring schedule. The

Table 11.1 Example post-lung transplant routine monitoring schedule

Routine monitoring	0–3 months posttransplant	3–6 months posttransplant	6–12 months posttransplant	>12 months posttransplant
Clinic visit at lung transplant center (including vitals sign measurements such as blood pressure and weight)	Every 1–4 weeks (generally weekly for 4–6 weeks, slowly spacing out to 2–4 weeks depending on clinical course)	Every 4–8 weeks	Every 2–3 months	Every 4–12 months (depending on transplant center distance and patient access to local medical care where studies may be performed and communicated to the transplant center)
PFT (spirometry) and CXR	Every 1–4 weeks (generally weekly for 4–6 weeks, slowly spacing out to 2–4 weeks depending on clinical course)	Every 4–8 weeks	Every 2–3 months	Every 4 months
CBC, BMP (includes glucose)—blood	Every 1–4 weeks (generally weekly for 4–6 weeks, slowly spacing out to 2–4 weeks depending on clinical course)	Every 4 weeks	Every 4–6 weeks	Every 4–12 weeks (depending on clinical course, medical complications, etc.)
Tacrolimus or cyclosporine and/or sirolimus levels—blood	Every 1–4 weeks (generally weekly for 4–6 weeks, slowly spacing out to 2–4 weeks depending on clinical course)	Every 4 weeks	Every 4–6 weeks	Every 4–12 weeks (depending on dose and drug level stability)
CMV PCR (preferably IU/mL)—blood	Duration of prophylaxis may differ among transplant programs—once prophylaxis is discontinued, CMV PCR weekly for 4 weeks, every 2 weeks for 8 weeks, and then monthly for 3–6 months			With every clinic visit
EBV PCR (preferably IU/mL)—blood	For recipients whose serologic status is donor-positive/recipient-negative (D+/R−), EBV PCR every 2–12 weeks			As needed
LFT, Mg, Ca, PO₄—blood	Every 1–4 weeks (generally weekly for 4–6 weeks, slowly spacing out to 2–4 weeks depending on clinical course)	Every 4 weeks	Every 2–3 months	With every clinic visit

Table 11.1 (continued)

Routine monitoring	0–3 months posttransplant	3–6 months posttransplant	6–12 months posttransplant	>12 months posttransplant
Lipid panel	As needed	As needed	As needed	At 1 year posttransplant then every 1–2 years depending on results
Cancer screening	Annual skin exam for skin cancer (more frequent follow-up to be determined by dermatology if needed) and routine cancer screening for age/sex/risk factors			
Bone density testing	As needed	As needed	As needed	At 1 year posttransplant then every 1–5 years depending on bone density status

PFTs pulmonary function testing, *CXR* chest radiograph, *CBC* complete blood count with differential, *BMP* basic metabolic panel, *CMV PCR* cytomegalovirus polymerase chain reaction, *IU/mL* international units per milliliter, *EBV* Epstein-Barr virus, *LFT* liver function testing, *Mg* magnesium, *Ca* calcium, *PO₄* phosphorus

transplant pulmonologist must assume the role of a very thorough internist for the lung transplant recipient in order to monitor and address the many complications occurring after lung transplantation. This chapter focuses on the medical management of non-pulmonary issues in the lung transplant recipient.

Renal Complications

Renal disease is a common and an increasingly recognized complication following lung transplantation. According to data collected by the International Society for Heart and Lung Transplantation (ISHLT), at 1 year following lung transplantation, over 20% of recipients have an abnormal creatinine and nearly 2% require dialysis. At 5 years posttransplant, nearly 50% of recipients have an abnormal creatinine with an additional 3% requiring dialysis and 0.8% having undergone renal transplantation [1]. Ojo and colleagues found that over 15% of lung transplant recipients by 5 years met the criteria for chronic renal failure as defined by a glomerular filtration rate (GFR) of ≤ 29 mL/min/1.73 m^2 of body surface area [2]. Not only is chronic renal disease common following lung transplantation, but it also has a significant impact on overall survival. Within a group of nonrenal solid organ transplant recipients, chronic renal failure was associated with a 4.5-fold increased risk of death [2].

Calcineurin inhibitors, namely, cyclosporine and tacrolimus, are a mainstay of the immunosuppression regimen for lung transplant recipients, but they unfortunately have the known side effect of nephrotoxicity [3]. Increasing age, female gender, and presence of pretransplant diabetes or hypertension have also been found to be risk factors for the development of chronic renal disease following lung transplantation. In addition, hepatitis C has been associated with the development of chronic renal failure in liver transplant recipients, but insufficient data are available to assess if the same is true for lung transplant recipients [2].

Chronic renal disease significantly increases the overall complexity of the medical management of lung transplant recipients. Given the substantial prevalence of renal disease following lung transplantation and the impact of chronic renal disease on long-term outcomes, special care must be taken to minimize kidney injury during all phases of the transplant process. Full assessment of pretransplant renal function, minimization of nephrotoxic medications, and treatment of modifiable cardiovascular risk factors are all strategies to reduce long-term risk of chronic renal disease in lung transplant recipients.

Hematologic Complications

Various hematologic alterations may arise following lung transplantation, including anemia, thrombocytopenia, and leukopenia. Postoperative hemorrhage is one cause of early anemia following lung transplant surgery. One study found over

13% of recipients with pulmonary fibrosis and nearly 17% of recipients with emphysema experienced significant postoperative hemorrhage, defined as blood loss requiring transfusion of ≥2 units of packed red blood cells (PRBCs) to maintain a hematocrit of >30% [4]. Another early cause of anemia is immune-mediated hemolysis, known as passenger lymphocyte syndrome (PLS), due to antibody production against recipient red blood cells (RBCs) by donor lymphocytes carried by the transplanted organ. PLS appears to be more common in lung and heart transplant recipients as opposed to other solid organ transplant recipients [5].

Drug-induced hematologic abnormalities following lung transplantation are wide-ranging. Bone marrow suppression can occur with a variety of posttransplant medications including tacrolimus, cyclosporine, mycophenolate, trimethoprim-sulfamethoxazole, ganciclovir, and valganciclovir [5]. In addition, immune-mediated hemolytic anemia and thrombotic microangiopathy (encompassing thrombotic thrombocytopenic purpura [TTP] and hemolytic uremic syndrome [HUS]) have both been reported with the use of calcineurin inhibitors [6, 7]. There is also a subset of patients with idiopathic pulmonary fibrosis (IPF) and other interstitial pneumonias who have telomerase mutations that can manifest pancytopenia, resulting in intolerance of lymphocyte antiproliferative agents after lung transplantation [8]. Telomerase dysfunction has been shown to be a critical factor driving myelodysplastic syndrome (MDS) and leukemia; thus, these patients should be monitored closely for the development of myelodysplasia [9, 10].

Finally, infectious causes such as Epstein-Barr virus (EBV), cytomegalovirus (CMV), and parvovirus B19 as well as infiltrative causes such as posttransplant lymphoproliferative disorder (PTLD) may also cause hematologic aberrations following lung transplantation [5]. Given the myriad of possible contributing factors to hematologic alterations in lung transplant recipients, special care must be taken to monitor appropriate laboratory values closely and attention paid to the diverse etiologies of abnormalities as they present.

Gastrointestinal Complications

Gastroesophageal reflux disease (GERD) appears to be common in patients with advanced lung disease. In a US Veterans Administration case-control study, patients with erosive esophagitis and/or esophageal stricture were more likely to have concurrent pulmonary disease [11]. Patients with IPF and cystic fibrosis (CF) have been found to have particularly high rates of GERD, 87% and 80%, respectively, as measured by a 24-h esophageal pH testing [12, 13]. There has also been found to be a link between pulmonary symptoms and GERD with concurrent esophageal dysmotility, which is the result of delayed clearance of reflux contents from the esophagus [14]. While the association between GERD and lung disease is apparent, it is still unclear if GERD contributes to the development of advanced pulmonary disease or if the pulmonary disease predisposes to GERD.

In the lung transplant population, GERD is thought to be a marker of possible micro aspiration, resulting in pulmonary graft injury and leading to chronic lung allograft dysfunction (CLAD). Several studies have shown that the occurrence of GERD increases after lung transplantation and may increase with time following transplant surgery [15–17]. Although no studies have found a causative link between GERD and CLAD, several studies have evaluated the impact of posttransplant fundoplication surgery and the development or progression of CLAD. Lung transplant recipients who undergo early posttransplant fundoplication for documented GERD have been found to have a better forced expiratory volume in 1 s (FEV$_1$) at 1 year posttransplant, higher peak FEV$_1$, and longer survival [18, 19]. In addition, Davis and colleagues found fundoplication in lung transplant recipients with documented GERD resulted in improvement in FEV$_1$ following the reflux surgery [20]. Greater than 80% of study participants had an improvement in FEV$_1$ with an average improvement of 24%. Of lung transplant recipients who met the criteria for bronchiolitis obliterans syndrome (BOS), 77% no longer met the criteria for BOS following fundoplication surgery. The impact of fundoplication on

FEV_1 appeared to be greatest in those with lower grades of BOS as patients with BOS grade 3 ($\geq 50\%$ decrease from peak posttransplant FEV_1) had only a 17% improvement in the BOS grade.

GERD appears to have the potential for a significant impact on posttransplant graft function likely due to the predisposition to aspiration of gastroesophageal reflux contents. Fundoplication surgery may be able to reverse this effect, particularly if performed early in the development of graft function. Evaluation and management of GERD are therefore critical in lung transplant recipients who present with graft dysfunction, particularly if no immunologic etiology is found.

Diarrhea is a common complaint in lung transplant recipients, occurring in nearly 30% of patients in one study [21]. Magnesium supplementation is frequently required after a lung transplant; see the section in this chapter on "Cardiovascular, Metabolic, and Electrolyte Complications" for further discussion. As some magnesium formulations are used for laxative purposes, patients using magnesium supplements may consequently experience diarrhea, particularly at higher doses. Another common cause of diarrhea after lung transplantation is related to immunosuppression, in particular the immunosuppressive agent mycophenolate, which has been found to have an incidence of diarrhea in solid organ transplant recipients ranging from nearly 1/3 to over 1/2 of patients [22]. Furthermore, there may be many infectious causes of diarrhea after lung transplantation, including diarrhea caused by CMV disease (see Chap. 15 for further discussion regarding CMV, its manifestations, and treatment) or a wide array of enteric pathogens. A careful history, examination, and evaluation must be done in the lung transplant recipient presenting with diarrhea to help determine the etiology and appropriate management.

Neurologic Complications

The range of neurologic complications following lung transplantation is broad, encompassing encephalopathy, cerebrovascular events, seizures, headaches, and neuromuscular complications. Reports have indicated an incidence of neurologic complications between 68 and 79% with severe neurologic complications in up to 38% of lung transplant recipients [23, 24]. Complications occur early with a median time of 9.6mo following transplantation [21]. There are conflicting data regarding the impact of neurologic complications on overall survival; however, Mateen and colleagues found an association with death in lung transplant recipients with neurologic complications (HR 4.3), but Živković and colleagues did not [23, 24].

Encephalopathy is the most common neurologic complication following lung transplantation and in most cases (90%) is severe enough to require urgent attention and/or prolonged hospitalization [23, 24]. Medication-induced neurotoxicity (e.g., calcineurin inhibitors, prednisone, or narcotics) and metabolic disturbances are most common [23, 24]. Posterior reversible encephalopathy syndrome (PRES) is a severe drug-induced toxicity occurring following lung transplantation and is characterized by a combination of headache, seizures, visual disturbances, and/or altered mental status with characteristic findings on magnetic resonance imaging (MRI) [25]. Hypertension is frequently present but not necessary for the diagnosis as 20–30% of patients may be normotensive [26]. In lung transplant recipients, calcineurin inhibitors have been recognized as a potential etiology of PRES. [27] Bartynski and colleagues found an incidence of PRES of 0.5% among all solid organ transplant recipients and an average time of occurrence in lung transplant recipients of 90 days following transplant surgery (range 64–104 days) [26]. Treatment for PRES has not been well-studied particularly in the solid organ transplant population, but measures are generally supportive in nature, with a decrease or cessation of the calcineurin inhibitor in addition to management of hypertension. In a single-center study of patients with hematologic disorders or allogenic transplantation, 44% of patients with PRES were able to be continued on the same calcineurin inhibitor, 37% were changed to a different calcineurin inhibitor, and 7% were switched from a calcineurin inhibitor to sirolimus [28]. With this management strategy, only 8% experienced recurrence of PRES, requiring a further change in immunosuppression.

Of the other neurologic complications following lung transplantation, seizures occur in approximately 8% of recipients, headaches in 20%, and neuromuscular complications ranging from 4 to 21% [23, 24]. Headaches are most commonly an exacerbation of pre-existing migraines in 35%, followed by calcineurin inhibitor toxicity in 27% of lung transplant recipients [24]. Neuromuscular complications following lung transplantation are varied, including polyneuropathies (such as peripheral neuropathy due to medications or diabetes), mononeuropathies (such as phrenic nerve neuropathy following surgery), myopathies (such as critical care myopathies), and plexopathies (such as brachial plexopathy) [24].

As discussed above, the range of neurologic complications following lung transplantation is broad with a variety of etiologies. While morbidity is increased with these complications, it is unclear if there is an overall impact on mortality in lung transplant recipients.

Oncologic Complications

Malignancy following lung transplantation is common and increases with time after transplant. According to the ISHLT, nearly 11% of deaths after the first year posttransplant are attributable to non-lymphoma malignancy. In addition, posttransplant lymphoproliferative disorder (PTLD) is responsible for 2% of deaths following the first 30 days after transplant [1].

Skin cancer accounts for the majority of malignancy following lung transplantation, with squamous cell carcinoma (SCC) predominating over basal cell carcinoma (BCC) [29]. Lung and heart transplant recipients are more likely to develop skin cancer than other solid organ transplant recipients, likely due to the increased overall intensity of immunosuppression required. In addition, older age, duration and level of immunosuppression, and previous pretransplant SCCs are all risk factors for the development of skin cancer following lung transplantation [30]. Not all immunosuppressants may contribute to this increased risk, however, as both mycophenolate and sirolimus may reduce the incidence of skin cancer following solid organ transplantation [31, 32].

Immunosuppression alone is not the only posttransplant medication contributing to the development of skin cancer. Voriconazole exposure has also been found to significantly impact the occurrence of skin cancer. A retrospective study of over 300 lung transplant recipients found a 2.6-fold increased risk for SCC in patients who had any exposure to voriconazole, with a cumulative effect showing a 5.6% increase in risk for every 60-day exposure [33]. Certain viral infections may also predispose lung transplant recipients to develop various skin cancers. SCC has been linked to human papillomavirus (HPV), Kaposi's sarcoma to *Human herpesvirus 8* (HHV8), and Merkel cell carcinoma to *Merkel cell polyomavirus* [29, 34, 35].

PTLD is a broad category that contains several distinct processes and is characterized by the proliferation of immune cells in the setting of posttransplant immunosuppression. A large review of the United Network of Sharing database, a database of solid organ transplants performed in the United States, found the incidence of PTLD in lung transplant recipients to be 3.7% [36]. Other studies have reported higher incidences with ranges of 6.2–9.4% [37]. PTLD is more common in lung transplant recipients, occurring twice as frequently as in other solid organ transplant recipients [37]. EBV serostatus is the biggest risk factor for the development of PTLD, with a EBV seropositive donor organ transplanted into a EBV seronegative recipient having the highest risk. Lung transplant recipients in this category have a 20-fold increase risk of developing PTLD than lung transplant recipients who were seropositive prior to transplantation [37]. An additional significant risk factor for PTLD is the intensity of posttransplant immunosuppression [38].

Treatment of PTLD is dependent upon the category of diagnosis and may range from reduction of immunosuppression to combination chemotherapy. The World Health Organization categorizes PTLD as plasmacytic hyperplasia and infectious mononucleosis-like PTLD, polymorphic PTLD, monomorphic PTLD, or classical Hodgkin lymphoma-like PTLD [39]. Prognosis following treatment of PTLD also likely depends on the category of diagnosis as well as the timing of occurrence following lung transplantation. While some studies have found worse survival following the diagnosis of PTLD, others have not [40, 41].

Colon cancer has been found to be generally increased in patients with CF. In a recent review of the US cystic fibrosis foundation registry during the years 1990–2009, the standardized incidence ratio (SIR), defined as the number of observed cases of colon cancer divided by the number of expected cases of colon cancer, was 6.2 in all patients with CF. [42] In patients who underwent organ transplantation, the SIR for colon cancer was 30.1. Several additional studies have found a similar increased risk for patients with CF following lung transplantation [43, 44]. The increased risk does not appear to be limited to lung transplant recipients with CF alone, however. Safaeian and colleagues found lung transplant recipients as a whole had a significantly increased risk of colon cancer, SIR 2.34 [43]. Screening recommendations for colon cancer in lung transplant recipients do not exist currently; however, the data imply screening may need to be performed diligently, particularly in patients with CF.

Telomerase dysfunction has been shown to be a critical factor driving myelodysplastic syndrome (MDS) and leukemia; thus, these patients who undergo lung transplantation should be monitored closely for the development of myelodysplasia and other associated hematologic disorders [9, 10]. Consideration should be taken for lung transplant recipients with telomerase dysfunction to be proactively followed by hematologists-oncologists who are familiar with the evaluation and management of hematologic disorders associated with telomeropathies.

Lung cancer also appears to occur more frequently following lung transplantation. Several studies have shown an increased risk of lung cancer, particularly in the native lung in COPD and IPF recipients of a single-lung transplant [45–47]. These patients have been found to have prevalence of native lung cancer ranging from 1.5 to 8.9% [47]. There are no current guidelines for screening for lung cancer in lung transplant recipients. Consideration should be given to screening patients who may be at high risk such as recipients of single-lung transplants due to COPD and IPF.

Malignancy is a common complication following lung transplantation, and routine screening regimens should be considered.

Cardiovascular, Metabolic, and Electrolyte Complications

Several cardiovascular and metabolic alterations can occur following lung transplantation, most commonly due to side effects related to the immunosuppressive medications. Hypertension, hypercholesterolemia, diabetes mellitus, and osteoporosis are all potential complications in lung transplant recipients. Several studies have evaluated the prevalence of these cardiovascular and metabolic alterations. Hypertension has been found to be present in 45% of lung transplant recipients at 1 year posttransplant, 65% by 3 years posttransplant, and 67% by 5 years posttransplant [48]. Similarly, hypercholesterolemia is present in 16% of lung transplant recipients at 1 year posttransplant, 33% by 3 years posttransplant, and 48% by 5 years posttransplant [48]. The estimated prevalence of diabetes mellitus following lung transplantation has varied among studies, with 6–23% by 1 year posttransplant and 7–39% by 3 years posttransplant [48–50]. The prevalence of metabolic syndrome is also increased, with 24% of lung transplant recipients meeting the criteria by 1 year posttransplant.

Diabetes mellitus, in particular, appears to result in significant morbidity and mortality following lung transplantation. Hackman and colleagues found that respiratory infections and

Aspergillus infections occur more frequently in lung transplant recipients with diabetes [51]. More importantly, lung transplant recipients with new-onset diabetes had a median survival of 4.3 years as compared to 10.1 years in patients without diabetes. Patients with pretransplant diabetes also had lower survival with a median of 5.0 years. Risk factors for the development of posttransplant diabetes include older age ≥ 50, cystic fibrosis diagnosis, male gender, body mass index (BMI) ≥ 30, and tacrolimus use at discharge [48, 52].

Loss of bone mineral density also appears to be a common complication following lung transplantation, although many patients have pre-existing bone mineral density alterations prior to transplant. Wang and colleagues found that 36% of lung transplant candidates had osteopenia based on bone mineral density testing and that 31% had osteoporosis [53]. This increased prevalence is likely due to the common use of corticosteroids in advanced lung disease management, a known risk factor for loss of bone mineral density. Significant bone loss is common following lung transplantation, again primarily to the use of corticosteroids as a mainstay of the transplant immunosuppressive regimen. As such, prevention of bone loss with posttransplant administration of calcium and vitamin D as well as appropriate monitoring for bone loss and treatment when needed is essential to preserve bone health.

As has been found with normal subjects, resistance training may prevent and even increase bone density following lung transplantation. Mitchell and colleagues randomized lung transplant recipients at 2 months following transplantation to a control group and a group that performed 6 months of resistance training [54]. Both groups lost significant but comparable amounts of lumbar bone density at 2 months posttransplant (−14.5%), but the group who performed resistance training was able to increase lumbar bone density significantly after 6 months (+9.2%) and returned to values that were within 5% of their baseline levels. The control group continued to lose lumbar bone density and

decreased to values that were 19.5% less than pretransplant values.

The immunosuppressant medications used following lung transplantation can produce profound metabolic derangements in lung transplant recipients. Careful monitoring is necessary to prevent long-term sequelae and morbidity due to these complications.

Conclusions

Many non-pulmonary complications occur following lung transplantation, a large number of which are related to immunosuppressant effects or toxicities. Non-pulmonary complications include but are not limited to renal dysfunction, hematologic abnormalities, gastrointestinal complications, neurologic sequelae, oncologic manifestations, and metabolic derangements. While monitoring lung allograft function following transplantation is critical to overall survival, monitoring for the subsequent non-pulmonary complications is also important to avoid increased morbidity and mortality in lung transplant recipients. The lung transplant pulmonologist must assume the role of a very thorough internist for the lung transplant recipient in order to monitor and address the many complications occurring after lung transplantation.

References

1. Yusen RD, Edwards LB, Kucheryavaya AY, Benden C, Dipchand AI, Goldfarb SB, et al. The Registry of the International Society for Heart and Lung Transplantation: thirty-second official adult lung and heart-lung transplantation report—2015; focus theme: early graft failure. J Heart Lung Transplant. 2015;34:1264–77.
2. Ojo AO, Held PJ, Port FK, Wolfe RA, Leichtman AB, Young EW, et al. Chronic renal failure after transplantation of a nonrenal organ. N Engl J Med. 2003;349:931–40.
3. Bloom RD, Doyle AM. Kidney disease after heart and lung transplantation. Am J Transplant. 2006;6:671–9.
4. Vicente R, Morales P, Ramos F, Solé A, Mayo M, Villalain C. Perioperative complications in lung transplantation in patients with emphysema and

fibrosis: experience from 1992-2002. Transplant Proc. 2006;38:2560–2.

5. Modrykamien A. Anemia post-lung transplantation: mechanisms and approach to diagnosis. Chron Respir Dis. 2010;71(1):29–34.

6. McMillan MA, Muirhead CS, Lucie NP, Briggs JD, Junor BJ. Autoimmune haemolytic anaemia related to cyclosporine with ABO-compatible kidney donor and recipient. Nephrol Dial Transplant. 1991;6:57–9.

7. Sing N, Gayowski T, Marino IR. Hemolytic uremic syndrome in solid-organ transplant recipients. Transpl Int. 1996;9:68–75.

8. Tokman S, Singer JP, Devine MS, Westall GP, Aubert JD, Tamm M, Snell GI, Lee JS, Goldberg HJ, Kukreja J, Golden JA, Leard LE, Garcia CK, Hays SR. Clinical outcomes of lung transplant recipients with telomerase mutations. J Heart Lung Transplant. 2015;34(10):1318–24.

9. Colla S, Ong DS, Ogoti Y, Marchesini M, Mistry NA, Clise-Dwyer K, Ang SA, Storti P, Viale A, Giuliani N, Ruisaard K, Ganan Gomez I, Bristow CA, Estecio M, Weksberg DC, Ho YW, Hu B, Genovese G, Pettazzoni P, Multani AS, Jiang S, Hua S, Ryan MC, Carugo A, Nezi L, Wei Y, Yang H, D'Anca M, Zhang L, Gaddis S, Gong T, Horner JW, Heffernan TP, Jones P, Cooper LJ, Liang H, Kantarjian H, Wang YA, Chin L, Bueso-Ramos C, Garcia-Manero G, DePinho RA. Telomere dysfunction drives aberrant hematopoietic differentiation and myelodysplastic syndrome. Cancer Cell. 2015;27(5):644–57.

10. Townsley DM, Dumitriu B, Young NS. Bone marrow failure and the telomeropathies. Blood. 2014;124(18):2775–83.

11. el-Serag HB, Sonnenberg A. Comorbid occurrence of laryngeal or pulmonary disease with esophagitis in United States military veterans. Gastroenterology. 1997;113:755–60.

12. Raghu G, Freudenberger TD, Yang S, Curtis JR, Spada C, Hayes J, et al. High prevalence of abnormal acid gastroesophageal reflux in idiopathic pulmonary fibrosis. Eur Respir J. 2006;27:136–42.

13. Ledson MJ, Tran J, Walshaw MJ. Prevalence and mechanisms of gastro-oesophageal reflux in adults cystic fibrosis patients. J R Soc Med. 1998;158:1804–8.

14. Pellegrini CA, DeMeester TR, Johnson LF, Skinner DB. Gastroesophageal reflux and pulmonary aspiration: incidence, functional abnormality, and results of surgical therapy. Surgery. 1979;86:110–9.

15. D'Ovidio F, Mura M, Ridsdale R, Takahashi H, Waddell TK, Hutcheon M, et al. The effect of reflux and bile acid aspiration on the lung allograft and its surfactant and innate immunity molecules SP-A and SP-D. Am J Transplant. 2006;6(8):1930.

16. Young LR, Hadjiliadis D, Davis RD, Palmer SM. Lung transplantation exacerbates gastroesophageal reflux disease. Chest. 2003;124:1689–93.

17. Hadjiliadis D, Duane Davis R, Steele MP, Messier RH, Lau CL, Eubanks SS, et al. Gastroesophageal reflux disease in lung transplant recipients. Clin Transpl. 2003;17:363–8.

18. Hartwig MG, Anderson DJ, Onaitis MW, Reddy S, Snyder LD, et al. Fundoplication after lung transplantation prevents the allograft dysfunction associated with reflux. Ann Thorac Surg. 2011;92(2):462–8.

19. Cantu EIII, Appel JZIII, Hartwig MG, Woreta H, Green C, et al. J. Maxwell Chamberlain Memorial Paper. Early fundoplication prevents chronic allograft dysfunction in patients with gastroesophageal reflux disease. Ann Thorac Surg. 2004;78(4):1142–51.

20. Davis RD Jr, Lau CL, Eubanks S, Messier RH, Hadjiliadis D, et al. Improved lung allograft function after fundoplication in patients with gastroesophageal reflux disease undergoing lung transplantation. J Thorac Cardiovasc Surg. 2003;125(3):533–42.

21. Bravo C, Gispert P, Borro JM, de la Torre M, Cifrián Martinez JM, et al. Prevalence and management of gastrointestinal complications in lung transplant patients: MITOS Study Group. Transplant Proc. 2007;39(7):2409–12.

22. Product Information: CELLCEPT® oral capsules, tablets, suspension, powder for IV injection, mycophenolate mofetil oral capsules, tablets, suspension, powder for IV injection. Nutley, NJ: Roche Laboratories, Inc; 2007.

23. Mateen FJ, Dierkhising RA, Rabinstein AA, van de Beek D, Wijdicks EFM. Neurological complications following adult lung transplantation. Am J Transplant. 2010;10:908–14.

24. Živković SA, Jumaa M, Barišić N, McCurry K. Neurologic complications following lung transplantation. J Neurol Sci. 2009;280:90–3.

25. Hinchey J, Chaves C, Appignani B, Breen J, Pao L, et al. A reversible posterior leukoencephalopathy syndrome. N Engl J Med. 1996;334:494–500.

26. Bartynski WS, Tan HP, Boardman JF, Shapiro R, Marsh JW. Posterior reversible encephalopathy syndrome after solid organ transplantation. Am J Neuroradiol. 2008;29:92–30.

27. Thyagarajan GK, Cobanoglu A, Johnston W. FK506-induced fulminant leukoencephalopathy after single-lung transplantation. Ann Thorac Surg. 1997;64(5):1461–4.

28. Cerejo MC, Barajas RF, Cha S, Logan AC. Management strategies for posterior reversible encephalopathy syndrome (PRES) in patients receiving calcineurin-inhibitor or sirolimus therapy for hematologic disorders and allogeneic transplantation. Abstract presented at the 56th annual meeting of the American Society of Hematology, San Francisco, CA, USA, 6–9 Dec 2014.

29. Robbins HY, Arcasoy SM. Malignancies following lung transplantation. Clin Chest Med. 2011;32:343–55.

30. Zwald FO, Brown M. Skin cancer in solid organ transplant recipients: advances in therapy and management: part 1. Epidemiology of skin cancer in solid organ transplant recipients. J Am Acad Dermatol. 2011;65:253–61.

31. Crespo-Leiro MG, Alonso-Pulpón L, Vázquez de Prada JA, Almenar L, Arizón JM, Brossa V, et al. Malignancy after heart transplantation: incidence, prognosis and risk factors. Am J Transplant. 2008;8:1031–9.

32. Campistol JM, Eris J, Oberbauer R, Friend P, Hutchison B, Morales JM, et al. Sirolimus therapy after early cyclosporine withdrawal reduces the risk for cancer in adult renal transplantation. J Am Soc Nephrol. 2006;17:581–9.

33. Singer JP, Boker A, Metchnikoff C, Binstock M, Boettger R, Golden JA, et al. High cumulative dose exposure to voriconazole is associated with cutaneous squamous cell carcinoma in lung transplant recipients. J Heart Lung Transplant. 2012;31:694–9.

34. Chang Y, Cesarman E, Pessin MS, Lee F, Culpepper J, Knowles DM, et al. Identification of herpesvirus-like DNA sequences in AIDS-associated Kaposi's sarcoma. Science. 1994;266:1865–9.

35. Feng H, Shuda M, Chang Y, Moore PS. Clonal integration of a polyomavirus in human Merkel cell carcinoma. Science. 2008;319:1096–100.

36. Dharnidharka VR, Tejani AH, Ho PL, Harmon WE. Post-transplant lymphoproliferative disorder in the United States: young Caucasian males are at highest risk. Am J Transplant. 2002;2(10):993–8.

37. Aris RM, Maia DM, Neuringer IP, Gott K, Kiley S, Gertis K, et al. Post-transplantation lymphoproliferative disorder in the Epstein-Barr virus-naïve lung transplant recipient. Am J Respir Crit Care Med. 1996;154(6 Pt 1):1712–7.

38. Penn I. Cancers complicating organ transplantation. N Engl J Med. 1990;323(5):1767–9.

39. Swerdlow SH, Campo E, Harris NL, Jaffe ES, Pileri SA, Stein H, et al. World Health Organization classification of tumours of haematopoietic and lymphoid tissues. Lyon: IARC Press; 2008.

40. Wheless SA, Gulley ML, Raab-Traub N, McNeillie P, Neuringer IP, Ford HJ, et al. Post-transplantation lymphoproliferative disease: Epstein-Barr virus DNA levels, HLA-A3, and survival. Am J Respir Crit Care Med. 2008;178(10):1060–5.

41. Paranjothi S, Yusen RD, Kraus MD, Lynch JP, Patterson GA, Trulock EP. Lymphoproliferative disease after lung transplantation: comparison of presentation and outcome of early and late cases. J Heart Lung Transplant. 2001;20(10):1054–63.

42. Maisonneuve P, Marshall BC, Knapp EA, Lowenfels AB. Cancer risk in cystic fibrosis: a 20-year nation-wide study from the United States. J Natl Cancer Inst. 2013;105(2):122–9.

43. Safaeian M, Robbins HA, Berndt SI, Lynch CF, Faumeni JF Jr, Engels EA. Risk of colorectal cancer after solid organ transplantation in the United States. Am J Transplant. 2016;16:960–7.

44. Meyer KC, Fancois ML, Thomas HK, Radford KL, Hayes DS, Mack TL, et al. Colon cancer in lung transplant recipients with CF: increase risk and results of screening. J Cyst Fibros. 2011;10:366–9.

45. Grewal AS, Padera RF, Boukedes S, Divo M, Rosas IO, Camp PC, et al. Prevalence and outcome of lung cancer in lung transplant recipients. Respir Med. 2015;109(3):427–33.

46. Olland AB, Falcoz PE, Santelmo N, Kessler R, Massard G. Primary lung cancer in lung transplant recipients. Ann Thorac Surg. 2014;98(1):362–71.

47. Belli EV, Landolfo K, Keller C, Thomas M, Odell J. Lung cancer following lung transplant: single institution 10 year experience. Lung Cancer. 2013;81(3):451–4.

48. Silverborn M, Jeppsson A, Mårtensson G, Nilsson F. New-onset cardiovascular risk factors in lung transplant recipients. J Heart Lung Transplant. 2005;24:1536–43.

49. Ollech JE, Kramer MR, Peled N, Ollech A, Amital A, et al. Post-transplant diabetes mellitus in lung transplant recipients: incidence and risk factors. Eur J Cardiothorac Surg. 2008;33(5):844–8.

50. Savioli G, Surbone S, Giovi I, Salinaro F, Preti P, et al. Early development of metabolic syndrome in patients subjected to lung transplantation. Clin Transpl. 2013;27(3):E237–43.

51. Hackman KL, Bailey MJ, Snell GI, Bach LA. Diabetes is a major risk factor for mortality after lung transplantation. Am J Transplant. 2014;14:438–45.

52. Ye X, Kuo H-T, Sampaio MS, Jiang Y, Bunnaradist S. Risk factors for development of new-onset diabetes mellitus after transplant in adult lung transplant recipients. Clin Transpl. 2011;25:885–91.

53. Wang TKM, O'Sullivan S, Gamble GD, Ruygrok PN. Bone density in heart or lung transplant recipients—a longitudinal study. Transplant Proc. 2013;45:2357–65.

54. Mitchell MJ, Baz MA, Fulton MN, Lisor CF, Braith RW. Resistance training prevents vertebral osteoporosis in lung transplant recipients. Transplantation. 2003;76:557–62.

Management of Cellular and Humoral Rejection: Prevention, Diagnosis, and Treatment

12

Erika D. Lease and Ganesh Raghu

Abbreviations

ACR	Acute cellular rejection
AMR	Antibody-mediated rejection
ATG	Antithymocyte globulin
BAL	Bronchoalveolar lavage
BOS	Bronchiolitis obliterans syndrome
CDC	Complement-dependent cytotoxicity
CLAD	Chronic lung allograft dysfunction
CMV	Cytomegalovirus
cPRA	Calculated panel reactive antibody
DSA	Donor-specific antibody
ELISA	Enzyme-linked immunosorbent assay
FEV1	Forced expiratory volume in 1 second
FVC	Forced vital capacity
GERD	Gastroesophageal reflux disease
HLA	Human leukocyte antigen
HRCT	High-resolution computed tomography
ISHLT	International Society for Heart and Lung Transplantation
IVIG	Intravenous immunoglobulin
MFI	Mean fluorescent intensity
OKT3	Muromonab-CD3
PRA	Panel reactive antibody
TBBX	Transbronchial biopsy
UNOS	United network of sharing

E. D. Lease (✉)
Division of Pulmonary, Critical Care, and Sleep Medicine, University of Washington, Seattle, WA, USA
e-mail: edlease@uw.edu

G. Raghu
Division of Pulmonary, Critical Care, and Sleep Medicine, Department of Medicine University of Washington, Seattle, WA, USA

Center for Interstitial Lung Disease, ILD, Sarcoid and Pulmonary Fibrosis Program, University of Washington Medicine, Seattle, WA, USA

Scleroderma Clinic, University of Washington Medicine, Seattle, WA, USA
e-mail: graghu@uw.edu

Introduction

Acute cellular and antibody-mediated (humoral) rejections are two forms of acute rejection seen following lung transplantation. The management of acute cellular and antibody-mediated rejection is complex and may be individualized based on the unique situation of each patient but is guided by early diagnosis and prompt treatment that includes augmentation of immunosuppression among a variety of additional medical strategies. Treatment of acute cellular rejection and antibody-mediated rejection is important due to the associations with the development of chronic lung allograft dysfunction (CLAD), the primary cause of mortality following lung transplantation. With optimal management and further study, the goal is for a decreased incidence of CLAD with

© The Author(s) 2018
G. Raghu, R. G. Carbone (eds.), *Lung Transplantation*, https://doi.org/10.1007/978-3-319-91184-7_12

an improved survival and quality of life for all lung transplant recipients.

Patients who present with new respiratory symptoms concerning for rejection or a decline in spirometry despite the presence or absence of symptoms should undergo formal evaluation for diagnosis. Possible etiologies include, but are not limited to, acute cellular or antibody-mediated rejection, infection, anastomotic and/or airway stenoses, or the onset of CLAD. Testing should include formal spirometry (if initial decline in spirometry is reported from a home monitoring device), testing for donor-specific antibodies (DSA), as well as bronchoscopy to evaluate for anastomotic and/or airway stenoses and to obtain specimens via bronchoalveolar lavage (BAL) and transbronchial biopsies (TBBX). Additional evaluation and testing may be warranted depending on the clinical presentation. Please see an example algorithm for the evaluation and management of lung function decline and ACR in Fig. 12.1.

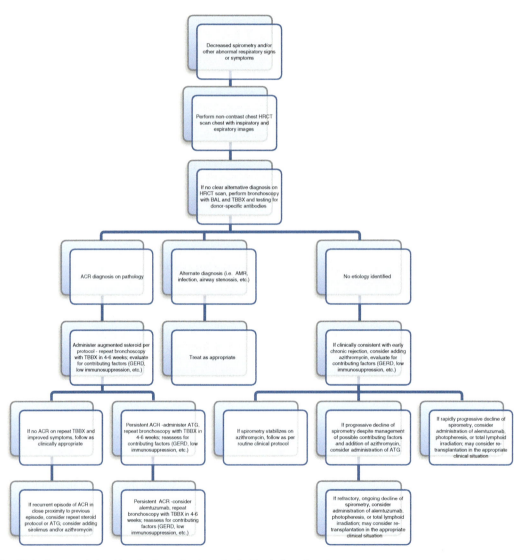

Fig. 12.1 Suggested algorithm for the evaluation of a decline in lung function

Acute Cellular Rejection

Definition/Diagnosis

The International Society for Heart and Lung Transplantation (ISHLT) formulated a diagnosis of acute cellular rejection (ACR) based exclusively on the pathologic presence of perivascular and interstitial mononuclear cell infiltrates [1]. The intensity and extension of the infiltrating cells form the basis of the histologic grade (Table 12.1). Please see Chap. 13. Airway inflammation (lymphocytic bronchiolitis) is determined by the presence and extent of mononuclear cells in the bronchiolar submucosa. Tissue specimens for diagnosis of acute cellular rejection are generally obtained via bronchoscopy and transbronchial biopsies (TBBX). Laboratory, radiographic, and clinical findings may be helpful in the consideration of ACR following lung transplantation but add little diagnostic value due to the variable and nonspecific findings seen in patients with ACR.

Table 12.1 Classification and grading of acute pulmonary allograft rejection

A: Acute rejection
A0—None
A1—Minimal
A2—Mild
A3—Moderate
A4—Severe
B: Airway inflammation ("R" denotes revised grade to avoid confusion with 1996 scheme)
B0—None
B1R—Low grade
B2R—High grade
BX—Ungradeable
C: Chronic airway rejection—Obliterative bronchiolitis
C0—Absent
C1—Present
D: Chronic vascular rejection—Accelerated graft vascular sclerosis

Adapted with permission from Elsevier from Stewart S, Fishbein MC, Snell GI, Berry GJ, Boehler A, Burke MM et al. Revision of the 1996 working formulation for the standardization of nomenclature in the diagnosis of lung rejection. J Heart Lung Transplant 2007;26:1229–42

Prevention

Induction Immunosuppression

Induction immunosuppression is a treatment intended to deplete circulating T cells with the purpose of reducing acute cellular rejection following lung transplantation, particularly until maintenance immunosuppression has reached full effect. The use of induction immunosuppression appears to be increasing with time with more than half of lung transplant programs reporting use of induction immunosuppressive agents in 2010 [2]. A large Cochrane Database systematic review compared a variety of combinations of no induction, polyclonal or monoclonal T-cell antibody induction, interleukin-2 receptor (IL-2) antagonist induction, or muromonab-CD3 (OKT3) induction and found no differences in mortality, acute rejection, adverse effects (including infection), or bronchiolitis obliterans syndrome (BOS) [3]. A more recent analysis of data from the United Network of Sharing (UNOS) in the USA found the use of antibody-based induction immunosuppression to have a positive impact on survival and decreased rates of acute rejection within the first year [4]. More studies are needed to delineate the impact of induction immunosuppression on acute rejection and the optimal induction regimen.

Monitoring/Spirometry

As a decline in forced expiratory volume in 1 second (FEV_1) is often the first sign of acute rejection and/or CLAD, close monitoring of spirometry is essential for early identification [5]. Lung transplant recipients are encouraged to utilize home spirometers to monitor lung function parameters such as the FEV_1 and the forced expiratory capacity (FVC). Monitoring of daily home spirometry has been shown to improve detection of a sustained decline for 3 days or more of FEV_1 by ≥20% from the lung transplant recipient's baseline best FEV_1 by an average of 276 days earlier than without daily home monitoring [6]. Despite this significantly earlier detection, no studies have demonstrated a benefit in survival with home spirometry monitoring although several have shown a non-statistically significant positive trend for freedom from BOS and reduced rates of re-transplantation [7].

Monitoring/Surveillance Bronchoscopy

Despite being commonly performed, there are little data to support the utilization of surveillance screening for ACR via bronchoscopy and TBBX [8]. The intention of surveillance monitoring by TBBX is to attempt to identify subclinical ACR before the onset of symptoms or graft dysfunction and to intervene therapeutically with the belief that early and prompt treatment of ACR is beneficial for improving outcomes and decreasing the risk of CLAD in lung transplant recipients. ACR (A-grade) and more likely lymphocytic bronchiolitis (B-grade) do appear to be associated with the development of CLAD/BOS [8–10]. However, there is no definitive evidence that earlier identification of these abnormalities in an asymptomatic patient with preserved lung function alters the treatment course or overall outcome in lung transplant recipients. Bronchoscopy can result in many complications including but not limited to pneumothorax, bleeding, and complications of sedation; therefore, further studies are needed to determine if there is a benefit in performing surveillance bronchoscopy with TBBX in lung transplant recipients and if the benefit outweighs the procedural risks.

Maintenance Immunosuppression

Significant improvements in immunosuppressants have been made since the beginnings of solid organ transplantation; however, the optimal post-transplant immunosuppression regimen remains unclear. In the 2012 ISHLT annual registry report, unadjusted data showed lower rates of ACR within the first year post-transplant in patients who receive maintenance immunosuppression therapy with tacrolimus and mycophenolate mofetil, followed by tacrolimus and azathioprine, then cyclosporine and mycophenolate mofetil, and finally cyclosporine and azathioprine [11]. However, a multicenter randomized trial comparing tacrolimus and cyclosporine found no difference in rates of ACR at 1 year and 3 years post-transplant although tacrolimus was associated with a lower risk of BOS [12]. In addition, another single-center randomized trial showed no difference between mycophenolate mofetil and azathioprine in rates of grade 2 (A2) ACR within the first 6 months post-transplant [13]. As with induction immunosuppression, further studies are needed to determine the optimal maintenance immunosuppression regimen.

Regardless of maintenance immunosuppression regimen, however, optimization of the prescribed regimen should be assured by adherence, avoidance of interacting medications or foods, and close monitoring of drug trough levels when available. Medication nonadherence is a complicating factor in lung transplant recipients as with all patients. One single-center study found an average individual medication timing adherence (± 30 min from prescribed timing) of 98.1% although the range was 31.2–100% [14]. Overall, medication adherence, defined as having an individual timing-adherence score of $\geq 80\%$, was seen in 92.3% of recipients. However, over 14% of patients missed one or more 24-hour period of medication, with over 40% in the nonadherent group (an individual timing-adherence score of $\leq 80\%$) missing one or more 24-h period of medication. Instruction and emphasis on the importance of taking immunosuppressant medication regularly and at the prescribed time are an important factor to assure adequate immunosuppression levels.

Risk Factors for Allograft Dysfunction and Rejection

At times, an identifiable trigger can be found contributing to the development of ACR and CLAD. Recognition and management of these triggers may be helpful to prevent future episodes of ACR.

Gastroesophageal Reflux Disease

Gastroesophageal reflux disease (GERD) appears to have the potential for a significant impact on post-transplant graft function, likely due to the predisposition to aspiration of gastroesophageal reflux contents and the subsequent injury that occurs. In an animal model of lung transplant, chronic aspiration of gastric contents led to a higher grade of acute rejection than in those without aspiration of gastric contents [15]. Several studies in lung transplant recipients have found that GERD diagnosed by 24-h pH study or 24-h pH-impedance study is associated with an earlier onset of ACR, higher rate of ACR, and multiple episodes of ACR [16, 17]. In addition, one study found that anti-reflux surgery performed either pre-transplant or within the first 6 months following lung transplantation resulted in a decreased risk of ACR in the first year [18].

Infections

Chronic sinusitis in cystic fibrosis patients is not uniformly thought to be a risk factor for ACR following lung transplantation; however, there are some data regarding the risk of recolonization of the lung allograft from the sinuses with *Pseudomonas aeruginosa* and the development of BOS. In one study, 65% of cystic fibrosis lung transplant recipients had persistent sinus colonization with *Pseudomonas aeruginosa* following lung transplantation [19]. Patients who did not have persistent colonization of the sinuses or recolonization of the lung allograft had a significantly better survival rate and decreased incidence of BOS as compared to those who had colonization. Attempts to reduce sinus colonization have not been successful as pre-transplant sinus surgery has not been found to reduce recolonization of the lung allograft or improve overall survival [20].

Whether persistent bacterial colonization of the sinuses or recolonization of the lung allograft plays a role in the development of ACR is unknown. However, infections with bacterial organisms commonly found as sinus and pulmonary colonizers have been implicated in the development of ACR. In an animal model of lung transplant, *Pseudomonas* pulmonary infection was found to possibly contribute to the development of ACR through the disruption of established lung tolerance [21]. Additionally, *Staphylococcus aureus* infections within the first 90 days following lung transplantation have been associated with increased 1-year and 3-year mortality as well as rates of ACR and CLAD [22]. *Chlamydia pneumoniae* infection following lung transplantation, whether donor-derived, de novo, or reactivation, has also been implicated with early mortality, ACR, and CLAD [23]. Further elucidation of the impact of bacterial infections on the development of ACR following lung transplantation and potential pre-transplant prevention are warranted.

Respiratory viruses have also been found to possibly play a role in the development of ACR although data are mixed. Kumar and colleagues found a significant association with symptomatic or asymptomatic lower respiratory tract viral infections and a subsequent diagnosis of ACR ($\geq$A2) and/or a $\geq 20\%$ decline in FEV_1 within the ensuing 3 months following the respiratory viral infection [24]. While Soccal and colleagues did not find an association with lower respiratory tract viral infection and the development of ACR in the subsequent 3 months, they did find that respiratory viral infections when present concurrently with ACR caused more severe lung dysfunction with a slower short-term recovery [25].

Cytomegalovirus (CMV) is another infection that may contribute to the development of ACR following lung transplantation. Solidoro and colleagues provided evidence that CMV-specific prophylaxis resulted in decreased rates of ACR, including lymphocytic bronchiolitis [26]. ACR has been found to be associated with high levels of CMV-specific CD8+ T-cell activity and presence of CMV in the lung allograft, indicating activated CMV-specific CD8+ T cells in the lung may play a role in promoting ACR [27]. Whether CMV actively contributes to the development of ACR or is a bystander in the setting of immune activation due to ACR is yet to be determined.

Treatment

As no randomized studies or standardized clinical practice guidelines exist regarding optimal treatments for ACR, there is significant variability among providers regarding the decision to treat certain pathologic grades despite evidence that both A1 and B1 are individually associated with the development of BOS [9, 28]. Gordon and colleagues surveyed pulmonologists at lung transplant centers in the USA in 2009 and found 65% would not treat asymptomatic A1 rejection and 20% would not treat symptomatic A1 rejection [29]. In addition, 50% of transplant pulmonologists who responded would not treat asymptomatic B1R lymphocytic bronchiolitis and 15% would not treat symptomatic B1R lymphocytic bronchiolitis.

If treatment is warranted, methylprednisolone is generally considered the first-line therapy although the dosing regimen and need for subsequent prednisone taper are unclear as data are lacking for the most effective treatment regimen for ACR. Although no clinical trials or comparative studies exist, early studies suggested clinical as well as pathologic response following pulse corticosteroids for treatment of ACR [30–32]. Regimens for treatment of ACR generally incorporate IV methylprednisolone, 500–1000 mg for 3 days, followed by an oral prednisone taper at many lung transplant centers.

Refractory (persistent ACR despite appropriate treatment) or recurrent (repeated ACR in close proximity to recently treated and cleared ACR) rejection despite administration of pulse corticosteroids necessitates further consideration of possible triggers as well as further treatment options. Depending on the timing of the subsequent episode of rejection, a repeat course of pulse corticosteroids may be considered if deemed clinically appropriate. The T-cell-depleting agent polyclonal antithymocyte globulin (ATG) is used frequently by many lung transplant centers for the treatment of refractory or recurrent ACR. ATG has been shown to reduce episodes of ACR when used as an induction agent although there are no studies of its use in the treatment of documented ACR in lung transplant recipients [33]. The anti-CD52 monoclonal antibody alemtuzumab has been shown to be effective in the treatment of ACR refractory to ATG [34, 35]. Alemtuzumab targets all cells that express CD52, but, for the purposes of treating ACR, it results in a rapid and sustained depletion of lymphocytes. Lastly, muromonab-CD3 (OKT3) has been shown to be effective for the treatment of ACR refractory to pulse corticosteroids, after a second recurrence of ACR following taper of oral corticosteroids, or as primary treatment for ≥A3 ACR. A variety of other treatments have been reported for refractory ACR including inhaled cyclosporine [36, 37], methotrexate [38], extracorporeal photopheresis [39], and total lymphoid irradiation [40].

Following treatment for ACR, augmentation or alteration of the maintenance immunosuppressive regimen may be helpful to prevent further episodes of ACR. Substituting tacrolimus for cyclosporine has been shown to be helpful in the treatment for refractory ACR [41, 42]. Also, an animal model has shown the addition of sirolimus to cyclosporine potentiates the immunosuppressive effects and reverses ACR [43].

After treatment for ACR has been completed, it has been found to be useful to repeat TBBX to assure resolution of ACR and determine if further treatment is warranted [44]. Sibley and colleagues found, despite rapid clinical improvement, changes of ACR remained persistent on histologic samples up to 30 days following treatment [45]. As such, the literature supports that repeat TBBX should be delayed until 30–45 days following the initial bronchoscopy [44, 45].

Antibody-Mediated Rejection

Definition/Diagnosis

Antibody-mediated rejection (AMR) following lung transplantation has been increasingly recognized in the last decade, yet clarity as to how to confidently recognize AMR remains elusive and a diagnostic challenge. Unlike in renal and heart transplant recipients where AMR is well-recognized and defined, the concept of AMR in lung transplant recipients is still evolving. At the core, AMR is a process by which recipient immune cells produce antibodies directed toward antigens in the allograft. The antigen-antibody complex leads to a cascade of both complement-dependent and complement-independent pathways resulting in graft injury and dysfunction.

Table 12.2 Classification of antibody-mediated rejection

	Allograft dysfunction	Other causes excluded	Lung histology	Lung biopsy C4d	DSA
Definite					
Clinical	+	+	+	+	+
Subclinical	N/A	N/A	+	+	+
Probable					
Clinical	+	+	+/−[a]	+/−[a]	+/−[a]
		−	+	+	+
Subclinical	N/A	N/A	+/−[a]	+/−[a]	+/−[a]
Possible					
Clinical	+	+	+/−[b]	+/−[b]	+/−[b]
		−	+/−[a]	+/−[a]	+/−[a]
Subclinical	N/A	N/A	+/−[b]	+/−[b]	+/−[b]

N/A not applicable, *DSA* donor-specific antibodies
Adapted with permission of Elsevier from Levine DJ, Glanville AR, Aboyoun C, Belperio J, Benden C, Berry GJ et al. Antibody-mediated rejection of the lung: A consensus report of the International Society for Heart and Lung Transplantation. J Heart Lung Transplant 2016;35(4):397–406
[a]Only 1 missing element of lung histology, lung biopsy C4d, or DSA
[b]Only 2 missing elements of lung histology, lung biopsy C4d, or DSA

A consensus document was recently put forth by the ISHLT outlining a working definition for AMR [46]. Pulmonary AMR has been divided into clinical AMR (diagnostic findings *with* graft dysfunction) and subclinical AMR (diagnostic findings *without* graft dysfunction). Each group is then divided into definite, probable, or possible AMR depending on the constellation of clinical and diagnostic findings including consistent lung histology, presence of positive lung biopsy C4d staining (a marker of activation of the classical pathway of the complement system), presence of circulating DSA, and the exclusion of other causes of graft dysfunction (i.e., ACR, pulmonary infection, etc.) (Table 12.2).

The Pathology Council of the ISHLT issued a separate document with the purpose of formulating a more consistent histologic characterization in the evaluation of pulmonary AMR [47]. The group elected to use the terms "neutrophilic capillaritis" and "neutrophilic margination" as findings suggestive of pulmonary AMR. Neutrophilic capillaritis was defined as a "patchy or diffuse process composed of dense neutrophilic septal infiltrates associated with neutrophilic karyorrhetic debris and fibrin with or without platelet–fibrin thrombi in the microvasculature, alveolar hemorrhage and flooding of neutrophils into adjacent airspaces."

Neutrophilic margination was defined as "neutrophilic infiltrates within the interstitial capillaries and septa in the absence of karyorrhetic changes and fibrinous accumulations." The authors recognize, however, that these histologic findings are nonspecific and can be seen in a variety of disorders. As imaging and the clinical presentation of AMR are also nonspecific, diagnosis of AMR remains a clinical diagnosis within the context of suggestive clinical and diagnostic findings.

The presence of DSA in the setting of pulmonary graft dysfunction with no other known cause (i.e., ACR, infection, etc.) is a frequent scenario in the clinical presentation of AMR. The measurement of DSA is generally performed using newer solid-phase assays that report antibody detection as a mean fluorescent intensity (MFI). Unfortunately there has been no consensus as to what level of MFI constitutes a clinically relevant antibody production for either pre- or posttransplant monitoring and if the clinically relevant MFI should be the same for all human leukocyte antibodies (HLA). Additionally, there are limited data for management of the presence of DSA in the setting of no clinical symptoms and preserved lung function; see the section in this chapter on "Prevention: Monitoring/Surveillance HLA."

Prevention

Pre-transplant Desensitization

Pre-transplant sensitization to HLA, which is the pre-transplant production of antibodies to HLA, is a significant limiting factor for some patients and their access to suitable organs. Pre-transplant HLA antibodies may be present in patients who have received prior blood transfusions, pregnancy, prior transplantation, or at times due to no clear etiology. Recent advances in technology have led to changes in the detection of HLA antibodies, with newer solid-phase assays used more commonly than the older complement-dependent cytotoxicity (CDC) assays. With the more sensitive newer assays, there have been variable reports as to the percentage of lung transplant recipients who present with pre-transplant HLA antibodies. As there is no consensus as to what level of MFI constitutes a clinically relevant HLA antibody, the literature cites the presence of HLA antibodies using a variety of MFI cutoff points. For example, using a MFI of $\geq$300, 62–89% of lung transplant recipients are found to have the presence of HLA antibodies [48]. If a MFI of $\geq$1000 is used, 58.5 of lung transplant recipients are found to have the presence of HLA antibodies with a median calculated panel reactive antibody test (cPRA, a clinical estimate of the effective donor pool but not a marker of the number or intensity of antibody production) of 3% with MFI between 1000 and 3000 and 21% with MFI $\geq$3000 [49].

In an attempt to determine the appropriate MFI cutoff for clinical significance, one study found a MFI $\geq$3000 was associated with longer waiting times pre-transplant as well as increased post-transplant AMR regardless of the negative pre-transplant CDC crossmatch results [49]. Another study found in a retrospective review of blood samples after the development of the newer solid-phase assays, despite a negative CDC crossmatch, lung transplant recipients who had pre-transplant donor-specific HLA antibodies of MFI >5000 had a 1-year survival of 33% as compared to 71% for MFI 2000–5000 [50]. Unfortunately, the appropriate MFI cutoff point is still not clear and is dependent on individual center practices.

In patients who are particularly sensitized, attention has been focused on whether a pre-transplant desensitization protocol is helpful to improve the potential donor pool for a recipient. The appropriate level of cPRA to consider a patient highly sensitized is unclear, however, as a cPRA of as little as 10% has been found to result in worse outcomes [51]. Desensitization studies have generally focused on patients with much higher cPRA given the limited donor pool available to these patients. One study evaluated a desensitization protocol of plasmapheresis, Solu-Medrol, bortezomib, rituximab, and intravenous immunoglobulin (IVIG) in patients with a cPRA of $\geq$80% [52]. The protocol did not result in changes in the cPRA, and survival was similar to other sensitized patients who had not undergone desensitization. Another study evaluated the use of a perioperative desensitization protocol initiated at the time of transplantation and continued through the immediate post-transplant period that included plasmapheresis, IVIG, ATG, and mycophenolic acid [53]. The desensitization protocol was utilized in recipients with a panel reactive antibody (PRA) of $\geq$30%, regardless of whether the HLA antibody was donor-specific. Sensitized patients had 30-day and 1-year survival similar to patients who were not sensitized prior to transplant, but no comparison was made to sensitized patients who did not undergo the desensitization protocol. Further studies are needed to evaluate the efficacy, feasibility, and timing of desensitization protocols in highly sensitized lung transplant candidate.

Monitoring/Spirometry

As with ACR, graft dysfunction associated with AMR is best to be discovered early for prompt evaluation and treatment. However, a decline in spirometry is nonspecific and can be the result of many processes. As many lung transplant recipients perform home monitoring of spirometry, AMR must be considered in any patient presenting with lung function decline.

Monitoring/Surveillance HLA

In the guidelines outlined by the ISHLT, the presence of DSA without graft dysfunction or pathologic findings can be considered as a diagnosis of possible subclinical AMR [46]. As such, several studies have evaluated the utility of surveillance screening of HLA and DSA antibodies rather than only when graft dysfunction occurs. Snyder and colleagues performed HLA testing on lung transplant recipients at 1, 3, 6, 9, and 12 months post-transplant as well as when clinically indicated [54]. They found 32% (139/441) of patients had positive testing for HLA antibodies, 78% of which occurred within the first year post-transplant and 39% (54/139) of which developed DSA. The presence of post-transplant HLA was associated with the development of BOS (HR 1.54; $p = 0.04$) as well as death (HR 1.53; $p < 0.0001$). The presence of post-transplant DSA was associated with death (HR 2.42; $p < 0.0001$) but not the development of BOS, although the authors felt the study may not have been powered to detect an association of post-transplant DSA and BOS due to the small numbers of patients with DSA.

Another study evaluated the finding of de novo post-transplant DSA in lung transplant recipients in relation to the association with BOS and mortality [55]. Lung transplant recipients underwent surveillance HLA monitoring every 2–3 months (with each surveillance bronchoscopy) for the first 2 years post-transplant as well as when clinically indicated. The initial HLA testing was performed with an enzyme-linked immunosorbent assay (ELISA), and, if positive, subsequent testing was performed with a solid-phase assay. The authors found 13% of lung transplant recipients developed de novo DSA which was associated with all stages of BOS (HR 6.59; $p < 0.001$) and with high-grade BOS (Stage ≥ 2) (HR 5.76; $p < 0.001$). Patients who developed de novo DSA had a significantly reduced survival ($p < 0.001$) with a particular association with death due to BOS (HR 9.86; $p < 0.001$).

Although these studies show an association between HLA antibodies and DSA with the development of BOS and mortality, no studies have evaluated the appropriate course of action in patients who are found to have post-transplant HLA antibodies or de novo DSA particularly in the absence of graft dysfunction. It remains unclear if intervention or treatment in patients with post-transplant HLA antibodies or de novo DSA in the absence of graft dysfunction will alter the association with BOS or mortality. Further studies are needed to further delineate the appropriate use of HLA surveillance testing and subsequently the most beneficial interventions or treatments.

Treatment

There are limited data for the treatment of AMR following lung transplantation; thus, the information available is based on small case reports and case series with heavy reliance on the available data from the treatment of other solid organ transplant recipients. As discussed above, it remains unclear which treatments, if any, should be given to which patients among the various diagnostic groups outlined by the ISHLT [46]. For example, it is uncertain if a patient with possible subclinical AMR as defined by the presence of DSA without graft dysfunction or pathologic changes should receive treatment for AMR and, if so, if the treatment should be the same as for a patient with definite clinical AMR as defined by graft dysfunction, presence of DSA, and clear pathologic changes. Additionally, there are no data to direct if the treatment regimen should differ depending on which diagnostic findings are present and to what degree (e.g., very low MFI of DSA vs. very high MFI of DSA). It is important to note that, despite the presence of more evidence in the literature for treatment of AMR in the kidney transplant population, a recent systematic review found insufficient evidence to provide recommendations for treatment [56].

The available treatment modalities for AMR center primarily on removing antibodies from the circulation and preventing further antibody development and production by B cells and plasma cells. Generally, some combinations of plasmapheresis, IVIG, rituximab, and bortezomib are the most commonly used agents in the treatment of AMR following lung transplantation. Plasmapheresis is a mechanism by which antibodies can be physically removed from the circulation. Clinical experience suggests that, although plasmapheresis does not remove all antibodies, it does generally reduce the number and intensity of DSA, the degree of which may be helpful in predicting clinical outcomes [57, 58]. IVIG has immunomodulatory properties that help to neutralize circulating antibodies as well as promote downregulation of the humoral immune response [59]. Rituximab is a monoclonal antibody against CD20 expressed on B cells which have not yet differentiated into antibody-producing plasma cells. Rituximab results in apoptosis of B cells that express CD20; however, it is unclear the clinical effect, if any, this has in the management of AMR [60–62]. Bortezomib is a newer agent that acts as a proteasome inhibitor which targets and results in apoptosis of plasma cells, differentiated antibody-producing B cells. The use of bortezomib in the treatment of AMR following lung transplantation is limited to clinical experience and case reports [63]. Similarly, the use of eculizumab, an anti-C5 monoclonal antibody that inhibits terminal complement activation, is limited to a single case report in a lung transplant recipient, although more experience is available in the kidney transplant population [64, 65].

Overall, there are little data to direct the management of AMR following lung transplantation. Further studies are needed in order to advance understanding of AMR and its treatments as well to improve outcomes following treatment.

Conclusions

Acute cellular and antibody-mediated rejections are two forms of acute rejection seen following lung transplantation. The management of ACR and AMR is complex and may be individualized based on the unique situation of each patient. Through prevention strategies, the incidence of ACR and AMR may be reduced, although more study is needed regarding strategies to prevent acute rejection. The mainstay of treatment for ACR as well as for AMR is through the augmentation of immunosuppression through a variety of medical strategies. Management of ACR and AMR is important due to the associations with the

development of CLAD, the primary cause of mortality following lung transplantation. With optimal management and further study, the goal is for improved survival and quality of life for all lung transplant recipients.

References

1. Stewart S, Fishbein MC, Snell GI, Berry GJ, Boehler A, Burke MM, et al. Revision of the 1996 working formulation for the standardization of nomenclature in the diagnosis of lung rejection. J Heart Lung Transplant. 2007;26:1229–42.
2. Hertz MI, Aurora P, Benden C, Christie JD, Dobbels F, Edwards LB, et al. Scientific Registry of the International Society for Heart and Lung Transplantation: introduction to the 2011 annual reports. J Heart Lung Transplant. 2011;30:1071–7.
3. Penninga L, Møller CH, Penninga EI, Iversen M, Gluud C, Steinbrüchel DA. Antibody induction therapy for lung transplant recipients. Cochrane Database Syst Rev. 2013;11:CD008927.
4. Whitson BA, Lehman A, Wehr A, Hayes D Jr, Kirkby S, Pope-Harman A, et al. To induce or not to induce: a 21st century evaluation of lung transplant immunosuppression's effect on survival. Clin Transpl. 2014;28:450–61.
5. Bjotuft O, Johansen B, Boe J, Foerster A, Holter E, Geiran O. Daily home spirometry facilitates early detection of rejection in single lung transplant recipients with emphysema. Eur Respir J. 1993;6:705–8.
6. Finkelstein SM, Snyder M, Stibbe CE, Lindgren B, Sabati N, Killoren T, et al. Staging of bronchiolitis obliterans syndrome using home spirometry. Chest. 1999;116:120–6.
7. Robson KS, West AJ. Improving survival outcomes in lung transplant recipients through early detection of bronchiolitis obliterans: daily home spirometry versus standard pulmonary function testing. Can J Respir Ther. 2014;50(1):17–22.
8. Glanville AR. The role of surveillance bronchoscopy post–lung transplantation. Semin Respir Crit Care Med. 2013;34:414–20.
9. Glanville AR, Aboyoun CL, Havryk A, Plit M, Rainer S, Malouf MA. Severity of lymphocytic bronchiolitis predicts long-term outcome after lung transplantation. Am J Respir Crit Care Med. 2008;177:1033–40.
10. Burton CM, Iversen M, Scheike T, Carlsen J, Andersen CB. Is lymphocytic bronchiolitis a marker of acute rejection? An analysis of 2,697 transbronchial biopsies after lung transplantation. J Heart Lung Transplant. 2008;27:1128–34.
11. Christie JD, Edwards LB, Kucheryavaya AY, Benden C, Dipchand AI, Dobbels F, et al. The Registry of the International Society for Heart and Lung Transplantation: 29th adult lung and heart-lung

transplant report-2012. J Heart Lung Transplant. 2012;31:1073–86.

12. Treede H, Glanville AR, Klepetko W, Aboyoun C, Vettorazzi E, Lama R, et al., European and Australian Investigators in Lung Transplantation. Tacrolimus and cyclosporine have differential effects on the risk of development of bronchiolitis obliterans syndrome: results of a prospective, randomized international trial in lung transplantation. J Heart Lung Transplant. 2012;31:797–804.

13. Palmer SM, Baz MA, Sanders L, Miralles AP, Lawrence CM, Rea JB, et al. Results of a random-ized, prospective, multicenter trial of mycopheno-late mofetil versus azathioprine in the prevention of acute lung allograft rejection. Transplantation. 2001;71:1772–6.

14. Bosma OH, Vermeulen KM, Verschuuren EA, Erasmus ME, van der Bij W. Adherence to immu-nosuppression in adult lung transplant recipients: prevalence and risk factors. J Heart Lung Transplant. 2011;30:1275–80.

15. Hartwig MG, Appel JZ, Li B, et al. Chronic aspira-tion of gastric fluid accelerates pulmonary allograft dysfunction in a rat model of lung transplantation. J Thorac Cardiovasc Surg. 2006;131(1):209–17.

16. Lo WK, Burakoff R, Goldberg HJ, Feldman N, Chan WW. Pre-transplant impedance measures of reflux are associated with early allograft injury after lung trans-plantation. J Heart Lung Transplant. 2015;34:26–35.

17. Shah N, Force SD, Mitchell PO, Lin E, Lawrence EC, Easley K, et al. Gastroesophageal reflux disease is associated with an increased rate of acute rejec-tion in lung transplant allografts. Transplant Proc. 2010;42:2702–6.

18. Lo WK, Goldberg HJ, Wee J, Fisichella PM, Chan WW. Both pre-transplant and early post-transplant antireflux surgery prevent development of early allograft injury after lung transplantation. J Gastrointest Surg. 2016;20:111–8.

19. Vital D, Hofer M, Benden C, Holzmann D, Boehler A. Impact of sinus surgery on pseudomonal airway colonization, bronchiolitis obliterans syndrome and survival in cystic fibrosis lung transplant recipients. Respiration. 2013;86:25–31.

20. Leung MK, Rachakonda L, Weill D, Hwang PH. Effects of sinus surgery on lung transplan-tation outcomes in cystic fibrosis. Am J Rhinol. 2008;22:192–6.

21. Yamamoto S, Nava RG, Zhu J, Huang HJ, Ibrahim M, Mohanakumar T, et al. Cutting edge: Pseudomonas aeruginosa abolishes established lung transplant tol-erance by stimulating B7 expression on neutrophils. J Immunol. 2012;189:4221–5.

22. Shields RK, Clancy CJ, Minces LR, Kwak EJ, Silveira FP, Abdel Massih RC, et al. Staphylococcus aureus infections in the early period after lung trans-plantation: epidemiology, risk factors, and outcomes. J Heart Lung Transplant. 2012;31:1199–206.

23. Glanville AR, Gencay M, Tamm M, Chhajed P, Plit M, Hopkins P, et al. Chlamydia pneumoniae infection after lung transplantation. J Heart Lung Transplant. 2005;24:131–6.

24. Kumar D, Husain S, Hong Chen M, Moussa G, Himsworth D, Manuel O, et al. Study evaluating the clinical impact of community-acquired respiratory viruses in lung transplant recipients. Transplantation. 2010;89:1028–33.

25. Soccal PM, Aubert J-D, Bridevaux P-O, Garbino J, Thomas Y, Rochat T, et al. Upper and lower respi-ratory tract viral infections and acute graft rejec-tion in lung transplant recipients. Clin Infect Dis. 2010;51:163–70.

26. Solidoro P, Libertucci D, Delsedime L, Ruffini E, Bosco M, Costa C, et al. Combined cytomegalovi-rus prophylaxis in lung transplantation: effects on acute rejection, lymphocytic bronchitis/bronchiol-itis, and herpesvirus infections. Transplant Proc. 2008;40:2013–4.

27. Roux A, Mourin G, Fastenackels S, Almeida JR, Candela Iglesias M, Boyd A, et al. CMV driven CD8 + T-cell activation is associated with acute rejection in lung transplantation. Clin Immunol. 2013;148(1):16–26.

28. Hopkins PM, Aboyoun CL, Chhajed PN, Malouf MA, Plit ML, Rainer SP, et al. Association of mini-mal rejection in lung transplant recipients with oblit-erative bronchiolitis. Am J Respir Crit Care Med. 2004;170(9):1022–6.

29. Gordon IO, Bhorade S, Vigneswaran WT, Garrity ER, Husain AN. SaLUTaRy: survey of lung transplant rejection. J Heart Lung Transplant. 2012;31(9):972.

30. Hutter JA, Despins P, Higenbottam T, Stewart S, Wallwork J. Heart-lung transplantation: better use of resources. Am J Med. 1988;85(1):4–11.

31. Yousem SA, Martin T, Paradis IL, Keenan R, Griffith BP. Can immunohistological analysis of transbron-chial biopsy specimens predict responder status in early acute rejection of lung allografts? Hum Pathol. 1994;25(5):525–9.

32. Clelland C, Higenbottam T, Stewart S, et al. Bronchoalveolar lavage and transbronchial lung biopsy during acute rejection and infection in heart-lung transplant patients. Studies of cell counts, lym-phocyte phenotypes, and expression of HLA-DR and interleukin-2 receptor. Am Rev Respir Dis. 1993;147(6 Pt 1):1386–92.

33. Palmer SM, Miralles AP, Lawrence CM, Gaynor JW, Davis RD, Tapson VF. Rabbit antithymocyte globulin decreases acute rejection after lung transplantation: results of a randomized, prospective study. Chest. 1999;116(1):127–33.

34. Reams BD, Musselwhite LW, Zaas DW, Steele MP, Garantziotis S, Eu PC, et al. Alemtuzumab in the treatment of refractory acute rejection and bronchiol-itis obliterans syndrome after human lung transplanta-tion. Am J Transplant. 2007;7(12):2802–8.

35. Reams BD, Davis RD, Curl J, Palmer SM. Treatment of refractory acute rejection in a lung trans-plant recipient with campath 1H. Transplantation. 2002;74(6):903–4.

36. Keenan RJ, Iacono A, Dauber JH, Zeevi A, Yousem SA, Ohori NP, et al. Treatment of refractory acute allograft rejection with aerosolized cyclosporine in lung transplant recipients. J Thorac Cardiovasc Surg. 1997;113(2):335–40.

37. Iacono A, Dauber J, Keenan R, Spichty K, Cai J, Grgurich W, et al. Interleukin 6 and interferon gamma gene expression in lung transplant recipients with refractory acute cellular rejection: implications for monitoring and inhibition by treatment with aerosolized cyclosporine. Transplantation. 1997;64(2):263–9.

38. Cahill BC, O'Rourke MK, Strasburg KA, Savik K, Jessurun J, Bolman RM III, et al. Methotrexate for lung transplant recipients with steroid-resistant acute rejection. J Heart Lung Transplant. 1996;15(11):1130–7.

39. Benden C, Speich R, Hofbauer GF, Irani S, Eich-Wanger C, Russi EW, et al. Extracorporeal photopheresis after lung transplantation: a 10-year single-center experience. Transplantation. 2008;86:1625–7.

40. Valentine VG, Robbins RC, Wehner JH, Patel HR, Berry GJ, Theodore J. Total lymphoid irradiation for refractory acute rejection in heart-lung and lung allografts. Chest. 1996;109(5):1184–9.

41. Vitulo P, Oggionni T, Cascina A, Arbustini E, D'Armini AM, Rinaldi M, et al. Efficacy of tacrolimus rescue therapy in refractory acute rejection after lung transplantation. J Heart Lung Transplant. 2002;21(4):435–9.

42. Sarahrudi K, Estenne M, Corris P, Niedermayer J, Knoop C, Glanville A, et al. International experience with conversion from cyclosporine to tacrolimus for acute and chronic lung allograft rejection. J Thorac Cardiovasc Surg. 2004;127(4):1126–32.

43. Hausen B, Boeke K, Berry GJ, Christians U, Schüler W, Morris RE. Successful treatment of acute, ongoing rat lung allograft rejection with the novel immunosuppressant SDZ-RAD. Ann Thorac Surg. 2000;69(3):904–9.

44. Aboyoun CL, Tamm M, Chhajed PN, Hopkins P, Malouf MA, Rainer S, et al. Diagnostic value of follow-up transbronchial lung biopsy after lung rejection. Am J Respir Crit Care Med. 2001;164(3):460–3.

45. Sibley RK, Berry GJ, Tazelaar HD, Kraemer MR, Theodore J, Marshall SE, et al. The role of transbronchial biopsies in the management of lung transplant recipients. J Heart Lung Transplant. 1993;12(2):308–24.

46. Levine DJ, Glanville AR, Aboyoun C, Belperio J, Benden C, Berry GJ, et al. Antibody-mediated rejection of the lung: a consensus report of the International Society for Heart and Lung Transplantation. J Heart Lung Transplant. 2016;35(4):397–406.

47. Berry G, Burke M, Andersen C, Angelini A, Bruneval P, Calabrese F, et al. Pathology of pulmonary antibody-mediated rejection: 2012 update from the Pathology Council of the ISHLT. J Heart Lung Transplant. 2013;32(1):14–21.

48. Brugière O, Suberbielle C, Thabut G, Lhuillier E, Dauriat G, Metivier AC, et al. Lung transplantation in patients with pretransplantation donor-specific antibodies detected by Luminex assay. Transplantation. 2013;95(5):761–5.

49. Kim M, Townsend KR, Wood IG, Boukedes S, Guleria I, Gabardi S, et al. Impact of pretransplant anti-HLA antibodies on outcomes in lung transplant candidates. Am J Respir Crit Care Med. 2014;189(10):1234–9.

50. Smith JD, Ibrahim MW, Newell H, Danskine AJ, Soresi S, Burke MM, et al. Pre-transplant donor HLA-specific antibodies: characteristics causing detrimental effects on survival after lung transplantation. J Heart Lung Transplant. 2014;33(10):1074–82.

51. Lau CL, Palmer SM, Posther KE, Howell DN, Reinsmoen NL, Massey HT, et al. Influence of panel-reactive antibodies on posttransplant outcomes in lung transplant recipients. Ann Thorac Surg. 2000;69:1520–4.

52. Snyder LD, Gray AL, Reynolds JM, Arepally GM, Bedoya A, Hartwig MG, et al. Antibody desensitization therapy in highly sensitized lung transplant candidates. Am J Transplant. 2014;14:849–56.

53. Tinckam KJ, Keshavjee S, Chaparro C, Barth D, Azad S, Binnie M, et al. Survival in sensitized lung transplant recipients with perioperative desensitization. Am J Transplant. 2015;15:417–26.

54. Snyder LD, Wang Z, Chen DF, Reinsmoen NL, Finlen-Copeland CA, Davis WA, et al. Implications for human leukocyte antigen antibodies after lung transplantation: a 10-year experience in 441 patients. Chest. 2013;144(1):226–33.

55. Morrell MR, Pilewski JM, Gries CJ, Pipeling MR, Crespo MM, Ensor CR, et al. De novo donor-specific HLA antibodies are associated with early and high-grade bronchiolitis obliterans syndrome and death after lung transplantation. J Heart Lung Transplant. 2014;33(12):1288–94.

56. Roberts DM, Jiang SH, Chadban SJ. The treatment of acute antibody-mediated rejection in kidney transplant recipients: a systematic review. Transplantation. 2012;94:775–83.

57. Jackups R Jr, Canter C, Sweet SC, Mohanakumar T, Morris GP. Measurement of donor-specific HLA antibodies following plasma exchange therapy predicts clinical outcome in pediatric heart and lung transplant recipients with antibody-mediated rejection. J Clin Apher. 2013;28(4):301–8.

58. Otani S, Davis AK, Cantwell L, Ivulich S, Pham A, Paraskeva MA, et al. Evolving experience of treating antibody-mediated rejection following lung transplantation. Transpl Immunol. 2014;31(2):75–80.

59. Shehata N, Palda VA, Meyer RM, Blydt-Hansen TD, Campbell P, Cardella C, et al. The use of immunoglobulin therapy for patients undergoing solid organ transplantation: an evidence-based practice guideline. Transfus Med Rev. 2010;24(Suppl 1):S7–S27.

60. Yilmaz VT, Suleymanlar G, Koksoy S, Ulger BV, Ozdem S, Akbas H, et al. Therapy modalities for antibody mediated rejection in renal transplant patients. J Investig Surg. 2016;22:1–7.
61. Sautenet B, Blancho G, Büchler M, Morelon E, Toupance O, Barrou B, et al. One-year results of the effects of rituximab on acute antibody-mediated rejection in renal transplantation: RITUX ERAH, a multicenter double-blind randomized placebo-controlled trial. Transplantation. 2016;100(2): 391–9.
62. Hachem RR, Yusen RD, Meyers BF, Aloush AA, Mohanakumar T, Patterson GA, et al. Anti-human leukocyte antigen antibodies and preemptive antibody-directed therapy after lung transplantation. J Heart Lung Transplant. 2010;29(9):973–80.
63. Neumann J, Tarrasconi H, Bortolotto A, Machuca T, Canabarro R, Sporleder H, et al. Acute humoral rejection in a lung recipient: reversion with bortezomib. Transplantation. 2010;89(1):125–6.
64. Dawson KL, Parulekar A, Seethamraju H. Treatment of hyperacute antibody-mediated lung allograft rejection with eculizumab. J Heart Lung Transplant. 2012;31(12):1325–6.
65. Eskandary F, Wahrmann M, Mühlbacher J, Böhmig GA. Complement inhibition as potential new therapy for antibody-mediated rejection. Transpl Int. 2016;29(4):392–402.

Pathology of Lung Rejection: Cellular and Humoral Mediated

13

Anja C. Roden and Henry D. Tazelaar

Introduction

Acute rejection is the host's response to the recognition of the graft as foreign. It can occur days, months, or even years after transplantation. Rejection can be divided into cellular and humoral forms. Acute cellular rejection is the predominant type of acute rejection of lung allografts. It is mediated by T lymphocytes that recognize foreign human leukocyte antigens (HLA) or other antigens [1, 2]. Humoral rejection is mediated by preformed or de novo recipient antibodies (therefore, also referred to as antibody-mediated rejection [AMR]) against antigens of the donor organ cells.

Acute rejection is an important complication in patients with lung allografts. Twenty-nine percent of adult patients have at least one episode of treated acute rejection between discharge from the hospital and 1 year after transplantation [3]. Moreover, 3.6% and 1.8% of all deaths that occur within the first 30 days or between 30 days and 1 year following lung transplantation are due to acute rejection, respectively [3]. In addition, the

frequency and severity of acute rejections are thought to represent the major risk factor for the subsequent development of bronchiolitis obliterans syndrome (BOS) [1, 4–6].

HLA mismatch, genetic and recipient factors, type of immunosuppression, vitamin D deficiency, and infection are risk factors of acute rejection. For instance, the recipient alloimmune response is thought to be related to the recognition of differences to donor antigens leading to acute lung allograft rejection. Indeed a higher degree of HLA mismatch has been shown to increase the risk of acute rejection although this effect is not consistent across all HLA loci or studies [4, 7–10]. Mismatches at the HLA-DR, HLA-B [7], and HLA-A [8] loci, as well as a combination of all three loci [9], appear specifically important. For instance, acute rejection within 2 months after transplantation has been shown to be associated with HLA-DR mismatch, while acute rejection at 4 years has been found to be associated with HLA-B mismatch [11].

Several host genetic characteristics have been studied that may modulate acute lung rejection. For instance, a genotype leading to increased IL1- production may protect against acute rejection [12], while a multidrug-resistant genotype (MDR1 C3435T) appears to predispose to persistent acute rejection that is resistant to immunosuppressive treatment [13].

The incidence of acute rejection appears to be age-dependent, with the lowest incidence of

A. C. Roden (✉)
Department of Laboratory Medicine and Pathology,
Mayo Clinic Rochester, Rochester, MN, USA
e-mail: Roden.anja@mayo.edu

H. D. Tazelaar
Department of Laboratory Medicine and Pathology,
Mayo Clinic Arizona, Scottsdale, AZ, USA
e-mail: tazelaar.henry@mayo.edu

© The Author(s) 2018
G. Raghu, R. G. Carbone (eds.), *Lung Transplantation*, https://doi.org/10.1007/978-3-319-91184-7_13

acute rejection in infants (< age 2) [14]. However, children have a higher risk for acute rejection than adults [15]. Furthermore, the registry of the International Society of Heart and Lung Transplantation (ISHLT) showed that the incidence of acute rejection between discharge and 1-year follow-up was slightly higher in younger adult lung allograft recipients (age 18–34 years) (36%) [16] when compared to the entire adult population in which 29% had at least one acute rejection episode [3]. The incidence of acute rejection does not seem to change in older lung transplant recipients (age 65 and higher) [17].

Regimens of immunosuppression might also play a role in acute rejection. For instance, the rate of acute rejection in the first year after transplantation was highest among recipients who were on cyclosporine-based regimens and lowest among those on tacrolimus-based regimens [18].

Vitamin D deficiency might also play a role in acute rejection. A study found that 80% of lung recipients were 25(OH)D deficient around the time of transplantation and that vitamin D-deficient recipients had more episodes of acute cellular rejection and infection [19]. A similar association between vitamin D deficiency and acute rejection has been described in other solid organ recipients including the liver, kidney, and heart. Although the exact mechanism for this phenomenon is not entirely clear, it is speculated that (1) vitamin D might slow down the maturation of antigen-presenting cells as in vitro studies have shown, (2) vitamin D might induce dendritic cells to acquire tolerance, and/or (3) a synergistic effect between vitamin D analogs and immunosuppressants occurs [19].

Viral infections have also been thought to modulate the immune system and to increase alloreactivity. Indeed, a high incidence of acute rejection has been found in lung transplant recipients after community-acquired respiratory tract infections with human influenza virus, respiratory syncytial virus, rhinovirus, coronavirus, and parainfluenza virus [20–22]. *Chlamydia pneumoniae* infection has also been linked to the development of acute rejection in one study [23]. The significance of CMV infections and the impact of CMV prophylaxis

strategies on acute rejection frequency are not clear at this time [24].

The clinical course of acute rejection can be variable. Acute rejection is often identified on surveillance transbronchial biopsy in an asymptomatic patient. If symptoms occur, they might be non-specific and overlap with those seen in other complications and diseases in this patient population. These symptoms might include dyspnea, fever, leukocytosis, and a widened alveolar-arterial oxygen gradient. Higher-grade rejection appears to cause more severe symptoms and can lead to acute respiratory distress [17]. In patients with rejection, pulmonary function testing may show a decrease in forced expiratory volume in 1 s (FEV_1) and vital capacity (VC). Although spirometry has a sensitivity of greater than 60% for detecting infection or rejection of Grade A2 and higher, it cannot differentiate between the two [25]. Furthermore, the usefulness of spirometry is diminished in single lung transplant recipients, as the dysfunction of the native lung confounds the pulmonary function test results [26].

Although in approximately half of the cases of acute rejection, chest X-ray studies are normal, ill-defined perihilar and lower lobe opacities, along with septal lines and pleural effusions, may be seen. Findings on CT scan might include ground-glass opacities, septal thickening, volume loss, nodules and consolidation, and pleural effusions. Infiltrates observed on imaging studies during the first week after lung transplantation are usually caused by the reimplantation response, i.e., reperfusion edema and other factors. Infiltrates that persist beyond the first week following transplantation suggest acute rejection or infection. However, although early, the authors of small studies have attempted to demonstrate the usefulness of chest X-rays and chest CT scans in the diagnosis of rejection, more recent data show a very low sensitivity for acute rejection (as low as 35%) and no discriminatory value between rejection and other processes [27].

Exhaled nitric oxide (NO) can also serve as a marker of lung injury; it is often increased in patients with lymphocytic bronchiolitis and acute rejection [28–30]. Furthermore, in a study of inert gas single-breath washout, the slope of alveolar plateau for helium had a sensitivity of 68% for acute rejection [25].

Although the presentation of the patient and several ancillary studies may suggest the presence of acute allograft rejection, none of these findings are specific. Therefore, tissue diagnosis is necessary for a definitive diagnosis. Histopathology of adequate lung biopsy samples obtained from transbronchial biopsy is currently the gold standard to assess lung allografts for rejection and to distinguish rejection from its clinical mimickers such as aspiration, infection, drug toxicity, and recurrent disease.

Recently, the transbronchial cryobiopsy technique was introduced which yields larger biopsies containing more alveoli, small airways, and veins and venules while exhibiting less procedural alveolar hemorrhage and crush artifact than conventional forceps transbronchial allograft biopsies [31–33]. Although cryobiopsies appear to be as safe as forceps biopsies, complications can occur which is one of the reasons that this technique has so far not been universally performed for this purpose [31].

Other lung tissue specimens from lung allografts include wedge biopsies, explants for retransplant, or autopsy specimens from lung transplant recipients. Wedge biopsies, although seldom obtained in clinical practice, and specimens from explants provide useful histopathologic insights into the etiology of lung allograft dysfunction in advanced stages following all possible medical interventions.

Morphologic Features of Cellular Rejection

Cellular alloreactive injury to the donor lung affects both the vasculature and the airways [34]. Perivascular mononuclear cell infiltrates are the hallmark of acute cellular rejection. These infiltrates may be accompanied by subendothelial chronic inflammation (e.g., endotheliitis or intimitis) and also by lymphocytic bronchiolitis, which is characteristic of small airway rejection. The histologic changes are divided into grades based on intensity of the cellular infiltrate and the occurrence of an accompanying acute lung injury pattern.

In 1990, the ISHLT sponsored the Lung Rejection Study Group (LRSG), a workshop to develop a "working formulation" for the diagnosis of lung rejection by transbronchial biopsy [35]. Since then the grading scheme has been revised twice, in 1996 [36] and 2007 [34]. The grading scheme is strictly pathologic, based on morphologic features recognized in transbronchial biopsies of the allograft. Clinical parameters are not considered.

Due to overlapping histologic features between acute rejection and infection, the grading scheme relies on the absence of concurrent infection. Furthermore, infection and rejection may occur together. Therefore, the LRSG recommends grading rejection only after the rigorous exclusion of infection [34].

The most recent classification of lung allograft biopsies is the 2007 ISHLT consensus classification of allograft rejection [34] (Table 13.1). An attempt should be made to accurately distinguish the grade of rejection since treatment is largely dependent on the histologic grade assessed by an experienced pulmonary pathologist familiar with the histopathologic features and criteria used for grading. However, inter- and intra-observer variability in grading can impact treatment and outcome [37, 38]. Two studies using the 1996 grading system found relatively good interobserver agreements for the A grades (kappa of 0.65 and 0.73) [37, 38]; however, these results could not be replicated in another study in which the kappa was 0.47 in spite of dichotomization of the A grades to A0/A1 versus A2-4 [39]. Intraobserver agreement for acute rejection has been found to be good with kappa values of 0.65 and 0.79 [37, 39]. Using the revised 2007 ISHLT classification, Bhorade and colleagues showed an overall concordance rate of 74% for Grade A and 89% for Grade B specimens between a site pathologist and a central pathologist [40]. However, the weighted kappa scores in that study showed only fair to moderate agreement for A grades (kappa values varied between 0.22 and 0.48) and less than a chance agreement to moderate agreement for B grades (kappa values varied

Table 13.1 Classification of cellular allograft rejection according to the 2007 revised ISHLT consensus classification of lung allograft rejection

Type of rejection	ISHLT grade	Histomorphologic features
Acute rejection	A0 None	Normal pulmonary parenchyma
	A1 Minimal	Occasional blood vessels are surrounded by a thin chronic mononuclear cell infiltrate
	A2 Mild	Multiple blood vessels are surrounded by a more prominent mononuclear cell infiltrate Infiltrate confined to the perivascular adventitia Endotheliitis may occur
	A3 Moderate	Dense mononuclear cell infiltrates surround blood vessels and extend into interstitium Endotheliitis common Eosinophils and occasional neutrophils common Acute lung injury may be apparent
	A4 Severe	Diffuse perivascular, interstitial, and air space infiltrates of mononuclear cells Prominent alveolar pneumocyte damage and endotheliitis Intra-alveolar necrotic epithelial cells, macrophages, eosinophils, hemorrhage, and neutrophils may occur Acute lung injury
Small airway inflammation—Lymphocytic bronchiolitis	B0 None	Unremarkable small airways
	B1R[a] Low grade	Lymphocytes within the submucosa of the bronchioles
	B2R High grade	Marked lymphocytic infiltrate of the airway epithelium and airway wall Greater numbers of eosinophils and plasmacytoid cells Epithelial damage including necrosis, metaplasia, and marked intraepithelial lymphocytic infiltration Epithelial ulceration, fibrinopurulent exudate, cellular debris, and neutrophils can occur
	BX Ungradeable	Grading hampered by lack of definite small airways, presence of infection, tangential cutting, artifact, etc.
Chronic airway rejection—Obliterative bronchiolitis	C0 None	Small airways similar in size to the accompanying artery No fibrosis
	C1 Present	Fibrosis in the wall of small airways
Chronic vascular rejection	D0 None	No arterial or venous changes
	D1 Present	Pulmonary arteries and/or veins are thickened by fibrointimal connective tissue

Adapted with permission of Elsevier from Stewart S, Fishbein MC, Snell GI, Berry GJ, Boehler A, Burke MM, Glanville A, Gould FK, Magro C, Marboe CC, et al. Revision of the 1996 working formulation for the standardization of nomenclature in the diagnosis of lung rejection. J Heart Lung Transplant 2007; 26:1229–1242
[a]R denotes the revised 2007 classification

between −0.04 and 0.46). Interestingly, the kappa values for A and B grades were dependent on the time that had elapsed between transplantation and biopsy. The best agreement occurred in biopsies taken within 6 weeks of transplant. Slightly higher agreements (81% and 93%, for A and B grades, respectively) were shown in a study that evaluated the interobserver agreement between two transplant pathologists from the same institution using the 2007 revision grading Scheme [31]. Although cryobiopsies are larger and appear to be easier interpretable, interobserver reproducibility did not improve with the use of cryobiopsies in that study [31].

2007 ISHLT Revised Consensus Classification of Lung Allograft Rejection

Acute Rejection: A Grade

Acute rejection is defined by the presence of perivascular mononuclear cell infiltrates with or without endotheliitis [34]. With progression, this infiltrate becomes more widespread and extends into the alveolar septa and, subsequently, into the alveoli. The majority of the mononuclear cells in acute rejection are T cells, although a few studies have described increased populations of B cells or eosinophils [34, 41, 42]. The histologic features of rejection are summarized in Table 13.1.

No Acute Rejection (ISHLT Grade A0)

Features of acute cellular rejection are lacking, although the biopsy may not be entirely normal.

Minimal Acute Rejection (ISHLT Grade A1)

Scattered infrequent blood vessels, particularly venules, in the alveolated lung parenchyma are surrounded by a relatively thin (ring of two to three layers) chronic mononuclear cell infiltrate (Fig. 13.1a, b). The lymphocytic rim can be loose or compact and is in general circumferential but does not spill into the adjacent interstitium. Endotheliitis and eosinophils are absent. In adequately alveolated and artifact-free specimens, the lymphocytic infiltrates may be detected at low magnification, but often higher power study is needed to identify the infiltrates.

Mild Acute Rejection (ISHLT Grade A2)

Although in mild acute rejection the perivascular infiltrate of lymphocytes is still confined to the perivascular adventitia without infiltrating the adjacent interstitium or air spaces, there are more layers of lymphocytes surrounding vessels (Fig. 13.2a, b). In addition, the perivascular mononuclear infiltrates surrounding venules and arterioles are more frequent than in Grade A1. They are typically recognizable at low magnification. These infiltrates usually consist of a mixture of small round lymphocytes, activated lymphocytes, plasmacytoid lymphocytes, macrophages, and eosinophils. The cellular infiltrates can be compact or loose. Subendothelial infiltration by mononuclear cells may be noted which can be associated with hyperplastic or regenerative changes in the endothelium. Concurrent lymphocytic bronchiolitis may be seen.

Moderate Acute Rejection (ISHLT Grade A3)

Venules and arterioles are cuffed by easily recognizable dense perivascular mononuclear cell infiltrates that are commonly associated with endotheliitis (Fig. 13.3a–c). Eosinophils and even occasional neutrophils are common. In

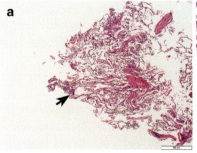
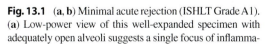
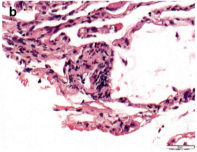

Fig. 13.1 (a, b) Minimal acute rejection (ISHLT Grade A1). (a) Low-power view of this well-expanded specimen with adequately open alveoli suggests a single focus of inflammatory infiltrate (arrow). (b) High magnification confirms a small vessel almost completely surrounded by a few layers of mononuclear cells. Magnification, ×40 (a), ×400 (b)

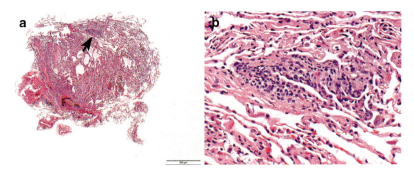

Fig. 13.2 (**a**, **b**) Mild acute rejection (ISHLT Grade A2). (**a**) At low magnification, an inflammatory infiltrate is easily identified (arrow) even though this specimen has crush artifact. (**b**) This mononuclear infiltrate completely surrounds a small vessel and is comprised of more than three layers without extending into the surrounding interstitium. Magnification, ×40 (**a**), ×400 (**b**)

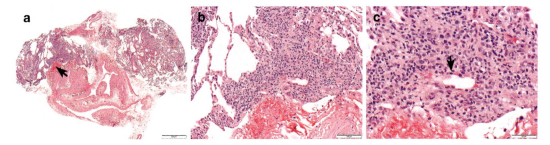

Fig. 13.3 (**a–c**) Moderate acute rejection (ISHLT Grade A3). (**a**) A prominent inflammatory infiltrate is apparent at low power (arrow). (**b**) This mononuclear infiltrate surrounds multiple small vessels and extends into the surrounding interalveolar septa. (**c**) Eosinophils are present, and a few lymphocytes within the endothelial lining are suggestive of endotheliitis (arrow). Magnification, ×40 (**a**), ×200 (**b**), ×400 (**c**)

moderate acute rejection, the inflammatory cell infiltrate extends into the adjacent alveolar septa where it can be associated with type II pneumocyte hyperplasia. The inflammatory infiltrate can also extend into adjacent airspaces and be associated with collections of intra-alveolar macrophages and lymphocytes. Histologic features of acute lung injury may become apparent in the form of airspace fibrin.

Severe Acute Rejection (ISHLT Grade A4)

In severe rejection, there are diffuse perivascular, interstitial, and air space infiltrates of mononuclear cells with prominent alveolar pneumocyte damage and endotheliitis (Fig. 13.4a–f). This may be associated with necrotic intra-alveolar epithelial cells, hemorrhage and neutrophils, and usually morphologic evidence of acute lung injury in the form of organizing pneumonia,

fibrin deposition, or hyaline membranes. Parenchymal necrosis, infarction, or necrotizing vasculitis may be identified; however, these features are more evident on surgical rather than transbronchial lung biopsies. It should be noted that a paradoxical diminution of perivascular infiltrates can occur as cells extend into interalveolar septa and air spaces where they are admixed with macrophages.

Protocol surveillance biopsies of lung allografts are performed in many institutions. Even though these patients are in general asymptomatic and clinically stable, one study showed that 39% of surveillance biopsies reveal acute cellular rejection with 43% showing features of minimal rejection, 49% mild rejection, and 8% moderate rejection [43]. A more recent prospective study identified morphologic findings of acute cellular rejection only in 6% of surveillance biopsies [44], while a retrospective study of 592

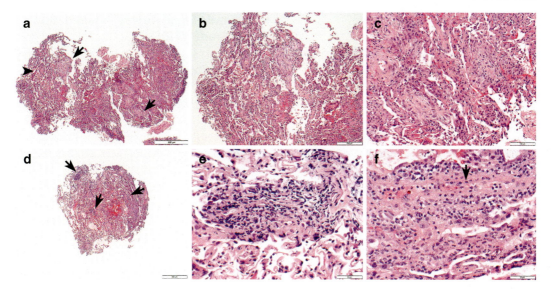

Fig. 13.4 (**a–f**) Severe acute rejection (ISHLT Grade A4). (**a**) At low magnification, organizing pneumonia (arrows) and interstitial thickening (arrowhead) are identified. (**b**) Intra-alveolar fibrin and blood with organization with proliferating fibroblasts are also present. (**c**) High-power view reveals more organizing pneumonia and interstitial thickening predominantly due to type II pneumocyte hyperplasia and scattered chronic inflammatory cells. Foamy macrophages and fibroblasts are forming clusters within alveolar spaces. (**d**) Another piece from the same biopsy reveals foci of inflammation (arrows). (**e**) These foci represent perivascular mononuclear cell infiltrates further suggestive of acute rejection. (**f**) Endotheliitis is also apparent (arrow points towards lymphocytes in between endothelial cells). Magnification, ×40 (**a**, **d**), ×100 (**b**), ×200 (**c**), ×400 (**e**, **f**)

surveillance biopsies taken within 400 days of transplantation revealed histologic findings of either acute cellular rejection or obliterative bronchiolitis in 31% of biopsies with 36% within the first 100 days and 25% between 100 and 400 days following transplantation [45].

Evidence suggests that acute cellular rejection is an important risk factor for the development of BOS [24]. Indeed, studies have demonstrated an increased risk of BOS with single episodes, increased frequencies, and increased severity of acute cellular rejection. Moreover, patients with multiple episodes of even minimal acute cellular rejection were shown to be at increased risk for BOS [46], and yet a single episode of minimal acute rejection without recurrence or subsequent progression to a higher grade has been identified as an independent significant predictor of BOS [47]. Because of these findings, patients who are asymptomatic but are found to have acute cellular rejection (even minimal acute cellular rejection) on a surveillance allograft biopsy might be treated accordingly. However, several centers do not utilize surveillance transbronchial lung biopsies and/or treat asymptomatic patients with no clinical evidence of allograft dysfunction. Prospective well-designed clinical studies are needed to provide evidence to support surveillance transbronchial lung biopsies and therapeutic interventions.

Small Airway Inflammation: Lymphocytic Bronchiolitis—B Grade

This grade applies only to small airways such as terminal or respiratory bronchioles. Bronchi, if present, should be described separately. It is important to mention in the pathology report whether or not small airways are present. If no small airways are identified or the biopsy has obvious infection, the grade "BX" should be used. The R behind grades 1 and 2 denotes the revised 2007 version.

No Airway Inflammation (ISHLT Grade B0)

The small airways appear unremarkable without evidence of bronchiolar inflammation.

Low-Grade Small Airway Inflammation (ISHLT Grade B1R)

Low-grade inflammation is characterized by lymphocytes within the submucosa of the bronchioles (Fig. 13.5a–c). The lymphocytic infiltrates can be infrequent and scattered or form a circumferential band; however, intraepithelial lymphocytic infiltration is not present. Occasional eosinophils may be seen within the submucosa. There is no evidence of epithelial damage, neutrophils, necrosis, ulceration, or significant amount of nuclear debris.

High-Grade Small Airway Inflammation (ISHLT Grade B2R)

In high-grade small airway inflammation, there is marked lymphocytic infiltrate of the airway epithelium and airway wall. The mononuclear cells in the submucosa appear larger, and a greater number of eosinophils and plasmacytoid cells can be seen (Fig. 13.6a–c). In addition, there is evidence of epithelial damage including necrosis, metaplasia, and marked intraepithelial lymphocytic infiltration. In its most severe form, high-grade airway inflammation is associated with epithelial ulceration, fibrinopurulent exudate, cellular debris, and neutrophils. It is important to exclude an infectious process, especially if the number of neutrophils is disproportionally high when compared to other mononuclear cells within the airway wall.

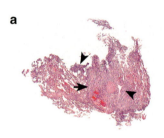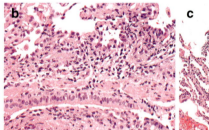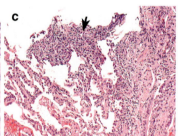

Fig. 13.5 (**a–c**) Low-grade small airway inflammation and moderate acute rejection (ISHLT Grade A3, B1R). (**a**) A small airway is surrounded by an inflammatory infiltrate (arrow). This biopsy also shows patchy inflammatory infiltrates away from the airway (arrowheads). (**b**) The mononuclear cell infiltrate is centered on the submucosa of the small airway, while the mucosa appears unremarkable consistent with low-grade small airway inflammation. (**c**) This biopsy also shows a marked mononuclear cell infiltrate around small vessels (arrow) and extending into the surrounding interstitium consistent with moderate acute rejection. Magnification, ×40 (**a**), ×400 (**b**), ×200 (**c**)

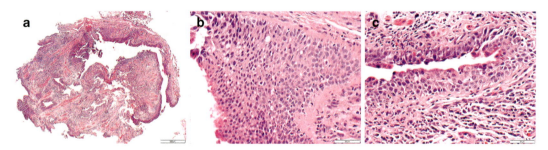

Fig. 13.6 (**a–c**) High-grade small airway inflammation (ISHLT Grade B2R). (**a**) A marked inflammatory infiltrate is noted within the wall of a small airway. (**b**) This chronic inflammatory infiltrate extends into the mucosa. (**c**) Squamous metaplasia is focally present. Magnification, ×40 (**a**), ×400 (**b, c**)

Ungradeable Small Airway Inflammation (ISHLT Grade BX)

Small airways might not be evaluable for several reasons including lack of small airways due to sampling problems, infection, tangential cutting, artifact, etc. In patients who are known to have an infection that could cause lymphocytic bronchiolitis, the allograft biopsy should also be classified as ungradeable for small airway rejection.

Chronic Airway Rejection: Obliterative Bronchiolitis—C Grade

Chronic airway rejection is restricted to submucosal and intraluminal scarring of small airways including terminal and respiratory bronchioles. When large tissue sections of the lung are examined, obliterative bronchiolitis may be recognized as a panlobar process but is usually patchy.

No Chronic Airway Rejection (ISHLT Grade C0)

The small airways appear similar in size to the accompanying artery with a ragged inner surface. Fibrosis is not present.

Chronic Airway Rejection (ISHLT Grade C1)

Narrowing of the small airways due to fibrosis in the airway wall is the hallmark of chronic airway rejection. The fibrosis may be eccentric or concentric. The type of fibrosis depends on the acuteness of the process, the degree of organization, and the amount of accompanying inflammation. The fibrosis can range from loose myxoid granulation tissue with variable numbers of inflammatory cells filling or partially obstructing the airway lumen in the more acute phase (Fig. 13.7a) to dense hyalinized collagen in the wall of bronchioles that is a characteristic of the chronic phase (Fig. 13.7b).

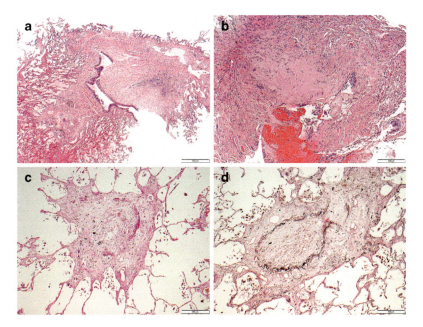

Fig. 13.7 (**a–d**) Chronic airway rejection (obliterative bronchiolitis) (ISHLT Grade C1). (**a**) Loose fibroblast proliferation with a patchy chronic inflammatory infiltrate is noted eccentric within the submucosa of a small airway narrowing its lumen. (**b**) In this example, submucosal collagen fibrosis eccentrically narrows the lumen of a small airway. (**c**) In this autopsy case of an allograft recipient, some airways are completely replaced by scar tissue. Focal smooth muscle might be suggestive of an airway. (**d**) A Verhoeff-Van Gieson stain highlights the remaining elastic fibers which helps to identify this scar replacing a former small airway. Magnification, ×40 (**a**), ×100 (**b–d**)

Metaplastic squamous or cuboidal epithelium may overly the bronchiolar fibrosis. Sometimes, only a slit-like lumen of the airway may remain as a result of a confluent submucosal scar or intraluminal polyps of scar tissue. There may be rather prominent capillaries supplying the intraluminal fibrotic areas. Ultimately, the bronchiolar lumen might be entirely occluded by dense scar tissue (Fig. 13.7c, d). In these cases, only an elastic stain highlighting residual elastic tissue, the vicinity of the scar to a pulmonary artery, and residual smooth muscle may indicate that a small airway has been replaced by fibrotic scar. In the chronic phase, inflammation may be minimal or absent. Usually, the scarring process is confined exclusively to respiratory bronchioles and terminal bronchioles, although it may occasionally involve adjacent alveoli.

Obliterative bronchiolitis is only infrequently identified in lung allografts by transbronchial biopsy, and the sensitivity of this morphologic finding for the presence of chronic rejection is only between 15 and 28% [48–50]. In a recent study, all seven conventional transbronchial biopsies that were included from patients clinically known to have BOS, the clinical equivalent to morphologic obliterative bronchiolitis, failed to reveal morphologic findings of obliterative bronchiolitis [31]. Although cryobiopsies contained more small airways, all nine cryobiopsies that were also included in that study from patients with clinically proven BOS did not reveal obliterative bronchiolitis in the tissue [31]. This low sensitivity is largely due to sampling and its patchy nature. Therefore, BOS is used and more reliable for the clinical assessment of chronic airway rejection. BOS is calculated as <80% FEV_1 in at least two consecutive lung function tests of the patient's maximum FEV_1 posttransplantation [51]. Despite the low sensitivity of transbronchial biopsies for obliterative bronchiolitis, the specificity of this morphologic finding in an allograft biopsy is high, ranging from 75 to 94% [49, 50]. Therefore, an attempt to diagnose obliterative bronchiolitis should be made in lung allograft biopsies.

Chronic Vascular Rejection: D Grade

No Chronic Vascular Rejection (ISHLT Grade D0)

The pulmonary arteries appear of a similar size as the accompanying airways. The intima is slender and the media not thickened.

Chronic Vascular Rejection (ISHLT Grade D1)

Chronic vascular rejection rarely is identified on biopsies since they usually lack vessels of sufficient size. Wedge biopsies, explants, or autopsy material may reveal it. Therefore, according to the ISHLT, the D grade of rejection is not applicable to allograft transbronchial biopsies. Although cryobiopsies contain a higher number of venules and small veins, in a recent small study, no difference was found in the number of cases with possible vascular rejection when compared to transbronchial biopsies [31].

Vascular rejection is characterized by thickened pulmonary arteries and more often veins, due to fibrointimal connective tissue (Fig. 13.8a, b). Also, thickening is usually concentric. Chronic vascular rejection may be patchy. Chronic vascular rejection usually starts with intimal proliferation. Subsequently, the internal elastic lamina may become fragmented and discontinuous. Occasionally the underlying muscular wall becomes thinned. In approximately half of the reported cases, a concurrent endovasculitis has been observed. The process is similar in pulmonary veins, although the intimal deposits may be less cellular and more waxy, eosinophilic, and sclerotic. Recanalized thrombi may mimic chronic vascular rejection. In contrast to heart allografts, chronic vascular rejection in lung transplants has not resulted in graft loss; however, some patients develop pulmonary hypertension particularly those with BOS [52, 53].

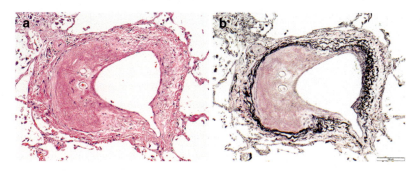

Fig. 13.8 (**a**, **b**) Chronic vascular rejection (ISHLT Grade D1). (**a**) A small vessel shows slightly eccentric intimal fibrosis. (**b**) A Verhoeff-Van Gieson stain delin-eates the internal elastic lamina which helps to better identify the extent of the intimal fibrosis. Magnification, ×200 (**a**, **b**)

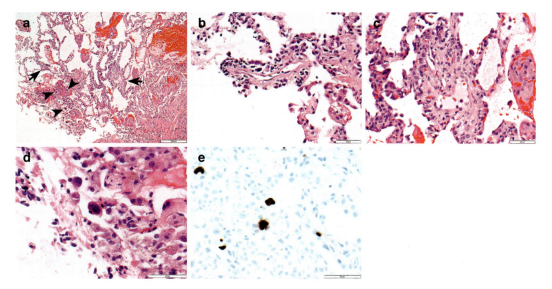

Fig. 13.9 (**a**–**e**) Cytomegalovirus (CMV) infection mim-icking acute rejection. (**a**) This biopsy shows small chronic inflammatory infiltrates surrounding small vessels (arrows). In addition, large atypical cells are identified (arrowheads). (**b**, **c**) High-power view confirms mononu-clear cells forming only a few layers around small vessels as can be seen in minimal acute rejection. (**d**) The large atypical cells have pink nuclear and cytoplasmic inclu-sions suggestive of CMV inclusions which were con-firmed by a CMV immunostain (**e**). Magnification, ×100 (**a**), ×400 (**b**, **c**), ×600 (**d**, **e**)

Mimickers of Cellular Rejection

Infection can mimic acute cellular rejection. For instance, viral infection, particularly CMV (Fig. 13.9a–e) but also *pneumocystis jirovecii* pneumonia, can be associated with perivascular mononuclear cell inflammation mimicking acute cellular rejection [54]. Infection can also cause small airway inflammation imitating lympho-cytic bronchiolitis.

Mimickers of severe acute rejection include conditions that might present with acute lung injury or diffuse alveolar damage. These condi-tions include infection, drug toxicity, aspiration,

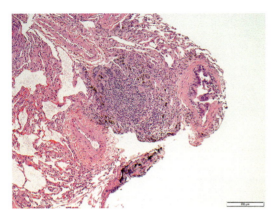

Fig. 13.10 Bronchiolar-associated lymphatic tissue (BALT). A nodule comprised of lymphocytes and anthracotic pigment is identified in the vicinity to an unremarkable small airway. Magnification, ×100

AMR, or harvest/reperfusion injury. The presence of perivascular inflammation is helpful in establishing the diagnosis of rejection. However, perivascular inflammation is not entirely specific for acute rejection, and many other conditions may simulate or mimic alloreactive lung injury [54].

Marked perivascular and/or peribronchiolar mononuclear infiltrates might also raise the possibility of posttransplantation lymphoproliferative disease (PTLD), and in such cases, an appropriate workup should be performed, including doing studies for Epstein-Barr virus, which is ubiquitous in PTLD. Further differential diagnosis of perivascular and interstitial infiltrates include recurrent primary diseases.

Small airway rejection and the perivascular infiltrates of Grade A rejection should be distinguished from bronchiolar-associated lymphatic tissue (BALT) . BALT is found in the vicinity of airways, usually contains black anthracotic pigment, and presents as a rather nodular collection of chronic inflammatory cells which does not surround a vessel (Fig. 13.10). Epithelial injury, neutrophils, or eosinophils should not be seen in BALT collections [34].

Antibody-Mediated Rejection

Originally recognized in kidney transplant patients who presented with acute allograft rejection, anti-donor antibodies, and poor prognosis

[55], AMR is now well established in kidney and heart allografts. In lung transplantation, AMR is still an evolving concept but likely explains acute and chronic graft dysfunction/failure in a subset of patients. Evidence suggests that AMR occurs due to circulating antibodies that are either (1) preformed because of pregnancy, blood transfusion, or previous organ transplantation or (2) arise de novo after transplantation due to HLA mismatch. Furthermore, the recent development of very sensitive and specific solid-phase flow cytometry and Luminex-based methodologies has allowed for more accurate detection of antibody specificities in sensitized recipients, and it has become clear that more patients than previously expected have or develop preformed anti-HLA antibodies. Immune stimulation by prior infections or autoimmunity may also contribute to the development of antibodies in those patients with no identifiable risk factors.

Overall, these preexisting or de novo antibodies can react with donor antigens, leading to immediate graft loss (hyperacute rejection), accelerated humoral rejection, and/or BOS [56]. In addition, recent studies have consistently demonstrated an increased incidence of acute rejection (a threefold increase in one study) [57], persistent rejection, increased BOS [58], or worse overall survival [59] in patients with anti-HLA antibodies. This effect is seen both with pretransplant HLA sensitization and with the development of de novo anti-HLA donor-specific antibodies after transplantation [58].

About 10–15% of lung transplant recipients are pre-sensitized to HLA antigens [60].

Even though "unacceptable antigens" are avoided during the virtual crossmatch, patients with positive pretransplant PRA are at higher risk for posttransplant complications. Their posttransplant PRA can stay stable or increase via generation of either donor-specific or non-donor-specific anti-HLA antibodies. Similarly, patients that had negative PRA screening tests before transplantation can develop de novo non-donor-specific or donor-specific anti-HLA antibodies after transplantation.

The mechanisms by which antibodies promote lung allograft injury remain poorly understood. Antibody binding to allo-HLA or other endothelial or epithelial targets in the lung allograft can activate the complement cascade. Complement deposits lead to endothelial cell injury, production of proinflammatory molecules, and recruitment of inflammatory cells. Complement-independent antibody-mediated mechanisms can also induce endothelial cell activation without cell injury, leading to increased gene expression and subsequent proliferation [56]. Furthermore, as demonstrated by in vitro studies, anti-HLA antibodies can cause proliferation of airway epithelial cells as well, producing fibroblast-stimulating growth factors [61], potentially contributing to the generation of obliterative bronchiolitis.

Although the diagnosis of AMR in lung allograft biopsies remains challenging, when the triple test criteria are met (graft dysfunction, positive panel reactive antibodies, and evidence of complement deposition in the graft), the disease can be life-threatening, and prognosis can be poor. Although the optimal treatment of AMR in the lung is currently not known due to the lack of clinical trials, treatment is typically comprised of plasmapheresis, possibly intravenous immunoglobulin (IVIG), and medications such as rituximab and bortezomib, among others. As such, the associated histopathologic and clinical parameters are the subject of intense investigation. Deposition of complement 4d (C4d), a complement split product, on the capillary endothelium has been suggested as a surrogate marker for AMR in heart, kidney, and pancreas transplants [62–71]. However, the role of C4d deposition in the diagnosis of AMR in lung allografts is still unclear. Moreover, reproducibility of C4d deposition in allograft lung TBBx is problematic, even among pathologists who routinely evaluate C4d in lung allograft biopsies [72]. Furthermore, there are currently no specific or sensitive morphologic features of AMR in lung allografts, although some features that are more commonly identified in these patients have emerged in some recent studies [73]. Studies have attempted to evaluate immunoglobulins (Ig) and complement deposits in the subendothelial space. Septal capillary deposits of Igs and complement products such as C1q, C3d, C4d, and C5b-9 have been described in association with anti-HLA antibod-

ies [74, 75] as well as allograft dysfunction and BOS [76, 77]. However, except for C4d and in some institutions C3d, these studies have in general not been implemented for the workup of lung transplant biopsies for possible AMR. One of the reasons for the difficulties in lung is the relatively high background that is encountered in immunohistochemical as well as immunofluorescence studies. Often, C4d binds to the vascular elastic lamina or shows other non-specific binding such as intracapillary serum. Staining is commonly only focal, and, therefore, sensitivity and specificity have not been established. Only linear, continuous luminal endothelial staining of capillaries, arterioles, and/or venules by C4d should be interpreted as positive. In addition, C4d is not specific to AMR but also can be seen in infection, and harvest/reperfusion injury, or any process that is associated with complement activation.

In general, the concept of specific histopathologic features associated with AMR remains controversial in lung transplantation. The 2007 ISHLT revised consensus classification [34] did propose histopathologic features that might be specific for AMR. Because of the lack of specific histologic findings of AMR, a multidisciplinary approach to the diagnosis was recommended that includes the following: (1) the presence of circulating antibodies (HLA antibodies, anti-endothelial and anti-epithelial antibodies), (2) focal or diffuse C4d deposition (Fig. 13.11a–c), (3) histologic features of acute lung injury or hemorrhage (diffuse alveolar damage, capillary injury associated with neutrophils and nuclear debris, i.e., capillaritis), and (4) clinical signs of graft dysfunction [78]. In 2013, the Pathology Council of the ISHLT published findings in a summary statement with recommendations for the pathologic evaluation of AMR [78]. This report included suggestions for protocol biopsies with serologic evaluation for donor-specific antibodies (DSAs) at or near time of biopsy. In addition, this statement included recommendations for histopathologic patterns in AMR (Fig. 13.12a–e) and indications for immunohistochemical or immunofluorescence studies to further elucidate findings in AMR (Box 13.1). The morphologic features were confirmed by the 2016 consensus report of the ISHLT [79].

Fig. 13.11 (**a–c**)
Complement 4d (C4d).
Diffuse C4d deposition
is defined by continuous
subendothelial staining
in more than 50% of
capillaries either by
immunohistochemistry
(**a**) or immunofluo-
rescence (**b**, arrows
point toward capillary
loops) often forming
donut-shaped structures.
The interpretation of
C4d deposition can be
complicated by
non-specific staining
including intracapillary
serum (arrows)
(**c**). Magnification,
×400 (**a–c**)

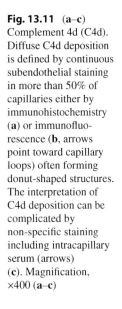
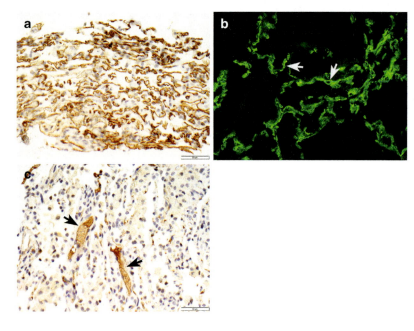

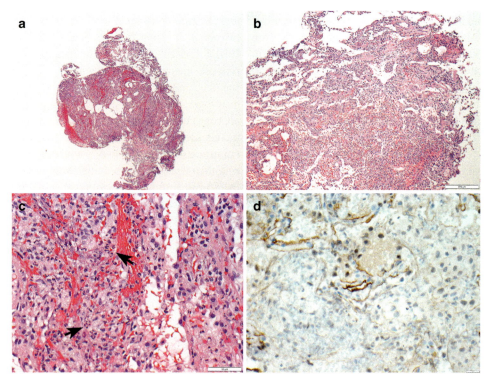

Fig. 13.12 (**a–e**) Possible antibody-mediated rejection (AMR). This patient presented with shortness of breath. Anti-DQ2 donor-specific antibodies were identified. The patient had undergone heart-lung transplantation 1 month prior to this biopsy. (**a**) A low-power view shows patchy inflammatory infiltrates and thickened interstitium. (**b**) At medium magnification, it becomes apparent that the inter-stitial thickening is due to neutrophilic inflammation and macrophages. Some alveoli are also filled with clusters of macrophages, scattered neutrophils, and blood. (**c**) There is neutrophilic margination in capillaries and neutrophilic capillaritis (arrows). (**d**, **e**) Complement 4d deposition was found in approximately 10–20% of capillaries by immunohistochemistry (**d**) and immunofluorescence (arrows) (**e**). Magnification, ×40 (**a**), ×100 (**b**), ×400 (**c–e**)

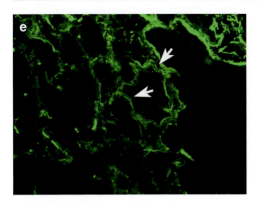

Fig. 13.12 (continued)

The 2016 consensus report confirmed the need for a multidisciplinary approach to establish a diagnosis of AMR in the lung that "integrates the clinical presentation with available immunologic and pathologic diagnostic tools" [79]. An AMR staging was also proposed (Table 13.2) [79].

Recently, Wallace and colleagues reported findings of the Banff study of the pathology of allograft lungs with DSA [73]. Nine experienced lung transplant pathologists from multiple institutions performed digital slide interpretation to study transbronchial biopsy specimens from patients with known antibody status (established within 30 days of biopsy) and negative infectious workup. The study demonstrated that biopsies from patients with DSA more commonly showed morphologic features of acute lung injury with or without diffuse alveolar damage than biopsies from patients with non-DSA or no circulating antibodies. Endotheliitis was more common in patients with DSA than patients without circulating antibodies. However, there was no difference in occurrence of endotheliitis between biopsies from patients with circulating non-DSA vs DSA or non-DSA vs no circulating antibodies. Specimens associated with DSA had a significant higher frequency of capillary inflammation, including neutrophilic margination, increased neutrophils, or capillaritis with karyorrhexis than patients with non-DSA or no circulating antibodies. C4d staining was positive in less than 50% of capillaries in 14% of biopsies and in more than 50% of capillaries in 7% of biopsies. While there was no difference between the groups in biopsies

Table 13.2 Staging of antibody-mediated rejection as proposed by the International Society for Heart and Lung Transplantation

Clinical antibody-mediated rejection	
Definite clinical AMR[a]	Allograft dysfunction DSA[b] present Histology suggestive of AMR C4d deposition Other causes of graft dysfunction were excluded except ACR[c] which can occur concurrently
Probable clinical AMR	Allograft dysfunction Two of the following 3 criteria: 　DSA present 　Histology suggestive of AMR 　C4d deposition When all 3 diagnostic criteria are identified, this grade can be applied even if infection or ACR is also present
Possible clinical AMR	Allograft dysfunction One of the following 3 criteria: 　DSA present 　Histology suggestive of AMR 　C4d deposition When 2 diagnostic criteria are identified, this grade can be applied even if infection or ACR is also present

Subclinical antibody-mediated rejection

Histologic criteria of AMR identified on surveillance transbronchial biopsy with or without
　C4d deposition
　DSA present
No allograft dysfunction

Data from: Levine DJ, Glanville AR, Aboyoun C, Belperio J, Benden C, Berry GJ, Hachem R, Hayes D, Neil D, Reinsmoen NL, et al. Antibody-mediated rejection of the lung: A consensus report of the International Society for Heart and Lung Transplantation. The Journal of Heart and Lung Transplantation: 2016; 35:397–406
[a]*AMR* antibody-mediated rejection
[b]*DSA* donor-specific antibodies
[c]*ACR* acute cellular rejection

with <50% staining, biopsies with DSA more often had over 50% capillaries staining for C4d than biopsies without any circulating antibodies. There were no significant differences identified between HLA classes of the DSA and any of the evaluated pathologic findings. Taken together, this study identified capillary inflammation, acute lung injury, and endotheliitis as morphologic features in lung allograft biopsies that correlate with the presence of circulating DSA. However, none

of these histopathologic features were specific to patients with DSA. Morphologic findings of acute lung injury with diffuse alveolar damage had the highest odds ratio for the presence of circulating DSA. This study also cautioned the usefulness of C4d immunohistochemical stain for the diagnosis of AMR in lung allografts because of its infrequent diffuse positivity. Although the study shows that some morphologic features correlate with the presence of circulating DSA and, therefore, might be histopathologic markers to at least suggest the possibility of AMR, the reproducibility of these morphologic features is quite problematic even among experienced lung transplant pathologists. In fact, the interobserver reproducibility kappa values ranged between 0.14 and 0.4, indicating a less than a chance to moderate agreement. The lowest agreement was noted for suspicion for aspiration (median kappa, 0.14) and the highest for acute cellular rejection, alveolar hemosiderosis, and C4d staining (median kappa, 0.4, all).

Although a definite diagnosis of AMR seems to elude pathologic interpretation at the current time, in a fully contextualized clinical environment, the findings from the biopsy specimen may aid the clinician to make a reasonable diagnosis of AMR if other relevant clinical and serologic features are present. The proposed "triple test" [78] of clinical features, serologic evidence of DSA, and pathologic findings supportive of AMR including capillary inflammation, acute lung injury with or without diffuse alveolar damage, and endotheliitis may currently be the best guide to the diagnosis of AMR.

There is no IHSLT recommendation at this time regarding the coexistence of AMR and acute rejection, but it clearly does occur.

Hyperacute Rejection

Hyperacute rejection is a severe form of AMR mediated by preexisting antibodies to ABO blood groups, HLA class I or II, or other antigens on graft vascular endothelial cells. This rejection occurs within minutes to a few hours after the transplanted organ begins to be perfused. As in any form of AMR, the preexisting antibodies can result from previous pregnancies, blood transfusions, or previous transplant, and their binding to donor antigens provokes complement and cytokine activation resulting in endothelial cell damage and platelet activation with subsequent vascular thrombosis and graft destruction. The outcome is commonly fatal.

In hyperacute rejection, lungs are edematous, cyanotic, and heavy, have a firm consistency, lack crepitation, and show red hepatization [80–83]. The cut surface reveals patchy poorly defined areas of hemorrhagic consolidation. Anastomoses are intact and typically widely patent. Histologically, alveolar hemorrhage, platelet and fibrin thrombi, neutrophilic infiltration, necrosis of vessel walls, and diffuse alveolar damage are observed [76–80, 83, 84]. C4d deposition has been described.

Although hyperacute rejection is a well-known complication in kidney and heart transplantations, in lung transplantation, it appears to be rather rare with only eight cases reported. Six patients died within 1 h and 13 days after transplantation [80–85]. Only two patients survived [86, 87]. One of these two patients was treated with plasmapheresis, antithymocyte globulin, and cyclophosphamide immediately after hyperacute rejection was diagnosed [86]. The other patient was highly presensitized when he underwent double lung transplantation [87]. This patient was treated with multiple plasma exchanges and intravenous immunoglobulin pre- and posttransplantation together with posttransplant rituximab and bortezomib and later with anti-C5 antibody and eculizumab. Although in pretransplant, panel reactive antibodies (PRAs) were negative in four of the eight reported patients, crossmatch was positive in all reported cases.

Collectively, although hyperacute rejection is rare after lung transplantation, one should keep this reaction in mind given that false-negative PRAs may occur and pretransplantation crossmatch is not often possible [80].

Specimen Requirements

At least five pieces of well-expanded alveolated parenchyma are required for adequate evaluation of a transbronchial lung allograft biopsy specimen for acute rejection by the LRSG [34]. This specimen requirement was based on the "uniform opinion of the consensus meeting." To ensure that the minimum number of required pieces of alveolated lung parenchyma is available for pathology review, it is recommended that the bronchoscopist needs to take more than five pieces. Even more pieces might be necessary to provide small airways for review. Interestingly, a prospective 12-month single-operator study by Scott and colleagues [88] including 219 transbronchial allograft biopsies with 6 to 56 samples per procedure (mean 17.3 samples per procedure) taken from 3 lobes (or 2 lobes and the lingula of 1 lung) of 54 heart-lung transplant and 2 single lung transplant recipients revealed a sensitivity of 94% and a specificity of 90% for identification of rejection by histopathology. This study estimated that 18 samples per procedure are needed to have a 95% confidence of finding rejection. Therefore, false-negative results due to patchy distribution of acute rejection are likely not uncommon. The absence of histologic and immunophenotypic features of acute rejection or antibody-mediated rejection requires clinicopathologic correlation as a negative biopsy does not necessary rule out rejection. Furthermore, the bronchoscopist should be familiar with imaging studies, especially high resolution computed tomography studies if available, and aim to sample radiologically abnormal bronchopulmonary segments. If such imaging was not recently performed or the results are normal, then samples should be obtained from different lobes to try to minimize sampling error.

Specimens should be gently agitated in formalin to open up the alveoli. There is currently no recommendation for cryobiopsies. In a recent study using cryobiopsies to evaluate rejection in lung allografts, a median of three pieces provided twice as many alveoli and small airways than a median of ten pieces by conventional forceps biopsy [31].

The ISHLT recommends a minimum of three levels from the paraffin block for hematoxylin and eosin (H&E) staining for histologic examination [34]. In addition, "connective tissue stains" such as trichrome or Verhoeff-Van Gieson (VVG) stain are recommended to evaluate airways for the presence of submucosal fibrosis and vessels for graft vascular disease. Stains for microorganisms including Gomori-Grocott methenamine silver stain (GMS) and acid fast bacilli (AFB) may be added. While silver stains are routinely performed on lung allograft biopsies in some institutions, they are currently not mandated by the LRSG because many microbiologic, serologic, and molecular techniques are available and used to identify infections in these patients [34, 89]. BAL may be performed at the time of biopsy and is useful for the exclusion of infection but currently has no clinical role in the diagnosis of acute rejection.

Summary

The transbronchial allograft biopsy is currently the gold standard to evaluate the graft for cellular rejection and to exclude its clinical mimickers in lung transplant patients. When reviewing transbronchial biopsy material of these patients, attention must be paid not only to features of rejection but also to its morphologic mimickers, especially infection, PTLD, and abnormal drug effect. Before a diagnosis of acute cellular rejection can be rendered, an infectious process should be excluded by using stains for microorganisms and/or clinical tests including cultures of BAL and/or tissue and serology. While studies to identify histopathologic and immunophenotypic features of AMR are evolving, there are currently no specific morphologic findings, and clinical and serologic correlations are required for the diagnosis. Prospective, well-designed long-term studies with longitudinal data of therapeutic intervention of ACR on histopathology in totally asymptomatic patients with no physiological or HRCT evidence of allograft dysfunction are needed to determine the clinical significance and relevance of such interventions.

References

1. Martinu T, Chen DF, Palmer SM. Acute rejection and humoral sensitization in lung transplant recipients. Proc Am Thorac Soc. 2009;6:54–65.
2. Haque MA, Mizobuchi T, Yasufuku K, Fujisawa T, Brutkiewicz RR, Zheng Y, Woods K, Smith GN, Cummings OW, Heidler KM, et al. Evidence for immune responses to a self-antigen in lung transplantation: role of type V collagen-specific T cells in the pathogenesis of lung allograft rejection. J Immunol. 2002;169:1542–9.
3. Yusen RD, Edwards LB, Kucheryavaya AY, Benden C, Dipchand AI, Goldfarb SB, Levvey BJ, Lund LH, Meiser B, Rossano JW, Stehlik J. The Registry of the International Society for Heart and Lung Transplantation: thirty-second official adult lung and heart-lung transplantation report—2015; focus theme: early graft failure. J Heart Lung Transplant. 2015;34:1264–77.
4. Martinu T, Pavlisko EN, Chen DF, Palmer SM. Acute allograft rejection: cellular and humoral processes. Clin Chest Med. 2011;32:295–310.
5. Glanville AR, Aboyoun CL, Havryk A, Plit M, Rainer S, Malouf MA. Severity of lymphocytic bronchiolitis predicts long-term outcome after lung transplantation. Am J Respir Crit Care Med. 2008;177:1033–40.
6. Verleden SE, Ruttens D, Vandermeulen E, Vaneylen A, Dupont LJ, Van Raemdonck DE, Verleden GM, Vanaudenaerde BM, Vos R. Bronchiolitis obliterans syndrome and restrictive allograft syndrome: do risk factors differ? Transplantation. 2013;95:1167–72.
7. Schulman LL, Weinberg AD, McGregor C, Galantowicz ME, Suciu-Foca NM, Itescu S. Mismatches at the HLA-dr and HLA-b loci are risk factors for acute rejection after lung transplantation. Am J Respir Crit Care Med. 1998;157:1833–7.
8. Quantz MA, Bennett LE, Meyer DM, Novick RJ. Does human leukocyte antigen matching influence the outcome of lung transplantation? An analysis of 3,549 lung transplantations. J Heart Lung Transplant. 2000;19:473–9.
9. Wisser W, Wekerle T, Zlabinger G, Senbaclavaci O, Zuckermann A, Klepetko W, Wolner E. Influence of human leukocyte antigen matching on long-term outcome after lung transplantation. J Heart Lung Transplant. 1996;15:1209–16.
10. Christie JD, Edwards LB, Kucheryavaya AY, Aurora P, Dobbels F, Kirk R, Rahmel AO, Stehlik J, Hertz MI. The Registry of the International Society for Heart and Lung Transplantation: twenty-seventh official adult lung and heart-lung transplant report—2010. J Heart Lung Transplant. 2010;29:1104–18.
11. Mangi AA, Mason DP, Nowicki ER, Batizy LH, Murthy SC, Pidwell DJ, Avery RK, McCurry KR, Pettersson GB, Blackstone EH. Predictors of acute rejection after lung transplantation. Ann Thorac Surg. 2011;91:1754–62.

12. Zheng HX, Burckart GJ, McCurry K, Webber S, Ristich J, Iacono A, Dauber J, McDade K, Grgurich W, Zaldonis D, et al. Interleukin-10 production genotype protects against acute persistent rejection after lung transplantation. J Heart Lung Transplant. 2004;23:541–6.

13. Zheng HX, Zeevi A, McCurry K, Schuetz E, Webber S, Ristich J, Zhang J, Iacono A, Dauber J, McDade K, et al. The impact of pharmacogenomic factors on acute persistent rejection in adult lung transplant patients. Transpl Immunol. 2005;14:37–42.

14. Ibrahim JE, Sweet SC, Flippin M, Dent C, Mendelhoff E, Huddleston CB, Trinkaus K, Canter CE. Rejection is reduced in thoracic organ recipients when transplanted in the first year of life. J Heart Lung Transplant. 2002;21:311–8.

15. Scott JP, Whitehead B, de Leval M, Helms P, Smyth RL, Higenbottam TW, Wallwork J. Paediatric incidence of acute rejection and obliterative bronchiolitis: a comparison with adults. Transpl Int. 1994;7:S404–6.

16. Yusen RD, Christie JD, Edwards LB, Kucheryavaya AY, Benden C, Dipchand AI, Dobbels F, Kirk R, Lund LH, Rahmel AO, Stehlik J. The Registry of the International Society for Heart and Lung Transplantation: thirtieth adult lung and heart-lung transplant report—2013; focus theme: age. J Heart Lung Transplant. 2013;32:965–78.

17. De Vito Dabbs A, Hoffman LA, Iacono AT, Zullo TG, McCurry KR, Dauber JH. Are symptom reports useful for differentiating between acute rejection and pulmonary infection after lung transplantation? Heart Lung. 2004;33:372–80.

18. Christie JD, Edwards LB, Kucheryavaya AY, Benden C, Dipchand AI, Dobbels F, Kirk R, Rahmel AO, Stehlik J, Hertz MI. The Registry of the International Society for Heart and Lung Transplantation: 29th adult lung and heart-lung transplant report-2012. J Heart Lung Transplant. 2012;31:1073–86.

19. Lowery EM, Bemiss B, Cascino T, Durazo-Arvizu RA, Forsythe SM, Alex C, Laghi F, Love RB, Camacho P. Low vitamin D levels are associated with increased rejection and infections after lung transplantation. J Heart Lung Transplant. 2012;31:700–7.

20. Kumar D, Erdman D, Keshavjee S, Peret T, Tellier R, Hadjiliadis D, Johnson G, Ayers M, Siegal D, Humar A. Clinical impact of community-acquired respiratory viruses on bronchiolitis obliterans after lung transplant. Am J Transplant. 2005;5:2031–6.

21. Vilchez RA, Dauber J, McCurry K, Iacono A, Kusne S. Parainfluenza virus infection in adult lung transplant recipients: an emergent clinical syndrome with implications on allograft function. Am J Transplant. 2003;3:116–20.

22. Garantziotis S, Howell DN, McAdams HP, Davis RD, Henshaw NG, Palmer SM. Influenza pneumonia in lung transplant recipients: clinical features and association with bronchiolitis obliterans syndrome. Chest. 2001;119:1277–80.

23. Glanville AR, Gencay M, Tamm M, Chhajed P, Plit M, Hopkins P, Aboyoun C, Roth M, Malouf M. Chlamydia pneumoniae infection after lung transplantation. J Heart Lung Transplant. 2005;24:131–6.

24. Sharples LD, McNeil K, Stewart S, Wallwork J. Risk factors for bronchiolitis obliterans: a systematic review of recent publications. J Heart Lung Transplant. 2002;21:271–81.

25. Van Muylem A, Melot C, Antoine M, Knoop C, Estenne M. Role of pulmonary function in the detection of allograft dysfunction after heart-lung transplantation. Thorax. 1997;52:643–7.

26. Becker FS, Martinez FJ, Brunsting LA, Deeb GM, Flint A, Lynch JP III. Limitations of spirometry in detecting rejection after single-lung transplantation. Am J Respir Crit Care Med. 1994;150:159–66.

27. Gotway MB, Dawn SK, Sellami D, Golden JA, Reddy GP, Keith FM, Webb WR. Acute rejection following lung transplantation: limitations in accuracy of thin-section CT for diagnosis. Radiology. 2001;221:207–12.

28. Silkoff PE, Caramori M, Tremblay L, McClean P, Chaparro C, Kesten S, Hutcheon M, Slutsky AS, Zamel N, Keshavjee S. Exhaled nitric oxide in human lung transplantation: a noninvasive marker of acute rejection. Am J Respir Crit Care Med. 1998;157:1822–8.

29. Gashouta MA, Merlo CA, Pipeling MR, McDyer JF, Hayanga JW, Orens JB, Girgis RE. Serial monitoring of exhaled nitric oxide in lung transplant recipients. J Heart Lung Transplant. 2015;34:557–62.

30. De Soyza A, Fisher AJ, Small T, Corris PA. Inhaled corticosteroids and the treatment of lymphocytic bronchiolitis following lung transplantation. Am J Respir Crit Care Med. 2001;164:1209–12.

31. Roden AC, Kern RM, Aubry MC, Jenkins SM, Yi ES, Scott JP, Maldonado F. Transbronchial cryobiopsies in the evaluation of lung allografts: do the benefits outweigh the risks? Arch Pathol Lab Med. 2016;140(4):303–11.

32. Yarmus L, Akulian J, Gilbert C, Illei P, Shah P, Merlo C, Orens J, Feller-Kopman D. Cryoprobe transbronchial lung biopsy in patients after lung transplantation: a pilot safety study. Chest. 2013;143:621–6.

33. Fruchter O, Fridel L, Rosengarten D, Raviv Y, Rosanov V, Kramer MR. Transbronchial cryobiopsy in lung transplantation patients: first report. Respirology. 2013;18:669–73.

34. Stewart S, Fishbein MC, Snell GI, Berry GJ, Boehler A, Burke MM, Glanville A, Gould FK, Magro C, Marboe CC, et al. Revision of the 1996 working formulation for the standardization of nomenclature in the diagnosis of lung rejection. J Heart Lung Transplant. 2007;26:1229–42.

35. Berry GJ, Brunt EM, Chamberlain D, Hruban RH, Sibley RK, Stewart S, Tazelaar HD. A working formulation for the standardization of nomenclature in the diagnosis of heart and lung rejection: Lung Rejection Study Group. The International Society for Heart Transplantation. J Heart Transplant. 1990;9:593–601.

36. Yousem SA, Berry GJ, Cagle PT, Chamberlain D, Husain AN, Hruban RH, Marchevsky A, Ohori NP,

Ritter J, Stewart S, Tazelaar HD. Revision of the 1990 working formulation for the classification of pulmonary allograft rejection: Lung Rejection Study Group. J Heart Lung Transplant. 1996;15:1–15.

37. Chakinala MM, Ritter J, Gage BF, Aloush AA, Hachem RH, Lynch JP, Patterson GA, Trulock EP. Reliability for grading acute rejection and airway inflammation after lung transplantation. J Heart Lung Transplant. 2005;24:652–7.

38. Colombat M, Groussard O, Lautrette A, Thabut G, Marrash-Chahla R, Brugière O, Mal H, Lesèche G, Fournier M, Degott C. Analysis of the different histologic lesions observed in transbronchial biopsy for the diagnosis of acute rejection. Clinicopathologic correlations during the first 6 months after lung transplantation. Hum Pathol. 2005;36:387–94.

39. Stephenson A, Flint J, English J, Vedal S, Fradet G, Chittock D, Levy RD. Interpretation of transbronchial lung biopsies from lung transplant recipients: inter- and intraobserver agreement. Can Respir J. 2005;12:75–7.

40. Bhorade SM, Husain AN, Liao C, Li LC, Ahya VN, Baz MA, Valentine VG, Love RB, Seethamraju H, Alex CG, et al. Interobserver variability in grading transbronchial lung biopsy specimens after lung transplantation. Chest. 2013;143:1717–24.

41. Yousem SA, Martin T, Paradis IL, Keenan R, Griffith BP. Can immunohistological analysis of transbronchial biopsy specimens predict responder status in early acute rejection of lung allografts? Hum Pathol. 1994;25:525–9.

42. Reams BD, Musselwhite LW, Zaas DW, Steele MP, Garantziotis S, Eu PC, Snyder LD, Curl J, Lin SS, Davis RD, Palmer SM. Alemtuzumab in the treatment of refractory acute rejection and bronchiolitis obliterans syndrome after human lung transplantation. Am J Transplant. 2007;7:2802–8.

43. Trulock EP, Ettinger NA, Brunt EM, Pasque MK, Kaiser LR, Cooper JD. The role of transbronchial lung biopsy in the treatment of lung transplant recipients: an analysis of 200 consecutive procedures. Chest. 1992;102:1049–54.

44. Hopkins PM, Aboyoun CL, Chhajed PN, Malouf MA, Plit ML, Rainer SP, Glanville AR. Prospective analysis of 1,235 transbronchial lung biopsies in lung transplant recipients. J Heart Lung Transplant. 2002;21:1062–7.

45. Chakinala MM, Ritter J, Gage BF, Lynch JP, Aloush A, Patterson GA, Trulock EP. Yield of surveillance bronchoscopy for acute rejection and lymphocytic bronchitis/bronchiolitis after lung transplantation. J Heart Lung Transplant. 2004;23:1396–404.

46. Hopkins PM, Aboyoun CL, Chhajed PN, Malouf MA, Plit ML, Rainer SP, Glanville AR. Association of minimal rejection in lung transplant recipients with obliterative bronchiolitis. Am J Respir Crit Care Med. 2004;170:1022–6.

47. Hachem RR, Khalifah AP, Chakinala MM, Yusen RD, Aloush AA, Mohanakumar T, Patterson GA, Trulock EP, Walter MJ. The significance of a single episode of minimal acute rejection after lung transplantation. Transplantation. 2005;80:1406–13.

48. Kramer MR, Stoehr C, Whang JL, Berry GJ, Sibley R, Marshall SE, Patterson GM, Starnes VA, Theodore J. The diagnosis of obliterative bronchiolitis after heart-lung and lung transplantation: low yield of transbronchial lung biopsy. J Heart Lung Transplant. 1993;12:675–81.

49. Chamberlain D, Maurer J, Chapparo C, Idolor C. Evaluation of transbronchial biopsy in the diagnosis of bronchiolitis obliterans after lung transplantation. J Heart Lung Transplant. 1994;13:963–71.

50. Pomerance A, Madden B, Burke MM, Yacoub MH. Transbronchial biopsy in heart and lung transplantation: clinicopathologic correlations. J Heart Lung Transplant. 1995;14:761–73.

51. Meyer KC, Raghu G, Verleden GM, Corris PA, Aurora P, Wilson KC, Brozek J, Glanville AR. An international ISHLT/ATS/ERS clinical practice guideline: diagnosis and management of bronchiolitis obliterans syndrome. Eur Respir J. 2014;44:1479–503.

52. Saggar R, Ross DJ, Saggar R, Zisman DA, Gregson A, Lynch JP III, Keane MP, Weigt SS, Ardehali A, Kubak B, et al. Pulmonary hypertension associated with lung transplantation obliterative bronchiolitis and vascular remodeling of the allograft. Am J Transplant. 2008;8:1921–30.

53. Nathan SD, Shlobin OA, Ahmad S, Barnett SD, Burton NA, Gladwin MT, Machado RF. Pulmonary hypertension in patients with bronchiolitis obliterans syndrome listed for retransplantation. Am J Transplant. 2008;8:1506–11.

54. Tazelaar HD. Perivascular inflammation in pulmonary infections: implications for the diagnosis of lung rejection. J Heart Lung Transplant. 1991;10:437–41.

55. Takemoto SK, Zeevi A, Feng S, Colvin RB, Jordan S, Kobashigawa J, Kupiec-Weglinski J, Matas A, Montgomery RA, Nickerson P, et al. National conference to assess antibody-mediated rejection in solid organ transplantation. Am J Transplant. 2004;4:1033–41.

56. Colvin RB, Smith RN. Antibody-mediated organ-allograft rejection. Nat Rev Immunol. 2005;5:807–17.

57. Girnita AL, McCurry KR, Iacono AT, Duquesnoy R, Corcoran TE, Awad M, Spichty KJ, Yousem SA, Burckart G, Dauber JH, et al. HLA-specific antibodies are associated with high-grade and persistent-recurrent lung allograft acute rejection. J Heart Lung Transplant. 2004;23:1135–41.

58. Palmer SM, Davis RD, Hadjiliadis D, Hertz MI, Howell DN, Ward FE, Savik K, Reinsmoen NL. Development of an antibody specific to major histocompatibility antigens detectable by flow cytometry after lung transplant is associated with bronchiolitis obliterans syndrome. Transplantation. 2002;74:799–804.

59. Hadjiliadis D, Chaparro C, Reinsmoen NL, Gutierrez C, Singer LG, Steele MP, Waddell TK, Davis RD,

Hutcheon MA, Palmer SM, Keshavjee S. Pre-transplant panel reactive antibody in lung transplant recipients is associated with significantly worse post-transplant survival in a multicenter study. J Heart Lung Transplant. 2005;24:S249–54.

60. Appel JZ III, Hartwig MG, Davis RD, Reinsmoen NL. Utility of peritransplant and rescue intravenous immunoglobulin and extracorporeal immunoadsorption in lung transplant recipients sensitized to HLA antigens. Hum Immunol. 2005;66:378–86.

61. Jaramillo A, Smith CR, Maruyama T, Zhang L, Patterson GA, Mohanakumar T. Anti-HLA class I antibody binding to airway epithelial cells induces production of fibrogenic growth factors and apoptotic cell death: a possible mechanism for bronchiolitis obliterans syndrome. Hum Immunol. 2003;64:521–9.

62. Choi J, Cho YM, Yang WS, Park TJ, Chang JW, Park SK. Peritubular capillary C4d deposition and renal outcome in post-transplant IgA nephropathy. Clin Transpl. 2007;21:159–65.

63. Herman J, Lerut E, Van Damme-Lombaerts R, Emonds MP, Van Damme B. Capillary deposition of complement C4d and C3d in pediatric renal allograft biopsies. Transplantation. 2005;79:1435–40.

64. Moll S, Pascual M. Humoral rejection of organ allografts. Am J Transplant. 2005;5:2611–8.

65. Fedson SE, Daniel SS, Husain AN. Immunohistochemistry staining of C4d to diagnose antibody-mediated rejection in cardiac transplantation. J Heart Lung Transplant. 2008;27:372–9.

66. Mauiyyedi S, Crespo M, Collins AB, Schneeberger EE, Pascual MA, Saidman SL, Tolkoff-Rubin NE, Williams WW, Delmonico FL, Cosimi AB, Colvin RB. Acute humoral rejection in kidney transplantation: II. Morphology, immunopathology, and pathologic classification. J Am Soc Nephrol. 2002;13:779–87.

67. Mauiyyedi S, Pelle PD, Saidman S, Collins AB, Pascual M, Tolkoff-Rubin NE, Williams WW, Cosimi AA, Schneeberger EE, Colvin RB. Chronic humoral rejection: identification of antibody-mediated chronic renal allograft rejection by C4d deposits in peritubular capillaries. J Am Soc Nephrol. 2001;12:574–82.

68. Rodriguez ER, Skojec DV, Tan CD, Zachary AA, Kasper EK, Conte JV, Baldwin WM III. Antibody-mediated rejection in human cardiac allografts: evaluation of immunoglobulins and complement activation products C4d and C3d as markers. Am J Transplant. 2005;5:2778–85.

69. Smith RN, Brousaides N, Grazette L, Saidman S, Semigran M, Disalvo T, Madsen J, Dec GW, Perez-Atayde AR, Collins AB. C4d deposition in cardiac allografts correlates with alloantibody. J Heart Lung Transplant. 2005;24:1202–10.

70. Tan CD, Baldwin WM III, Rodriguez ER. Update on cardiac transplantation pathology. Arch Pathol Lab Med. 2007;131:1169–91.

71. de Kort H, Munivenkatappa RB, Berger SP, Eikmans M, van der Wal A, de Koning EJ, van Kooten C, de Heer E, Barth RN, Bruijn JA, et al. Pancreas allograft biopsies with positive c4d staining and anti-donor antibodies related to worse outcome for patients. Am J Transplant Off J Am Soc Transplant Am Soc Transplant Surg. 2010;10:1660–7.

72. Roden AC, Maleszewski JJ, Yi ES, Jenkins SM, Gandhi MJ, Scott JP, Christine Aubry M. Reproducibility of Complement 4d deposition by immunofluorescence and immunohistochemistry in lung allograft biopsies. J Heart Lung Transplant. 2014;33:1223–32.

73. Wallace WD, Li N, Andersen CB, Arrossi AV, Askar M, Berry GJ, DeNicola MM, Neil DA, Pavlisko EN, Reed EF, et al. Banff study of pathologic changes in lung allograft biopsy specimens with donor-specific antibodies. J Heart Lung Transplant. 2016;35:40–8.

74. Ionescu DN, Girnita AL, Zeevi A, Duquesnoy R, Pilewski J, Johnson B, Studer S, McCurry KR, Yousem SA. C4d deposition in lung allografts is associated with circulating anti-HLA alloantibody. Transpl Immunol. 2005;15:63–8.

75. Miller GG, Destarac L, Zeevi A, Girnita A, McCurry K, Iacono A, Murray JJ, Crowe D, Johnson JE, Ninan M, Milstone AP. Acute humoral rejection of human lung allografts and elevation of C4d in bronchoalveolar lavage fluid. Am J Transplant. 2004;4:1323–30.

76. Magro CM, Abbas AE, Seilstad K, Pope-Harman AL, Nadasdy T, Ross P Jr. C3d and the septal microvasculature as a predictor of chronic lung allograft dysfunction. Hum Immunol. 2006;67:274–83.

77. Westall GP, Snell GI, McLean C, Kotsimbos T, Williams T, Magro C. C3d and C4d deposition early after lung transplantation. J Heart Lung Transplant. 2008;27:722–8.

78. Berry G, Burke M, Andersen C, Angelini A, Bruneval P, Calbrese F, Fishbein MC, Goddard M, Leone O, Maleszewski J, et al. Pathology of pulmonary antibody-mediated rejection: 2012 update from the Pathology Council of the ISHLT. J Heart Lung Transplant. 2013;32:14–21.

79. Levine DJ, Glanville AR, Aboyoun C, Belperio J, Benden C, Berry GJ, Hachem R, Hayes D, Neil D, Reinsmoen NL, et al. Antibody-mediated rejection of the lung: a consensus report of the International Society for Heart and Lung Transplantation. J Heart Lung Transplant. 2016;35:397–406.

80. de Jesus Peixoto Camargo J, Marcantonio Camargo S, Marcelo Schio S, Noguchi Machuca T, Adélia Perin F. Hyperacute rejection after single lung transplantation: a case report. Transplant Proc. 2008;40:867–9.

81. Campo-Canaveral de la Cruz JL, Naranjo JM, Salas C, Varela de Ugarte A. Fulminant hyperacute rejection after unilateral lung transplantation. Eur J Cardiothorac Surg. 2012;42:373–5.

82. Choi JK, Kearns J, Palevsky HI, Montone KT, Kaiser LR, Zmijewski CM, Tomaszewski JE. Hyperacute rejection of a pulmonary allograft. Immediate clinical and pathologic findings. Am J Respir Crit Care Med. 1999;160:1015–8.

83. Scornik JC, Zander DS, Baz MA, Donnelly WH, Staples ED. Susceptibility of lung transplants to pre-

formed donor-specific HLA antibodies as detected by flow cytometry. Transplantation. 1999;68:1542–6.

84. Frost AE, Jammal CT, Cagle PT. Hyperacute rejection following lung transplantation. Chest. 1996;110:559–62.

85. Masson E, Stern M, Chabod J, Thevenin C, Gonin F, Rebibou JM, Tiberghien P. Hyperacute rejection after lung transplantation caused by undetected low-titer anti-HLA antibodies. J Heart Lung Transplant. 2007;26:642–5.

86. Bittner HB, Dunitz J, Hertz M, Bolman MR III, Park SJ. Hyperacute rejection in single lung transplantation—case report of successful management by means of plasmapheresis and antithymocyte globulin treatment. Transplantation. 2001;71:649–51.

87. Dawson KL, Parulekar A, Seethamraju H. Treatment of hyperacute antibody-mediated lung allograft rejection with eculizumab. J Heart Lung Transplant. 2012;31:1325–6.

88. Scott J, Fradet G, Smyth R, et al. Prospective study of transbronchial biopsies in the management of heart-lung and single lung transplant patients. J Heart Lung Transplant. 1991;10:626–37.

89. Troxell ML, Lanciault C. Practical applications in immunohistochemistry: evaluation of rejection and infection in organ transplantation. Arch Pathol Lab Med. 2016;140(9):910–25.

Prevention and Treatment Regimens for Non-viral Infections in the Lung Transplant Recipient

14

Martin R. Zamora

Introduction

The obligate requirement for potent immunosuppressive agents necessary to reduce the incidence of allograft rejection places the lung transplant (LTX) recipient at high risk for infectious complications. Compared to other solid organ transplant recipients, LTX recipients are generally more aggressively immunosuppressed and have more frequent and severe infections. Additional factors including transmission of infectious organisms from the donor organs; preoperative microbial colonization of the recipient's lungs; posttransplant factors such as a decreased cough reflex due to airway denervation, poor mucociliary clearance, and airway ischemia; and the continued environmental exposure of the lung allograft contribute to the high risk of infections post-lung transplantation [1, 2]. Infectious complications remain the leading cause of morbidity and mortality across all time points following LTX and are the most common cause of death in patients with chronic lung rejection. Pulmonary infections and airway colonization with *Pseudomonas aeruginosa* or *Aspergillus* species, particularly in cystic fibrosis patients, may cause ongoing innate immune activation and have been associated with the development of chronic lung

allograft dysfunction [3]. Therefore, a thorough understanding of the prevention, diagnosis, and treatment of non-viral infection is critical for the optimal management of the LTX recipient.

Perioperative Period

The risk for and types of infections vary with the time posttransplant [2]. Given the intensity of the immunosuppression and higher incidence of acute allograft rejection, the greatest risk tends to occur in the perioperative period and the first few months posttransplant.

In the immediate perioperative period, LTX recipients are at risk for both bacterial and fungal infections and occasionally reactivation of latent mycobacterial infections. Gram-negative organisms such as *Pseudomonas* and gram-positive organisms such as methicillin-resistant *Staphylococcus aureus* (MRSA) are often seen [4]. Infections due to the latter include catheter-related bacteremia, sepsis, ventilator- or hospital-acquired pneumonia, and surgical wound infection. These may be a result of preoperative lung colonization as commonly seen in recipients transplanted for cystic fibrosis or non-cystic fibrosis bronchiectasis. Other sources include donor colonization or infection or recipient nosocomial infection due to mechanical ventilation, indwelling catheters, or intravenous lines. Recipient-derived organisms also include

M. R. Zamora
Division of Pulmonary Sciences and Critical Care Medicine, University of Colorado, Aurora, CO, USA
e-mail: marty.zamora@ucdenver.edu

© The Author(s) 2018
G. Raghu, R. G. Carbone (eds.), *Lung Transplantation*, https://doi.org/10.1007/978-3-319-91184-7_14

vancomycin-resistant *Enterococcus*, MRSA, multidrug-resistant (MDR) gram-negative organisms, and *Clostridium difficile*. Prophylactic strategies should not only cover some of these organisms but should also consider the recipient's history of exposure to infection. The choice of empiric antibiotics must provide coverage against potentially MDR gram-negative organisms and MRSA. Based on local antipseudomonal sensitivity patterns, most centers employ an antibiotic regimen including an antipseudomonal B-lactam such as cefepime, meropenem, or piperacillin-tazobactam along with vancomycin. This regimen is typically used for 3 days when it can be tailored based on donor cultures or when another indication for prolonged antibiotial therapy arises in the early perioperative period.

Donor respiratory specimens are typically obtained by bronchoscopy with bronchoalveolar lavage (BAL) and cultured prior to explantation and implantation. The results of donor sputum or BAL gram stains and cultures can then be utilized to tailor the antibiotic regimen after the initial empiric choices. For LTX recipients who are colonized prior to transplant, antibiotic prophylaxis should target known culture results and sensitivities. Perioperative antibiotics can be selected at the time of being placed on the waiting list using these results and can be updated based on new cultures and sensitivities, while a patient remains on the waiting list. This is critical in cystic fibrosis patients or those with non-cystic fibrosis bronchiectasis as they typically harbor MDR gram-negative organisms which are an emerging problem posttransplant and have been associated with suboptimal outcomes in LTX recipients.

Surgical wound and chest tube or line infections are usually caused by skin flora, most commonly *Staphylococcus aureus*. Pleural or mediastinal infections may occur particularly in patients colonized preoperatively with gram-negative organisms or those with an airway anastomotic dehiscence. The ischemic airways are also a major risk factor for *Aspergillus* tracheobronchitis [3, 5]. Surgical site infection has also been reported in patients colonized with MDR organisms. Although not evidenced-based, patients colonized with MDR organisms should probably receive longer courses of antibiotics in the perioperative period.

Clostridium difficile colitis is also higher in the perioperative period presenting as diarrhea or in its severest form, toxic megacolon [6]. Oral vancomycin is used for the treatment of mild to moderate disease, but intravenous Flagyl may be required in patients with nausea and vomiting who cannot tolerate oral agents. In addition to intravenous antibiotics, severe disease such as toxic megacolon may require rectal vancomycin slurries, fecal transplantation, or colectomy. Fidaxomicin, a new macrocyclic antibiotic, has been shown to be effective in mild to moderate *C. difficile* infection, but controlled evidence is lacking in LTX recipients.

Lung transplant recipients are at high risk for airway colonization with fungal organisms due to their continuous exposure to environmental infectious agents. Infections due to *Candida* or *Aspergillus* species complicate the perioperative period. While *C. albicans* is the most common *Candida* species in LTX recipients, non-albicans species are increasingly reported post- LTX. These organisms may be more resistant to azole therapy. It has been estimated that 86% of LTX recipients become colonized with *Candida* species and 23% with *Aspergillus* species and 15–35% develop invasive fungal infections [7]. Infections due to *Aspergillus* species are increased in patients colonized pretransplant with *Aspergillus* and those with ongoing airway ischemia [5]. Early *Candida* prophylaxis typically involves the use of nystatin 5 cm^3 swish and swallow QID or fluconazole 100 mg po QD. If *Aspergillus* is a concern, an oral azole, either voriconazole 200 mg po BID or itraconazole 100 mg po BID, with or without inhaled amphotericin-B 20–40 mg QD, is employed. Prophylaxis for *Pneumocystis jirovecii* is provided by trimethoprim-sulfamethoxazole (TMP-SMX) 160 mg/180 mg po Q MWF.

It should be noted that any lung transplant recipient who demonstrates respiratory dysfunction requires a full and thorough evaluation of BAL specimens for a complete battery of stains and cultures each time the procedure is done (Table 14.1).

Table 14.1 Routine BAL specimen stains, cultures, and PCR for lung transplant recipients demonstrating respiratory dysfunction[a]

Organisms	Stains	Culture	PCR
Bacteria	Gram stain	X	
Fungi	Giemsa stain	X	
Mycobacteria	Acid-fast stain	X	
Nocardia	Partial acid-fast stain	X	
Cytomegalovirus	Immunohistochemistry	X	
Pneumocystis jirovecii	Direct fluorescent antibody		
Community-acquired respiratory viruses	Rapid antigen test	X	X

[a]The microbiology laboratory should be notified that this BAL specimen is from a lung transplant recipient as they may harbor multiresistant organisms and/or currently receiving antibiotic therapy. Request for CFU/mL from BAL must be included

Bacterial Infections

Gram-negative organisms, particularly *Pseudomonas aeruginosa*, remain the most common cause of bacterial pneumonia in the LTX recipient [8]. Other gram-negative organisms causing infection and pneumonia include *Escherichia coli*, *Klebsiella pneumoniae*, *Acinetobacter baumannii*, *Stenotrophomonas maltophilia*, *Alcaligenes xylosoxidans*, *Burkholderia cepacia*, and *Serratia marcescens*. These are particularly an issue in recipients transplanted for cystic fibrosis [9]. Airway colonization with *Pseudomonas aeruginosa* posttransplant has been associated with the development of chronic lung allograft dysfunction through stimulation of innate immunity [3]. *Staphylococcus aureus* is the second most common cause of bacterial pneumonia in these patients. In LTX recipients presenting with presumed pneumonia, empiric antibiotic coverage should be directed against MRSA, *Pseudomonas*, and atypical organisms. Bronchoscopy with bronchoalveolar lavage should be performed to obtain cultures (colony-forming units) and/or protected brush specimens for cultures from visualized airway secretions and transbronchial biopsy as it is prudent to differentiate infection from acute cellular rejection. Patients should receive 14 days of antibiotic therapy, and the regimen should be tailored based on culture results and sensitivity data [10].

Patients with cystic fibrosis may also develop chronic sinus infections posttransplant. Sinus colonization with MDR gram-negative organisms persist following transplant and can predispose these patients to pulmonary infections. For these reasons, some programs aggressively treat sinus disease prior to transplant with surgery and inhaled antibiotics. Similar measures may need to be employed posttransplant.

Several organisms require special consideration: the MDR gram-negative bacteria and *Burkholderia cepacia*.

Multidrug-Resistant (MDR) Gram-Negative Bacteria

The MDR gram-negative organisms are becoming increasingly problematic posttransplant [10]. While typically described in LTX recipients with cystic fibrosis (due to airway injury, the requirement for intense immunosuppression, and recurrent antibiotic exposure), all LTX recipients are at increased risk for the development of MDR organisms. The MDR organisms commonly include *Pseudomonas aeruginosa*, *Acinetobacter baumannii*, *Stenotrophomonas maltophilia*, *Enterobacteriaceae*, and the *Burkholderia cepacia complex* which will be discussed below. It has been shown that greater than 50% of cystic fibrosis patients are colonized with MDR *Pseudomonas aeruginosa* at the time of listing for LTX [11, 12]. While these patients have been reported to have worse survival posttransplant than those with susceptible strains, this is not consistently seen. MDR *Acinetobacter* species are increasing in prevalence and have been reported in cohorts of

LTX recipients. These patients had more severe infections, sepsis, and mortality compared to non-transplant [13]. Furthermore, prolonged infection was associated with allograft fibrosis and death from respiratory failure. *Stenotrophomonas* has been reported to colonize up to 10% of cystic fibrosis patients, may cause posttransplant pneumonia, and is highly MDR [14]. The *Enterobacteriaceae*, including *Klebsiella pneumoniae* and *Escherichia coli*, have developed a number of resistance mechanisms. Extended spectrum B-lactamases or the AmpC B-lactamase accounts for carbapenem resistance and is becoming a global problem. While infrequent in LTX recipients in North America, knowledge of emerging resistance patterns and local antibiotic resistance mechanisms is critical as LTX recipients are at increasing risk of acquiring these highly resistant organisms [15].

A high level of suspicion and early combination antibiotic therapy is essential for the treatment of the MDR organisms. This strategy allows the patient to be exposed to at least one antibiotic with efficacy against the offending organism. A B-lactam and a quinolone are often prescribed but should be chosen based on local antibiotic resistance patterns [16]. Synergy studies, as performed by the checkerboard assay, may identify therapeutic antibiotic combinations. However, studies using synergy to guide antibiotic therapy have shown mixed results. The agents of choice for *Acinetobacter* are the carbapenems. If carbapenem resistance is identified, ampicillin-sulbactam, colistin or polymyxin B, and tigecycline are options. In non-transplant patients, rifampin has been added to these agents. However, there is marked drug-drug interaction between rifampin and immunosuppressive agents, so it is not commonly prescribed in transplant recipients. *Stenotrophomonas* is usually treated with TMP-SMX, but fluoroquinolones, ceftazidime, or tigecycline may be used as alternative agents or in those patients with severe sulfa allergies.

Burkholderia cepacia complex

The genus *Burkholderia* consists of several species (genomovars), the largest of which is now known as the *Burkholderia cepacia complex*. It is increasingly recognized that individual genomovars confer varying risks of infection and effect on survival posttransplant [17–20]. *B. cenocepacia* (genomovar III) and *B. gladioli* have been associated with a very high risk of posttransplant mortality compared to patients with other genomovars or those not infected with the *Burkholderia cepacia complex* at all. Furthermore, patients with *B. cepacia* species other than *B. cenocepacia* did not have any decrement in survival compared to non-*Burkholderia cepacia complex*-infected patients. The *B. cepacia* syndrome is more likely to occur in *B. cenocepacia* patients and involves a sepsis-like picture with bacteremia, pneumonia, antibacterial resistance, and increased mortality. For these reasons, many centers consider *B. cenocepacia* an absolute contraindication to transplant. Candidates with other *Burkholderia* genomovars appear to have acceptable outcomes and may be considered for LTX. It should be noted that the most recent LTX recipient selection guidelines do not consider *B. cenocepacia* an absolute contraindication to lung transplantation [21]. Treatment of *Burkholderia cepacia complex* is very difficult, and triple antibiotic coverage is recommended [22]. Meropenem, an aminoglycoside, and either ceftazidime or TMP-SMX are a typical regimen. Outcomes in the early pretransplant period are very poor, but some success has been reported in the later posttransplant period.

Nocardia

Lung transplant recipients are at greater risk for *Nocardia* than other solid organ transplant recipients. This is most likely due to continuous exposure of the lung allograft to the environment. Infection due to *Nocardia* species is acquired through inhalation of aerosolized organisms in the environment. Dissemination is characteristic of *Nocardia*, most often to the brain, skin, bones, and eye [23]. *Nocardia* presents as a pulmonary nodule or nodules or a subacute pneumonia in either the transplanted lung or the native lung in the case of single LTX. Signs and symptoms are nonspecific, and patients may present with an asymptomatic, incidentally discovered pulmonary nodule

[24]. In approximately 50% of cases, *Nocardia* disseminates to the central nervous system or skin. The combination of pulmonary and central nervous system (CNS) lesions should alert the clinician to the likelihood of *Nocardia* infection. Other infectious considerations with this combination include mycobacterial or fungal infection, *Cryptococcus* or *Rhodococcus*. The diagnosis of *Nocardia* is made by isolation from the respiratory tract or skin or other involved sites. *Nocardia* appears as a branching gram-positive rod with a beaded pattern which is partially acid-fast. Polymerase chain reaction important for speciation as antibiotic susceptibility varies across *Nocardia* species. Sulfonamides are the drugs of choice for most *Nocardia* species particularly *N. asteroides*.

Management strategies are based on susceptibility data and expert opinion as randomized controlled trials are lacking in transplant recipients. Determining the species and susceptibility patterns is critical for optimal *Nocardia* therapy. Combination empiric therapy utilizing three different classes of antibiotics is recommended until speciation and antibiotic susceptibility are determined. TMP-SMX has high oral bioavailability and excellent pulmonary and CNS penetration and is highly effective against most *Nocardia* species. Further recommendations include the addition of a carbapenem, either imipenem or meropenem, which provides excellent CNS penetration. Concern for a higher seizure risk from imipenem in patients with CNS involvement has led many experts to favor meropenem, with a lower seizure risk, over imipenem. Amikacin is highly effective against all *Nocardia* species except *N. transvalensis* [23, 25, 26], but due to an increased risk of nephrotoxicity, its use should be balanced against the efficacy and availability of less toxic agents. Linezolid has been identified as a highly effective alternative; however, its long-term use may be limited by bone marrow suppression.

Once the speciation and susceptibilities are known, the antibiotic regimen can be adjusted. Induction therapy generally lasts 3–6 weeks but may need to be longer based on the severity of the disease and the presence of dissemination.

Following the induction phase, a consolidation phase is required. TMP-SMX generally results in cure rates approaching 90% for pulmonary disease [27]. Minocycline is a useful second-line agent but may have variable CNS penetration [28]. Alternative oral agents include clarithromycin, ciprofloxacin, moxifloxacin, and amoxicillin-clavulanic acid. Linezolid has efficacy, but its long-term use may be limited by bone marrow suppression. Some experts recommend the use of two agents for severe *Nocardia* infections particularly those with CNS involvement. Six months of therapy is common for isolated pulmonary disease, but many clinicians continue for 12 months [29]. Patients with CNS disease are typically treated for 9–12 months, and some experts recommend suppressive therapy for the length of time the patient remains immunosuppressed.

Preventive strategies include covering exposed skin and/or using a mask during gardening or during exposure to construction sites. During periods of augmented immunosuppression, avoidance of these areas or high-risk activities is recommended. While TMP-SMX use for *Pneumocystis jirovecii* is effective against *Nocardia*, breakthrough infections have been reported [30].

Fungal Infections

Prophylaxis

Fungal colonization and infections are common following LTX occurring in up to 15–35% of patients. Other commonly encountered molds include *Fusarium*, *Scedosporium*, *Acremonium*, *Paecilomyces*, *Scopulariopsis*, *Trichosporon*, *Penicilium*, and *Zygomycota*. Mortality rates from fungal infections range from 20 to 60% [31, 32]. Therefore, antifungal prophylaxis in some form has become universal in LTX centers. A survey of LTX centers revealed marked variability in antifungal prophylaxis regimens across centers. Common approaches were universal prophylaxis or targeted prophylaxis against *Aspergillus* colonization. Inhaled amphotericin-B and concomitant use of an azole or an azole alone were the most common regimens employed. The use of voriconazole has been shown to decrease invasive *Aspergillus* during the first year posttransplant as compared to itraconazole +/− inhaled amphotericin-B. However, long-term voriconazole use is associated with increased liver function tests and the risk of developing skin cancer.

Mold Infections

Aspergillus Infection

Aspergillus fumigatus is the leading cause of fungal pneumonia in LTX recipients [33, 34]. However, other *Aspergillus* species including *A. flavus*, *A. niger*, and *A. terreus* have been reported as causing invasive fungal disease. *Proven* invasive fungal infection is confirmed by histologic or cytologic identification of fungal elements in tissue samples or isolation of non-*Aspergillus* species from the blood. The serum *Aspergillus* galactomannan assay has poor reported sensitivity in lung transplant recipients particularly those with tracheobronchitis. The use of this assay is more sensitive when applied to BAL fluid rather than serum in patients with tracheobronchitis or invasive pulmonary infection. Most centers do not routinely send the serum or BAL galactomannan assay due to these sensitivity issues. A *probable* invasive fungal infection should be suspected in the presence of CT findings in the appropriate clinical setting. Invasive pulmonary *aspergillosis* commonly presents radiographically with focal or multifocal consolidation and infiltrates or nodules with or without cavitation. The characteristic "halo sign" is not regularly seen.

Aspergillus infections may be localized as an airway colonizer or may be invasive manifesting as tracheobronchitis, invasive pulmonary *aspergillosis*, or disseminated *aspergillosis* [34]. *Aspergillus* tracheobronchitis is characterized by necrosis, ulcerations, and pseudomembrane formation. It typically occurs at the main stem anastomosis or in the ischemic large airways. Diagnosis is confirmed by bronchoscopy. It is most likely to occur in the first few months posttransplant, and many centers employ inhaled amphotericin-B prophylaxis in recipients colo-

nized preoperatively with *Aspergillus* species. The treatment of tracheobronchitis is with inhaled amphotericin-B plus systemic antifungal agents. For invasive *Aspergillus* infections, treatment typically involves the use of azoles, echinocandins, or liposomal amphotericin-B. Voriconazole is more effective than itraconazole and is the drug of choice for invasive *Aspergillus*. Posaconazole also has activity against most *Aspergillus* species. Recent reports also suggest that voriconazole in combination with an echinocandin is superior to azole therapy alone [35]. The duration of therapy should be for a minimum of 6–12 weeks for pulmonary aspergillosis; longer duration is dictated by clinical response and monitoring.

Other Molds

The *Zygomycetes* and *Scedosporium* species typically cause local disease requiring surgery and antifungal therapy with posaconazole for the *Zygomycetes* and voriconazole for *Scedosporium*. However, disseminated disease is also likely particularly with *Scedosporium*. It is important to identify patients colonized with *Scedosporium* prior to transplant to allow the clinician the chance to treat the patient with voriconazole in order to alleviate the risk of infection posttransplant.

Yeast Infections

Candida Infection

While *C. albicans* is the most common species causing *candidal* infections in LTX recipients, an increase in *non-albicans* species has been reported [34]. Invasive *candidiasis* tends to occur in the first 3 months posttransplant. *Candidemia*, associated with indwelling catheters, prolong ICU stay, and the use of total parenteral nutrition is the most common form of *candidal* infection during the perioperative period. Infection at the airway anastomosis and in the pleural space, esophagus, oropharynx, or urinary tract can also be seen. Prophylaxis with nystatin swish and swallow is typically employed. The diagnosis of invasive candidiasis is made by isolation of the *Candida* species from a usually sterile body site or identification of invasive organisms in a tissue biopsy. While *C. albicans* is typically sensitive to the azoles, as stated previously, *non-albicans* species are more likely to be fluconazole resistant. Therefore, the echinocandins should be considered the drug of choice for invasive *candidiasis* pending identification of the specific organism involved. Liposomal amphotericin-B may also be utilized but may have more toxicity than the echinocandins.

Cryptococcus Neoformans

Cryptococcosis is a rare cause of invasive fungal infection in LTX recipients. It tends to occur after the first posttransplant year. Manifestations include pulmonary disease presenting as cavitary nodules or pneumonia, meningitis, fungemia, necrotizing cellulitis, or pericarditis [36]. The diagnosis is made by culture of *Cryptococcus* from respiratory samples or other body fluids or a positive *cryptococcal* antigen. A lumbar puncture should be performed in patients with *Cryptococcus* regardless of whether CNS symptoms are present. The immune reconstitution syndrome has been reported during therapy of *cryptococcal* disease in solid organ transplant recipients. Treatment recommendations include the use of liposomal amphotericin-B with the addition of flucytosine if CNS disease is present. A complete review of these recommendations was recently published by the Infectious Disease Society of America [37].

Endemic Mycoses

The endemic fungi (*histoplasmosis, coccidiomycosis,* and *blastomycosis*) can cause pneumonia or disseminated disease in LTX recipients [34]. The occurrence is variable depending on the organism: the onset of *coccidiomycosis* can be as early as several months posttransplant, whereas *histoplasmosis* tends to occur after the first posttransplant year. The diagnosis of endemic mycosis infection can be made by the *Histoplasma* urinary antigen, fungal isolator blood culture tubes, or histology on bone marrow or other tissue biopsies. Treatment is with liposomal Amphotericin-B. Lifelong prophylaxis is recommended for patients in endemic areas for *coccid-*

iomycosis or in those with a prior history of *coccidiomycosis.*

Pneumocystis jirovecii

P. jirovecii, previously *Pneumocystis carinii*, was more common in the absence of prophylaxis and can cause pneumonia in immunosuppressed patients. Patients typically present with hypoxemia at rest or with exertion, dyspnea, or a nonproductive cough. Chest X-ray findings are nonspecific and mimic other common illnesses in the lung transplant recipient. Diagnosis is made by examining induced sputum or BAL fluid. Prophylaxis with TMP-SMX is quite effective in preventing *P. jirovecii* pneumonia (PJP). Evidence suggests that LTX recipients are at risk for PJP throughout their lives. Therefore, prophylaxis should be continued throughout the life of the LTX recipient [8]. In patients who are severely sulfa allergic, inhaled pentamidine, dapsone, or atovaquone are effective alternatives. It should be noted that these alternative agents do not provide protection against *Listeria, Nocardias* or *Toxoplasma* species. Treatment of *P. jirovecii* pneumonia involves high-dose TMP-SMX and an oral steroid taper in patients with exercise or resting hypoxemia. Desensitization can be employed in patients with mild to moderate sulfa allergy for treatment of *P. jirovecii* pneumonia.

Mycobacterial Infections

Mycobacterium tuberculosis

Lung transplant recipients are at greater risk for TB than other solid organ transplant recipients. Infection due to *Mycobacterium tuberculosis* may be due to reactivation of latent disease in the recipient or through donor transmission of active or latent disease and by new exposure to *M. tuberculosis* [38]. Donor risk factors associated with increased transmission include travel to an endemic region/country with a high TB incidence, a high TB incidence in the donor's country of origin, household exposure to active TB, and a history of incarceration. In donors with these risk factors, additional screening with a chest CT scan and AFB smears and cultures on BAL fluid are warranted [39, 40]. Rates of infection have been reported to range from <1 to 6% in Spain and in US series [41–44]. TB tends to occur in the first year posttransplant but can occur at any time. Once infected, LTX recipients frequently develop disseminated disease to extrapulmonary sites [45]. Patients typically present with cough, fever, weight loss, and night sweats, but disseminated disease may present with a sepsis-like syndrome and multiorgan failure. Extrapulmonary sites of involvement include the lymph nodes, bone marrow, joints, skin, central nervous system, kidneys, liver, pleural space, and gastrointestinal tract. Positive cultures are diagnostic of TB and allow susceptibility testing which is important in endemic areas which may have higher rates of drug resistance. Treatment of active *Mycobacterium tuberculosis* is the same as in the non-transplant patient, but it should be noted that rifampin has significant drug-drug interactions with the calcineurin inhibitors. A typical regimen involves the use of three to four bactericidal drugs for the first 2 months of therapy. The regimen can then be tailored to two drugs based on susceptibility patterns to complete the course of therapy. The LTX recipient may require a prolonged course of therapy particularly for cavitary or disseminated disease [46].

Potential LTX recipients should be screened and evaluated for latent *Mycobacterium tuberculosis* using the tuberculin skin test with appropriate controls. If the skin test is positive and there is no evidence of active TB on chest X-ray, therapy with isoniazid for 6–9 months is warranted.

Nontuberculous Mycobacterial Infection

The *nontuberculous mycobacterial* (NTM) organisms most commonly associated with clinical disease in LTX recipients are *M. avium complex*, *M. abscessus*, and *M. haemophilum*. *M. fortuitum*, *M. chelonae*, *M. xenopi*, *M. kansasii*, and *M. marinum* less commonly cause disease [47]. The presentation of infectious signs and symptoms is similar to that of pulmonary TB. Isolation of the organism from a single sputum sample may be a contaminant, a colonizer, or an infection. At our center, upon isolation of NTM from a single sample, we obtain a high-resolution CT scan of the chest to look for nodularity or cavitation and then perform a bronchoscopy for BAL, histologic examination, and tissue culture from transbronchial biopsies. Treatment depends on the type of NTM isolated, the location of the infection, and the overall health of the host. The treatment of *Mycobacterium avium-intracellulare* may be challenging in LTX recipients but is similar to non-immunosuppressive patients. Clarithromycin and ethambutol plus a third drug for a minimum 6–9 months are a typical regimen. Longer-term therapy is required for disseminated or cavitary disease. *M. abscessus* may infect surgical wounds or joints and require surgical debridement and resection of infected tissue in order to control the infection. The immune reconstitution syndrome may be seen with treatment of *M. avium*, can be quite severe, and may require augmented immunosuppression [48]. The use of chronic azithromycin to prevent or to slow the progression of chronic lung allograft dysfunction may be associated with macrolide-resistant NTM. Special consideration should be given to cystic fibrosis and non-cystic fibrosis bronchiectasis patients who may be colonized with or have an infection due to NTM organisms prior to transplant. Recurrence is possible but is most likely to occur with *M. abscessus*. This has led many LTX centers to consider the latter a contraindication to transplant. However, a recent report found no difference in posttransplant outcomes, so the approach to patients colonized with *M. abscessus* should be individualized [49].

Summary

Bacterial, fungal, and mycobacterial infections continue to be an important cause of morbidity and mortality following LTX. Acute infections have significant adverse effects on long-term allograft function and outcomes. Chronic airway colonization with bacteria and fungi has been associated with the development of chronic lung allograft dysfunction. The emergence of MDR gram-negative organisms and fungi with antimicrobial resistance patterns is a growing problem in the transplant population. Significant drug-drug interactions occur between antimicrobials and immunosuppressive agents. The development of the immune reconstitution syndrome during treatment of certain infections can be severe and may require augmented immunosuppression. All of these factors complicate the optimal management of infections on LTX recipients.

References

1. Len O, Gavalda J, Blanes M, Montejo M, San Juan R, Moreno A, et al. Donor infection and transmission to the recipient of a solid allograft. Am J Transplant. 2008;8:2420–5.
2. Fishman JA. Infection in solid organ transplant recipients. N Engl J Med. 2007;357:2601–14.
3. Weigt SS, Elashoff RM, Huang C, Ardehali A, Gregson AL, Kubak B, et al. Aspergillus colonization of the lung allograft is a risk factor for bronchiolitis obliterans syndrome. Am J Transplant. 2009;9:1903–11.
4. Lease ED, Zaas DW. Complex bacterial infections pre- and post-transplant. Semin Respir Crit Care Med. 2010;31:234–42.
5. Hsu JL, Khan MA, Sobel RA, Jiang X, Clemons KV, Nguyen TT, et al. Aspergillus fumigatus invasion increases with progressive airway ischemia. PLoS One. 2013;14:e77136.
6. Gunderson CC, Gupta MR, Lopez F, Lombard GA, LaPlace SG, Taylor DE, et al. Clostridium difficile colitis in lung transplantation. Transpl Infect Dis. 2008;10:245–51.
7. Singh N. Fungal infections in the recipients of solid organ transplantation. Infect Dis Clin N Am. 2003;17:113–34.
8. Avery RK. Infections after lung transplantation. Semin Respir Crit Care Med. 2006;27:544–51.
9. Lynch JP, Sayah DM, Belperio JA, Weigt SS. Lung transplantation for cystic fibrosis: results, indications, complications and controversies. Semin Respir Crit Care Med. 2015;36:299–320.
10. Shoham S, Shah PD. Impact of multidrug-resistant organisms on patients considered for lung transplantation. Infect Dis Clin N Am. 2013;27:343–58.
11. Dobbin C, Maley M, Harkness J, Benn R, Malouf M, Glanville A, et al. The impact of pan-resistant bacterial pathogens on survival after lung transplantation in cystic fibrosis: results from a single large referral center. J Hosp Infect. 2004;56:277–82.
12. Hadjiliadis D, Steele MP, Chaparro C, Singer LG, Waddell TK, Hutcheon MA, et al. Survival of lung transplant patients with cystic fibrosis harboring pan-resistant bacteria other than Burkholderia cepacia, compared with patients harboring sensitive bacteria. J Heart Lung Transplant. 2007;26(8):834.
13. Nunley DR, Bauldoff GS, Mangino JE, Pope-Harman AL. Mortality associated with Acinetobacter baumanii infections experienced by lung transplant recipients. Lung. 2010;188(5):381.
14. Denton M, Kerr KG. Microbiological and clinical aspects of infection associated with Stenotrophomonas maltophilia. Clin Microbiol Rev. 1998;11:57–80.
15. Van Delden C, Blumberg EA. Multidrug resistant gram-negative bacteria in solid organ transplant recipients. Am J Transplant. 2009;9(Suppl 4):S27–34.
16. Peleg AY, Hooper DC. Hospital-acquired infections due to gram negative bacteria. N Engl J Med. 2010;362:1804–13.
17. Boussaud V, Guillerrmain R, Grenet D, Coley N, Souilamas R, Bonnette P, et al. Clinical outcome following lung transplantation in patients with cystic fibrosis colonized with Burkholderia cepacia complex: results from two French centres. Thorax. 2008;63:732–7.
18. Alexander BD, Petzold EW, Reller LB, Palmer SM, Davis RD, Woods CW, et al. Survival after lung transplantation of cystic fibrosis patients infected with Burkholderia cepacia complex. Am J Transplant. 2008;8:1025–30.
19. Murray S, Charbeneau J, Marshall BC, LiPuma JJ. Impact of Burkholderia infection on lung transplantation in cystic fibrosis. Am J Respir Crit Care Med. 2008;178:363–71.
20. Hafkin J, Blumberg E. Infections in lung transplantation: new insights. Curr Opin Organ Transplant. 2009;14:483–7.
21. Weill D, Benden C, Corris PA, Dark JH, Davis RD, Keshavjee S, et al. A consensus document for the selection of lung transplant candidates: 2014—an update from the pulmonary transplantation council of the International Society for Heart and Lung Transplantation. J Heart Lung Transplant. 2015;34:1–15.
22. Chaparro C, Maurer J, Gutierrez C, Krajden M, Chan C, Winton T, et al. Infection with Burkholderia cepacia in cystic fibrosis: outcome following lung transplantation. Am J Respir Crit Care Med. 2001;163:43–8.
23. Clark NM. Nocardia in solid organ transplant recipients. Am J Transplant. 2009;9(Suppl 4):S70–7.
24. Tripodi MF, Adinolfi LE, Andreana A, Sarnataro G, Durante Mangoni E, Gambardella M, et al. Treatment of pulmonary nocardiosis in heart-transplant patients: importance of susceptibility studies. Clin Transpl. 2001;15:415–20.
25. Minero MV, Marin M, Cercenado E, Rabadan PM, Bouza E, Munoz P. Nocardiosis at the turn of the century. Medicine. 2009;88:250–61.
26. Lopez FA, Johnson F, Novosad DM, Beaman BL, Holodniy M. Successful management of disseminated

Nocardia transvalensis infection in a heart transplant recipient after development of sulfonamide resistance: case report and review. J Heart Lung Transplant. 2003;22:492–7.

27. Wallace RJ Jr, Septimus EJ, Williams TW Jr, Conklin RH, Satterwhite TK, Bushby MB, et al. Use of trimethoprim-sulfamethoxazole for treatment of infections due to nocardia. Rev Infect Dis. 1982;4:315–25.

28. Weber L, Yium J, Hawkins S. Intracranial Nocardia dissemination during minocycline therapy. Transpl Infect Dis. 2002;4:108–12.

29. Lerner PI. Nocardiosis. Clin Infect Dis. 1996;22:891–903.

30. Peleg AY, Husain S, Qureshi ZA, Silveira FP, Sarumi M, Shutt KA, et al. Risk factors, clinical characteristics, and outcomes of nocardia infection in organ transplant recipients: a matched case-control study. Clin Infect Dis. 2007;44:1307–14.

31. Sole A, Salavert M. Fungal infections after lung transplantation. Transplant Rev. 2008;22:89–104.

32. Neoh CF, Snell G, Levvey B, Morrissey CO, Stewart K, Kong DCM. Antifungal prophylaxis in lung transplantation. Intl J Antimicrobial Agents. 2014;44:194–202.

33. Geltner C, Lass-Florl C. Invasive pulmonary aspergillosis in organ transplants—focus on lung transplants. Resp Invest. 2016;54:76–84.

34. Chambers DC, Sole A. Mold infections in cardiothoracic transplantation. In: Mooney ML, Hannan MM, Husain S, Kirklin JK, editors. Diagnosis and management of infectious diseases in cardiothoracic transplantation and mechanical circulatory support. Philadelphia: Elsevier; 2011. p. 195–209.

35. Elefanti A, Mouton JW, Verweij PE, Tsakris A, Zerva L, Meletiades J. Amphotericin B- and voriconazole-echinocandin combinations against Aspergillus species: effect of serum on inhibitory and fungicidal interactions. Antimicrob Agents Chemother. 2013;57:4656–63.

36. Wu G, Vilchez RA, Eidelman B, Fung J, Kormos R, Kusne S. Cryptococcal meningitis: an analysis among 5521 consecutive organ transplant recipients. Transplant Infect Dis. 2022;4:183–8.

37. Perfect JR, Dismukes WE, Dromer F, Goldman DL, Graybill JR, Hamill RJ, et al. Clinical practice guidelines for the management of cryptococcal disease: 2010 update by the Infectious Diseases Society of America. Clin Infect Dis. 2010;50:291–322.

38. Winthrop KL, Kubak BM, Pegues DA, Hufana C, Costamagna P, Desmond E, et al. Transmission of mycobacterium tuberculosis via lung transplantation. Am J Transplant. 2004;4:1529–33.

39. Morris MI, Daly JS, Blumberg E, Kumar D, Sester M, Schluger N, et al. Diagnosis and management of tuberculosis in transplant donors: a donor-derived infections consensus conference report. Am J Transplant. 2012;12:2288–300.

40. Mortenen E, Hellinger C, Keller C, Cowan LS, Shaw T, Hwang S, et al. Three cases of donor-derived pulmonary tuberculosis in lung transplant recipients and review of 12 previously reported cases: opportunities for early diagnosis and prevention. Transplant Infect Dis. 2014;16:67–75.

41. Torre-Cisneros J, Doblas A, Aguado JM, San Juan R, Blanes M, Montejo M, et al. Tuberculosis after solid organ transplant: incidence, risk factors and clinical characteristics in the RESITRA (Spanish Network in Infection in Transplantation) cohort. Clin Infect Dis. 2009;48:1657–65.

42. Morales P, Briones A, Torres JJ, Sole A, Perez D, Pastor A. Pulmonary tuberculosis in lung and heart-lung transplantation: fifteen years of experience in a single center in Spain. Transplant Proc. 2005;37:4050–5.

43. Bravo C, Roldan J, Roman A, Degracia J, Majo J, Guerra J, et al. Tuberculosis in lung transplant recipients. Transplantation. 2005;79:59–64.

44. Schulman LL, Scully B, McGregor CC, Austin JH. Pulmonary tuberculosis after lung transplantation. Chest. 1997;111:1459–62.

45. Singh N, Paterson DL. Mycobacterium tuberculosis infection in solid-organ transplant recipients: impact and implications for management. Clin Infect Dis. 1998;27:1266–77.

46. American Thoracic Society, CDC and Infectious Diseases Society of America. Treatment of tuberculosis. MMWR Morb Mortal Wkly Rep. 2003;52:1–77.

47. Morales P, Santos M, Hadjiliadis D, Aris RM. Mycobacterial infections in cardiothoracic transplantation. In: Mooney ML, Hannan MM, Husain S, Kirklin JK, editors. Diagnosis and management of infectious diseases in cardiothoracic transplantation and mechanical circulatory support. Philadelphia: Elsevier; 2011. p. 161–73.

48. Field SK, Cowie RL. Lung disease due to the more common nontuberculous mycobacteria. Chest. 2006;129:1653–72.

49. Lobo LJ, Chang LC, Esther CR Jr, Gilligan PH, Tulu Z, Noone PG. Lung transplant outcomes in cystic fibrosis patients with preoperative mycobacterium abscessus respiratory infections. Clin Transpl. 2013;27:523–9.

Respiratory Viruses and Other Relevant Viral Infections in the Lung Transplant Recipient

15

Ali Abedi, Reed Hall, and Deborah Jo Levine

Introduction

As advances occur in surgical technique, postoperative care, and immunosuppressive therapy, the rate of mortality in the early postoperative period following lung transplantation continues to decline [1].

With the improvements in immediate and early posttransplant mortality, infections and their sequel as well as rejection and chronic allograft dysfunction are increasingly a major cause of posttransplant mortality [2–5].

This chapter will focus on infections by respiratory viruses and other viral infections relevant to lung transplantation, including data regarding the link between viral infections and allograft dysfunction.

Factors Related to Risk of Respiratory Viral Infections

Lungs are the most prone to infection of all solid organ transplantations [2, 4]. This reality is based on multiple factors related and unique to lung transplantation [1, 2]. The lungs are continually exposed to both new environmental pathogens and the colonized native upper airways. Furthermore, many of the natural defense mechanisms of the respiratory system are made ineffective by both the technical aspects of lung transplantation and the relatively increased degree of immunosuppression required to minimize high rates of acute and chronic rejection seen in lung transplantation compared to other solid organs [1, 2, 6, 7].

The usual physical barriers of the respiratory tract against infections include the presence of the mucociliary escalator that traps and expels infectious organisms. These mechanisms are facilitated by the integrity of the epithelium lining the trachea, bronchi, and small airways. The complete disruption of the bronchial circulation during lung transplantation can cause a loss of epithelium integrity and associated mucociliary action, which may not fully recover despite development of collateral flow in the future [1, 2, 6, 8, 9]. Additional compromise of the anatomical barrier to infection is created by the potential suppression of the cough reflex caused by denervation of the allograft [4, 7]. Disruption of the normal lymphatic flow of

A. Abedi
Department of Pulmonary and Critical Care Medicine, University of Texas Health San Antonio, San Antonio, TX, USA

R. Hall
Pharmacy, University Hospital—University Health System, San Antonio, TX, USA
e-mail: Reed.hall@uhs-sa.com

D. J. Levine (✉)
Department of Pulmonary and Critical Care Medicine, University of Texas Health Science Center San Antonio, San Antonio, TX, USA
e-mail: levinedj@uthscsa.edu

© The Author(s) 2018
G. Raghu, R. G. Carbone (eds.), *Lung Transplantation*, https://doi.org/10.1007/978-3-319-91184-7_15

the lung during transplantation also increases the risk of infections by creating edema and stasis of interstitial fluids [4, 7].

The incidence of allograft dysfunction due to both acute and chronic rejection in lung transplantation is among the highest in solid transplantation, requiring relatively high levels of immunosuppression targeting multiple lines of immune cells and their associated cytokine pathways.

The use of induction and high levels of maintenance of immunosuppression creates a significant risk for development of viral infection, with higher tacrolimus levels having been specifically associated with increased rates of CARV infections [2]. Prevention and suppression of infection by respiratory viruses involves the activities of cellular and antibody-mediated immunity, which are impaired by immunosuppression targeting adaptive T-cell-mediated processes. This point is highlighted by relatively weak antibody response to vaccines directed against certain respiratory viruses in recipients of solid organ transplantation [3, 10–13].

The transmission of donor-harbored infections at the time of transplantation is another factor that increases the likelihood of viral infection in the LTR [1, 4, 5]. With many viruses, the highest risk for development active disease exists in circumstances when a recipient with no prior exposure or established humoral immunity to a virus is "mismatched" with a donor whose tissues harbor the active infection or latent form of the virus. Viral infections that have previously been documented as originating from donor lung tissue include CMV, Epstein-Barr virus, varicella-zoster, adenovirus, influenza, hepatitis B and C, and human immunodeficiency virus, in addition to others [2, 4, 14, 15]. Therefore, at most centers, the evaluation of a donor for lung transplantation routinely includes serologic screening for common viruses, as well as bronchoscopic assessment with PCR analysis of BAL samples for common respiratory viruses [1, 2].

Reactivation of latent virus previously introduced to the LTR following induction and maintenance of immunosuppressive therapy is another risk factor for clinically significant viral infection [16–18]. For this reason the initial pretransplant candidate evaluation process includes a thorough screening for many of the same viruses listed above. In addition to helping to determine a patient's candidacy for transplantation, this screening can help determine the need and duration of antiviral prophylaxis to specific viruses in the posttransplantation period [19, 20].

Infections with previously latent viruses in donor or recipient tissues are of significant concern early in the posttransplantation period. However, the period after several months posttransplantation represents its own risks for viral infection [2, 4, 5, 14, 15]. This phenomenon is related primarily to the return to community life by LTRs who have recovered from the initial surgical course and any subsequent physiologic or infectious insults. Evidence suggests LTRs who are greater than 1 year from surgery are five times more likely to present with CARV infections compared to those less than 1 year from transplantation [2, 14, 21].

Changing Epidemiology of Viral Infections in Lung Transplantation

Respiratory viruses and some members of the *Herpesviridae* family frequently cause clinically significant infections with potentially severe complications after solid organ transplantation (SOT).

Advancement in the field of diagnostic virology, primarily based on new molecular assays, has greatly improved the breadth and sensitivity of detection methods for viral infections. Multiplex PCR assays have now been available and FDA-approved for nearly a decade; they have provided a significantly larger number of small laboratories without expertise in viral culture techniques the opportunity to participate in real time diagnosis of a wide array of respiratory viral pathogens [22–24]. Furthermore, these new multiplex PCR-based assays are able to provide more rapid and sensitive identification of respiratory viruses than traditional viral culture and immunofluorescence testing [22, 25, 26].

Just in the last decade, several new viral respiratory tract pathogens have been identified, including human metapneumovirus (hMPV), human bocavirus (HBoV), new strains of human coronavirus (HCoV-NL63 and HCoV-HKU1), and new species of rhinovirus (HRV-C) [27, 28].

Respiratory and Other Viral Infections and Lung Allograft Dysfunction

The development of chronic lung allograft rejection (CLAD), encountered as bronchiolitis obliterans syndrome (BOS) or restrictive chronic lung allograft dysfunction (R-CLAD), continues to be the primary driver of mortality in LTR after the first 2 years following transplantation. Obliterative bronchiolitis, the hallmark of BOS, appears to be the pathologic end-stage of a process initially beginning with airway epithelial injury and leading to inflammatory reactions that promote airway obliteration. The inciting injury to the epithelium may be initiated as an exposure to toxic chemicals or drugs, infection including to viral agents, or an autoimmune process [3, 29, 30]. Airway inflammation and injury resulting from both the number and severity of episodes of acute rejection are also thought to play an important role in the development of CLAD [3, 30].

Viral infection as a process leading to allograft rejection has been previously documented in other solid organ transplants, such as renal allograft dysfunction caused by infections with BK virus and CMV. Similarly, multiple studies over the last two decades have indicated that respiratory viral infections play a major role in the development of acute rejection and chronic lung allograft dysfunction, manifested both as BOS and R-CLAD [3, 19, 29–37]. And these findings apply to both CMV and non-CMV respiratory viruses, with symptomatic or asymptomatic respiratory virus infection (RVI) [3, 19, 30, 32, 38–42].

In the past, remarkably high rates of pathologically documented graft changes suggestive of acute rejection have been reported in the setting of active respiratory viral infections. In some series as many as 62% of cases of respiratory virus infection in LTR were noted to have varying degrees of perivascular mononuclear cell infiltrates, as are seen in acute cellular rejection [3, 35, 36, 41, 43]. These findings are further supported by cohort studies where higher incidences of BOS have been noted in LTR who suffered CARV infections and have been reproduced in different settings where the acute and long-term outcomes of respiratory viral infection on declining allograft function have been documented [3, 33–35, 37, 39, 41, 42].

In cases where this relationship is seen, factors more likely to be associated with the development of graft dysfunction include respiratory virus infection involving the lower respiratory tract and infection with viruses known to cause more severe respiratory illness in general such as influenza and the paramyxoviruses [3, 33–35, 37, 39, 41].

The relationship between viral infection of the respiratory tract and development of allograft rejection would seem to be based on the similarity in pathogenesis of these processes. During the acute phase of a viral infection, as well as during the prolonged viral shedding often seen in the setting of lung transplantation, chemotactic cytokines released by injured parenchymal cells in the inflamed graft recruit alloreactive leukocytes. This process is further augmented by immune response specifically targeting the virus [44].

During this process, Th-1 and Th-2 CD4 T-cell subtypes and their associated cytokines interleukin (IL)-1, tumor necrosis factor, IL-6, and IL-8 are upregulated. The resulting alloreactive environment in the transplanted lung may lead to immune-mediated injury to the airway and subsequent rejection and graft dysfunction [45–51].

In recent lung transplant literature, the activity of the CXCR3 receptor expressed on the surface of activated lymphocytes provides further evidence supporting the role of viral infection in the development of lymphocyte-mediated allograft dysfunction [52, 53]. The CXCR3 receptor and its ligands, CXCL9-11, have roles both in the immune response to viruses and in the development of BOS [54–56]. In the setting of CARV infection in LTRs, the concentrations of each

CXCR3 ligand are increased and associated with larger decline in FEV^1 at 6 months [52].

In the case of CMV specifically, which is not a member of the CARV group, the interplay of viral-associated changes and host immune factors forms a pathophysiologic relationship that promotes development of allograft dysfunction. Here the cytokine cascades induced by the activity of CMV infection, as well as cytokines involved in the pathophysiology of rejection, promote the progression of one another [57–60].The release of tumor necrosis factor-alpha during allograft rejection, which acts as a key reactivation signal for latent CMV, facilitates viral replication and progression to active infection. Meanwhile the activity of CMV within the vascular endothelium and smooth muscle induces the upregulation of adhesion molecules which promote further proliferation and activity of inflammatory cells in the graft, leading to development of rejection. CMV has been thought to play an additional role in the development of rejection by the process of molecular mimicry, where the immune response against viral antigens leads to the production of anti-endothelial antibodies within the graft [2, 42, 57, 58, 60, 61].

Respiratory Viruses and Viral Infections Relevant to Lung Transplantation

Community-Acquired Respiratory Viruses (CARVs)

CARVs represent a diverse group of human pathogenic viruses, which belong to several distinct families. These include the *Paramyxoviridae* (RSV, hMPV, and PIV), *Orthomyxoviridae* (influenza A and B), *Picornaviridae* (rhinovirus and enteroviruses), *Adenoviridae* (adenovirus), and *Coronaviridae* (coronaviruses) [27, 28].

These viruses represent the most common causes of human respiratory infections and are most commonly acquired from contact with infected individuals or secretions left in the environment by an infected person [62–64].

Modes of transmission include contact with secretions followed by autoinoculation of mucosal membranes versus direct inoculation large droplets or aerosols.

Infection patterns for some of these organisms follow typical seasonal or temporal patterns and in these cases tend to mirror patterns in the general community. Healthcare-associated infections can also occur, even exhibiting cases of outbreaks within hospitals [65].

CARV infections can lead to serious complications in those with predisposing factors such as immunosuppression and altered pulmonary anatomical defense mechanisms, with LTR at particularly high risk of developing severe infections. Infections of the respiratory tract by CARVS in LTR can be further complicated by the occurrence of secondary bacterial infections and increased incidence of associated acute and chronic rejection [4, 21, 42, 64, 66, 67].

Picornaviruses, primarily RhV, are the most common viruses found in nasopharyngeal and BAL samples collected from LTR bit at routine screening and healthcare visits specifically for respiratory and infectious symptoms [14, 42, 67, 68]. Common CARVs and other RhV are much more likely to be isolated during emergency visits than routine screening, suggesting a higher incidence of symptomatic infection [14]. In general the LTR population can have as high as a 10% incidence of positive tests for CARV infection at surveillance screening without symptoms, with nearly double this rate when tested while presenting with symptoms of an acute respiratory illness [4, 14, 69].

The spectrum of disease severity for CARV infection in LTR varies significantly and does so depending on the specific infectious agent. RhV infections which are the most common of CARVs can often present with limited symptoms or be found on asymptomatic screening in one third of cases [14]. The most common symptoms of RhV infection include rhinorrhea and nasal congestion, with fevers and myalgias being relatively uncommon. Meanwhile, infections with influenza and paramyxoviruses (RSV and PIV) are almost always associated with symptoms and much more likely to be febrile illnesses [14, 67,

70]. Lower respiratory tract involvement with radiographic manifestation is typically rare except in the case of influenza. Infections with influenza and paramyxoviruses are also more than twice as likely to result in hospitalization compared with RhV and coronavirus, with nearly 50% of cases requiring admission [14, 21, 70].

In nearly all cases of symptomatic infection with CARVs, lower FEV_1 and FVC can be seen when compared to preinfection values for patients [14].

Respiratory Syncytial Virus (RSV)

RSV is an almost universally common respiratory tract infection of early childhood. It carries an incomplete pattern of natural immunity and frequent reinfections [45, 71]. It is the most charcterstic virus of the *Paramyxoviridae*. RSV is among the most commonly isolated CRVs and clinically ranges from mild upper respiratory infection symptoms such as rhinorrhea and cough to life-threatening lower respiratory tract infections with bronchiolitis and pneumonia similar to influenza. Risk factors for more severe disease include higher levels of immunosuppression, infection immediately following transplantation, and pre-existing pulmonary pathology. In LTR, RSV infection can cause significant morbidity and can be associated with acute and chronic graft dysfunction [72, 73]. RSV has been shown to significantly increase the risk of graft dysfunction, with as much as a mean FEV_1 decline of 30% in some series and associated mortality ranging from 10 to 15% [74–76].

Reverse transcription-polymerase chain reaction (RT- PCR)-based assays are the current mainstay of diagnosis with excellent sensitivity in symptomatic patients, while fluorescent antibody and serologic testing as well as viral culture can also be used to diagnose acute infection [76].

In the normal host, RSV infection primarily affects airway epithelial cells. The subsequent immune response, mediated in part by the IL-2-mediated T-helper 1 (Th1) activity, can clear the infection and prevent a prolonged inflammatory response leading to reactive airways disease [69, 77–80]. Th1 deficiency, meanwhile, can be asso-

ciated with viral persistence and chronic airway inflammation, with a Th2-driven interleukin-10-associated response [81]. Suppression of the IL-2 pathway in LTR and the associated alterations in mucosal immunity may influence the pathogenesis of RSV infection in LTR and subsequent allograft dysfunction.

Prophylaxis and Treatment

Currently, there is no vaccine or antiviral prophylactic regimen for RSV, but there are multiple clinical trials assessing the effectiveness of innovative RSV vaccines. Pavilizumab is recommended for prophylaxis in children meeting treatment criteria, but the use of this medication for the prevention of RSV in older transplant recipients is not recommended [82].

There are limited data regarding the role of antiviral therapy to treat RSV in lung transplant recipients. Currently, the drug of choice is ribavirin with or without corticosteroids, which can be administered intravenous, orally, or inhaled (Table 15.1) [82, 83, 85–87]. Treatment decisions are commonly dependent on the severity of disease, and inhaled ribavirin is most often the route of choice for severe RSV infections. Inhaled ribavirin has many drawbacks: administration requires a hospital admission and an extended inhalation interval, and it can be teratogenic to women of child-bearing age. Because of these factors of the medication, appropriate precautions should be taken [82]. Intravenous ribavirin has reported success, although it is only available through compassionate use in the United States

Table 15.1 Ribavirin treatment regimens

Dosage form	Regimen	Duration
Inhaled ribavirin	6 g over 12–18 h	3–7 days
IV ribavirin [83, 84]	Day 1: 33 mg/kg in three divided doses (q8h) Maintenance: 20 mg/kg/day in three divided doses every 8 h	7 days + negative swab
PO ribavirin [84, 85]	400 mg three times daily ± loading dose Or 20 mg/kg/day divided every 8 h	5–10 days

Data from References [83–86]

[82, 83]. Adjunctive therapy using pavilizumab and intravenous immunoglobulin has been used, with little published efficacy [82, 88]. Lastly, presatovir and ALN-RSV01 are medications undergoing phase II clinical trials to assess the efficacy of these novel antiviral agents for the treatment of RSV infections in lung transplant patients [89].

Parainfluenza Virus (PIV)

The PIV family includes four major serotypes that have been found to cause human disease, with serotype 3 most commonly isolated from LTRs. Incidence of respiratory infection with parainfluenza virus ranges from 2 to 10% of all LTRs. As a community-acquired infection, the majority of cases occur more than 1 year following transplantation, with seasonal peaks in the warmer months of spring and summer [69, 90]. Parainfluenza virus infections have been associated with high rates acute cellular rejection, up to 82% in one series. Furthermore in this series, a significant portion, nearly one third of cases, progressed to develop BOS [90].

Prophylaxis and Treatment

There are no known vaccines or prophylactic antiviral medications known to prevent parainfluenza. Currently, there are no proven treatments for parainfluenza viral infections. Ribavirin, steroids, and IVIG have been used to treat parainfluenza infections in transplant recipients but have not been proven to provide benefit [91]. DAS181, a novel sialidase fusion protein, has been used through compassionate use and is currently in phase II trials for treatment of parainfluenza in immunocompromised patients [92, 93].

Human Metapneumovirus (hMPV)

hMPV is a relatively new addition to the paramyxovirus family. hMPV presents with a clinical spectrum of disease similar to RSV, albeit typically less severe. Disease severity can range from asymptomatic infection to severe lower respiratory tract infection [94, 95]. Current data do not support an association with hMPV infection and the development of persistent allograft dysfunction as is the case with RSV [96]. However, evidence of acute decline in lung function following hMPV infection does exist [69, 74, 75].

Influenza A and B Virus

Influenza A and B viruses are associated with seasonal infections, most common in the winter months and accounting for up to 5% of viral infections in LTRs [97]. Compared to normal hosts, where influenza infection is typically a self-limited upper respiratory syndrome with myalgias and fever, the risk of lower respiratory tract involvement is higher for LTRs and immunocompromised populations in general [35, 43].

Consequently, the Centers for Disease Control recommend annual influenza vaccination and chemoprophylaxis for the immunocompromised during community outbreaks [98].

In some series a majority of LTR patients with active influenza had concomitant acute allograft rejection, and seasonal increases in BOS have been suggested to have association with influenza outbreaks [36, 41, 99, 100]. Despite this, unlike paramyxovirus infections, serious influenza disease does not appear to be very common in LTR [72]. Rapid diagnostic methods using antigen-based assays or PCR amplification of target nucleic acid sequences can be performed on nasopharyngeal swabs or BAL samples.

Prophylaxis

The immunogenicity of the influenza vaccine in lung transplant recipients is unknown [82]. Even so, seasonal influenza vaccine is recommended for transplant patients [101]. Along with immunizing transplant patients themselves, herd immunity is a very important strategy when it comes to posttransplant patient care. Therefore, it is essential to ensure all close contacts of lung transplant recipients are also vaccinated. There are two types of influenza vaccines available: the intranasal live attenuated influenza vaccine and the intramuscular inactivated vaccine. Live attenuated vaccines are contraindicated in transplant recipients; therefore, the inactivated vaccine is to be administered. Due to the intensity of immunosuppression directly posttransplant and concern of decreased immunogenicity, vaccinations are often withheld directly after transplantation. According to the American Society of Transplantation, a reasonable time frame is to wait at least 3 months after transplant before influenza vaccine administration [82] .

Postexposure prophylaxis with oseltamivir or zanamivir may be indicated in transplant recipients exposed to influenza, primarily if it is an exposure of someone living in their household [82]. Prophylaxis should be initiated if patient presents within 48 h of exposure for oseltamivir and 36 h of exposure for zanamivir [102, 103]. See Table 15.2 for prophylaxis dosing and duration.

Treatment

There are two classes of antivirals that have been used to treat influenza: the M2 inhibitors (amantadine and rimantadine) and neuraminidase inhibitors (oseltamivir, zanamivir, and peramivir). The neuraminidase inhibitors are preferred agents to treat influenza [82]. M2 inhibitors are no longer recommended due to increased resistance and inactivity to influenza A and B, respectively [82]. Oseltamivir is commercially available as a capsule and suspension; zanamivir is administered as an inhalation and peramivir as an infusion [102–104]. Currently, the IV formulation of

zanamivir and oseltamivir are only available as an investigational use, and not commercially available. Oseltamivir is the most used antiviral to treat influenza in the lung transplant population; zanamivir and peramivir lack data for severe disease and for treatment of hospitalized patients [101, 105]. The usual duration of therapy for influenza A or B treatment is 5 days, although immunosuppressed patients, including lung transplant recipients, may have prolonged viral replication and also have an increased risk of developing antiviral resistance; therefore, longer duration of therapy can be considered [82, 105]. Dosing and duration of therapy is presented in Table 15.2.

Rhinoviruses (RhV)

RhVs are the most common cause of colds in adults and are members of the *Picornaviridae* family [66]. Much like in the general population, RhVs are increasingly recognized as the most common cause of respiratory viral illness in the LTR [66, 106–111]. In addition, as many as 50% of PCR-documented cases of RhV infections in transplant recipients have few to no symptoms at the time of surveillance testing [106, 108, 112]. The typical clinical presentation involves an afebrile upper respiratory illness with rhinorrhea and sinus congestion. It is sometimes associated with sore throat and cough. Coinfections with

Table 15.2 Dosing of anti-influenza medications

	CrCl (mL/min)	Treatment	Duration	Prophylaxis	Duration
Oseltamivir	≥60	75 mg twice daily	≥5 days	75 mg once daily	7–10 days
	30–60	30 mg twice daily		30 mg once daily	
	10–30	30 mg once daily		30 mg every other day	
	HD/CrCl<10	30 mg after each HD session	5 days	30 mg after every other HD cycle	
Zanamivir	N/A	Two inhalations (10 mg) twice daily	≥5 days	Two inhalations (10 mg) once daily	10 days
Peramivir (IV)	≥ 50	600 mg	Single dose	N/A	
	30–49	200 mg			
	10–29	100 mg			
	< 10/HD	Dose after dialysis, adjusted based on creatinine clearance			

Data from References [102–105]

other pathogens complicate many cases of RhV infection in LTR and may contribute significantly to the relatively high morbidity and mortality rates observed [110].

The incidence of RhV-associated lower respiratory tract infection in LTR has been documented in contrast to typically mild and self-limited disease in the general population. These events are associated with risk of both acute and chronic rejection and increased mortality [106, 110].

There a currently no specific prophylactic or treatment options available for RhV.

Adenovirus

Adenovirus is a non-enveloped DNA virus ubiquitous in the community. Adenovirus causes a primary infection in all individuals typically in the first few years of life and counts for about 10% of all childhood respiratory illness. From there the virus may remain in lymphoepithelial tissues in latent form and subsequently create disease by reactivation [70, 113].

The mode of transmission of adenovirus in general involves inhalation of aerosolized droplets, direct contact with conjunctival secretions, feco-oral contamination, or contact with infected blood [66]. In the immunocompromised, speculation exists regarding adenovirus disease as either a primary infection from the environment or the result of transmission from the donor tissue and reactivation of previously latent virus epithelia of the pharynx, intestinal tract, and urinary tract [13, 114, 115].

In the immune competent host, symptoms associated with infection are usually self-limited, including cough, pharyngitis, keratoconjunctivitis, gastroenteritis, and fevers.

Disease in the immunocompromised, including LTR, has a wide range of severity. Although asymptomatic infection is reported, severe disease with significant morbidity and mortality can also occur. Infection sites in the immunocompromised are typically comprised of the urinary tract, gastrointestinal tract, lung, and liver [116]. More severe disease and poorer outcomes can be predicted based on higher number of affected sites and organ systems involved, as well as pathologically determined invasive disease [116–118].

The more feared complications of adenovirus infection for the recipients of solid organ transplants include pneumonia and hepatitis, with mortality rates of up to 50% documented [70].

Severe pulmonary infections have specifically been documented in LTR, with many of these cases progressing to respiratory failure with high mortality rates. In these instances, pathologic assessments at autopsy have revealed necrotizing hemorrhagic pneumonia with diffuse alveolar damage, as well as invasive disease represented by basophilic inclusions within bronchial epithelial cell consistent with adenovirus infection [114]. These severe infections have been documented to occur both in the first few weeks following transplantation and less frequently years after returning to the community [114, 119].

Prophylaxis and Treatment

There are no vaccines or established chemoprophylaxis to prevent adenovirus in solid organ transplant recipients.

Currently, there are no randomized controlled trials regarding the treatment of severe adenovirus infections. The current preferred therapy for most centers is minimization of immunosuppression. If an antiviral is needed cidofovir can be considered [120]. This drug should be utilized with caution; cidofovir administration is associated with significant adverse reactions, primarily neutropenia and nephrotoxicity, both of which are pronounced with lung transplant [120, 121]. In order to mitigate nephrotoxicity caused by cidofovir, probenacid and hydration should be added to the regimen [121]. Probenacid is administered 3 h before, 3 h after, and 8 h after cidofovir, along with hydration with normal saline [120, 121]. As adjunct to reduced immunosuppression with or without cidofovir, immunoglobulin may be considered, primarily in patients with hypogammaglobinemia [120], although the benefits of IVIG in the setting of adenovirus infection with or without hypogammaglobinemia are still not clear. In the future, brincidofovir (CMX001), a lipid conjugate of cidofovir which is currently in clinical trials, may be a viable option. Benefits of this dosage form may include an oral formulation, higher potency, and less nephrotoxicity.

Coronaviruses

Coronaviruses are a frequent cause of the common cold with currently an unclear role in infections affecting LTR [14, 21, 68]. New sensitive molecular assays for detection of coronavirus infection can help to detect this virus, which can range from simple upper respiratory illness to severe lower respiratory tract infections [122]. Severe infections in the immunocompromised can present as pneumonia and bronchiolitis [123, 124].

Similar to RhV infections, no current pharmacologic options for prophylaxis or treatment are available.

Human Bocavirus (HBoV)

HBoV, a recently identified member of the *Parvoviridae* family, can cause respiratory disease in humans with typically seasonal pattern in winter [125, 126]. Although a great deal of data regarding infections in the immunocompromised has not yet been compiled, case reports have documented severe respiratory and disseminated infections in the setting of lung transplantation [127].

β-Herpesviruses

The *Herpesviridae* are a heterogeneous family of morphologically similar double-stranded DNA viruses that can infect humans and other animals. Humans act as primary hosts for eight members of this virus family and are typically transmitted through direct person-to-person contact.

Cytomegalovirus (CMV)

CMV is the most common and important among the opportunistic infections that complicate lung transplantation. Its association to morbidity and mortality posttransplant has been well documented and increasingly shown to be mediated by elevated risk of acute and chronic allograft dysfunction [2, 32, 128–131].

CMV exposure and seropositivity are ubiquitous in the general population, ranging from 30 to 97% [59]. Exposure to and infection with the virus confer a life-long carrier status with risk of future reactivation in the setting of a compromised immune system [2, 69, 132]. The overall incidence of CMV infection in LTR has been reported as the highest among all solid organ transplants, with figures ranging from 30 to 86% of patients, in part due to the relatively higher-level immunosuppression required in the post-lung transplantation setting [57, 59]. The high incidence rates and associated complications of CMV infection exact a high price on the LTR population, with mortality rates reported at 2–12% [2, 57, 69].

Unlike community-acquired infections, the primary risk factor development of CMV infection appears to be a mismatch between the serostatus of donor and recipient [57, 59, 131]. The highest risk category is that of a seropositive donor with seronegative recipient, in which case the transplant recipient who lacks previously formulated immunity to CMV receives exposure to the virus harbored within the allograft at a time when immunosuppression is at its most aggressive [59]. The intensity of the immunosuppression regimen, both at induction and maintenance, is also an important risk factor for CMV infection, as are host factors such as age medical comorbidities [57, 59]. Other modes of infection include transfusion of blood products from a seropositive donor and reactivation of latent infection in a seropositive LTR.

Clinical Manifestations

CMV infection and disease are distinct clinical entities. Replication of CMV with or without symptoms is regarded as infection, while the presence of symptoms or physiologic changes attributable to CMV is required to meet a definition of disease. The hallmarks of CMV disease include fevers and malaise, myalgias and arthralgias, leukopenia and thrombocytopenia, as well as tissue invasive manifestations [20, 59].

Tissue invasive disease most commonly manifests as a pneumonitis. This syndrome can present with subtle fevers, nonproductive cough, and dyspnea associated with decline in pulmonary function tests. Other manifestations of tissue invasive disease include incidences of hepatitis associated with abnormal liver function tests, and gastroenteritis and colitis typically presenting with nausea, vomiting, and diarrhea [20].

Diagnosis

Quantitative nucleic acid-based amplification assays utilizing polymerase chain reaction (PCR) technology for the identification of viremia have largely replaced previously used methods of diagnosis relying on antigen detection for viral particles. Monitoring and diagnosis of CMV infection is now used in the overwhelming majority of transplant center [133]. Despite this, there is no current consensus on threshold values of CMV viral load considered to be an indicator of infection. Viral culture performed on blood, urine, and BAL samples is no longer routinely recommended for detection of CMV [42].

The presence of cell-mediated immunity to CMV, as determined by quantiferon-CMV assay measuring the presence of a CD8 T-cell response to the virus, holds promise as a marker to determine risk of CMV disease. Patients with positive CMV interferon-gamma release assays have been shown to more frequently clear viremia without progression to clinical disease, while those with negative assays suffer higher rates of late onset CMV disease after discontinuation of prophylactic therapy [134, 135].

Treatment General

Intravenous ganciclovir has historically been the treatment of choice for the treatment of CMV [136]. The IV formulation is still the drug of choice for severe life-threatening disease and in patients who have severe diarrhea or cannot tolerate medications by mouth [137]. In 2007, the Victor Study group concluded that oral valganciclovir is also a treatment option in select solid organ transplant recipients with mild to moderate disease [138], although it should be noted that less than 10% of the patients in the Victor Study were lung transplant recipients, and these patients did not have severe disease [138]. Whether using intravenous ganciclovir or oral valganciclovir treatment should be continued for 14–21 days plus viral clearance [136]. If virus is not cleared after 21 days, there is a high risk for recurrent disease; therefore, longer duration may be necessary if resolution of viremia is not accomplished [136–138]. Table 15.3 outlines dosing guidelines adjusted for renal function for both ganciclovir and valganciclovir.

Prophylaxis

Chemoprophylaxis for CMV should be started as soon as possible, and always within 10 days after transplantation for those at risk for CMV [136]. Recommendations for prophylaxis of CMV disease in lung transplant recipients are based on donor and recipient IGG serostatus (Table 15.4). For patients at the highest risk for developing CMV disease, donor IGG positive and recipient IGG negative (D+/R−), prophylaxis with IV ganciclovir, valganciclovir, or a combination of both is recommended [136]. The duration of prophylaxis varies, but at least 12 months of prophylaxis is recommended, with some centers extending prophylaxis beyond 12 months [136, 142]. As adjunct to chemoprophylaxis, CMV immune globulin can also be considered for the D+/R− high-risk group of patients [136]. For moderate-risk recipient IGG seropositive recipients, IV ganciclovir or valganciclovir is recommended for 6–12 months [136, 142, 143]. For low-risk donor and recipient IGG seronegative negative patients, no CMV-specific prophylaxis is necessary [136, 142]. HSV prophylaxis with acyclovir is still indicated, but neither ganciclovir nor valganciclovir is required [35, 142, 144] (Table 15.4). Preemptive therapy, i.e., withholding valganciclovir or IV ganciclovir prophylaxis and monitoring patients on a weekly basis for CMV viremia then treating to prevent disease progression, is generally not recommended in lung transplant recipients [136].

Table 15.3 CMV treatment

Estimated CrCl	Valganciclovir		Estimated CrCl	Ganciclovir	
	Prophylaxis/maintenance	Treatment/induction		Prophylaxis/maintenance	Treatment/induction
CrCl ≥60 mL/min	900 mg daily	900 mg twice daily	CrCl ≥70 mL/min	5 mg/kg daily	5 mg/kg twice daily
CrCl 40–59 mL/min	450 mg daily	450 mg twice daily	CrCl 50–69 mL/min	2.5 mg/kg daily	2.5 mg/kg twice daily
CrCl 25–39 mL/min	450 mg every other day	450 mg daily	CrCl 25–49 mL/min	1.25 mg/kg daily	2.5 mg/kg daily
CrCl 10–24 mL/min	450 mg twice weekly	450 mg every other day	CrCl 10–24 mL/min	0.625 mg/kg daily	1.25 mg/kg daily
CrCl <10 mL/min	Use not recommended consider ganciclovir		CrCl <10 mL/min	0.625 mg/kg three times weekly following dialysis	1.25 mg/kg three times weekly following dialysis
Alternative dosing valganciclovir in dialysis	Solution 100 mg three times weekly following dialysis	Solution 200 mg three times weekly following dialysis			

Data from References [139–141]

Table 15.4 CMV prophylactic regimens

Risk level		Recommended medication therapy	Duration
High	D+/R-	IV ganciclovir Or Valganciclovir +/− CMV IVIG	At least 12 months
Moderate	D+/R+ D−/R+	IV ganciclovir Or Valganciclovir	6–12 months
Low	D−/R-	CMV-specific chemoprophylaxis not recommended	

Data from References [136, 139, 140, 142]

Resistance

An emerging concern is the management of ganciclovir-resistant CMV disease. Ganciclovir resistance is associated with high morbidity and mortality, and there are few options when it comes to treatment [145]. Current drugs of choice are either foscarnet or cidofovir, both of which are highly toxic and require extended hospitalizations when initiating therapy. Resistance is usually due to a mutation of the UL97 gene and less commonly the UL54 gene [136, 145]. The UL97 mutation does not confer resistance to cidofovir or foscarnet, but the UL54 mutation may confer resistance to all three medications and is therefore more difficult to treat [136, 145]. Many times as adjunct to cidofovir or foscarnet transplant, centers consider discontinuation of the current antimetabolite and initiating leflunomide, which has both antiviral and antimetabolite properties [146, 147]. Future options for treatment of CMV include maribavir and brincidofovir (CMX001), both of which are currently in clinical trials and not available for use [148, 149]. No matter the situation, treatment of ganciclovir-resistant CMV should be undertaken with caution and on a case by case basis.

Epstein-Barr Virus (EBV)

EBV, an oncogenic virus, holds a strong association for the development of post-lymphoproliferative disease (PTLD). Encompassing a heterogeneous group of lymphoproliferative disorders, PTLD ranges from a reactive polyclonal lymphoid hyperplasia to aggressive non-Hodgkin's lymphomas. A deficient EBV-specific cellular immune response caused by immunosuppressant regimens is considered to be at the etiology of PTLD [68, 150]. In the setting of lung transplantation, the incidence of PTLD has been noted to range from 1 to 20%, with intense prolonged immunosuppression and EBV mismatch (EBV positive donor and EBV negative recipient) considered major risk factors [150–152]. In the setting of EBV mismatch, monitoring of viral load can be clinically useful as a continuous increase of EBV load may indicate pending development of PTLD [153].

Prophylaxis and Prevention

Overall immunosuppression plays a vital role in EBV and PTLD occurrence [154]. The use of lymphocyte-depleting therapy has been linked to increased PTLD cases [154]. This should be considered with discussing the use of lymphocyte-depleting induction and treatment approaches in order to prevent rejection and minimize the risk of PTLD [154]. Both acyclovir and ganciclovir have in vitro activity against EBV lytic replication and have been used as prophylaxis, although efficacy is not proven [154].

Another approach is monitoring of EBV viral load with serial PCRs during posttransplant follow up. This allows centers to preemptively add chemoprophylaxis, decrease immunosuppression, and trend the viral load. As with other prophylactic strategies, the efficacy of EBV monitoring and preemptive intervention to decreases the occurrence of PTLD posttransplant has is not established.

Treatment

Minimization of immunosuppression is a mainstay in management of EBV and PTLD. With reduced immunosuppression, the reconstituted cytotoxic T-Cell population is thought to control the EBV infected B-cell population [154]. The addition of antiviral medication in combination to reduced immunosuppression for patients with PTLD is controversial. This is primarily due to the majority of EBV within a PTLD mass not undergoing lytic infection; therefore, the utility of antiviral therapy is not well defined [154]. IVIG has also been considered as an adjunctive therapy to the treatment regimen, although the benefit of the addition of IVIG is not established.

Anti-CD20 treatment with rituximab with or without traditional chemotherapy is an option depending on severity of the disease and patients response to reduced immunosuppression [154]. Usual regimens are those similar to B-cell lymphoma, often requiring CHOP [154]. Even with treatment options, PTLD in lung transplant recipients remains a high cause of morbidity and mortality. Recently a single center reported approximately 50% of patients treated with a rituximab-based therapy had full remission of disease and 22% with no response to treatment and a 5-year survival of only 29% after PTLD diagnosis [155].

Due to the complexity of the transplant and severity of PTLD, a multidisciplinary approach is often beneficial. Patients, transplant care providers, along with a cancer treatment center can devise a plan that would best fit each individual patient and maximize outcome and quality of life.

Herpes Simplex Virus (HSV) 1 and 2 and Varicella-Zoster Virus (VZV)

HSV and VZV are members of the *Alphaherpesvirinae* which previously represented opportunistic infectious agents in first week post-lung transplantation. Infection with HSV in particular was a cause of severe pneumonitis in up to 10% LTR and associated with high mortality rates [4, 68]. However, severe HSV infection has since become a relatively rare complication with improved antiviral prophylaxis in the posttransplant setting.

Herpes zoster, caused by the reactivations of dormant VZV infection, presents with painful vesicular dermatomal skin lesions. Development of zoster in LTR bears a cumulative probability of approximately 20% after 5 years posttransplantation, with over 5% of cases progressing to disseminated cutaneous infection. Following occurrence of herpes zoster, the post-herpetic neuralgia syndrome can be observed in nearly one of five of those effected [151].

Prophylaxis

Prior to listing, transplant candidates should be evaluated for varicella seropositivity [156]. Seronegative patients are commonly considered for the varicella vaccine, administered least 14 days prior to transplantation [156]. The varicella vaccine is a live-attenuated vaccine and should not be administered after transplantation; therefore, every effort should be made to vaccinate appropriate patients prior to transplantation [156].

All lung transplant recipients should receive prophylaxis for herpes viruses directly after transplantation [156, 157]. Most patients will be receiving prophylaxis with valganciclovir for CMV; this is sufficient herpes virus prophylaxis [156, 157]. For patients who do not require CMV prophylaxis (donor and recipient are seronegative for CMV), acyclovir or valacyclovir is the drug of choice for prophylaxis [156, 157], although famciclovir is also acceptable (Table 15.5).

Treatment

Treatment as an outpatient with oral antivirals is appropriate for mucocutaneous and mild to moderate disease in lung transplant recipients. Patients with moderate to severe disease who are hospitalized require more aggressive therapy [156, 157]. For these transplant recipients, primarily those diagnosed with disseminated or

Table 15.5 Herpes simplex/herpes zoster (VZV) prophylaxis and treatment table

| Medication | Indication | | |
	Prophylaxis	Treatment (outpatient) Duration: 7–14 days	Treatment (moderate to severe/CNS) Duration: 21 days
Acyclovir (PO)	400–800 mg 2× daily	HSV: 400 mg 3× daily VZV: 800 mg 5× daily	N/A
Valacyclovir (PO)	500 mg 2× daily	HSV: 1 g 2× daily VZV: 1 g 3× daily	N/A
Famciclovir (PO)	500 mg 2× daily	HSV: 500 mg 2× daily VZV: 500 mg 3× daily	N/A
Acyclovir (IV)	N/A	5 mg/kg 3× daily (if unable to tolerate PO)	10 mg/kg 3× daily

All medications are adjusted for renal function; refer to individual product labeling
Data from References [158–161]

CNS disease, intravenous acyclovir is the drug of choice (Table 15.5) [156, 157].

Duration of therapy ranges from 7 to 21 days depending on the severity of disease [156, 157]. For localized herpes zoster infections, therapy should be continued for at least 7 days *AND* until the lesions are crusted over [156]. It should be noted that a delay in lesion crusting is commonly seen in transplant recipients, which often extends the duration of therapy. In general, duration of treatment for mild to moderate HSV and VZV disease is recommended to for 7–14 days, and 21 days in severe and central nervous system infections [156, 157].

Human Herpes Virus (HHV) 6 and 7

HHV-6 and HHV-7 are lymphotropic viruses belonging to the same subfamily as CMV. They can cause primary infections during early childhood. Patients who have undergone solid organ transplantation have been noted to suffer reactivation of disease typically early in the posttransplantation period [162].

The clinical syndrome associated with HHV-6 can consist of skin rashes, hepatitis, bone marrow suppression, pneumonitis, and encephalopathy, although severity of infection varies and the majority of cases are thought to be asymptomatic [68, 162].

The clinical impact of HHV-7 is less well characterized.

Human Herpes Virus (HHV) 8

HHV-8 is the virus associated with the development of Kaposi's sarcoma (KS), which is a well-characterized entity following SOT in heart, renal, and liver transplant recipients. The incidence of KS after transplantation in the United States is approximately 0.4%, with the majority of cases occurring in renal transplant recipients. In about 60% of cases, KS lesions are confined to skin and mucosa of the oropharynx, while the remainder can exhibit involvement of internal organs and lymph nodes [163]. In the last few decades, a mounting number of cases of KS in LTR have brought recognition to HHV 8 as an important pathogen in the setting of lung transplantation [163, 164]. KS, considered a rare malignancy in LTR, can manifest with involvement of the allograft as bronchial and pleural disease, as well as cutaneous lesions or involvement of other viscera such as the gastric or intestinal tracts [163–166]. It should be considered in patients with characteristic skin lesions and pulmonary disease, including hemorrhagic pleural effusions that are typically rich in HHV-8 viral particles and DNA when tested [166]. Furthermore, an association between increasing HHV-8 viremia and progression of pulmonary KS has been previously described [163].

Although data on the management of this rare entity in LTR are limited, most cases appear to have full or partial response to reduction in immunosuppression, with small case series showing response to therapy with sirolimus

[163]. Other therapies traditionally used in the treatment of KS include conventional chemotherapies with bleomycin, vincristine, and doxorubicin in addition to radiation, although there are no data regarding these therapeutic modalities in the setting of lung transplantation.

HHV-8 is susceptible in vitro to the anti-*Herpesviridae* agents cidofovir, foscarnet, and ganciclovir, with data from the management of KS in the setting of HIV suggesting a reduced risk of developing KS [167–169]. However, data on the use of these agents in the management of KS following SOT are again limited.

Other Viruses

Several other viral infections have been documented to create complications in the course of lung transplantation. Although largely out of the scope of this chapter, a few examples are briefly discussed below.

BK Virus

BK virus is a member of the human polyomavirus family, almost universally infecting healthy adults with seroprevalence in up to 100%. Data from kidney transplant recipients provde the largest source of information regarding clinically infection with BK virus, where reactivation of BK virus occurs in up to 45% and may cause parenchymal and obstructive renal allograft disease. In the setting of lung transplantation, only rare cases of BK virus-associated nephropathy of native kidneys have been reported [170–172].

Prevention and Treatment
Standard of prevention and treatment of BK virus in lung transplantation is not well established. Although BK virus may be detected in the urine of over 25% of lung transplants, viuria has not shown to have an effect on renal function [170, 173, 174]. Therefore, decreasing immunosuppression or the use of other treatment modalities, such as leflunomide for BK virus in lung transplantation, is not established as a standard of care.

Parvovirus B19

Parvovirus B19 can cause pure red cell aplasia, more commonly seen in renal transplant recipients. It has been shown to occur as a very rare complication after lung transplantation, in isolated case reports [68, 175]. Despite the relative lack of data in the literature on this subject, the ubiquity of parvovirus exposure in the community warrants investigation of this possibility in cases of unexplained isolated anemia in LTRs [176, 177].

Summary

Chronic lung allograft dysfunction (CLAD) continues to be the major causes of morbidity and mortality after lung transplantation. Viruses, especially the community respiratory viruses (CRV), are common and have also been a major source of morbidity in lung transplant recipients. An important and newly intense area of focus for research has been the interface between respiratory viruses, the respiratory virome, and chronic rejection. With improved techniques to study the pathogenesis of all types of chronic rejection as well as recent advances in metagenomics, we are no doubt in a place now when we can move forward in not only understanding the relationship between viruses and lung allograft rejection but also being able to work toward a solution.

References

1. Kotloff RM, Thabut G. Lung transplantation. Am J Respir Crit Care Med. 2011;184(2):159–71.
2. Burguete SR, Maselli DJ, Fernandez JF, Levine SM. Lung transplant infection. Respirology. 2013;18(1):22–38.
3. Vilchez RA, Dauber J, Kusne S. Infectious etiology of bronchiolitis obliterans: the respiratory viruses connection—myth or reality? Am J Transplant. 2003;3(3):245–9.
4. Speich R, van der Bij W. Epidemiology and management of infections after lung transplantation. Clin Infect Dis. 2001;33(Suppl 1):S58–65.
5. Witt CA, Meyers BF, Hachem RR. Pulmonary infections following lung transplantation. Thorac Surg Clin. 2012;22(3):403–12.

6. Norgaard MA, Andersen CB, Pettersson G. Airway epithelium of transplanted lungs with and without direct bronchial artery revascularization. Eur J Cardiothorac Surg. 1999;15(1):37–44.

7. Jordan S, Mitchell JA, Quinlan GJ, Goldstraw P, Evans TW. The pathogenesis of lung injury following pulmonary resection. Eur Respir J. 2000;15(4):790–9.

8. Verleden GM, Vos R, van Raemdonck D, Vanaudenaerde B. Pulmonary infection defense after lung transplantation: does airway ischemia play a role? Curr Opin Organ Transplant. 2010;15(5):568–71.

9. Gade J, Qvortrup K, Andersen CB, Thorsen S, Svendsen UG, Olsen PS. Bronchial arterial devascularization. An experimental study in pigs. Scand Cardiovasc J. 2001;35(3):212–20.

10. Blumberg EA, Albano C, Pruett T, Isaacs R, Fitzpatrick J, Bergin J, Crump C, Hayden FG. The immunogenicity of influenza virus vaccine in solid organ transplant recipients. Clin Infect Dis. 1996;22(2):295–302.

11. Fraund S, Wagner D, Pethig K, Drescher J, Girgsdies OE, Haverich A. Influenza vaccination in heart transplant recipients. J Heart Lung Transplant. 1999;18(3):220–5.

12. Kumar SS, Ventura AK, VanderWerf B. Influenza vaccination in renal transplant recipients. JAMA. 1978;239(9):840–2.

13. Humar A, Kumar D, Mazzulli T, Razonable RR, Moussa G, Paya CV, Covington E, Alecock E, Pescovitz MD, PV16000 Study Group. A surveillance study of adenovirus infection in adult solid organ transplant recipients. Am J Transplant. 2005;5(10):2555–9.

14. Bridevaux PO, Aubert JD, Soccal PM, Mazza-Stalder J, Berutto C, Rochat T, Turin L, Van Belle S, Nicod L, Meylan P, Wagner G, Kaiser L. Incidence and outcomes of respiratory viral infections in lung transplant recipients: a prospective study. Thorax. 2014;69(1):32–8.

15. Sims KD, Blumberg EA. Common infections in the lung transplant recipient. Clin Chest Med. 2011;32(2):327–41.

16. Allen U, et al. Discipline of transplant infectious diseases (ID). Foreword. Am J Transplant. 2009;9(Suppl 4):S1–2.

17. Smyth RL, Higenbottam TW, Scott JP, Wreghitt TG, Stewart S, Clelland CA, McGoldrick JP, Wallwork J. Herpes simplex virus infection in heart-lung transplant recipients. Transplantation. 1990;49(4):735–9.

18. Ljungman P, Griffiths P, Paya C. Definitions of cytomegalovirus infection and disease in transplant recipients. Clin Infect Dis. 2002;34(8):1094–7.

19. Fischer SA, Avery RK, AST Infectious Disease Community of Practice. Screening of donor and recipient prior to solid organ transplantation. Am J Transplant. 2009;9(Suppl 4):S7–18.

20. Humar A, Michaels M, AST ID, Working Group on Infectious Disease Monitoring. American Society of Transplantation recommendations for screening, monitoring and reporting of infectious complications in immunosuppression trials in recipients of organ transplantation. Am J Transplant. 2006;6(2):262–74.

21. Vu DL, Bridevaux PO, Aubert JD, Soccal PM, Kaiser L. Respiratory viruses in lung transplant recipients: a critical review and pooled analysis of clinical studies. Am J Transplant. 2011;11(5):1071–8.

22. Renaud C, Campbell AP. Changing epidemiology of respiratory viral infections in hematopoietic cell transplant recipients and solid organ transplant recipients. Curr Opin Infect Dis. 2011;24(4):333–43.

23. Krunic N, Yager TD, Himsworth D, Merante F, Yaghoubian S, Janeczko R. xTAG RVP assay: analytical and clinical performance. J Clin Virol. 2007;40(Suppl 1):S39–46.

24. Mahony JB. Nucleic acid amplification-based diagnosis of respiratory virus infections. Expert Rev Anti-Infect Ther. 2010;8(11):1273–92.

25. Kuypers J, Campbell AP, Cent A, Corey L, Boeckh M. Comparison of conventional and molecular detection of respiratory viruses in hematopoietic cell transplant recipients. Transpl Infect Dis. 2009;11(4):298–303.

26. Balada-Llasat JM, LaRue H, Kelly C, Rigali L, Pancholi P. Evaluation of commercial ResPlex II v2.0, MultiCode-PLx, and xTAG respiratory viral panels for the diagnosis of respiratory viral infections in adults. J Clin Virol. 2011;50(1):42–5.

27. Berry M, Gamieldien J, Fielding BC. Identification of new respiratory viruses in the new millennium. Viruses. 2015;7(3):996–1019.

28. Pavia AT. Viral infections of the lower respiratory tract: old viruses, new viruses, and the role of diagnosis. Clin Infect Dis. 2011;52(Suppl 4):S284–9.

29. Wright B, Gross JJ, Kilburn FL, Smith AC. State of the art: research in nursing education administration. J Nurs Educ. 1992;31(9):423–4.

30. Sharples LD, McNeil K, Stewart S, Wallwork J. Risk factors for bronchiolitis obliterans: a systematic review of recent publications. J Heart Lung Transplant. 2002;21(2):271–81.

31. Cooper JD, Billingham M, Egan T, Hertz MI, Higenbottam T, Lynch J, Mauer J, Paradis I, Patterson GA, Smith C, et al. A working formulation for the standardization of nomenclature and for clinical staging of chronic dysfunction in lung allografts. International Society for Heart and Lung Transplantation. J Heart Lung Transplant. 1993;12(5):713–6.

32. Keenan RJ, Lega ME, Dummer JS, Paradis IL, Dauber JH, Rabinowich H, Yousem SA, Hardesty RL, Griffith BP, Duquesnoy RJ, et al. Cytomegalovirus serologic status and postoperative infection correlated with risk of developing chronic rejection after pulmonary transplantation. Transplantation. 1991;51(2):433–8.

33. Palmer SM Jr, Henshaw NG, Howell DN, Miller SE, Davis RD, Tapson VF. Community respiratory viral

infection in adult lung transplant recipients. Chest. 1998;113(4):944–50.

34. Bridges ND, Spray TL, Collins MH, Bowles NE, Towbin JA. Adenovirus infection in the lung results in graft failure after lung transplantation. J Thorac Cardiovasc Surg. 1998;116(4):617–23.

35. Garantziotis S, Howell DN, McAdams HP, Davis RD, Henshaw NG, Palmer SM. Influenza pneumonia in lung transplant recipients: clinical features and association with bronchiolitis obliterans syndrome. Chest. 2001;119(4):1277–80.

36. Vilchez RA, McCurry K, Dauber J, Lacono A, Griffith B, Fung J, Kusne S. Influenza virus infection in adult solid organ transplant recipients. Am J Transplant. 2002;2(3):287–91.

37. Billings JL, Hertz MI, Savik K, Wendt CH. Respiratory viruses and chronic rejection in lung transplant recipients. J Heart Lung Transplant. 2002;21(5):559–66.

38. Massad MG, Ramirez AM. Influenza pneumonia in thoracic organ transplant recipients : what can we do to avoid it? Chest. 2001;119(4):997–9.

39. Faul JL, Akindipe OA, Berry GJ, Theodore J. Influenza pneumonia in a paediatric lung transplant recipient. Transpl Int. 2000;13(1):79–81.

40. Holt ND, Gould FK, Taylor CE, Harwood JF, Freeman R, Healy MD, Corris PA, Dark JH. Incidence and significance of noncytomegalovirus viral respiratory infection after adult lung transplantation. J Heart Lung Transplant. 1997;16(4):416–9.

41. Vilchez RA, McCurry K, Dauber J, Iacono A, Keenan R, Zeevi A, Griffith B, Kusne S. The epidemiology of parainfluenza virus infection in lung transplant recipients. Clin Infect Dis. 2001;33(12):2004–8.

42. Kotton CN, Kumar D, Caliendo AM, Asberg A, Chou S, Danziger-Isakov L, Humar A, Transplantation Society International CMV Consensus Group. International consensus guidelines on the management of cytomegalovirus in solid organ transplantation. Transplantation. 2010;89(7):779–95.

43. Vilchez R, McCurry K, Dauber J, Iacono A, Keenan R, Griffith B, Kusne S. Influenza and parainfluenza respiratory viral infection requiring admission in adult lung transplant recipients. Transplantation. 2002;73(7):1075–8.

44. Colvin BL, Thomson AW. Chemokines, their receptors, and transplant outcome. Transplantation. 2002;74(2):149–55.

45. Hall CB. Respiratory syncytial virus and parainfluenza virus. N Engl J Med. 2001;344(25):1917–28.

46. Skoner DP, Gentile DA, Patel A, Doyle WJ. Evidence for cytokine mediation of disease expression in adults experimentally infected with influenza A virus. J Infect Dis. 1999;180(1):10–4.

47. Arnold R, Humbert B, Werchau H, Gallati H, König W. Interleukin-8, interleukin-6, and soluble tumour necrosis factor receptor type I release from a human pulmonary epithelial cell line (A549) exposed to respiratory syncytial virus. Immunology. 1994;82(1):126–33.

48. Subauste MC, Jacoby DB, Richards SM, Proud D. Infection of a human respiratory epithelial cell line with rhinovirus. Induction of cytokine release and modulation of susceptibility to infection by cytokine exposure. J Clin Invest. 1995;96(1):549–57.

49. Matsukura S, Kokubu F, Noda H, Tokunaga H, Adachi M. Expression of IL-6, IL-8, and RANTES on human bronchial epithelial cells, NCI-H292, induced by influenza virus A. J Allergy Clin Immunol. 1996;98(6 Pt 1):1080–7.

50. Bruder JT, Kovesdi I. Adenovirus infection stimulates the Raf/MAPK signaling pathway and induces interleukin-8 expression. J Virol. 1997; 71(1):398–404.

51. Karp CL, Wysocka M, Wahl LM, Ahearn JM, Cuomo PJ, Sherry B, Trinchieri G, Griffin DE. Mechanism of suppression of cell-mediated immunity by measles virus. Science. 1996;273(5272):228–31.

52. Weigt SS, Derhovanessian A, Liao E, Hu S, Gregson AL, Kubak BM, Saggar R, Saggar R, Plachevskiy V, Fishbein MC, Lynch JP III, Ardehali A, Ross DJ, Wang HJ, Elashoff RM, Belperio JA. CXCR3 chemokine ligands during respiratory viral infections predict lung allograft dysfunction. Am J Transplant. 2012;12(2):477–84.

53. Kohlmeier JE, Cookenham T, Miller SC, Roberts AD, Christensen JP, Thomsen AR, Woodland DL. CXCR3 directs antigen-specific effector CD4+ T cell migration to the lung during parainfluenza virus infection. J Immunol. 2009;183(7):4378–84.

54. Lindell DM, Lane TE, Lukacs NW. CXCL10/CXCR3-mediated responses promote immunity to respiratory syncytial virus infection by augmenting dendritic cell and CD8(+) T cell efficacy. Eur J Immunol. 2008;38(8):2168–79.

55. Belperio JA, Keane MP, Burdick MD, Lynch JP III, Xue YY, Li K, Ross DJ, Strieter RM. Critical role for CXCR3 chemokine biology in the pathogenesis of bronchiolitis obliterans syndrome. J Immunol. 2002;169(2):1037–49.

56. Belperio JA, Keane MP, Burdick MD, Lynch JP III, Zisman DA, Xue YY, Li K, Ardehali A, Ross DJ, Strieter RM. Role of CXCL9/CXCR3 chemokine biology during pathogenesis of acute lung allograft rejection. J Immunol. 2003;171(9):4844–52.

57. Zamora MR. Cytomegalovirus and lung transplantation. Am J Transplant. 2004;4(8):1219–26.

58. Tullius SG, Tilney NL. Both alloantigen-dependent and -independent factors influence chronic allograft rejection. Transplantation. 1995;59(3):313–8.

59. Humar A, Snydman D, Snydman D, AST Infectious Diseases Community of Practice. Cytomegalovirus in solid organ transplant recipients. Am J Transplant. 2009;9(Suppl 4):S78–86.

60. SivaSai KS, Smith MA, Poindexter NJ, Sundaresan SR, Trulock EP, Lynch JP, Cooper JD, Patterson GA, Mohanakumar T. Indirect recognition of donor HLA class I peptides in lung transplant recipients with bronchiolitis obliterans syndrome. Transplantation. 1999;67(8):1094–8.

61. Lemstrom K Koskinen P, Krogerus L, Daemen M, Bruggeman C, Häyry P. Cytomegalovirus antigen expression, endothelial cell proliferation, and intimal thickening in rat cardiac allografts after cytomegalovirus infection. Circulation. 1995;92(9):2594–604.

62. Community-Acquired Respiratory Viruses. Am J Transplant. 2004;4(s10):105–9.

63. Garibaldi RA. Epidemiology of community-acquired respiratory tract infections in adults. Incidence, etiology, and impact. Am J Med. 1985;78(6B):32–7.

64. Kumar D, Erdman D, Keshavjee S, Peret T, Tellier R, Hadjiliadis D, Johnson G, Ayers M, Siegal D, Humar A. Clinical impact of community-acquired respiratory viruses on bronchiolitis obliterans after lung transplant. Am J Transplant. 2005;5(8):2031–6.

65. Raad I, Abbas J, Whimbey E. Infection control of nosocomial respiratory viral disease in the immuno-compromised host. Am J Med. 1997;102(3A):48–52; discussion 53–4.

66. Ison MG. Respiratory viral infections in transplant recipients. Antivir Ther. 2007;12(4 Pt B):627–38.

67. Chakinala MM, Walter MJ. Community acquired respiratory viral infections after lung transplantation: clinical features and long-term consequences. Semin Thorac Cardiovasc Surg. 2004;16(4):342–9.

68. Remund KF, Best M, Egan JJ. Infections relevant to lung transplantation. Proc Am Thorac Soc. 2009;6(1):94–100.

69. Shah PD, McDyer JF. Viral infections in lung transplant recipients. Semin Respir Crit Care Med. 2010;31(2):243–54.

70. Billings JL, Hertz MI, Wendt CH. Community respiratory virus infections following lung transplantation. Transpl Infect Dis. 2001;3(3):138–48.

71. Hall CB, Powell KR, MacDonald NE, Gala CL, Menegus ME, Suffin SC, Cohen HJ. Respiratory syncytial viral infection in children with compromised immune function. N Engl J Med. 1986;315(2):77–81.

72. Wendt CH, Fox JM, Hertz MI. Paramyxovirus infection in lung transplant recipients. J Heart Lung Transplant. 1995;14(3):479–85.

73. Wendt CH. Community respiratory viruses: organ transplant recipients. Am J Med. 1997;102(3A):31–6; discussion 42–3.

74. McCurdy LH, Milstone A, Dummer S. Clinical features and outcomes of paramyxoviral infection in lung transplant recipients treated with ribavirin. J Heart Lung Transplant. 2003;22(7):745–53.

75. Hopkins P, McNeil K, Kermeen F, Musk M, McQueen E, Mackay I, Sloots T, Nissen M. Human metapneumovirus in lung transplant recipients and comparison to respiratory syncytial virus. Am J Respir Crit Care Med. 2008;178(8):876–81.

76. Falsey AR, Formica MA, Walsh EE. Diagnosis of respiratory syncytial virus infection: comparison of reverse transcription-PCR to viral culture and serology in adults with respiratory illness. J Clin Microbiol. 2002;40(3):817–20.

77. Kurt-Jones EA, Popova L, Kwinn L, Haynes LM, Jones LP, Tripp RA, Walsh EE, Freeman MW, Golenbock DT, Anderson LJ, Finberg RW. Pattern recognition receptors TLR4 and CD14 mediate response to respiratory syncytial virus. Nat Immunol. 2000;1(5):398–401.

78. Sha Q, Truong-Tran AQ, Plitt JR, Beck LA, Schleimer RP. Activation of airway epithelial cells by toll-like receptor agonists. Am J Respir Cell Mol Biol. 2004;31(3):358–64.

79. Delgado MF, Coviello S, Monsalvo AC, et al. Lack of antibody affinity maturation due to poor Toll-like receptor stimulation leads to enhanced respiratory syncytial virus disease. Nat Med. 2009;15(1):34–41.

80. Graham BS, Rutigliano JA, Johnson TR. Respiratory syncytial virus immunobiology and pathogenesis. Virology. 2002;297(1):1–7.

81. Crowe JE Jr, Williams JV. Immunology of viral respiratory tract infection in infancy. Paediatr Respir Rev. 2003;4(2):112–9.

82. Manuel O, Estabrook M, Estabrook M, AST Infectious Diseases Community of Practice. RNA respiratory viruses in solid organ transplantation. Am J Transplant. 2013;13(Suppl 4):212–9.

83. Glanville AR, Scott AI, Morton JM, Aboyoun CL, Plit ML, Carter IW, Malouf MA. Intravenous ribavirin is a safe and cost-effective treatment for respiratory syncytial virus infection after lung transplantation. J Heart Lung Transplant. 2005;24(12):2114–9.

84. Hynicka LM, Ensor CR. Prophylaxis and treatment of respiratory syncytial virus in adult immunocompromised patients. Ann Pharmacother. 2012;46(4):558–66.

85. Pelaez A, Lyon GM, Force SD, Ramirez AM, Neujahr DC, Foster M, Naik PM, Gal AA, Mitchell PO, Lawrence EC. Efficacy of oral ribavirin in lung transplant patients with respiratory syncytial virus lower respiratory tract infection. J Heart Lung Transplant. 2009;28(1):67–71.

86. Li L, Avery R, Budev M, Mossad S, Danziger-Isakov L. Oral versus inhaled ribavirin therapy for respiratory syncytial virus infection after lung transplantation. J Heart Lung Transplant. 2012;31(8):839–44.

87. Burrows FS, Carlos LM, Benzimra M, Marriott DJ, Havryk AP, Plit ML, Malouf MA, Glanville AR. Oral ribavirin for respiratory syncytial virus infection after lung transplantation: efficacy and cost-efficiency. J Heart Lung Transplant. 2015;34(7):958–62.

88. Flynn JD, Akers WS, Jones M, Stevkovic N, Waid T, Mullett T, Jahania S. Treatment of respiratory syncytial virus pneumonia in a lung transplant recipient: case report and review of the literature. Pharmacotherapy. 2004;24(7):932–8.

89. ClinicalTrials.gov [Internet]. Bethesda (MD); National Library of Medicine (US). 2010 Feb 5. Identifier NCT01065935, Phase 2b Study of ALN-RSV01 in Lung Transplant Patients Infected With Respiratory Syncytial Virus (RSV); 2012

May; [3 page]. https://clinicaltrials.gov/ct2/show/NCT01065935?term=aln-rsv01&rank=2.

90. Vilchez RA, Dauber J, McCurry K, Iacono A, Kusne S. Parainfluenza virus infection in adult lung transplant recipients: an emergent clinical syndrome with implications on allograft function. Am J Transplant. 2003;3(2):116–20.

91. Liu V, Dhillon GS, Weill D. A multi-drug regimen for respiratory syncytial virus and parainfluenza virus infections in adult lung and heart-lung transplant recipients. Transpl Infect Dis. 2010;12(1):38–44.

92. Drozd DR, Limaye AP, Moss RB, Sanders RL, Hansen C, Edelman JD, Raghu G, Boeckh M, Rakita RM. DAS181 treatment of severe parainfluenza type 3 pneumonia in a lung transplant recipient. Transpl Infect Dis. 2013;15(1):E28–32.

93. ClinicalTrials.gov [Internet]. Bethesda (MD); National Library of Medicine (US). 2012 July. Identifier NCT01644877,A Phase II, Randomized, Double-blind, Placebo-controlled Study to Examine the Effects of DAS181 in Immunocompromised Subjects With Lower Respiratory Tract Parainfluenza Infection on Supplemental Oxygen (DAS181-2-05); 2012 July; [3 page]. https://clinicaltrials.gov/ct2/show/NCT01644877?term=das181&rank=5.

94. Englund JA, Boeckh M, Kuypers J, Nichols WG, Hackman RC, Morrow RA, Fredricks DN, Corey L. Brief communication: fatal human metapneumovirus infection in stem-cell transplant recipients. Ann Intern Med. 2006;144(5):344–9.

95. Kamboj M, Gerbin M, Huang CK, Brennan C, Stiles J, Balashov S, Park S, Kiehn TE, Perlin DS, Pamer EG, Sepkowitz KA. Clinical characterization of human metapneumovirus infection among patients with cancer. J Infect. 2008;57(6):464–71.

96. Chien JW, Martin PJ, Gooley TA, Flowers ME, Heckbert SR, Nichols WG, Clark JG. Airflow obstruction after myeloablative allogeneic hematopoietic stem cell transplantation. Am J Respir Crit Care Med. 2003;168(2):208–14.

97. Kim YJ, Boeckh M, Englund JA. Community respiratory virus infections in immunocompromised patients: hematopoietic stem cell and solid organ transplant recipients, and individuals with human immunodeficiency virus infection. Semin Respir Crit Care Med. 2007;28(2):222–42.

98. Harper SA, Bradley JS, Englund JA, File TM, Gravenstein S, Hayden FG, McGeer AJ, Neuzil KM, Pavia AT, Tapper ML, Uyeki TM, Zimmerman RK, Expert Panel of the Infectious Diseases Society of America. Seasonal influenza in adults and children—diagnosis, treatment, chemoprophylaxis, and institutional outbreak management: clinical practice guidelines of the Infectious Diseases Society of America. Clin Infect Dis. 2009;48(8):1003–32.

99. Kuo JH, Hwang R. Preparation of DNA dry powder for non-viral gene delivery by spray-freeze drying: effect of protective agents (polyethyleneimine and sugars) on the stability of DNA. J Pharm Pharmacol. 2004;56(1):27–33.

100. Hohlfeld J, Niedermeyer J, Hamm H, Schäfers HJ, Wagner TO, Fabel H. Seasonal onset of bronchiolitis obliterans syndrome in lung transplant recipients. J Heart Lung Transplant. 1996;15(9):888–94.

101. Armstrong C. ACIP releases recommendations for influenza vaccination, 2015-2016. Am Fam Physician. 2015;92(8):732–40.

102. Relenza® (zanamivir) [package insert]. Research Park, NC: GlaxoSmithKline; 2013.

103. Tamiflu® (oseltamivir) [package insert]. Foster City, CA: Roche; 2008.

104. Rapivab® (peramivir) [package insert]. Durham, NC: BioCryst Pharmaceuticals; 2014.

105. Centers for Disease Control and Prevention, N.C.f.I.a.R.D.N. Influenza antiviral medications: summary for clinicians. 2016 5/26/2016 6/27/2016.

106. Kaiser L, Aubert JD, Pache JC, Deffernez C, Rochat T, Garbino J, Wunderli W, Meylan P, Yerly S, Perrin L, Letovanec I, Nicod L, Tapparel C, Soccal PM. Chronic rhinoviral infection in lung transplant recipients. Am J Respir Crit Care Med. 2006;174(12):1392–9.

107. Martino R, Porras RP, Rabella N, Williams JV, Rámila E, Margall N, Labeaga R, Crowe JE Jr, Coll P, Sierra J. Prospective study of the incidence, clinical features, and outcome of symptomatic upper and lower respiratory tract infections by respiratory viruses in adult recipients of hematopoietic stem cell transplants for hematologic malignancies. Biol Blood Marrow Transplant. 2005;11(10):781–96.

108. van Kraaij MG, van Elden LJ, van Loon AM, Hendriksen KA, Laterveer L, Dekker AW, Nijhuis M. Frequent detection of respiratory viruses in adult recipients of stem cell transplants with the use of real-time polymerase chain reaction, compared with viral culture. Clin Infect Dis. 2005;40(5):662–9.

109. Roghmann M, Ball K, Erdman D, Lovchik J, Anderson LJ, Edelman R. Active surveillance for respiratory virus infections in adults who have undergone bone marrow and peripheral blood stem cell transplantation. Bone Marrow Transplant. 2003;32(11):1085–8.

110. Ison MG, Hayden FG, Kaiser L, Corey L, Boeckh M. Rhinovirus infections in hematopoietic stem cell transplant recipients with pneumonia. Clin Infect Dis. 2003;36(9):1139–43.

111. Hassan IA, Chopra R, Swindell R, Mutton KJ. Respiratory viral infections after bone marrow/peripheral stem-cell transplantation: the Christie hospital experience. Bone Marrow Transplant. 2003;32(1):73–7.

112. Ghosh S, Champlin R, Couch R, Englund J, Raad I, Malik S, Luna M, Whimbey E. Rhinovirus infections in myelosuppressed adult blood and marrow transplant recipients. Clin Infect Dis. 1999;29(3):528–32.

113. Michaels MG, Green M, Wald ER, Starzl TE. Adenovirus infection in pediatric liver transplant recipients. J Infect Dis. 1992;165(1):170–4.

114. Ohori NP, Michaels MG, Jaffe R, Williams P, Yousem SA. Adenovirus pneumonia in lung transplant recipients. Hum Pathol. 1995;26(10):1073–9.

115. Kojaoghlanian T, Flomenberg P, Horwitz MS. The impact of adenovirus infection on the immunocompromised host. Rev Med Virol. 2003;13(3):155–71.

116. Howard DS, Phillips GL II, Reece DE, Munn RK, Henslee-Downey J, Pittard M, Barker M, Pomeroy C. Adenovirus infections in hematopoietic stem cell transplant recipients. Clin Infect Dis. 1999;29(6):1494–501.

117. Carrigan DR. Adenovirus infections in immunocompromised patients. Am J Med. 1997;102(3A):71–4.

118. Ison MG. Adenovirus infections in transplant recipients. Clin Infect Dis. 2006;43(3):331–9.

119. Simsir A, Greenebaum E, Nuovo G, Schulman LL. Late fatal adenovirus pneumonitis in a lung transplant recipient. Transplantation. 1998;65(4):592–4.

120. Florescu DF, Hoffman JA, AST Infectious Diseases Community of Practice. Adenovirus in solid organ transplantation. Am J Transplant. 2013;13(Suppl 4):206–11.

121. Vistide® (cidofovir) [package insert]. Foster City, CA: Gilead Sciences; 2010.

122. Heugel J, Martin ET, Kuypers J, Englund JA. Coronavirus-associated pneumonia in previously healthy children. Pediatr Infect Dis J. 2007;26(8):753–5.

123. Pene F, Merlat A, Vabret A, Rozenberg F, Buzyn A, Dreyfus F, Cariou A, Freymuth F, Lebon P. Coronavirus 229E-related pneumonia in immunocompromised patients. Clin Infect Dis. 2003;37(7):929–32.

124. Campanini G, Rovida F, Meloni F, Cascina A, Ciccocioppo R, Piralla A, Baldanti F. Persistent human cosavirus infection in lung transplant recipient, Italy. Emerg Infect Dis. 2013;19(10):1667–9.

125. Bastien N, et al. Human Bocavirus infection, Canada. Emerg Infect Dis. 2006;12(5):848–50.

126. Schenk T, Strahm B, Kontny U, Hufnagel M, Neumann-Haefelin D, Falcone V. Disseminated bocavirus infection after stem cell transplant. Emerg Infect Dis. 2007;13(9):1425–7.

127. Miyakis S, van Hal SJ, Barratt J, Stark D, Marriott D, Harkness J. Absence of human Bocavirus in bronchoalveolar lavage fluid of lung transplant patients. J Clin Virol. 2009;44(2):179–80.

128. Snyder LD, Finlen-Copeland CA, Turbyfill WJ, Howell D, Willner DA, Palmer SM. Cytomegalovirus pneumonitis is a risk for bronchiolitis obliterans syndrome in lung transplantation. Am J Respir Crit Care Med. 2010;181(12):1391–6.

129. Patel N, Snyder LD, Finlen-Copeland A, Palmer SM. Is prevention the best treatment? CMV after lung transplantation. Am J Transplant. 2012;12(3):539–44.

130. Mitsani D, Nguyen MH, Girnita DM, Spichty K, Kwak EJ, Silveira FP, Toyoda Y, Pilewski JM, Crespo M, Bhama JK, Abdel-Massih R, Zaldonis D, Zeevi A, Clancy CJ. A polymorphism linked to elevated levels of interferon-gamma is associated with an increased risk of cytomegalovirus disease among Caucasian lung transplant recipients at a single center. J Heart Lung Transplant. 2011;30(5):523–9.

131. Duncan SR, Paradis IL, Yousem SA, Similo SL, Grgurich WF, Williams PA, Dauber JH, Griffith BP. Sequelae of cytomegalovirus pulmonary infections in lung allograft recipients. Am Rev Respir Dis. 1992;146(6):1419–25.

132. Torre-Cisneros J. Toward the individualization of cytomegalovirus control after solid-organ transplantation: the importance of the "individual pathogenic balance". Clin Infect Dis. 2009;49(8):1167–8.

133. Zuk DM, Humar A, Weinkauf JG, Lien DC, Nador RG, Kumar D. An international survey of cytomegalovirus management practices in lung transplantation. Transplantation. 2010;90(6):672–6.

134. Lisboa LF, Kumar D, Wilson LE, Humar A. Clinical utility of cytomegalovirus cell-mediated immunity in transplant recipients with cytomegalovirus viremia. Transplantation. 2012;93(2):195–200.

135. Kumar D, Chernenko S, Moussa G, Cobos I, Manuel O, Preiksaitis J, Venkataraman S, Humar A. Cell-mediated immunity to predict cytomegalovirus disease in high-risk solid organ transplant recipients. Am J Transplant. 2009;9(5):1214–22.

136. Razonable RR, Humar A, AST Infectious Diseases Community of Practice. Cytomegalovirus in solid organ transplantation. Am J Transplant. 2013;13(Suppl 4):93–106.

137. Clark NM, Lynch JP III, Sayah D, Belperio JA, Fishbein MC, Weigt SS. DNA viral infections complicating lung transplantation. Semin Respir Crit Care Med. 2013;34(3):380–404.

138. Asberg A, Humar A, Jardine AG, Rollag H, Pescovitz MD, Mouas H, Bignamini A, Töz H, Dittmer I, Montejo M, Hartmann A, VICTOR Study Group. Long-term outcomes of CMV disease treatment with valganciclovir versus IV ganciclovir in solid organ transplant recipients. Am J Transplant. 2009;9(5):1205–13.

139. Cytovene® (ganciclovir) [package insert]. San Francisco, CA: Genentech; 2010.

140. Valcyte® (valganciclovir) [package insert]. San Francisco, CA: Genentech; 2015.

141. Lucas GM, Ross MJ, Stock PG, Shlipak MG, Wyatt CM, Gupta SK, Atta MG, Wools-Kaloustian KK, Pham PA, Bruggeman LA, Lennox JL, Ray PE, Kalayjian RC, HIV Medicine Association of the Infectious Diseases Society of America. Clinical practice guideline for the management of chronic kidney disease in patients infected with HIV: 2014 update by the HIV Medicine Association of the Infectious Diseases Society of America. Clin Infect Dis. 2014;59(9):e96–138.

142. Palmer SM, Limaye AP, Banks M, Gallup D, Chapman J, Lawrence EC, Dunitz J, Milstone A, Reynolds J, Yung GL, Chan KM, Aris R, Garrity E, Valentine V, McCall J, Chow SC, Davis RD,

Avery R. Extended valganciclovir prophylaxis to prevent cytomegalovirus after lung transplantation: a randomized, controlled trial. Ann Intern Med. 2010;152(12):761–9.

143. Ramanan P, Razonable RR. Cytomegalovirus infections in solid organ transplantation: a review. Infect Chemother. 2013;45(3):260–71.

144. Carraro E, Perosa AH, Siqueira I, Pasternak J, Martino MD. Rotavirus infection in children and adult patients attending in a tertiary Hospital of Sao Paulo, Brazil. Braz J Infect Dis. 2008;12(1):44–6.

145. Le Page AK, Jager MM, Iwasenko JM, Scott GM, Alain S, Rawlinson WD. Clinical aspects of cytomegalovirus antiviral resistance in solid organ transplant recipients. Clin Infect Dis. 2013;56(7):1018–29.

146. Avery RK, Mossad SB, Poggio E, Lard M, Budev M, Bolwell B, Waldman WJ, Braun W, Mawhorter SD, Fatica R, Krishnamurthi V, Young JB, Shrestha R, Stephany B, Lurain N, Yen-Lieberman B. Utility of leflunomide in the treatment of complex cytomegalovirus syndromes. Transplantation. 2010;90(4):419–26.

147. Snydman DR. Leflunomide: a small step forward in meeting the urgent need for treatment of drug-resistant cytomegalovirus infection. Transplantation. 2010;90(4):362–3.

148. ClinicalTrials.gov [Internet]. Bethesda (MD); National Library of Medicine (US). 2012 Jun 1. Identifier NCT01611974, Maribavir for Treatment of Resistant or Refractory CMV Infections in Transplant Recipients; 2012 July; [3 page]. https://clinicaltrials.gov/ct2/show/study/NCT01611974?term=maribavir&rank=2.

149. ClinicalTrials.gov [Internet]. Bethesda (MD); National Library of Medicine (US). 2015 May 7. Identifier NCT02439957, SURPASS: a randomized, double-blind, multicenter study of the efficacy, safety, and tolerability of brincidofovir versus valganciclovir for the prevention of cytomegalovirus (CMV) disease in CMV seropositive kidney transplant recipients (BCV CMV vGCV) (BCV CMV vGCV) ; 2015 September; [3 page]. https://clinicaltrials.gov/ct2/show/record/NCT02439957?term=cmx001&rank=14.

150. Gottschalk S, Rooney CM, Heslop HE. Post-transplant lymphoproliferative disorders. Annu Rev Med. 2005;56:29–44.

151. Manuel O, Kumar D, Singer LG, Cobos I, Humar A. Incidence and clinical characteristics of herpes zoster after lung transplantation. J Heart Lung Transplant. 2008;27(1):11–6.

152. Reams BD, McAdams HP, Howell DN, Steele MP, Davis RD, Palmer SM. Posttransplant lymphoproliferative disorder: incidence, presentation, and response to treatment in lung transplant recipients. Chest. 2003;124(4):1242–9.

153. Stevens SJ, Verschuuren EA, Pronk I, van Der Bij W, Harmsen MC, The TH, Meijer CJ, van Den Brule AJ, Middeldorp JM. Frequent monitoring of Epstein-Barr virus DNA load in unfractionated whole blood is essential for early detection of posttransplant lymphoproliferative disease in high-risk patients. Blood. 2001;97(5):1165–71.

154. Green M, Michaels MG. Epstein-Barr virus infection and posttransplant lymphoproliferative disorder. Am J Transplant. 2013;13(Suppl 3):41–54; quiz 54.

155. Kumarasinghe G, Lavee O, Parker A, Nivison-Smith I, Milliken S, Dodds A, Joseph J, Fay K, Ma DD, Malouf M, Plit M, Havryk A, Keogh AM, Hayward CS, Kotlyar E, Jabbour A, Glanville AR, Macdonald PS, Moore JJ. Post-transplant lymphoproliferative disease in heart and lung transplantation: defining risk and prognostic factors. J Heart Lung Transplant. 2015;34(11):1406–14.

156. Pergam SA, Limaye AP, AST Infectious Diseases Community of Practice. Varicella zoster virus in solid organ transplantation. Am J Transplant. 2013;13(Suppl 4):138–46.

157. Wilck MB, Zuckerman RA, AST Infectious Diseases Community of Practice. Herpes simplex virus in solid organ transplantation. Am J Transplant. 2013;13(Suppl 4):121–7.

158. Zovirax® (acyclovir sodium) for Injection [package insert]. Research Triangle Park, NC: Glaxo Smith Kline; 2003.

159. Zovirax® (acyclovir) [package insert]. Research Tringle Park, NC: Glaxo Smith Kline; 2005.

160. Valtrex® (vlacyclovir) [package insert]. Research Tringle Park, NC: Glaxo Smith Kline; 2008.

161. Famvir® (famciclovir) [package insert]. East Hanover, NJ: Novartis; 2011.

162. Lehto JT, Halme M, Tukiainen P, Harjula A, Sipponen J, Lautenschlager I. Human herpesvirus-6 and -7 after lung and heart-lung transplantation. J Heart Lung Transplant. 2007;26(1):41–7.

163. Sathy SJ, Martinu T, Youens K, Lawrence CM, Howell DN, Palmer SM, Steele MP. Symptomatic pulmonary allograft Kaposi's sarcoma in two lung transplant recipients. Am J Transplant. 2008;8(9):1951–6.

164. Sleiman C, Mal H, Roué C, Groussard O, Baldeyrou P, Olivier P, Fournier M, Pariente R. Bronchial Kaposi's sarcoma after single lung transplantation. Eur Respir J. 1997;10(5):1181–3.

165. Kantor R, Mayan H, Shalmon B, Reichert N, Farfel Z. Kaposi's sarcoma after lung transplantation in a Sephardic Jewish woman. Dermatology. 2000;200(1):49–50.

166. Tereza Martinu DH, Reidy M, Palmer S. Disseminated Kaposi sarcoma in a lung transplant recipient with pulmonary, pleural, and cutaneous involvement. Chest conference 2006; 2006.

167. Kedes DH, Ganem D. Sensitivity of Kaposi's sarcoma-associated herpesvirus replication to antiviral drugs. Implications for potential therapy. J Clin Invest. 1997;99(9):2082–6.

168. Mocroft A, Youle M, Gazzard B, Morcinek J, Halai R, Phillips AN. Anti-herpesvirus treatment and risk of Kaposi's sarcoma in HIV infection. Royal Free/

Chelsea and Westminster Hospitals Collaborative Group. AIDS. 1996;10(10):1101–5.

169. Glesby MJ, Hoover DR, Weng S, Graham NM, Phair JP, Detels R, Ho M, Saah AJ. Use of antiherpes drugs and the risk of Kaposi's sarcoma: data from the Multicenter AIDS Cohort Study. J Infect Dis. 1996;173(6):1477–80.

170. Thomas LD, Vilchez RA, White ZS, Zanwar P, Milstone AP, Butel JS, Dummer S. A prospective longitudinal study of polyomavirus shedding in lung-transplant recipients. J Infect Dis. 2007;195(3):442–9.

171. Doucette KE, Pang XL, Jackson K, Burton I, Carbonneau M, Cockfield S, Preiksaitis JK. Prospective monitoring of BK polyomavirus infection early posttransplantation in nonrenal solid organ transplant recipients. Transplantation. 2008;85(12):1733–6.

172. Schwarz A, Mengel M, Haller H, Niedermeyer J. Polyoma virus nephropathy in native kidneys after lung transplantation. Am J Transplant. 2005;5(10):2582–5.

173. Thomas LD, Milstone AP, Vilchez RA, Zanwar P, Butel JS, Dummer JS. Polyomavirus infection and its impact on renal function and long-term outcomes after lung transplantation. Transplantation. 2009;88(3):360–6.

174. Viswesh V, Yost SE, Kaplan B. The prevalence and implications of BK virus replication in non-renal solid organ transplant recipients: a systematic review. Transplant Rev (Orlando). 2015;29(3):175–80.

175. Kariyawasam HH, Gyi K, Hodson M, Cohen B. Anaemia in lung transplant patient caused by parvovirus B19. Thorax. 2000;55(7):619–20.

176. Heegaard ED, Petersen BL, Heilmann CJ, Hornsleth A. Prevalence of parvovirus B19 and parvovirus V9 DNA and antibodies in paired bone marrow and serum samples from healthy individuals. J Clin Microbiol. 2002;40(3):933–6.

177. Jordan J, Tiangco B, Kiss J, Koch W. Human parvovirus B19: prevalence of viral DNA in volunteer blood donors and clinical outcomes of transfusion recipients. Vox Sang. 1998;75(2):97–102.

Lung Allograft Dysfunction (LAD) and Bronchiolitis Obliterans Syndrome

16

Bart Vanaudenaerde, Robin Vos, Stijn Verleden, Elly Vandermeulen, and Geert Verleden

Introduction

Survival after lung transplantation is substantially shorter than survival after transplantation of other solid organs [1]. This disparity in survival has been mainly attributed to chronic rejection, which represents a major complication limiting the 5-year survival to approximately 50% [2]. Initial examination of lung tissue from recipients with persistent decline in allograft function after lung transplantation showed a pathological narrowing or obliteration of the small airways (obliterative bronchiolitis, OB), which was perceived to be the histological manifestation of chronic rejection occurring through alloimmune mechanisms [3]. As histological diagnosis of OB on transbronchial lung biopsy has a low sensitivity and specificity, the International Society for Heart and Lung Transplantation (ISHLT) introduced bronchiolitis obliterans syndrome (BOS), defined as a persistent decline of the forced expiratory volume in 1 s (FEV_1) of at least 20% compared to the mean of the two best postoperative measurements [4]. However, a number of allograft abnormalities are also able to cause a persistent decline in FEV_1, as previously described in 2001 by Estenne and colleagues [4]. Within the last decade, the lung transplant community repeatedly acknowledged that a substantial cohort of patients had a chronic FEV_1 decline after lung transplantation for which the previous definition of BOS was not the best descriptor [5]. Additional presentations resulting in a chronic allograft dysfunction (FEV_1 decline) after lung transplantation led to the introduction of a new classification system that can help in recognizing distinct entities with important differences in their clinical manifestations and pathobiology [6]. An umbrella term chronic lung allograft dysfunction (CLAD) was introduced to facilitate diagnosis and treatment of chronic allograft dysfunction [7]. Chronic rejection is by definition CLAD, but not all CLAD is chronic rejection as

B. Vanaudenaerde (✉)
Laboratory of Respiratory Diseases, Department of Clinical and Experimental Medicine, Katholieke Universiteit Leuven, Leuven, Belgium
e-mail: bart.vanaudenaerde@med.kuleven.be

R. Vos
Laboratory of Respiratory Diseases, Department of Clinical and Experimental Medicine, Katholieke Universiteit Leuven, Leuven, Belgium

Lung Transplant and Respiratory Intermediate Care Unit, Department of Respiratory Medicine, University Hospitals Leuven, Leuven, Belgium
e-mail: robin.vos@uzleuven.be

S. Verleden · E. Vandermeulen
Department of Clinical and Experimental Medicine, Katholieke Universiteit Leuven, Leuven, Belgium
e-mail: stijn.verleden@med.kuleuven.be; elly.vandermeulen@kuleuven.be

G. Verleden
Lung Transplantation Unit, University Hospital Gasthuisberg, Leuven, Belgium
e-mail: geert.verleden@uzleuven.be

© The Author(s) 2018
G. Raghu, R. G. Carbone (eds.), *Lung Transplantation*, https://doi.org/10.1007/978-3-319-91184-7_16

there can be another distinctive cause of the persistent decline in pulmonary function.

Chronic Lung Allograft Dysfunction (CLAD)

Late persistent allograft dysfunction, with progressive loss of pulmonary function and finally graft loss, was originally described in the first long-term survivor following lung transplantation (LTx), performed by Derom and colleagues in 1969 [8]. It was and remains one of the major problems hampering long-term outcome with a prevalence of 50% 5 years after lung transplantation and an associated mortality of 50% at 5 years [9]. However, some confusion remained concerning the terminology "OB" as it is also used in the non-lung transplant setting with histopathological findings, including the presence of intraluminal tissue proliferation and polyp formation by (myo-)fibroblasts but also collagen deposition within the alveolar ducts and spaces with varying degrees of bronchiolar involvement, currently also named proliferative bronchiolitis; bronchiolitis obliterans with organizing pneumonia (BOOP); cryptogenic organizing pneumonia (COP); or subepithelial fibrosis with fibrotic narrowing of the bronchiolar lumen, also named constrictive bronchiolitis [5]. In 1993, BOS was defined as a persistent loss of allograft function following lung transplantation, which could not be explained by other potentially reversible complications, such as acute rejection, infection, or bronchial suture problems. A $\geq$ 20% decline in FEV_1 from the best postoperative baseline, assessed by 2 measurements with a $\geq$ 3 weeks interval, was considered to be diagnostic for BOS diagnosis, and a further classification of different disease severity was introduced: BOS grade 1 was defined as FEV_1 decline between 66 and 80% of baseline, BOS grade 2 as FEV_1 51–65% of baseline, and BOS grade 3 as $FEV_1 \leq$ 50% of baseline (Table 16.1). After a revision of the BOS concept, BOS grade 0p ("potential BOS") was added (FEV_1 81–90% and/or an FEF25–75 value of $\leq$75% of baseline) with the aim to start early diagnostic procedures and treatment [4]. During

Table 16.1 Diagnostic criteria/diagnostic staging for bronchiolitis obliterans syndrome and restrictive allograft syndrome

Diagnostic stage for BOS	Diagnostic criteria for BOS	Center
BOS 0	$FEV_1 >$ 90% of baseline	St Louis (Cooper JD et al.; 1993) [3]
BOS Op	FEV_1 between 81 and 90% and/or an FEF_{25-75} value of $\leq$75% of baseline	Brussels (Estenne M; 2002) [4]
BOS 1	FEV_1 decline between 66 and 80% of baseline	
BOS 2	FEV_1 51–65% of baseline	
BOS 3	$FEV_1 \leq$ 50% of baseline	
	Diagnostic criteria for RAS	**Center**
	TLC decline $\geq$10% vs baseline	Toronto (Sato M et al.; 2011) [11]
	FVC decline $\geq$20%	Duke (Todd J et al.; 2014) [37]
	TLC decline >10% or FEV1/FVC >0.70	Leuven (Verleden S et al.; 2014) [6]
	TLC > 10% or TLC > 20% + CT	Hannover (Suhling H et al.; 2012) [13]

the past decades, BOS was generally accepted to be the manifestation of chronic rejection, representing the immune response of the receptor to the foreign donor lung graft including an innate immune and adaptive immune involvement as described by fundamental transplant immunologists like Sir Peter Medawar and Sir Edward Donnall [9]. This immune involvement included both chronic humoral and cell-mediated responses of the recipient, leading to irreversible tissue fibrosis, failure of the organ, and, eventually, graft loss. Extensive research has focused on BOS since its first observation, yet its exact etiology and pathogenesis remain elusive. Terminologies, mechanisms, and diagnostic criteria have been introduced and evolved over the years trying to get a grip on this dysfunction, to facilitate adequate diagnosis and treatment and to maximize the outcome for the patient. Although much progress has been made, also a lot of confusion has been generated.

In analogy with CLAD following liver transplantation, in 2010 Allan Glanville introduced the term CLAD in the lung transplant literature as an overarching term embracing all forms of chronic lung dysfunction [7]. CLAD defines all lung allografts not achieving or no longer maintaining normal function for a defined period of time [6] (Fig. 16.1). Every effort should be made to identify the specific cause of the persistent decline in pulmonary function in the hope that appropriate and successful therapeutic interventions can be done to restore and optimize graft function [5]. Various conditions may underlie CLAD, and CLAD is therefore not restricted to chronic rejection. It is suggested that diagnosis of CLAD does not (and cannot) make any assumptions regarding the potential reversibility or irreversibility of the underlying causes of allograft dysfunction, nor is the term CLAD so specific as

to justify its use as a diagnosis. By definition, all cases of bronchiolitis obliterans syndrome (BOS) are included, which represents about 70% of the CLAD diagnoses without specific causes [10]. Patients with BOS demonstrate a strictly obstructive pulmonary function decline (Fig. 16.2a, b), with typical air trapping and mosaic attenuation on chest CT, while histopathology demonstrates almost exclusively OB surrounded by normal-appearing lung parenchyma (Table 16.2; Fig. 16.3a, b). On the other hand, approximately 30% of patients identified with CLAD without specific causes develop a restrictive pulmonary function defect (Fig. 16.2a, b) (rCLAD) or also described as restrictive allograft syndrome (RAS) by the Toronto group [11]. Typical radiological and histopathological characteristics of rCLAD include persistent infiltrates as well as (sub)pleural and septal thickening on chest computed tomography (CT) and pleuroparenchymal fibroelastosis and concurrent obliterative bronchiolitis (OB) on histopathological examination (Table 16.2; Fig. 16.3a, b) [10]. Patients with rCLAD suffer from a far worse prognosis

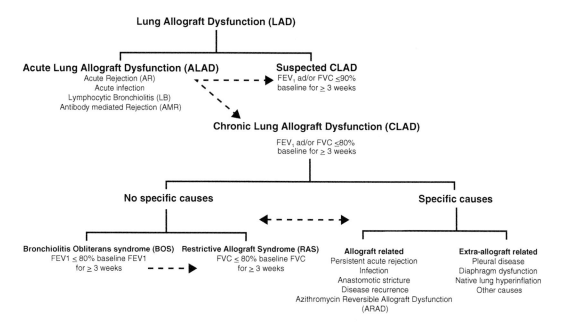

Fig. 16.1 A flow diagram demonstrating the diversity within chronic lung allograft dysfunction (CLAD) including the unknown causes including chronic rejection phenotype BOS and RAS and the known causes of CLAD including the allograft and non-allograft related

presentations (Adapted with permission of Elsevier from Verleden GM, Raghu G, Meyer KC, Glanville AR, Corris P. A new classification system for chronic lung allograft dysfunction. J Heart Lung Transplant 2014 Feb;33(2):127–33)

Fig. 16.2 (**a, b**) The lung function evolution of a lung transplant patient with BOS (**a**) and RAS (**b**) including FEV_1 and TLC. The red line represents the moment of diagnosis of CLAD

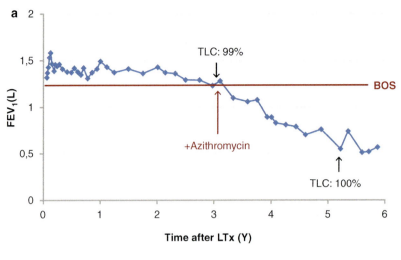

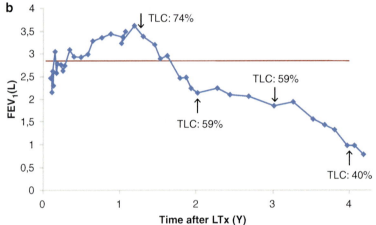

(6–18 months) after diagnosis versus patients with BOS (median survival 3 years) [12]. Some patients can evolve from BOS to RAS in a later stage [6] (Fig. 16.1), and therefore it is speculated that both BOS and RAS are in fact different phenotypes of chronic rejection.

Besides the predominant phenotypes, BOS and RAS (rCLAD) without specific causes, also other less frequent allograft- and extra-allograft-related reasons for a declining graft function are included within CLAD [6] (Fig. 16.1). Up to now the frequency of these different CLAD presentations is unknown. For example, chronic graft infection can also lead to a sustained decline in pulmonary function. Appropriate treatment of infection may lead to improved allograft function. Alternatively, patients may present a sustained pulmonary function decline and a restrictive

physiology (increased FEV_1/FVC ratio) due to size mismatch of the donor organ with the recipient chest cavity, obesity, or pleural problems, and hence these patients may be considered as having CLAD. Even a lung that does not achieve normal function (for instance, due to previously severe primary graft dysfunction) could be diagnosed with CLAD even if the FEV_1 is slowly improving but remains with a function that is significantly decreased when measured against predicted normal physiologic indices. Such a patient series with an early obstructive pulmonary function after bilateral lung transplantation was recently described by Suhling and colleagues [13]. Therefore, the term CLAD may also be used in this situation, although it would most often be used to describe loss of function from the best posttransplant FEV_1 achieved once the function

Table 16.2 The features of the different chronic lung allograft dysfunction phenotypes

	BOS	RAS
Clinically	No coarse crackles, minimal sputa	Minimal coarse crackles
	Typically progressive but may stabilize	Tends to be relentlessly progressive
	Recipients may have coexistent chronic bacterial infection	May start as or coincide with BOS
	May evolve to RAS	
Time of onset	Onset late after transplantation	Onset late after transplantation
Azithromycin	Irreversible	Irreversible
Pulmonary function	Obstructive ($FEV_1 \leq 80\%$ of baseline value)	Restrictive ($TLC \leq 90\%$ of baseline) and/or FEV_1/FVC normal or increased (with FEV_1 and/or FVC decline $\leq 80\%$ of baseline)
Radiology	Air trapping usually present	Consolidation, reticular pattern, infiltrates
	No/minimal infiltrates	With/without bronchiectasis
	With/without bronchiectasis	With/without air trapping
Histopathology	Obliterans bronchiolitis (OB) but (difficult to diagnose by transbronchial biopsy specimen)	Parenchymal/septal/pleural fibrosis with OB
Survival	Rapid progression (half a year)	Rapid progression (half a year)
Immune involvement	Moderate	Severe–organized
Other	Usually responds poorly to pharmacologic therapies	Correlates with the presence of early DAD posttransplant

Data from Verleden SE, Ruttens D, Vandermeulen E, Bellon H, Van Raemdonck DE, Dupont LJ, et al. Restrictive chronic lung allograft dysfunction: Where are we now? J Heart Lung Transplant. 2015 May;34 (5):625–30

Fig. 16.3 (**a**, **b**) An illustration of both phenotypes of CLAD being BOS (**a**) and RAS (**b**) by HRCT upper panel and microCT and histological imaging in the lower panels. In BOS, there is only OB lesions, with normal surrounding parenchyma, whereas in RAS there is scarring and thickening of the pleura, with fibrotic areas on CT and microCT scan and gross parenchymal fibrotic lesions on pathology

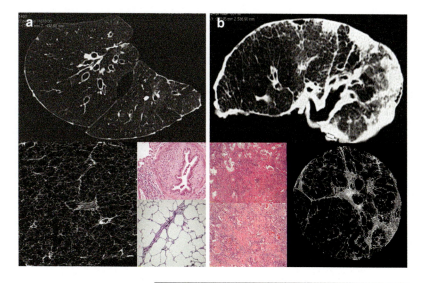

of the implanted allograft has stabilized. Also issues of persistent acute rejection, anastomotic stricture, disease recurrence, diaphragm dysfunction, native lung hyperinflation, and azithromycin-responsive airway neutrophilia (ARAD; previously considered as part of BOS) can be part of CLAD (Fig. 16.1). CLAD is more than just chronic rejection and may not "per se" be considered as irreversible.

Diagnosis and Clinical Presentation

After CLAD diagnosis, an evaluation to determine the reasons why the lung function has decreased is crucial (Fig. 16.1). Although the term "chronic" reflects a process that takes at least 3 weeks to develop, it is recommended to investigate the cause of the declining pulmonary function as soon as it was detected in order not to withheld potential therapies that might improve/restore lung function. As such, a decline of 10% in FEV_1 and/or FVC from stable baseline function (suspected CLAD) should already trigger further investigation to identify a possible cause. When CLAD is the likely cause of FEV_1 decline (>20% from baseline) by exclusion of other conditions, further investigation is definitely needed to gather additional information that facilitates the identification of specific CLAD phenotypes. Such investigations must include full pulmonary function testing, bronchoscopy with transbronchial and endobronchial biopsies, bronchoalveolar lavage (BAL) with viral/bacterial/fungal cultures and total and differential cell count, and CT thorax with inspiratory and expiratory imaging [6]. Only by this multidisciplinary approach, it will be possible to distinguish the different phenotypes of CLAD. Figure 16.1 gives a schematic overview of CLAD and its different subtypes.

For BOS/OB the only definite diagnosis is obliterative or constrictive bronchiolitis on pathologic analysis. Characteristic lesions of BO are patchily distributed throughout both lungs without any definite pattern, which may obscure definite diagnosis. BOS is a strictly clinical definition using serial pulmonary function testing to aid in the diagnosis of suspected lung allograft dysfunction. Signs of air trapping and mosaic attenuation on expiratory CT images are considered to be typical for BOS as well (Table 16.2; Fig. 16.3a, b).

Given the low specificity to detect small airway diseases and early interstitial changes using conventional imaging techniques, novel imaging techniques are being developed. One of these is microcomputed tomography (microCT), which allows (ex vivo) scanning of lung tissue specimens at very high resolution. MicroCT has confirmed that constrictive bronchiolitis in end-stage BOS mainly affects smaller conducting airways in a segmental pattern, while sparing larger airways as well as terminal bronchioles and the alveolar surface [14] (Fig. 16.3a, b). These findings were corroborated by histologic reconstruction of the bronchiolar lesions in BO. Another new imaging technique is parametric response mapping using high-resolution (helical) CT of inspiration and expiration, which permits visual representation of the lung affected by obstructive disease versus the lung tissue with normal aeration or restrictive disease [15]. This technique will likely become a valuable diagnostic tool in the future, especially in patients in whom lung function differences are difficult to interpret such as single-lung transplant patients or anastomosis dehiscence [16]. Similarly, magnetic resonance imaging, in which measurement of oxygen transfer function can be assessed, may serve as an early marker for detection of small airways obstruction [17].

Woodrow introduce the term restrictive BOS, based on a decrease of the FVC of at least 20% (accompanied by a concomitant decrease in FEV_1) [12]. His study, however, could not demonstrate a survival disadvantage for the patients suffering from a restrictive pulmonary function, probably due to exclusion of patients with persistent infiltrates which we now consider to be typical for restrictive CLAD patients. The Toronto group introduced restrictive allograft syndrome (RAS) for patients suffering from a persistent decline in FEV_1 (> 20% compared with the best postoperative values) and an associated restrictive pulmonary function defect, defined as a decline in total lung capacity (TLC) > 10% [11] (Table 16.1). As TLC is not routinely measured in most centers, the Duke group used the forced vital capacity (FVC), while we proposed to add the FEV_1/FVC ratio as a surrogate marker for restriction [18] (Table 16.1). If the latter remains stable while the FEV_1 drops, this may also point to a restrictive pulmonary function. In that respect, Sato and colleagues demonstrated a good correlation between FEV_1/FVC ratio and TLC decline [19]. Recently, the Hannover group have also proposed to add CT infiltrates as a diagnostic criteria as CT scan in RAS patients shows more interstitial opacities, ground-glass opacities, upper-lobe-dominant fibrosis, and honeycombing [13] (Table 16.1). RAS is further characterized by pleuroparenchymal fibroelastosis (PPFE) and OB on histopathology. In one of our recent studies, we found that patients with upper-lobe-dominant infiltrates have a superior survival compared to patients with lower lobe and diffuse infiltrates [20] (Table 16.1). Interestingly, there might be a large overlap between patients with diffuse parenchymal infiltrates and patients diagnosed with acute fibrinoid organizing pneumonia (AFOP) . This is a strictly pathological diagnosis and evident by acute fibrin deposition in the alveoli and is associated with a particular bad prognosis (0.3 year in the study by Paraskeva and colleagues) [21].

Risk Factors

Numerous studies established risk factors for BOS (currently regarded as CLAD) including immune factors and nonimmune factors [22], such as persistent elevated bronchoalveolar lavage (BAL) neutrophilia and interleukin (IL)-8 [23], acute rejection [24], lymphocytic bronchiolitis (LB) [25], infection [26], cytomegalovirus status [27], donor-specific antibodies [28], air pollution [29, 30], donor age, ischemic time, primary graft dysfunction, medication nonadherence [31], colonization with pseudomonas [32, 33], gastroesophageal reflux [34], and increased plasma C-reactive protein (CRP) [35]. However, all risk factors were established considering the old definition of BOS, incorporating all different phenotypes of CLAD, which most certainly will have a major impact on the results. Only recently some investigators tried to unravel specific risk factors for RAS for instance, although this was only investigated monocentric and includes gender, age, LB, acute rejection, pulmonary infection, pseudomonas colonization, and CMV mismatch [11, 36–38]. A new promising risk factor could be BAL eosinophilia. Indeed, in 82% of the patients with RAS, an increased BAL eosinophilia (>2%) was observed, which was associated with a rapid evolution toward RAS and death [39]. At diagnosis of RAS, an increased BAL IL-6 and CXCL10 was detected, whereas VEGF was downregulated, and these mediators correlated with survival after diagnosis [40]. Two studies identified late-onset DAD as a risk factor for RAS, whereas early-onset DAD rather predisposed to BOS. Within these studies, an involvement of the CXCR3 axis, controlling chemoattraction of mononuclear cells, was identified via increased concentrations of CXCL9, CXCL10, and CXCL11 (CXCR3 ligands) in BAL when DAD was diagnosed on biopsy, and prolonged increased levels of these chemokines predicted subsequent CLAD [41]. Recently, alarmins like S100 protein, which are important pro-inflammatory molecules, have also been demonstrated to be upregulated in BAL of RAS patients [42]. However, most risk factors for RAS have also been associated with BOS, and the abovementioned factors have not been validated yet to discriminate between BOS and RAS. It is clear that larger studies with uniform diagnostic criteria are necessary to identify risk factors for both RAS and BOS which might be able to discriminate between these two phenotypes of CLAD. One recent study from our group was able to discriminate RAS from BOS by increased levels of immunoglubulines in BAL which needs further investigation [43].

Mechanisms

The mechanisms of BOS (Fig. 16.4) causing the typical small airway obliterations have not been completely unraveled. Bronchioles typically do not have cartilage, glands, or goblet cells. Bronchioles are arranged in parallel, which maximizes cross-sectional area while minimizing their contribution to overall airflow resistance in the healthy lung. Recent evidence demonstrates that these obliterations are only segmental, that is, with a patent lumen more distal from the OB lesion, leading to normal terminal bronchioles and parenchyma, which may explain the low sensitivity of transbronchial biopsy procedures to detect OB. In lungs with end-stage BOS, 40–60% of the peripheral airways are affected by OB starting from the sixth generation of airway branching and increasing in more distal generations [14]. The current hypothesis proposes that an acute or repeated epithelial cell injury and innate immune responses to environmental insults (i.e., infection, particulate matter) is the most important driving factor, yet local mucosal inflammation, epithelial to mesenchymal transition, and also loss of epithelial progenitor cells (basal cells and clara cells)

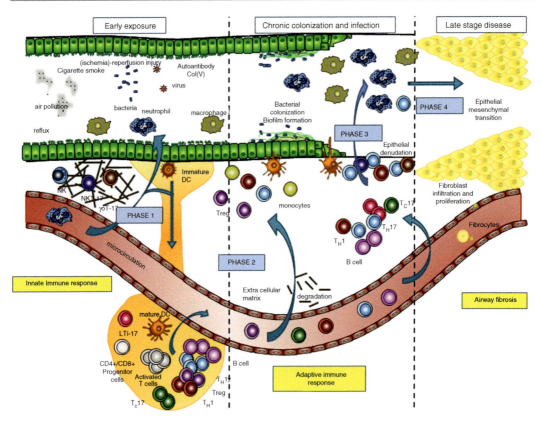

Fig. 16.4 The proposed mechanism of BOS starting with early innate involvement and mild adaptive involvement restricted to the small airway that will eventually turn into fibrotic plug and obliterated airways

have been implicated in abnormal re-epithelialization and subsequent fibrotic response [10, 44]. As such, injury and inflammation of the bronchiolar epithelium and subepithelial structures induces tissue repair mechanisms and activation of the adaptive immune system. However, this tissue repair is seemingly disproportionate and aberrant as it gives rise to excessive fibroproliferation within or around the bronchioles, causing airway dysfunction [10]. These OB lesions consist of fibroblasts, myofibroblasts, and extracellular matrix. The fibroblast may originate from proliferation or recruitment of resident fibroblasts; the dedifferentiation of airway epithelial cells to mesenchymal cells (epithelial to mesenchymal transition, EMT) or from circulating progenitors called fibrocytes [45, 46]. Apart from this fibroblast recruitment, activation of the immune system is also crucial in OB, which is considered to be the end result of overt innate and adaptive immune

responses with neutrophilic inflammation as a key player [23]. Stimulation of airway smooth muscle cells and bronchial epithelial cells with IL-17 induces IL-8 production, a key neutrophil chemoattractant, and matrix metalloproteinases (MMP-2, MMP-3, MMP-7, MMP-8, and MMP-9) leading to local oxidative stress, tissue damage, and airway remodeling [47–49]. Interestingly, recent studies indicate that infusion of mice with Ka1-tubulin or collagen type-V antibodies leads to an increase in IL-17 and graft inflammation and fibrosis, indicating that IL-17 might be an important link between the innate and adaptive immune responses (both cellular and humoral), eventually leading to graft loss [50]. Regulatory T (Treg) cells balance Th17 cells and serve as important players in maintaining tissue homeostasis and maintaining tolerance. A decrease in Treg cells is associated with BOS, although this could not be confirmed in biopsies [51, 52]. Despite the increasing evidence for the role of IL-17 [53], it is very unlikely to be the only mechanism inducing neutrophilic airway inflammation [54]. Interestingly, hyaluronan also promotes neutrophilic inflammation through stimulation of Toll-like receptors. Hyaluronan was elevated in the BAL fluid, blood, and tissue of patients with BOS, whereas inhibition of hyaluronan resulted in increased organ acceptance [55].

On the other hand, the mechanisms of RAS remain mostly elusive as mechanistic studies have not been performed yet. We recently reinvestigated important immunological cells and mediators in phenotypes of CLAD (BOS and RAS) by studying on the one hand end-stage human lung biopsies and on the other hand BAL samples at diagnosis of CLAD. Our findings support RAS as more representative of the true immune presentation of chronic rejection, characterized by a cellular and a humoral immune involvement (Fig. 16.5a, b). The immunological

mechanism of chronic rejection includes a variety of cellular and humoral processes, in which also antibody-mediated complement lysis, delayed-type hypersensitivity (DTH), and antibody-dependent cell-mediated cytotoxicity (ADCC) are involved [9]. In general, T-helper (CD4) and cytotoxic T (CD8) lymphocytes recognize alloantigens (primarily through major histocompatibility complex (MHC) molecules) present on cells of the foreign graft and proliferate in a sensitization phase. Activation of T-helper cells is the result of the interaction with an antigen-presenting cell (macrophages, dendritic cells, and B-cells) that expresses both appropriate alloantigen/MHC class II molecule complex and costimulatory molecules [9]. Dendritic cells are unique as they can cross-present exogenous alloantigens in class I MHC molecules to CD8+ T lymphocytes and induce direct cytotoxicity. Macrophages are not only antigen-presenting cells but can serve as effector cells by releasing

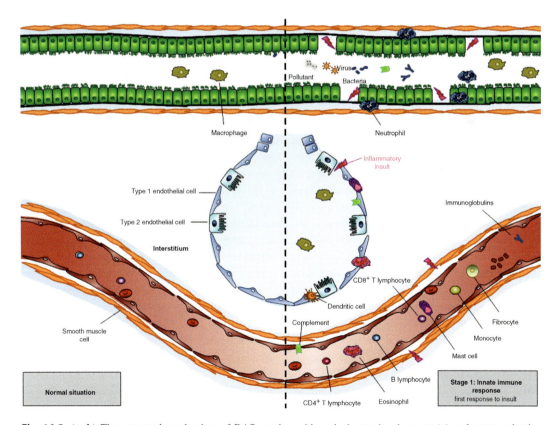

Fig. 16.5 (**a, b**) The proposed mechanism of RAS starting with early innate involvement (**a**) and severe adaptive involvement (**b**) all over the lung resulting in pleural/septal, parenchymal and, airway fibrosis

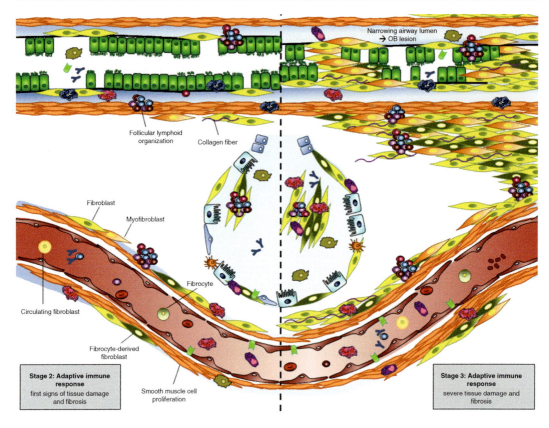

Narrowing airway lumen
→ OB lesion

Follicular lymphoid
organization   Collagen fiber

Fibroblast

Myofibroblast

Fibrocyte

Circulating fibroblast

Fibrocyte-derived
fibroblast

**Stage 2: Adaptive immune
response**
first signs of tissue damage
and fibrosis

Smooth muscle cell
proliferation

**Stage 3: Adaptive immune
response**
severe tissue damage and
fibrosis

Fig. 16.5 (continued)

lytic enzymes orchestrating ADCC [56]. Other effectors of the myeloid arm of the immune response of chronic rejection driven by T-helper cells (specific subsets) are neutrophils, eosinophils, and mast cells which can attack the allograft [9]. In general, a Th2 response is characterized by the release of IL-4, IL-5, IL-13, and CCL11/eotaxin promoting the activation of mast cells and eosinophils, which were demonstrated to be predominantly present in RAS [43]. Excessive pro-inflammatory mediators like histamine, oxygen radicals, cytotoxic cationic proteins, and cytokines cause pulmonary tissue damage. When this inflammatory response is persistent, tissue remodeling can occur via a pro-fibrotic Th2 polarized inflammation by the release of cytokines [57] and growth factors (TGF-β, PDGF, or GM-CSF) attracting fibroblasts to the site of inflammation [58, 59]. For these reasons, mast cells and eosinophils can be associated with fibrosis, being largely represented in

RAS. Eosinophils and mast cells may be attracted by *Aspergillus* species that release antigens promoting a Th2 response [60, 61]. In our own transplant cohort, we indeed noticed that most RAS patients were colonized with *Aspergillus* species (e.g., *Aspergillus fumigatus*). As already mentioned before, we have demonstrated that BAL eosinophilia is increased in RAS and was associated with worse survival [20]. In our explant biopsies, we could confirm that there is an increased tissue eosinophilia around the blood vessels in RAS compared to BOS, suggesting an increased migration rate of eosinophils out of the blood stream [62]. As explained earlier, the presence of neutrophils, which are also increased in BAL of RAS patients, can be triggered via pseudomonal airway colonization and subsequent IL-8 production [63]. Neutrophils can cause severe epithelial damage by release of airway remodeling proteins (MMP) consistent with our findings of the increased amount of neutrophils around the airways and MMPs, in both BOS and RAS [62]. T-helper cells can also activate B-cell maturation and proliferation into antibody-secreting plasma cells. The immunoglobulins can bind to specific Ig receptors, present on effector cells, causing antigen destruction via opsonization, neutralization, complement activation, or phagocytosis [64–66], depending on the specific function of the effector cell. Complement proteins complete the action of antibodies evolving to antibody-mediated rejection (AMR) [67]. Our findings demonstrated that complement proteins and immunoglobulins, including donor-specific antibodies (DSA), were predominantly increased in BAL of RAS patients, pointing to activation of B cells and additionally suggesting that there might be an overlap between RAS and AMR. The presence of DSA in the RAS phenotype might contribute to the increased mortality in RAS, as DSAs are associated with an increased risk of CLAD leading to a worse survival [68–70]. Experimental evidence concerning the role of B cells in lung transplant rejection is mostly derived from mouse models; B-cell knockout mice showed less obliterative airways disease following anti-MHC I administration [71], and in the mouse heterotopic trachea transplant model [72], an early increase in lymphocytes is seen before the tracheal lumen is obliterated with extracellular matrix, possibly mediated by an increased TGF-β production. Additional in vitro data demonstrated that HLA antibodies can activate airway epithelial cells and consequently induce the release of soluble growth factors, stimulate fibroblast proliferation, and induce epithelial cell apoptosis which participate in OB development [73, 74]. Besides epithelial cell damage, endothelial disruption occurs via interaction of DSAs to the graft endothelium promoting complement activation and deposition [64, 75, 76].

Inflammatory cells involved in the pathogenesis of BOS and RAS will produce a cascade of pro-inflammatory mediators leading to irreversible tissue remodeling causing airway (BOS/RAS) (Fig. 16.4), parenchymal (RAS), and perivascular fibrosis (RAS) [11, 77] (Fig. 16.5a, b). This tissue remodeling is characterized by collagen production of fibroblasts and extracellular matrix deposition that may be controlled by TGF-β, produced by cells of leukocyte lineage.

All cellular and humoral elements of chronic rejection together with extensive fibrosis are clearly present in RAS and to a much lesser degree in BOS, which was up to now considered to reflect chronic rejection. This possible change in concept, where chronic rejection may clinically present as RAS, raises the question what BOS exactly is and why it develops in transplanted lungs.

Therapy

Several therapies have been tested in the setting of BOS, however, with limited success. Only macrolide therapy (mostly azithromycin) has made it to the routine clinical practice, as this is able to reduce airway inflammation and more specifically IL-17, IL-8, and associated airway neutrophilia [54], leading to a stabilization or even increase in pulmonary function in a subset of patients. Other working mechanisms include strengthening of macrophages to resist oxidative damage and inhibition of EMT [78]. Therefore, it is recommended by a panel of experts to start azithromycin therapy as soon as BOS is suspected and a decline in FEV_1 is observed [68]. Prophylactic therapy with azithromycin also reduced the prevalence of BOS, suppressing airway and systemic inflammation [79]. A post hoc analysis of Vos and colleagues study demonstrated that the beneficial effects of prophylactic azithromycin treatment persisted up to 7 years after transplant with a prolonged BOS-free survival [80].

Other therapies aim to reduce existing autoantibodies and HLA antibodies. For example, preemptive depletion of HLA antibodies with rituximab (anti-CD20, depletes B cells) and/or intravenous immunoglobulins resulted in a lower incidence of BOS [28], and case reports with bortezomib (a proteasome inhibitor) [81] showed some FEV_1 stabilization. An aggressive desensitization approach using intravenous immunoglobulins, plasmapheresis, Solu-Medrol, bortezomib, and rituximab, however, did not lead to a significant reduction in pre-transplant HLA antibodies

[82]. A promising way to eliminate these antibodies may be extracorporeal photopheresis (ECP), a therapy during which leucocytes are treated ex vivo with 8-methoxypsoralen and UV light, which induces leukocyte apoptosis. A recent study showed that ECP was associated with a decreased level of donor-specific anti-HLA antibodies and auto-antibodies, while reducing the concentration of pro-inflammatory cytokines and increasing anti-inflammatory cytokines [83]. Clinically, ECP treatment results in attenuation of the decrease in FEV$_1$ following BOS onset and in some patients even an improvement, while it increases survival [84]. Especially those patients with azithromycin-resistant neutrophilia at BOS development had the most benefit of ECP treatment [84]. However, there are no randomized placebo-controlled trials to confirm that the observed effects are due to the therapy and not to the natural course of BOS. Other therapies are supported by an even lower body of evidence. Pilot or case studies demonstrated beneficial effects of montelukast [78] and pirfenidone [85], but their true value remains to be established. In the end, lung re-transplantation remains the only definitive treatment option in well-selected patients with end-stage BOS. However, the survival of those patients remains inferior compared to the survival after initial transplantation which is probably the reason why this procedure is only rarely performed [86].

Since RAS patients suffer from a poor prognosis after diagnosis, research to identify adequate treatment is urgently needed. In that perspective, several attempts have already been made to treat or at least slow down RAS progression, but most studies are based on only one or a few patients. Pirfenidone is an anti-fibrotic drug approved for treatment for idiopathic pulmonary fibrosis. Recently, a case report demonstrated that addition of pirfenidone may slow the evolution of RAS [87]. As inflammation plays an important role, depletion of T cells and B cells can be a way to treat RAS. A drug that could be beneficial is alemtuzumab (Campath-1H), which is an antagonist of CD52, a protein expressed on B cells, lymphocytes, dendritic cells, and monocytes. This drug was found to improve interstitial

changes and lung function in four patients who likely had RAS [88]. ECP is probably not a good treatment option as its use in RAS patients did not lead to a stabilization or increase in pulmonary function [84]. At present, these treatment options remain anecdotal, and other treatment options are necessary as preliminary evidence has shown that re-transplantation may not be an adequate therapeutic solution for patients with RAS, with a 3-year survival after re-transplantation limited to 34% compared with 68% in patients with BOS [89].

Conclusion

Chronic lung allograft dysfunction (CLAD) has entered the field of lung transplantation to embrace different causes of a persistent decrease in pulmonary function, including chronic rejection and its phenotyping BOS and RAS. Although BOS is very well described as a progressive obstructive pulmonary function defect, its exact pathophysiology and treatment options are still debatable. The diagnostic criteria for RAS as a restrictive pulmonary function defect need to be refined so that they can easily be used worldwide. Although the prevalence of RAS is some 25–30% among all patients with chronic rejection, reports are varying much between centers, which can so far not be explained. Although the prognosis of RAS is worse compared to BOS, this seems not to be the case for every patient with RAS. Specific risk factors and mechanistic clues for BOS and RAS are emerging; however, no real treatment options exist, although it became apparent that re-transplantation for RAS carries a worse prognosis compared to the re-transplantation for BOS. Subtyping of CLAD is also time-specific and can change along the course of the disease, as some patients may evolve from one phenotype to the other, especially from BOS to RAS. We definitely need prospective multicenter studies tackling all these questions about phenotyping, diagnosis, mechanisms, risk factors, and most of all treatment. Only then, we may further improve the outcome of our lung transplant patients with chronic rejection.

References

1. Sayegh MH, Carpenter CB. Transplantation 50 years later—progress, challenges, and promises. N Engl J Med. 2004;351(26):2761–6.
2. Goldfarb SB, Levvey BJ, Edwards LB, Dipchand AI, Kucheryavaya AY, Lund LH, et al. The Registry of the International Society for Heart and Lung Transplantation: nineteenth pediatric lung and heart-lung transplantation report-2016; focus theme: primary diagnostic indications for transplant. J Heart Lung Transplant. 2016;35(10):1196–205.
3. Cooper JD, Billingham M, Egan T, Hertz MI, Higenbottam T, Lynch J, et al. A working formulation for the standardization of nomenclature and for clinical staging of chronic dysfunction in lung allografts. International Society for Heart and Lung Transplantation. J Heart Lung Transplant. 1993;12(5):713–6.
4. Estenne M, Maurer JR, Boehler A, Egan JJ, Frost A, Hertz M, et al. Bronchiolitis obliterans syndrome 2001: an update of the diagnostic criteria. J Heart Lung Transplant. 2002;21(3):297–310.
5. Verleden GM, Vos R, Vanaudenaerde B, Dupont L, Yserbyt J, Van Raemdonck D, et al. Current views on chronic rejection after lung transplantation. Transpl Int. 2015;28(10):1131–9.
6. Verleden GM, Raghu G, Meyer KC, Glanville AR, Corris P. A new classification system for chronic lung allograft dysfunction. J Heart Lung Transplant. 2014;33(2):127–33.
7. Glanville AR. Bronchoscopic monitoring after lung transplantation. Semin Respir Crit Care Med. 2010;31(2):208–21.
8. Derom F, Barbier F, Ringoir S, Versieck J, Rolly G, Berzsenyi G, et al. Ten-month survival after lung homotransplantation in man. J Thorac Cardiovasc Surg. 1971;61(6):835–46.
9. Owen J, Punt J, Stranford S. Kuby immunology. 7th ed. New York: WH Freeman; 2013.
10. Verleden SE, Sacreas A, Vos R, Vanaudenaerde BM, Verleden GM. Advances in understanding bronchiolitis obliterans after lung transplantation. Chest. 2016;150(1):219–25.
11. Sato M, Waddell TK, Wagnetz U, Roberts HC, Hwang DM, Haroon A, et al. Restrictive allograft syndrome (RAS): a novel form of chronic lung allograft dysfunction. J Heart Lung Transplant. 2011;30(7):735–42.
12. Woodrow JP, Shlobin OA, Barnett SD, Burton N, Nathan SD. Comparison of bronchiolitis obliterans syndrome to other forms of chronic lung allograft dysfunction after lung transplantation. J Heart Lung Transplant. 2010;29(10):1159–64.
13. Suhling H, Dettmer S, Rademacher J, Greer M, Mark G, Shin H-O, et al. Spirometric obstructive lung function pattern early after lung transplantation. Transplantation. 2012;93(2):230–5.
14. Verleden SE, Vasilescu DM, Willems S, Ruttens D, Vos R, Vandermeulen E, et al. The site and nature of airway obstruction after lung transplantation. Am J Respir Crit Care Med. 2014;189(3):292–300.
15. Galbán CJ, Han MK, Boes JL, Chughtai KA, Meyer CR, Johnson TD, et al. Computed tomography-based biomarker provides unique signature for diagnosis of COPD phenotypes and disease progression. Nat Med. 2012;18(11):1711–5.
16. Verleden SE, Vos R, Vandermeulen E, Ruttens D, Bellon H, Heigl T, et al. Parametric response mapping of bronchiolitis obliterans syndrome progression after lung transplantation. Am J Transplant. 2016;16(11):3262–9.
17. Renne J, Lauermann P, Hinrichs JB, Schönfeld C, Sorrentino S, Gutberlet M, et al. Chronic lung allograft dysfunction: oxygen-enhanced T1-mapping MR imaging of the lung. Radiology. 2015;276(1):266–73.
18. Verleden SE, de Jong PA, Ruttens D, Vandermeulen E, van Raemdonck DE, Verschakelen J, et al. Functional and computed tomographic evolution and survival of restrictive allograft syndrome after lung transplantation. J Heart Lung Transplant. 2014;33(3):270–7.
19. Sato M. Chronic lung allograft dysfunction after lung transplantation: the moving target. Gen Thorac Cardiovasc Surg. 2013;61(2):67–78.
20. Verleden SE, Ruttens D, Vandermeulen E, Bellon H, Dubbeldam A, De Wever W, et al. Predictors of survival in restrictive chronic lung allograft dysfunction after lung transplantation. J Heart Lung Transplant. 2016;35(9):1078–84.
21. Paraskeva M, McLean C, Ellis S, Bailey M, Williams T, Levvey B, et al. Acute fibrinoid organizing pneumonia after lung transplantation. Am J Respir Crit Care Med. 2013;187(12):1360–8.
22. Corris PA, Christie JD. Update in transplantation 2007. Am J Respir Crit Care Med. 2008;177(10):1062–7.
23. Neurohr C, Huppmann P, Samweber B, Leuschner S, Zimmermann G, Leuchte H, et al. Prognostic value of bronchoalveolar lavage neutrophilia in stable lung transplant recipients. J Heart Lung Transplant. 2009;28(5):468–74.
24. Davis WA, Finlen Copeland CA, Todd JL, Snyder LD, Martissa JA, Palmer SM. Spirometrically significant acute rejection increases the risk for BOS and death after lung transplantation. Am J Transplant. 2012;12(3):745–52.
25. Glanville AR, Aboyoun CL, Havryk A, Plit M, Rainer S, Malouf MA. Severity of lymphocytic bronchiolitis predicts long-term outcome after lung transplantation. Am J Respir Crit Care Med. 2008;177(9):1033–40.
26. Glanville AR, Gencay M, Tamm M, Chhajed P, Plit M, Hopkins P, et al. Chlamydia pneumoniae infection after lung transplantation. J Heart Lung Transplant. 2005;24(2):131–6.
27. Smith MA, Sundaresan S, Mohanakumar T, Trulock EP, Lynch JP, Phelan DL, et al. Effect of development of antibodies to HLA and cytomegalovirus mismatch on lung transplantation survival and development of bronchiolitis obliterans syndrome. J Thorac Cardiovasc Surg. 1998;116(5):812–20.

28. Hachem RR, Tiriveedhi V, Patterson GA, Aloush A, Trulock EP, Mohanakumar T. Antibodies to K-α 1 tubulin and collagen V are associated with chronic rejection after lung transplantation. Am J Transplant. 2012;12(8):2164–71.

29. Nawrot TS, Vos R, Jacobs L, Verleden SE, Wauters S, Mertens V, et al. The impact of traffic air pollution on bronchiolitis obliterans syndrome and mortality after lung transplantation. Thorax. 2011;66(9):748–54.

30. Bhinder S, Chen H, Sato M, Copes R, Evans GJ, Chow C-W, et al. Air pollution and the development of posttransplant chronic lung allograft dysfunction. Am J Transplant. 2014;14(12):2749–57.

31. Sharples LD, McNeil K, Stewart S, Wallwork J. Risk factors for bronchiolitis obliterans: a systematic review of recent publications. J Heart Lung Transplant. 2002;21(2):271–81.

32. Botha P, Archer L, Anderson RL, Lordan J, Dark JH, Corris PA, et al. Pseudomonas aeruginosa colonization of the allograft after lung transplantation and the risk of bronchiolitis obliterans syndrome. Transplantation. 2008;85(5):771–4.

33. Vos R, Vanaudenaerde BM, Geudens N, Dupont LJ, Van Raemdonck DE, Verleden GM. Pseudomonal airway colonisation: risk factor for bronchiolitis obliterans syndrome after lung transplantation? Eur Respir J. 2008;31(5):1037–45.

34. D'Ovidio F, Mura M, Ridsdale R, Takahashi H, Waddell TK, Hutcheon M, et al. The effect of reflux and bile acid aspiration on the lung allograft and its surfactant and innate immunity molecules SP-A and SP-D. Am J Transplant. 2006;6(8):1930–8.

35. Vos R, Vanaudenaerde BM, De Vleeschauwer SI, Willems-Widyastuti A, Scheers H, Van Raemdonck DE, et al. Circulating and intrapulmonary C-reactive protein: a predictor of bronchiolitis obliterans syndrome and pulmonary allograft outcome. J Heart Lung Transplant. 2009;28(8):799–807.

36. Verleden GM, Vos R, Verleden SE, De Wever W, De Vleeschauwer SI, Willems-Widyastuti A, et al. Survival determinants in lung transplant patients with chronic allograft dysfunction. Transplantation. 2011;92(6):703–8.

37. Todd JL, Jain R, Pavlisko EN, Finlen Copeland CA, Reynolds JM, Snyder LD, et al. Impact of forced vital capacity loss on survival after the onset of chronic lung allograft dysfunction. Am J Respir Crit Care Med. 2014;189(2):159–66.

38. Verleden SE, Ruttens D, Vandermeulen E, Vaneylen A, Dupont LJ, Van Raemdonck DE, et al. Bronchiolitis obliterans syndrome and restrictive allograft syndrome: do risk factors differ? Transplantation. 2013;95(9):1167–72.

39. Verleden SE, Ruttens D, Vandermeulen E, van Raemdonck DE, Vanaudenaerde BM, Verleden GM, et al. Elevated bronchoalveolar lavage eosinophilia correlates with poor outcome after lung transplantation. Transplantation. 2014;97(1):83–9.

40. Verleden SE, Ruttens D, Vos R, Vandermeulen E, Moelants E, Mortier A, et al. Differential cytokine,

chemokine and growth factor expression in phenotypes of chronic lung allograft dysfunction. Transplantation. 2015;99(1):86–93.

41. Shino MY, Weigt SS, Li N, Palchevskiy V, Derhovanessian A, Saggar R, et al. CXCR3 ligands are associated with the continuum of diffuse alveolar damage to chronic lung allograft dysfunction. Am J Respir Crit Care Med. 2013;188(9):1117–25.

42. Saito T, Liu M, Binnie M, Sato M, Hwang D, Azad S, et al. Distinct expression patterns of alveolar "alarmins" in subtypes of chronic lung allograft dysfunction. Am J Transplant. 2014;14(6):1425–32.

43. Vandermeulen E, Verleden SE, Bellon H, Ruttens D, Lammertyn E, Claes S, et al. Humoral immunity in phenotypes of chronic lung allograft dysfunction: a broncho-alveolar lavage fluid analysis. Transpl Immunol. 2016;38:27–32.

44. Kelly FL, Kennedy VE, Jain R, Sindhwani NS, Finlen Copeland CA, Snyder LD, et al. Epithelial clara cell injury occurs in bronchiolitis obliterans syndrome after human lung transplantation. Am J Transplant. 2012;12(11):3076–84.

45. Gilpin SE, Lung KC, Sato M, Singer LG, Keshavjee S, Waddell TK. Altered progenitor cell and cytokine profiles in bronchiolitis obliterans syndrome. J Heart Lung Transplant. 2012;31(2):222–8.

46. Andersson-Sjöland A, Erjefält JS, Bjermer L, Eriksson L, Westergren-Thorsson G. Fibrocytes are associated with vascular and parenchymal remodelling in patients with obliterative bronchiolitis. Respir Res. 2009;10:103.

47. Vanaudenaerde BM, Wuyts WA, Dupont LJ, Van Raemdonck DE, Demedts MM, Verleden GM. Interleukin-17 stimulates release of interleukin-8 by human airway smooth muscle cells in vitro: a potential role for interleukin-17 and airway smooth muscle cells in bronchiolitis obliterans syndrome. J Heart Lung Transplant. 2003;22(11):1280–3.

48. Murphy DM, Forrest IA, Corris PA, Johnson GE, Small T, Jones D, et al. Simvastatin attenuates release of neutrophilic and remodeling factors from primary bronchial epithelial cells derived from stable lung transplant recipients. Am J Physiol Lung Cell Mol Physiol. 2008;294(3):L592–9.

49. Vanaudenaerde BM, De Vleeschauwer SI, Vos R, Meyts I, Bullens DM, Reynders V, et al. The role of the IL23/IL17 axis in bronchiolitis obliterans syndrome after lung transplantation. Am J Transplant. 2008;8(9):1911–20.

50. Subramanian V, Ramachandran S, Banan B, Bharat A, Wang X, Benshoff N, et al. Immune response to tissue-restricted self-antigens induces airway inflammation and fibrosis following murine lung transplantation. Am J Transplant. 2014;14(10):2359–66.

51. Bhorade SM, Chen H, Molinero L, Liao C, Garrity ER, Vigneswaran WT, et al. Decreased percentage of CD4+FoxP3+ cells in bronchoalveolar lavage from lung transplant recipients correlates with development of bronchiolitis obliterans syndrome. Transplantation. 2010;90(5):540–6.

52. Krustrup D, Iversen M, Martinussen T, Schultz HHL, Andersen CB. The number of FoxP3+ cells in transbronchial lung allograft biopsies does not predict bronchiolitis obliterans syndrome within the first five years after transplantation. Clin Transpl. 2015;29(3):179–84.

53. Ruttens D, Wauters E, Kiciński M, Verleden SE, Vandermeulen E, Vos R, et al. Genetic variation in interleukin-17 receptor A is functionally associated with chronic rejection after lung transplantation. J Heart Lung Transplant. 2013;32(12):1233–40.

54. Verleden SE, Vos R, Vandermeulen E, Ruttens D, Vaneylen A, Dupont LJ, et al. Involvement of interleukin-17 during lymphocytic bronchiolitis in lung transplant patients. J Heart Lung Transplant. 2013;32(4):447–53.

55. Todd JL, Wang X, Sugimoto S, Kennedy VE, Zhang HL, Pavlisko EN, et al. Hyaluronan contributes to bronchiolitis obliterans syndrome and stimulates lung allograft rejection through activation of innate immunity. Am J Respir Crit Care Med. 2014;189(5):556–66.

56. Platzer B, Stout M, Fiebiger E. Antigen cross-presentation of immune complexes. Front Immunol. 2014;5:140.

57. Keane MP, Gomperts BN, Weigt S, Xue YY, Burdick MD, Nakamura H, et al. IL-13 is pivotal in the fibro-obliterative process of bronchiolitis obliterans syndrome. J Immunol. 2007;178(1):511–9.

58. Zagai U, Lundahl J, Klominek J, Venge P, Sköld CM. Eosinophil cationic protein stimulates migration of human lung fibroblasts in vitro. Scand J Immunol. 2009;69(4):381–6.

59. Hügle T. Beyond allergy: the role of mast cells in fibrosis. Swiss Med Wkly. 2014;144:w13999.

60. Bhatt NY, Allen JN. Update on eosinophilic lung diseases. Semin Respir Crit Care Med. 2012;33(5):555–71.

61. Kousha M, Tadi R, Soubani AO. Pulmonary aspergillosis: a clinical review. Eur Respir Rev. 2011;20(121):156–74.

62. Vandermeulen E, Lammertyn E, Verleden SE, Ruttens D, Bellon H, Ricciardi M, et al. Immunological diversity in phenotypes of chronic lung allograft dysfunction: a comprehensive immunohistochemical analysis. Transpl Int. 2017;30:134–43.

63. Borthwick LA, Suwara MI, Carnell SC, Green NJ, Mahida R, Dixon D, et al. Pseudomonas aeruginosa induced airway epithelial injury drives fibroblast activation: a mechanism in chronic lung allograft dysfunction. Am J Transplant. 2016;16(6):1751–65.

64. Dunkelberger JR, Song W-C. Complement and its role in innate and adaptive immune responses. Cell Res. 2010;20(1):34–50.

65. Bonilla FA, Oettgen HC. Adaptive immunity. J Allergy Clin Immunol. 2010;125(2 Suppl 2):S33–40.

66. Warrington R, Watson W, Kim HL, Antonetti FR. An introduction to immunology and immunopathology. Allergy Asthma Clin Immunol. 2011;7(1):1–8.

67. Zeevi A. Chronic antibody-mediated rejection: new diagnostic tools—clinical significance of C4d deposition and improved detection and characterization of human leucocyte antigen antibodies. Clin Exp Immunol. 2014;178(Suppl 1):52–3.

68. Meyer KC, Raghu G, Verleden GM, Corris PA, Aurora P, Wilson KC, et al. An international ISHLT/ATS/ERS clinical practice guideline: diagnosis and management of bronchiolitis obliterans syndrome. Eur Respir J. 2014;44(6):1479–503.

69. Jaramillo A, Smith MA, Phelan D, Sundaresan S, Trulock EP, Lynch JP, et al. Development of ELISA-detected anti-HLA antibodies precedes the development of bronchiolitis obliterans syndrome and correlates with progressive decline in pulmonary function after lung transplantation. Transplantation. 1999;67(8):1155–61.

70. Snyder LD, Wang Z, Chen D-F, Reinsmoen NL, Finlen-Copeland CA, Davis WA, et al. Implications for human leukocyte antigen antibodies after lung transplantation: a 10-year experience in 441 patients. Chest. 2013;144(1):226–33.

71. Fukami N, Ramachandran S, Takenaka M, Weber J, Subramanian V, Mohanakumar T. An obligatory role for lung infiltrating B cells in the immunopathogenesis of obliterative airway disease induced by antibodies to MHC class I molecules. Am J Transplant. 2012;12(4):867–76.

72. Neuringer IP, Mannon RB, Coffman TM, Parsons M, Burns K, Yankaskas JR, et al. Immune cells in a mouse airway model of obliterative bronchiolitis. Am J Respir Cell Mol Biol. 1998;19(3):379–86.

73. Hachem RR, Yusen RD, Meyers BF, Aloush AA, Mohanakumar T, Patterson GA, et al. Anti-human leukocyte antigen antibodies and preemptive antibody-directed therapy after lung transplantation. J Heart Lung Transplant. 2010;29(9):973–80.

74. Jaramillo A, Smith CR, Maruyama T, Zhang L, Patterson GA, Mohanakumar T. Anti-HLA class I antibody binding to airway epithelial cells induces production of fibrogenic growth factors and apoptotic cell death: a possible mechanism for bronchiolitis obliterans syndrome. Hum Immunol. 2003;64(5):521–9.

75. Levine DJ, Glanville AR, Aboyoun C, Belperio J, Benden C, Berry GJ, et al. Antibody-mediated rejection of the lung: a consensus report of the International Society for Heart and Lung Transplantation. J Heart Lung Transplant. 2016;35(4):397–406.

76. Feucht HE, Felber E, Gokel MJ, Hillebrand G, Nattermann U, Brockmeyer C, et al. Vascular deposition of complement-split products in kidney allografts with cell-mediated rejection. Clin Exp Immunol. 1991;86(3):464–70.

77. Verleden SE, Ruttens D, Vandermeulen E, Bellon H, Van Raemdonck DE, Dupont LJ, et al. Restrictive chronic lung allograft dysfunction: where are we now? J Heart Lung Transplant. 2015;34(5):625–30.

78. Banerjee B, Musk M, Sutanto EN, Yerkovich ST, Hopkins P, Knight DA, et al. Regional differences in susceptibility of bronchial epithelium to mesenchymal

transition and inhibition by the macrolide antibiotic azithromycin. PLoS One. 2012;7(12):e52309.

79. Vos R, Vanaudenaerde BM, Verleden SE, De Vleeschauwer SI, Willems-Widyastuti A, Van Raemdonck DE, et al. A randomised controlled trial of azithromycin to prevent chronic rejection after lung transplantation. Eur Respir J. 2011;37(1):164–72.

80. Ruttens D, Verleden SE, Vandermeulen E, Bellon H, Vanaudenaerde BM, Somers J, et al. Prophylactic azithromycin therapy after lung transplantation: post hoc analysis of a randomized controlled trial. Am J Transplant. 2016;16(1):254–61.

81. Baum C, Reichenspurner H, Deuse T. Bortezomib rescue therapy in a patient with recurrent antibody-mediated rejection after lung transplantation. J Heart Lung Transplant. 2013;32(12):1270–1.

82. Snyder LD, Gray AL, Reynolds JM, Arepally GM, Bedoya A, Hartwig MG, et al. Antibody desensitization therapy in highly sensitized lung transplant candidates. Am J Transplant. 2014;14(4):849–56.

83. Baskaran G, Tiriveedhi V, Ramachandran S, Aloush A, Grossman B, Hachem R, et al. Efficacy of extracorporeal photopheresis in clearance of antibodies to donor-specific and lung-specific antigens in lung transplant recipients. J Heart Lung Transplant. 2014;33(9):950–6.

84. Greer M, Dierich M, De Wall C, Suhling H, Rademacher J, Welte T, et al. Phenotyping established chronic lung allograft dysfunction predicts extracorporeal photopheresis response in lung transplant patients. Am J Transplant. 2013;13(4):911–8.

85. Ihle F, von Wulffen W, Neurohr C. Pirfenidone: a potential therapy for progressive lung allograft dysfunction? J Heart Lung Transplant. 2013;32(5):574–5.

86. King TE, Bradford WZ, Castro-Bernardini S, Fagan EA, Glaspole I, Glassberg MK, et al. A phase 3 trial of pirfenidone in patients with idiopathic pulmonary fibrosis. N Engl J Med. 2014;370(22):2083–92.

87. Vos R, Verleden SE, Ruttens D, Vandermeulen E, Yserbyt J, Dupont LJ, et al. Pirfenidone: a potential new therapy for restrictive allograft syndrome? Am J Transplant. 2013;13(11):3035–40.

88. Kohno M, Perch M, Andersen E, Carlsen J, Andersen CB, Iversen M. Treatment of intractable interstitial lung injury with alemtuzumab after lung transplantation. Transplant Proc. 2011;43(5):1868–70.

89. Verleden SE, Todd JL, Sato M, Palmer SM, Martinu T, Pavlisko EN, et al. Impact of CLAD phenotype on survival after lung retransplantation: a multicenter study. Am J Transplant. 2015;15(8):2223–30.

Gastroesophageal Reflux and Esophageal Dysmotility in Patients Undergoing Evaluation for Lung Transplantation: Assessment, Evaluation, and Management

17

Robert B. Yates, Carlos A. Pellegrini, and Brant K. Oelschlager

Abbreviations

BOS	Bronchiolitis obliterans
CTD	Connective tissue disease
DGE	Delayed gastric emptying
FEV_1	Forced expiratory volume in 1 s
GEJ	Gastroesophageal junction
GER	Gastroesophageal reflux
GERD	Gastroesophageal reflux disease
HRM	High-resolution esophageal manometry
IEM	Ineffective esophageal motility
IPF	Idiopathic pulmonary fibrosis
LES	Lower esophageal sphincter
PPI	Proton pump inhibitor

R. B. Yates (✉)
Department of Surgery, Northwest Hospital and Medical Center, University of Washington Medicine, Seattle, WA, USA
e-mail: rby2@uw.edu

C. A. Pellegrini
Department of Surgery, University of Washington, Seattle, WA, USA
e-mail: pellegri@uw.edu

B. K. Oelschlager
Division of General Surgery, Department of Surgery, University of Washington Medical Center, Seattle, WA, USA
e-mail: brant@uw.edu

Introduction

Gastroesophageal reflux disease (GERD) is defined as abnormal distal esophageal acid exposure that is associated with patient symptoms, and it is the most common benign condition of the stomach and esophagus. The majority of patients with GERD experience "typical symptoms" (i.e., heartburn and regurgitation), and their symptoms are managed effectively with medications, specifically proton pump inhibitors (PPIs). In fact, because PPIs are so effective at decreasing gastric acid production and provide improvement in typical GERD-related symptoms, most patients with GERD who take these medications never undergo a formal diagnostic evaluation. Consequently, an empiric trial of PPI therapy has become viewed as both "diagnostic and therapeutic" for most patients that present with typical GERD symptoms.

In the vast majority of patients, GERD is a disease that affects quality of life and is associated with a low risk of developing life-threatening complications. In these patients, the end point of treatment is symptom management, and in most patients medical therapy is successful at achieving that goal. More recently, however, it has become clear that GERD is a contributing

© The Author(s) 2018
G. Raghu, R. G. Carbone (eds.), *Lung Transplantation*, https://doi.org/10.1007/978-3-319-91184-7_17

factor to certain types of advanced lung disease presumably due to repetitive micro-aspiration of gastroduodenal contents. Compared to most GERD patients, patients with GERD-related lung disease are unique in two major ways. First, these patients infrequently experience typical symptoms of GERD; therefore, the decision to evaluate these patients for GERD should not be determined based exclusively on patient-reported gastroesophageal symptoms. In fact, many pulmonologists have adopted a liberal approach to testing, or even empirically treating, patients with specific types of pulmonary disease for GERD regardless of the presence of symptoms. Furthermore, improvement in gastroesophageal symptoms should not be the end point of treatment in patients with GERD and chronic lung disease. Second, while PPI therapy is very effective at suppressing gastric acid production, recent evidence suggests that micro-aspiration of pH-neutral gastric contents can cause pulmonary injury. As a result, PPI therapy alone is ineffective at correcting the pathophysiologic mechanism behind GERD-related lung disease – micro-aspiration. Traditionally, antireflux surgery has been employed almost exclusively in patients who experience persistent life-limiting GERD symptoms despite maximal medical therapy (i.e., PPI therapy). However, in patients with GERD-related lung disease, antireflux surgery may be more appropriate than PPI therapy because antireflux surgery is the treatment that comes closest to eradicating all forms of gastroesophageal reflux (GER) with the creation of a mechanical barrier.

The purpose of this chapter is to provide a comprehensive review of GERD in the context of chronic severe pulmonary disease and related conditions, including esophageal dysmotility, connective tissue disorders, and lung transplantation. We discuss the approach to clinical evaluation and management of patients with GERD and GERD-related lung disease, emphasizing the relevant diagnostic testing and treatment options, including antireflux surgery.

Gastroesophageal Reflux Disease: Relevant Anatomy, Physiology, and Pathophysiology

Normal function of the stomach and esophagus is necessary to prevent GERD. The three primary mechanisms that counteract GER are a competent lower esophageal sphincter (LES), effective spontaneous esophageal clearance, and normal gastric emptying. Failure of any of these processes can lead to GERD.

Lower Esophageal Sphincter

The LES is the first defense against preventing reflux of gastric contents into the esophagus. Rather than a distinct anatomic structure, the LES is a zone of high pressure located just cephalad to the gastroesophageal junction (GEJ). This high-pressure zone is readily identified during esophageal manometry (see the section on "Clinical Evaluation of Patients with Suspected Gastroesophageal Reflux Disease").

The LES is made up of four anatomic structures: (1) The *intrinsic musculature of the distal esophagus* is normally in a state of tonic contraction. With the initiation of a swallow, these smooth muscle fibers relax and then return to a state of tonic contraction. (2) *Sling fibers of the gastric cardia* are oriented diagonally from the cardia-fundus junction to the lesser curve of the stomach and contribute significantly to the high-pressure zone of the LES. (3) The *crura of the diaphragm* surround the esophagus as it passes through the esophageal hiatus. During inspiration, a pressure gradient is created as intrathoracic pressure decreases relative to intraabdominal pressure. To counteract this pressure gradient, the anteroposterior diameter of the crural opening is decreased, compressing the esophagus and increasing pressure at the LES. (4) With the GEJ firmly anchored in the abdominal cavity, increased *intraabdominal pressure* is transmitted to the GEJ, which increases the pressure on the distal esophagus and prevents reflux of gastric contents.

Gastroesophageal reflux develops when intragastric pressure surpasses the high-pressure zone of the distal esophagus. This occurs under three conditions: (1) LES resting pressure is too low to counteract normal intragastric pressures (i.e., hypotensive LES); (2) LES inappropriately relaxes in the absence of peristaltic contraction of the esophagus (i.e., spontaneous LES relaxation); and (3) intragastric pressure surpasses the normal LES resting pressure [1]. It is important to remember that GER is a normal physiologic process that occurs even in the setting of normal gastroesophageal anatomy and function. The distinction between physiologic reflux (i.e., GER) and pathologic reflux (i.e., GERD) hinges on the total amount of esophageal acid exposure, patient symptoms, and the presence of mucosal damage of the esophagus.

The presence of a hiatal hernia is a common anatomic abnormality that can significantly compromise the LES antireflux mechanism and predispose to GER. A hiatal hernia is the abnormal displacement of the GEJ cephalad to the esophageal hiatus and into the posterior mediastinum. This occurs due to a failure of the phrenoesophageal ligament, a continuation of the peritoneum that reflects onto the esophagus at the hiatus and normally anchors the GEJ in the abdominal cavity. When the GEJ becomes displaced into the distal mediastinum, the LES becomes compromised and is unable to maintain a high-pressure zone to prevent reflux. When a hiatal hernia is present, the most common symptoms attributable to this finding are typical symptoms of GERD. However, many small hiatal hernias are completely asymptomatic, and a hiatal hernia is neither necessary nor sufficient to make the diagnosis of GERD. Therefore, the presence of such a hernia does not constitute an indication for operative correction.

Ineffective Esophageal Motility

The primary functions of the esophagus are to transport liquid and food boluses into the stomach, to clear refluxed gastroduodenal contents back into the stomach, and to prevent abnormal reflux from occurring. For these to be accomplished, the esophagus must generate sufficiently forceful peristaltic contractions, and the lower esophageal sphincter must simultaneously relax. Esophageal dysmotility is a broad term that refers to discoordinated esophageal body contractions, low-amplitude coordinated esophageal contractions, or both. High-resolution esophageal manometry (HRM) (see the section on "Clinical Evaluation of Patients with Suspected Gastroesophageal Reflux Disease") is the best modality to evaluate for esophageal dysmotility. Based on manometric evaluation, ineffective esophageal motility (IEM) is defined by the Chicago Classification v3.0 of HRM as ≥50% of swallows resulting in a distal esophageal contractile pressure of <450 mmHg (Fig. 17.1a–c) [2]. When esophageal dysmotility is present, the functions of the esophagus may become compromised.

Ineffective esophageal motility and GERD are intimately related. When GER occurs, intrinsic esophageal motility should rapidly and effectively clear the refluxate from the distal esophagus back into the stomach. Spontaneous esophageal clearance reduces the amount of time that the distal esophageal mucosa is exposed to acid and other gastroduodenal contents that are caustic to the esophageal mucosa. Furthermore, esophageal motility prevents reflux to the proximal esophagus. With impaired esophageal body motility, this intrinsic clearance mechanism fails to evacuate the esophagus of these refluxed materials. As a result, relatively infrequent GER can lead to prolonged episodes of distal esophageal acid exposure. This can be demonstrated on 24-h pH monitoring (Fig. 17.2a, b). When a patient with IEM is upright, gravity aids in draining the distal esophagus of refluxed gastric contents; however, in the supine position, incomplete esophageal clearance results in a column of fluid that can passively move toward the oropharynx, resulting in severe regurgitation, water brash sensation, and even aspiration.

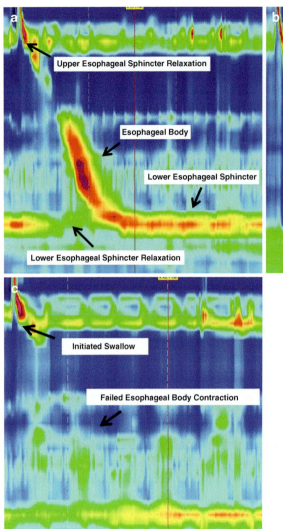

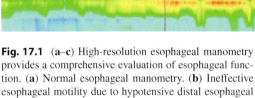

Fig. 17.1 (**a–c**) High-resolution esophageal manometry provides a comprehensive evaluation of esophageal function. (**a**) Normal esophageal manometry. (**b**) Ineffective esophageal motility due to hypotensive distal esophageal body contractility. (**c**) Ineffective esophageal motility due to failed swallows (**a–c**: Courtesy of the University of Washington Center for Esophageal and Gastric Surgery, Seattle, WA)

There is mounting evidence that esophageal dysmotility is prevalent among patients with GERD. In a study of over 1500 patients with abnormal distal esophageal acid exposure on 24-h pH monitoring, patients with abnormal esophageal body peristalsis demonstrated more severe GERD-related symptoms, worse esophagitis, and longer time to clearance of distal esophageal acid [3]. Furthermore, there appears to be an association between the presence of IEM and the severity of GERD: Esophageal dysmotility is more common in patients with esophagitis and Barrett's esophagus compared to patients with nonerosive reflux disease [4, 5]. Although esophageal dysmotility appears to increase GERD severity, GERD itself may potentiate—or even cause—esophageal dysmotility due to repeated exposure of the esophagus to caustic gastroduodenal contents. In support of this hypothesis, Heider and colleagues demonstrated improvement in esophageal dysmotility following antireflux surgery [6].

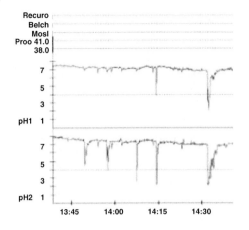

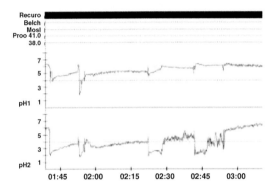

Fig. 17.2 (**a, b**) Representative portions of a 24-h esophageal pH monitoring tracing demonstrating episodes of reflux in the upright (**a**) and recumbent (**b**) positions. Note that in the presence of impaired esophageal clearance of gastric contents, a single episode of reflux can result in prolonged exposure of the distal esophagus to acidic gastric contents (**b**) (**a, b**: Courtesy of the University of Washington Center for Esophageal and Gastric Surgery, Seattle, WA)

There also appears to be a connection among IEM, GERD, and GERD-related respiratory conditions. In patients with GERD-related respiratory symptoms, IEM is the most commonly identified esophageal motility disorder. The logical explanation for this is that incomplete clearance of acid from the esophagus allows for proximal movement of the refluxate and eventual micro-aspiration. Pellegrini and colleagues were the first to systematically study this connection [7]. They evaluated 100 patients with elevated distal esophageal acid exposure on 24-h pH studies and defined aspiration as a drop in esophageal pH followed by patient-reported water brash

sensation and coinciding cough or wheeze. Ineffective esophageal motility was identified in 75% of patients who experienced aspiration based on these criteria. A study by Fouad and colleagues further supports the connection between prolonged distal esophageal acid exposure and respiratory symptoms [8]. They demonstrated that in patients with GERD-associated respiratory symptoms, the average duration of an episode of reflux was twice as long compared to patients with typical symptoms of GERD and no respiratory problems. They also found that 41% of patients with chronic cough and 53% of patients with asthma demonstrated IEM on esophageal manometry. Taken together, these findings suggest that IEM leads to longer esophageal acid exposure time, which in turn increases the risk of aspiration.

Since ineffective esophageal motility appears to facilitate aspiration and micro-aspiration is the underlying mechanism behind GERD-related respiratory symptoms and pulmonary disease, it should come as no surprise that the incidence of esophageal dysmotility is greater in patients with end-stage lung disease compared to normal healthy control subjects. In the most comprehensive evaluation of esophageal motor dysfunction in lung transplant candidates to date, Basseri and colleagues [9] performed HRM in 30 consecutive patients undergoing lung transplant evaluation. Compared to healthy control subjects, lung transplant candidates were found to have a higher incidence of hypotensive lower esophageal sphincter (63% vs. 20%, $p = 0.028$), which places these patients at increased risk for GER. Additionally, 77% of lung transplant candidates demonstrated some form of esophageal body dysfunction, and compared to healthy control subjects, these patients demonstrated fewer peristaltic contractions and a greater incidence of hypotensive peristaltic contractions and of complete esophageal body aperistalsis.

Finally, esophageal motility disorders are common in patients who undergo lung transplantation. Since the performance of the first pneumonectomy in the 1930s, it has been recognized that radical lung surgery is associated with postoperative anatomic and physiologic changes in the esophagus [10]. These changes include a shift of the esophagus to the ipsilateral side of the pneumonectomy, decreased distal esophageal body contractile amplitude, and decreased lower esophageal sphincter resting pressure. In lung transplantation, replacement of the removed organ prevents anatomic shift in the esophagus; however, esophageal dysmotility has been reported in up to 20% of patients following lung transplantation [11]. The reason for esophageal dysmotility following lung transplantation is thought to be due to inadvertent partial or complete vagal nerve injury that can occur during dissection and hemostasis within the posterior mediastinum during recipient pneumonectomy and implantation of the donor lung(s).

Delayed Gastric Emptying

Delayed gastric empting (DGE) is the ineffective clearance of gastric contents from the stomach. In some patients, DGE can result in significant symptoms, including nausea, early satiety, regurgitation, and vomiting. The three most common causes of DGE are diabetic, idiopathic, and postsurgical.

In any patient undergoing evaluation of GERD, it is important to consider whether delayed gastric emptying is present. First, DGE is a cause, albeit rare, of GERD: Delayed emptying of the stomach leads to increased intragastric pressure that overwhelms the antireflux mechanism of the LES and results in GER [12]. Second, in the setting of DGE, traditional GERD management strategies will likely be ineffective or even result in additional symptoms. For example, the performance of antireflux surgery in the setting of gastroparesis can result in severe upper abdominal bloating secondary to a distended stomach and inability to regurgitate or vomit. In this situation, reoperation to undo the fundoplication may be required. In patients without any symptoms of gastroparesis, generally no further testing is required. However, if there is any suspicion that gastric emptying may be abnormal, a radionuclide scintigraphy scan (i.e., gastric emptying study) should be performed.

There is mounting evidence that DGE is common in patients with chronic pulmonary disease, particularly when the pulmonary disease is associated with a connective tissue disorder, and following lung transplantation. Similar to posttransplant esophageal dysfunction, the likely mechanism underlying DGE following lung transplantation is vagal nerve injury incurred during transplantation. In one of the first reports of DGE in lung transplant patients, Berkowitz and colleagues published that 42% of lung transplant recipients reported persistent gastrointestinal symptoms and 24% of lung transplant recipients were ultimately diagnosed with DGE [13]. In the lung transplant population, DGE can easily be overlooked, because these patients require many medications, including immune suppression agents, which can cause gastroesophageal symptoms. Consequently, a high index of suspicion should be had for the presence of gastroparesis in lung transplant patients who present with any upper gastroesophageal symptoms. Identification of DGE in a lung transplant recipient is important, since DGE can lead to regurgitation and aspiration. The presence of delayed gastric emptying in the lung transplant population has led some surgeons to adding a gastric emptying procedure (pyloroplasty) during performance of laparoscopic antireflux surgery in these patients [14], although there is no consensus on whether this should be routinely performed during antireflux surgery.

Clinical Presentation of Gastroesophageal Reflux Disease

Typical Symptoms

Heartburn, regurgitation, and water brash are the three typical esophageal symptoms of GERD, and they are among the most common symptoms reported by patients with GERD (Table 17.1). Heartburn is very specific to GERD and described as epigastric and/or retrosternal caustic or stinging sensation. It is important to ask the patient about his or her symptoms in detail to differentiate typical heartburn from symptoms suggestive

Table 17.1 Prevalence of symptoms in 1000 patients with GERD symptom

	Prevalence (%)
Heartburn	80
Regurgitation	54
Abdominal pain	29
Cough	27
Dysphagia for solids	23
Hoarseness	21
Belching	15
Bloating	15
Aspiration	14
Wheezing	7
Globus	4

Box 17.1 Extraesophageal symptoms of GERD

Laryngeal symptoms of reflux:
1. Hoarseness/dysphonia
2. Throat clearing
3. Throat pain
4. Globus
5. Choking
6. Postnasal drip
7. Laryngeal and tracheal stenosis
8. Laryngospasm
9. Contact ulcers

Pulmonary symptoms of reflux:
1. Cough
2. Shortness of breath
3. Wheezing
4. Pulmonary disease (asthma, IPF, chronic bronchitis, and others)

of other disease processes, including pancreatitis, acute coronary syndrome, peptic ulcer disease, and cholelithiasis.

The presence of regurgitation often indicates progression of GERD. In severe cases, patients will be unable to bend over without experiencing an episode of regurgitation. Regurgitation of gastric contents to the oropharynx and mouth can produce a sour taste that patients will describe as either "acid" or "bile." This phenomenon is referred to as water brash. In patients who report regurgitation as a frequent symptom, it is important to distinguish between regurgitation of undigested and digested food. Regurgitation of undigested food is not common in GERD and suggests the presence of a different pathologic process, such as an esophageal diverticulum, achalasia, and gastroparesis.

Extraesophageal Symptoms

Extraesophageal symptoms of GERD arise from the respiratory tract and include both laryngeal and pulmonary symptoms (Box 17.1). Two proposed mechanisms may lead to extraesophageal symptoms of GERD [15]. First, proximal esophageal reflux and micro-aspiration of gastroduodenal contents cause direct caustic injury to the larynx and lower respiratory tract; this is probably the most common mechanism. Second, due to the common vagal innervation of the trachea and esophagus, distal esophageal acid exposure can trigger a vagal nerve reflex that results in bronchospasm and cough.

Unlike typical GERD symptoms (i.e., heartburn and regurgitation), extraesophageal symptoms of reflux are much less specific to GERD. Prior to attributing these symptoms to GERD, and certainly before proceeding with antireflux surgery, it is necessary to determine whether a patient's extraesophageal symptoms are due to abnormal GER or a primary laryngeal-bronchial-pulmonary etiology. This can be challenging. A lack of response of extraesophageal symptoms to a trial of PPI therapy cannot reliably refute GERD as the etiology of extraesophageal symptoms. Although PPI therapy can improve or completely resolve *typical* GERD symptoms, patients with *extraesophageal symptoms* experience variable response to medical treatment [16–18]. This may be explained by recent evidence that suggests acid is not the only underlying caustic agent that results in laryngeal and pulmonary injury [19–21]. PPI therapy will suppress gastric acid production, but micro-aspiration of non-acid refluxate, which contains caustic bile salts, pepsin, and other caustic agents, can cause ongoing injury and symptoms.

Therefore, in patients with extraesophageal symptoms of GERD, a mechanical barrier to reflux (i.e., esophagogastric fundoplication created during antireflux surgery) may be necessary to prevent ongoing laryngeal-tracheal-bronchial injury.

In patients who present with abnormal GER and bothersome extraesophageal symptoms, a thorough evaluation must be completed to rule out a primary disorder of their upper or lower respiratory tract. This should be completed whether or not typical GERD symptoms are also present. At the University of Washington Center for Esophageal and Gastric Surgery, we always collaborate with otolaryngologists and pulmonologists to determine if a non-gastrointestinal condition is present. Surgery is only considered as an option for patients in whom GERD is present and highly suspicious of being related to the patient's extraesophageal symptoms. Based on our results, we counsel these patients that they will have a 70% likelihood of improvement in extraesophageal symptoms following antireflux surgery. It should be noted that these results are inferior to those normally seen in patients treated only for typical symptoms of GERD [22].

Lung Conditions Related to Gastroesophageal Reflux Disease

Increasing evidence suggests GERD is a contributing factor to the pathophysiology of several pulmonary diseases [23, 24].

Asthma
In their extensive review, Bowrey and colleagues [25] examined medical and surgical antireflux therapy in patients with GERD and asthma. In these patients, the use of antisecretory medications was associated with improved respiratory symptoms in only 25–50% of patients with GERD-induced asthma. Furthermore, less than 15% of these patients experienced objective improvement in pulmonary function. One explanation for these results is that most of these studies lasted 3 months or less, which is potentially too short to see any improvement in pulmonary

function. Additionally, in several trials, gastric acid secretion was incompletely blocked by acid suppression therapy, and patients experienced ongoing GERD.

In patients with asthma and GERD, antireflux surgery appears to be more effective than medical therapy at managing pulmonary symptoms. Antireflux surgery is associated with improvement in respiratory symptoms in nearly 90% of children and 70% of adults with asthma and GERD. Several randomized trials have compared histamine-2 receptor antagonists and antireflux surgery in the management of GERD-associated asthma. Compared to patients treated with antisecretory medications, patients treated with antireflux surgery were more likely to experience relief of asthma symptoms, discontinue systemic steroid therapy, and improve peak expiratory flow rate. Thus, the presence of GERD in lung transplant recipient may induce airflow obstruction without overt manifestations of asthma and mimic bronchiolitis obliterans syndrome (BOS) and/or cause lung allograft dysfunction.

Idiopathic Pulmonary Fibrosis
Idiopathic pulmonary fibrosis (IPF) is a severe, chronic, and progressive lung disease that generally results in death within 5 years of diagnosis. Recently, the pathophysiology of IPF has been shown to hinge on alveolar epithelial injury followed by abnormal tissue remodeling. Proximal esophageal reflux and micro-aspiration of acid and non-acid gastric contents has been implicated as one possible cause of alveolar epithelial injury that can lead to IPF.

The incidence of GERD in patients with IPF has been reported to be between 35 and 94% [26–29]. Importantly, typical symptoms of GERD are not sensitive for abnormal reflux in patients with IPF, as many patients with IPF do not experience any heartburn, regurgitation, or acid brash despite having a very abnormal acid exposure [30]. Consequently, the threshold to test for GERD in patients with IPF should be low, as a result several authors have recommended ambulatory pH monitoring in all patients with IPF [31, 32]. It is important to appreciate, however, that several studies have demonstrated that the severity of reflux measured by ambulatory pH monitoring does not appear to be associated with severity of pulmonary disease in patients with IPF [33]. This should not discount the role that GERD plays in the pathophysiology of IPF, as multiple host-response factors are involved in the development of pulmonary dysfunction due to GERD, and the variability in pulmonary dysfunction may be related to one or more of these factors rather than the degree of GERD. This underscores the notion that a better test is needed to determine the relative contribution of GERD to lung dysfunction in patients with chronic lung disease.

Since IPF is a progressive, fatal disease, investigators have studied the effect of GERD treatment on pulmonary function and survival in patients with IPF. In reviewing the charts of 204 patients with IPF, Lee and colleagues [34] used logistic regression to show that both acid suppression therapy and history of Nissen fundoplication were associated with longer survival and slower pulmonary decline. Although PPI use suppresses gastric acid production, it does not prevent reflux of non-acid gastroduodenal contents. As previously stated, non-acid reflux has been implicated in both extraesophageal symptoms of reflux and IPF; thus, it is postulated that perhaps surgery may be more effective than medical treatment in this patient population. In 18 patients with IPF, Kilduff and colleagues [35] demonstrated PPI use was associated with fewer episodes of acid reflux on pH monitoring; however, these patients experienced no change in reported cough severity and were found to have persistent and significant non-acid reflux on esophageal impedance testing. Therefore, in IPF patients with significant GERD, the argument could be made that a mechanical barrier to both acid and non-acid reflux (i.e., antireflux surgery) is more appropriate than PPI therapy.

Antireflux surgery in patients with IPF appears to be safe, provides effective control of distal esophageal acid exposure, and may mitigate progression of pulmonary dysfunction. In the first report on this topic, Raghu and colleagues [36] published their experience with antireflux surgery in one patient with IPF and GERD. During 72 months of follow-up, they demonstrated stabilization of forced vital capacity, diffusion capacity of the lung to carbon monoxide, room air oxygen saturation, and exercise capacity on 6-min walk test. This observation led to a larger retrospective cohort study in which the same group studied the outcome of 27 patients with IPF who underwent laparoscopic antireflux surgery over a 14-year period [37]. Ninety-day mortality was zero, and there were no perioperative pulmonary complications. Distal esophageal acid exposure was normalized in 19 of 20 patients (95%), and only 1 patient underwent reoperation for recurrent GERD at 12 years after the initial antireflux surgery. The decline in pulmonary function (as measured by forced vital capacity [FVC]) was 102 mL over the first year following antireflux surgery. Compared with pulmonary decline published for two leading pharmacotherapies for IPF (nintedanib, 115 mL, and pirfenidone, 235 mL), this pulmonary decline following antireflux surgery was lesser but not statistically significant. With stronger evidence of the benefit of antireflux surgery in the mitigation of IPF-related pulmonary dysfunction and the relative safety of the procedure in these patients, an NIH-sponsored multicenter randomized controlled trial is underway to evaluate the safety and efficacy of laparoscopic antireflux surgery in the treatment of IPF (Treatment of IPF with Laparoscopic Antireflux Surgery [WRAP-IPF], NCT01982968).

Lung Transplantation

Despite advances in medical management, lung transplantation remains the only definitive treatment option for patients with end-stage lung disease. Unfortunately, patient survival following lung transplantation is short compared to survival after other solid organ transplantation. As of 2015, the median survival at 1, 3, and 5 years was 83.1%, 62.1%, and 46.2%, respectively [38].

The main reason for this inferior survival following lung transplantation is the development of bronchiolitis obliterans syndrome (BOS) in the transplanted lungs. BOS develops secondary to both immune and nonimmunologic chronic inflammatory responses to ongoing graft injury. At 5-year posttransplant, BOS can affect up to 80% of lung transplant patients, and by 3-year posttransplant, it accounts for up to 30% of all deaths [39]. Although the specific pathophysiology is incompletely understood, there is mounting evidence that GERD is a contributing factor to BOS. GERD is found in as many as 70% of patients after lung transplant [40], and it is now viewed as a modifiable risk factor for allograft deterioration. Additionally, it has been shown that a negative correlation exists between extent of esophageal acid exposure and graft function as measured by forced expiratory volume in 1 s [41].

Connective Tissue Disorders and Gastroesophageal Reflux Disease

Connective tissue disorders (CTD) are systemic rheumatologic diseases that affect protein-rich tissues, including the fat, bone, and cartilage. CTD typically involve the musculoskeletal system, including the skin, muscles, and joints, but they also can affect other organs, including the gastrointestinal tract and the lungs. Esophageal dysmotility and GERD are the two most common gastrointestinal manifestations of these diseases. Gastroparesis is also prevalent in this patient population. Patti and colleagues reported pathologic reflux in 70% of CTD patients evaluated by 24-h pH monitoring and 83% of CTD patients evaluated by esophageal manometry demonstrated low-amplitude peristalsis; nearly half of those patients had absent esophageal peristalsis [42]. Further, up to 60% of patients with scleroderma were found to have a complication of GERD, including Barrett's esophagus or peptic stricture [43].

Lung disease is also common in patients with CTD, and up to 60% of patients with CTD and lung involvement ultimately progress to end-stage lung disease and may be considered for transplantation [44]. As discussed in prior sections of this chapter, there is a strong association among esophageal dysmotility, GERD, and some pulmonary conditions, and it is now evident that a similar relationship exists in the CTD patient population. However, the CTD patient population is unique in that CTD patients also have a high prevalence of esophageal dysmotility. In patients with CTD and end-stage lung disease, Patti and colleagues reported an incidence of abnormal esophageal motility of 83%, and nearly half of those patients demonstrated absent peristalsis [45]. This was significantly more common than in patients with isolated CTD (36% abnormal peristalsis; 0% absent peristalsis) and normal healthy control patients with GERD (36% abnormal peristalsis; 0% absent peristalsis). Because of the high prevalence of esophageal dysmotility and severe chronic lung disease in patients with CTD, there has been hesitation to offer these patients lung transplantation due to concern for early graft dysfunction secondary to GERD-related BOS. Because antireflux surgery is very effective at controlling acid- and non-acid GERD, antireflux surgery may provide an opportunity to mitigate GERD-related BOS in this patient population.

Clinical Evaluation of Patients with Suspected GERD

The diagnosis of GERD is frequently made clinically based on the presence of typical GERD symptoms and improvement in those symptoms with PPI therapy. In patients without pulmonary disease or other symptoms that raise concern for an alternative diagnosis (i.e., esophageal stricture, achalasia, malignancy), this approach is acceptable. Since patients with GERD and coexisting pulmonary disease frequently lack gastroesophageal symptoms of GERD and stake of leaving GERD untreated is ongoing lung injury, a more definitive diagnosis of GERD is necessary. The diagnosis of GERD is confirmed by the presence of elevated distal esophageal acid exposure identified on ambulatory esophageal pH testing. Three additional tests—esophageal manometry, barium esophagram, and esophagogastroduodenoscopy—provide a comprehensive evaluation of gastroesophageal anatomy and function. In patients with abnormal esophageal pH testing who are also considering antireflux surgery, including patients with pulmonary disease, all four tests should be completed.

Ambulatory pH and Impedance Monitoring

Ambulatory pH monitoring quantifies distal esophageal acid exposure and is the gold standard test to diagnose GERD. Twenty-four-hour pH monitoring is conducted with a thin catheter that is passed into the esophagus via the patient's nose. The simplest catheter is a dual-probe pH catheter that is positioned 5 cm proximal to the LES based on esophageal manometry (see next section). Alternatively, 48-h ambulatory pH monitoring can be performed using an endoscopically placed wireless pH monitor. In one study, 48-h system increased sensitivity of detecting GERD by 22% [46].

Ambulatory pH monitoring generates a large amount of data concerning esophageal acid exposure (Fig. 17.3). A composite DeMeester score is calculated based on these data, and a score of

≥ 14.7 is abnormal. Importantly, patients undergoing esophageal pH monitoring should stop all acid suppression medications for 1 week prior to testing to avoid a false-negative test. Occasionally one may want to repeat the test—once the baseline is obtained—while the patient is on treatment with PPIs to determine the effect of treatment in esophageal acid exposure.

In addition to the objective data obtained with esophageal pH testing, the patient can keep track of reflux-related symptoms by pressing a button on an electronic data recorder. During the interpretation of the pH study, symptom index and symptom-associated probability are calculated based on the temporal relationship between the symptom event and episodes of distal esophageal acid exposure (Fig. 17.4). A symptom episode that occurs within 2 min of a reflux episode is defined as a close temporal relationship and suggests, but does not confirm, a cause and effect relationship between GER and patient symptoms. While the decision to perform antireflux surgery should not hinge on symptom correlation [47], it can help predict symptom improvement following antireflux surgery [48].

Esophageal impedance monitoring identifies episodes of non-acid reflux by detecting changes in the resistance to flow of an electrical current

---

24-H Dual-Probe Esophageal pH Study Report:

Distal channel placed 37 cm from the nares and 5 cm from the manometrically determined proximal border of the lower esophageal sphincter.

Duration of the test: 23 h 26 min

Acid Exposure (pH)

	Upright		Recumbent		Total	
Proximal Probe						
Time	44.6 min		9.2 min			
Percent Time	**6.7%**		**1.2%**			
Mean Acid Clearance Time	37 s		21 s			
Number of Episodes	72		26			
Longest Episode	8.0 min		1.4 min			
Distal Probe						
Time	79.2 min	Normal	110.3 min	Normal	189.5 min	Normal
Percent Time	**11.9%**	(<6.3%)	**14.8%**	(<1.2%)	**13.5%**	(<4.2%)
Mean Acid Clearance Time	49 s		65 s		57 s	
Number of Episodes	96		102		198	
Longest Episode	9.2 min		19.7 min		19.7 min	

DeMeester score: 56.3

Symptom Correlation: Good correlation for belch 58% (19 events). Very good for cough 82% (38 events). Very good for heartburn 94% (18 events).

Diagnosis: Abnormal 24-h esophageal pH study.

Fig. 17.3 Ambulatory 24-h esophageal pH monitoring report. In this patient, abnormal esophageal acid exposure was identified in the upright and recumbent positions and in both the distal and proximal esophagus. A complete report should include a calculated DeMeester composite score and symptom correlation (Courtesy of the University of Washington Center for Esophageal and Gastric Surgery, Seattle, WA)

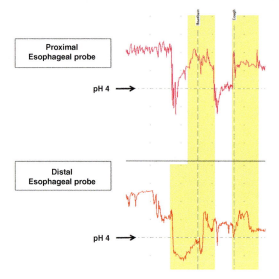

Fig. 17.4 Representative portion of a dual-probe 24-h esophageal pH study. Temporal correlation of reflux symptoms (e.g., heartburn and cough) with episodes of esophageal pH <4 is used to calculate symptom index, which can help predict symptom improvement after anti-reflux surgery (Courtesy of the University of Washington Center for Esophageal and Gastric Surgery, Seattle, WA)

(i.e., impedance). Impedance increases in the presence of air and decreases in the presence of a liquid bolus. Therefore, this technology can detect both gas and liquid movement in the esophagus. Some impedance catheters also have one or more pH sensor, allowing for the simultaneous detection of acid and non-acid reflux. There also exists a specialized pH-impedance catheter with a very proximal pH sensor that detects pharyngeal acid reflux. This catheter can be useful in the evaluation of patients with extra-esophageal symptoms such as cough, throat clearing, hoarseness, and wheezing.

Combined impedance-pH monitoring has been shown to identify reflux episodes with greater sensitivity than pH testing alone [49]. Although there is no consensus on whether impedance-pH testing should be performed on or off acid suppression therapy [50–53], our practice is to perform all impedance-pH testing off acid suppression. Furthermore, how impedance-pH monitoring should guide the management of GERD is unknown. Patel and colleagues attempted to determine the parameters on

esophageal impedance-pH monitoring that predict response of GERD symptoms to both medical and surgical treatment [54]. They showed that acid exposure time, and not the number of non-acid reflux events, best predicted symptom improvement to both medical and surgical therapy. Although the addition of impedance monitoring increased the sensitivity of the study, non-acid reflux measurements alone were unable to accurately predict symptom improvement to medical or surgical therapy for GERD.

Esophageal Manometry

Esophageal manometry is the most effective way to assesses function of the esophageal body and the lower esophageal sphincter. Standard esophageal manometry provides linear tracings of pressure waves of the esophageal body and LES (Fig. 17.5). High-resolution esophageal manometry gathers data using a 32-channel flexible catheter with pressure-sensing devices arranged at 1 cm intervals. The study generates a color contour plot of ten patients' swallows. It shows the response of the upper and lower esophageal sphincters as well as the esophageal body; time is on the x-axis, esophageal length is on the y-axis, and pressure is represented by a color scale (Fig. 17.6). In patients undergoing evaluation for GERD, esophageal manometry can exclude achalasia and identify patients with ineffective esophageal body peristalsis. Esophageal manometry also measures the LES resting pressure and assesses the LES for appropriate relaxation with deglutition. Because the LES is the major barrier to GER, a defective LES is common in patients with GERD [55].

Esophagogastroduodenoscopy

Endoscopy is an essential step in the evaluation of patients with GERD to evaluate for evidence of mucosal injury due to GER, including ulcerations, peptic strictures, and Barrett's esophagus. Endoscopic evaluation should also include an assessment of the integrity of the GEJ flap valve

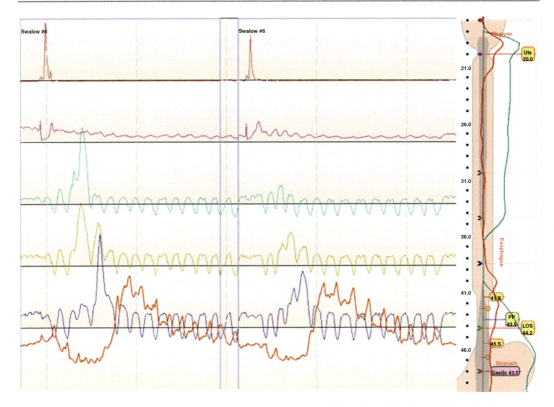

Fig. 17.5 Standard esophageal manometry tracing (Courtesy of the University of Washington Center for Esophageal and Gastric Surgery, Seattle, WA)

[56] as well as the presence of a hiatal hernia. The hernia should be measured in cranial-caudal, anteroposterior, and lateral dimensions.

Barium Esophagram

Barium esophagram provides a detailed anatomic evaluation of the esophagus and stomach that is useful during preoperative evaluation of patients with GERD. Of particular importance are the presence, size, and anatomic characteristics of a hiatal or paraesophageal hernia (Fig. 17.7). Despite its ability to identify episodes of GER, which can occur spontaneously or in response to patient positioning during the study, barium esophagram cannot confirm or refute the diagnosis of GERD. Additional gastroesophageal conditions that can be identified on barium esophagram are esophageal diverticula, tumors, peptic strictures, achalasia, dysmotility, and gastroparesis. If any one of these is found in a patient

undergoing evaluation for GERD, antireflux surgery should be delayed until appropriate evaluation of the unexpected findings is completed.

Additional Evaluations in Patients with Extraesophageal GERD Symptoms

While there is agreement among gastroenterologists, pulmonolgists, and surgeons that extraesophageal (laryngopharyngeal) reflux exists, a sensitive and specific test to diagnose this condition has yet to be developed. Despite this, in patients with isolated extraesophageal symptoms of GERD, clinical evaluation beyond the four major diagnostic evaluation tools noted above should be performed, particularly if antireflux surgery is being considered. Several questionnaires exist that assess the presence and severity of laryngopharyngeal symptoms. While these are easy to administer and score, they lack sensitivity

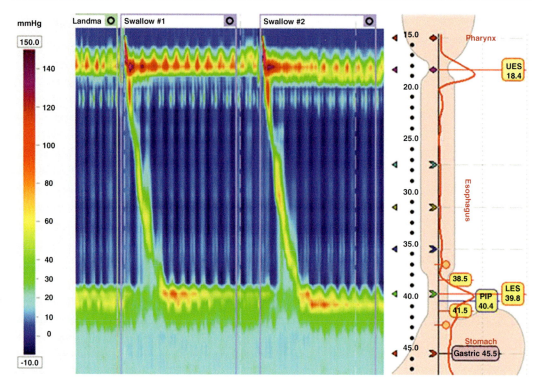

Fig. 17.6 High-resolution manometry tracing (Courtesy of the University of Washington Center for Esophageal and Gastric Surgery, Seattle, WA)

and specificity to GERD. Collaboration with an otolaryngologist is indispensable when vague, non-specific laryngopharyngeal symptoms are present, including throat clearing, hoarseness, throat pain, postnasal drainage, and globus sensation. Otolaryngologists are uniquely trained to perform a detailed history and examination that may identify a non-GERD etiology of the patient's symptoms. Furthermore, otolaryngologists can perform awake endoscopic evaluations of the upper aerodigestive tract. Laryngeal inflammation has been identified in patients with as few as three episodes a week of reflux [57], and these inflammatory changes can be identified on laryngoscopy and graded according to the reflux finding score [58]. Pathologic biomarkers, including pepsin, have been identified in laryngeal biopsy [21], bronchoalveolar lavage [59], and even sputum [60]. Additionally, laryngopharyngeal pH testing may identify the presence of proximal reflux of gastric contents. Although no single test may confirm or refute GERD as the cause of extraesophageal symptoms, taken

together the results of these studies can help guide treatment, including the decision to pursue antireflux surgery.

Treatment of Gastroesophageal Reflux Disease

Medical Management

For patients that present with typical symptoms of GERD, an 8-week course of PPI therapy is recommended [61, 62]. However, prior to empirically prescribing a PPI, it is necessary to ensure that the patient does not have symptoms that may indicate the presence of a gastroesophageal malignancy or other non-GERD diagnosis, including rapidly progressive dysphagia, regurgitation of undigested food, anemia, extraesophageal symptoms of GERD, or weight loss. If the symptoms improve with PPI therapy, then the trial is considered both diagnostic and therapeutic. If the symptoms persist after a trial of

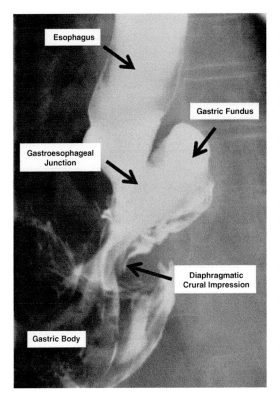

Fig. 17.7 Upper gastrointestinal series (esophagram) demonstrating a paraesophageal hernia. Note that the gastroesophageal junction and a portion of the gastric fundus are herniated cephalad to the diaphragmatic impression on the gastric body/fundus

medical therapy, a more extensive evaluation, as described above, is indicated. Although lifestyle modification has been advocated before or as an adjunct to medical therapy, the efficacy of such changes in the treatment of esophagitis has not been proved [63].

Proton pump inhibitors have revolutionized the pharmacologic treatment of GERD. As one of the most widely prescribed drugs worldwide, the annual expenditure on PPI therapy has reached approximately $24 billion [64]. These drugs stop gastric acid production by irreversibly binding the proton pump in the parietal cells of the stomach. The maximal pharmacological effect occurs approximately 4 days after initiation of therapy, and the effect lasts for the life of the parietal cell. For this reason, patients must stop PPI therapy 1 week prior to ambulatory pH monitoring to avoid a false-negative test result.

Proton pump inhibitors are well-tolerated medications. Immediate side effects of PPI therapy are relatively rare and generally mild, including headache, abdominal pain, flatulence, constipation, and diarrhea. This relatively safe side-effect profile and their effectiveness at controlling GERD symptoms have led to overprescription of these medications in both the outpatient and inpatient settings [65]. Although there are published evidence-based recommendations that might limit this practice of overprescription, including on-demand dosing and step-down therapy, clinicians frequently do not follow these guidelines.

Despite their short-term safety, there has been concern over the long-term effects of PPI use since their initial preclinical trials [66]. The most concerning long-term complication of PPI use is hypergastrinemia leading to enterochromaffin cell hyperplasia and ultimately carcinoid tumors. The first case of neuroendocrine tumor of the stomach in patient with 15-year history of PPI use has just been published [67], so it seems that the true risk of this is exceptionally low. However, additional associations have been made between PPI use and enteric infections, antiplatelet medication interactions, bone fractures, nutritional deficiencies, and community-acquired pneumonia [65]. Importantly, however, there have been no cause and effect relationship established, and patients prescribed with PPI therapy have more comorbid conditions than the general population, which may explain some of these associations. Therefore, until further studies better elucidate PPI as a contributing factor to these conditions, the results of these studies should be interpreted with caution.

One shortcoming of PPI therapy is that it actually does nothing to reduce gastroesophageal reflux (i.e., retrograde movement of gastric contents into the esophagus). Proton pump inhibitors render the gastric refluxate less acidic and consequently reduce the caustic injury to the esophagus during episodes of reflux. However, because GER still occurs (albeit with more alkaline gastric contents), patients with long-standing GERD frequently experience symptomatic regurgitation. Furthermore, proximal esophageal reflux of non-acid gastric contents can still be aspirated. This is an important consideration in generating a treatment plan for patients with chronic lung disease and patients undergoing lung transplant evaluation: Aspiration of non-acid refluxate is associated with lung injury that can lead to progression of lung disease or, in the case of a lung transplant patient, graft rejection and/or BOS. As such, surgical creation of a mechanical barrier to reflux may be more appropriate in these patient populations.

Surgical Management

For patients that exhibit elevated distal esophageal acid exposure and persistent typical GERD symptoms despite maximal medical therapy, antireflux surgery should be strongly considered. The application of laparoscopy to antireflux surgery has decreased patient morbidity and hospital length of stay. Furthermore, several studies have shown that antireflux surgery is cost-effective compared to prolonged PPI therapy [68, 69]. In patients that experience absolutely no improvement in their symptoms with the use of PPI, the diagnosis of GERD should be questioned, and surgeons must carefully consider alternative etiologies prior to offering surgical treatment. In patients with extraesophageal symptoms of GERD that do not improve with PPI therapy, consultation with an otolaryngologist and/or pulmonologist is necessary prior to proceeding with antireflux surgery to determine if a primary laryngeal, bronchial, or pulmonary cause of the symptoms is present. Endoscopic evidence of severe esophageal injury (e.g., ulcerations, peptic strictures, and Barrett's esophagus) can be considered evidence of abnormal distal esophageal acid exposure; however, endoscopic findings by themselves should not be considered an indication for operative therapy by themselves.

Several randomized trials with long-term follow-up have compared medical and surgical therapy for GERD. Spechler and colleagues [70] found that surgical therapy results in good symptom control after 10-year follow-up. Although they reported 62% of patients in the surgical group were taking antisecretory medications at long-term follow-up, the indications for this medication use were not necessarily GERD, and reflux symptoms did not change significantly when these patients stopped taking these medications.

Lundell and colleagues [71] randomized patients with erosive esophagitis into surgical or medical therapy. Treatment failure was defined as moderate or severe symptoms of heartburn, regurgitation, dysphagia, and/or odynophagia, recommencement of PPI therapy, reoperation, or grade 2 esophagitis. At 7-year follow-up, fewer treatment failures were seen in patients managed with fundoplication than omeprazole (33% vs. 53%, $p = 0.002$). In patients that did not respond to the initial dose of omeprazole, dose escalation was completed; however, surgical intervention remained superior. Patients treated with fundoplication experienced more obstructive and gas bloat symptoms (e.g., dysphagia, flatulence, inability to belch) compared with the medically treated cohort. At 12-year follow-up, the durability of these results remained: Patients who underwent fundoplication had fewer treatment failures compared with patients treated with medical therapy (47% vs. 55%, $p = 0.022$) [72].

Over the past 25 years, surgeon experience with antireflux surgery has increased dramatically. With increased experience, the durability of symptom improvement has increased, and perioperative complications have decreased. This is especially true in high-volume centers. In one single-institution study that followed 100 patients for 10 years after antireflux surgery, 90% of patients remained free of GERD symptoms [73]. We recently published our experience in a cohort of 288 patients undergoing antireflux surgery. With median follow-up of greater than 5 years, symptom improvement for heartburn was 90% and regurgitation was 92% [74]. These results confirm that antireflux surgery can provide excellent durable relief of GERD when patients are appropriately selected and excellent technique is employed. However, it should be noted that none of the studies mentioned above were limited to patients with GERD and pulmonary disease. While some of the patients in these studies did have respiratory symptoms, the majority did not, and the studies were not centered on the relationship between GERD and pulmonary disease.

Fisichella and associates were the first to comprehensively evaluate symptoms of GERD and gastroesophageal function (esophageal manometry, 24-h pH testing, UGI, EGD, and gastric emptying study) in patients who have undergone lung transplantation. In 35 consecutive lung transplant patients, 51% were found to have GERD (15 with typical symptoms and elevated distal esophageal acid exposure; 3 with typical symptoms and bronchoscopic evidence of aspiration). Although no differences in the manometric profile of the LES were demonstrated between the GERD and non-GERD groups, there were differences in the manometric results of the esophageal body. In GERD patients, the distal esophageal amplitude was significantly lower than in patients without GERD (median 46 mmHg vs. 90 mmHg, $P = 0.029$), and more patients with GERD demonstrated ineffective esophageal motility (36% vs. 6%, $P = 0.04$). While this study was performed prior to the adoption of the Chicago Classification v3.0, which is now considered diagnostic standard for high-resolution esophageal manometry, it still demonstrates that the presence of GERD is associated with manometric evidence of esophageal dysfunction. Finally, among all patients with GERD following lung transplantation, there were no hiatal hernias identified on UGI.

Two findings from this study point to interesting differences between lung transplant patients with GERD and those patients with GERD who have not undergone a lung transplant. First, although a hypotensive lower esophageal sphincter is frequently identified in patients with GERD, nearly all patients in this study had a normal LES resting pressure, regardless of the presence of GERD. Second, no hiatal hernias were identified in patients with GERD in this study, whereas type I sliding hiatal hernias are common among patients with GERD. These findings suggest that the pathophysiologic mechanism underlying GERD in lung transplant patients may be different than typical patients with GERD. Specifically, rather than have a baseline underlying low-

pressure LES, lung transplant patients may experience more transient LES relaxations that contribute to GER. Additionally, in this study, there was a higher prevalence of ineffective esophageal motility in the GERD patients compared to patients without GERD. From this observational study, it is not possible to determine if this ineffective esophageal motility is a contributing factor to GERD (inability to clear distal esophageal acid when reflux occurs) or a result of GERD (secondary to chronic distal esophageal inflammation). Further, it was not noted whether the patients with ineffective esophageal motility had an underlying disease, such as scleroderma, that could contribute to both lung disease and esophageal dysmotility.

Lung transplant patients are assumed to be at higher risk for an operation. Compared to a matched cohort of patients without pulmonary disease undergoing elective antireflux surgery, they have a higher overall comorbidity burden, higher rates of diabetes mellitus, and chronic renal disease, and pulmonary allografts do not function as well as healthy native lungs [75]. A single-center study found pulmonary transplant patients undergoing antireflux surgery have a longer postoperative length of stay (2.89 vs. 0.71 days) and higher readmission rate (25% vs. 3%) compared to the general population [76]. In a nationwide study using propensity-matched controls without history of lung transplant, Kilic and associates [75] found that lung transplant patients undergoing antireflux surgery had similar rates of postoperative mortality as well as overall and individual morbidity (cardiac, pulmonary, renal, wound, hollow viscous injury). Similar to single-center studies, hospital length of stay and estimated costs of care were higher in lung transplant patients.

In lung transplant patients with GERD, antireflux surgery is associated with improved objective measurement of allograft function. Hoppo and associates [77] retrospectively reviewed their experience with antireflux surgery in 22 lung transplant patients with GERD. After antireflux surgery, 91% of patients experienced significant improvement in forced expiratory volume in 1 s (FEV_1). In 12 patients that had decreasing FEV_1

before antireflux surgery, 11 patients experienced a reversal of this trend post-antireflux surgery. Additionally, following antireflux surgery, there were fewer episodes of pneumonia and rejection.

Considerations for Surgical Management of GERD in Patients with Ineffective Esophageal Motility and Lung Disease

Ineffective esophageal motility (IEM) refers to impaired distal esophageal contractility ("vigor") and is defined according to the Chicago Classification v3.0 of high-resolution esophageal manometry as ≥50% of peristaltic contractions having a distal esophageal contractile integral of <450 mmHg-s-cm [2]. At the most extreme end of the spectrum, the esophagus may exhibit *absent muscular contractility*. As discussed in prior sections, there is a clear association between IEM, GERD, and ESLD, especially among patients with mixed connective tissues disorders. There is a general consensus—emanated more from clinical judgment than scientific data—that impaired esophageal motility (in the most severe cases, absent esophageal contractility) decreases the ability of the esophagus to clear gastric refluxate from the esophagus and, consequently, reflux episodes may travel more proximally than in patients with normal esophageal motility. In theory, this places patients with IEM at increased risk for aspiration from refluxate, though with an intact oropharyngeal swallowing phase, IEM/absent contractility should not result in aspiration when eating or drinking. Therefore, remaining *nil* per os and receiving enteral nutrition through a gastrostomy tube do not necessarily solve this problem. As detailed in prior sections, aspiration is associated with some chronic lung diseases and BOS, the leading cause of graft failure following lung transplantation. Consequently, many lung transplant teams make IEM, particularly when severe (i.e., complete absence of esophageal body contractility), a contraindication to lung transplantation. Unfortunately, while the connections among these clinical entities appear to be logical, the current literature does not specifically answer the question: "Are IEM and absent esophageal contractility contraindications to lung transplantation?" At the University of Washington, we have observed (anecdotally) that patients with IEM who lack dysphagia do well after transplant. Therefore, in patients with IEM and absent esophageal contractility, we use dysphagia as a marker for the severity of esophageal dysfunction and as an additional criterion to determine whether the patient should remain in the transplant list. Furthermore, we have substantial experience with LARS in patients with IEM. Our studies [78] as well as those from Patti and associates [79] have shown that LARS is safe and effective at controlling GERD. These studies have a relatively small number of patients, and their outcomes are not based on mitigation of pulmonary decline in patients with lung disease. However, they do suggest indirectly that patients with IEM and GERD who are being considered for lung transplantation should not be declined transplantation based solely on the presence of IEM.

Summary

Gastroesophageal reflux disease is a very common condition that is associated with symptoms (like heartburn and regurgitation) that can significantly impair quality of life. Additionally, GERD appears to be a contributing factor to both end-stage lung disease and pulmonary failure after lung transplantation. For patients who experience life-limiting symptoms of GERD and for patients with severe pulmonary disease and GERD, diagnostic testing should be performed to confirm the diagnosis of GERD and evaluate for the presence of esophageal dysmotility. When medical therapy is ineffective or, in the case of GERD-related lung disease, insufficient, antireflux surgery should be considered. Laparoscopic antireflux surgery has a long-standing history of excellent control of typical symptoms of GERD. Recently, antireflux surgery has been shown to mitigate pulmonary decline in end-stage lung disease and prevent BOS in lung transplant recipients. Even in patients with severe pulmonary disease who are at relatively increased risk of undergoing an abdominal operation, antireflux surgery is safe in the hands of experienced gastroesophageal surgeons. For this reason, experienced gastroesophageal surgeons should be an integral member of the multidisciplinary team that manages these patients.

References

1. Galmiche JP, Janssens J. The pathophysiology of gastro-oesophageal reflux disease: an overview. Scand J Gastroenterol Suppl. 1995;211:7–18.
2. Kahrilas PJ, Bredenoord AJ, Fox M, Gyawali CP, Roman S, Smout AJPM, et al. The Chicago classification of esophageal motility disorders, v3.0. Neurogastroenterol Motil. 2015;27(2):160–74.
3. Diener U, Patti MG, Molena D, Fisichella PM, Way LW. Esophageal dysmotility and gastroesophageal reflux disease. J Gastrointest Surg. 2001;5(3):260–5.
4. Quigley EMM. Gastro-oesophageal reflux disease—spectrum or continuum? QJM. 1997;90(1):75–8.
5. Ho KY, Kang JY. Reflux esophagitis patients in Singapore have motor and acid exposure abnormalities similar to patients in the Western hemisphere. Am J Gastroenterol. 1999;94(5):1186–91.
6. Heider TR, Behrns KE, Koruda MJ, Shaheen NJ, Lucktong TA, Bradshaw B, et al. Fundoplication improves disordered esophageal motility. J Gastrointest Surg. 2003;7(2):159–63.
7. Pellegrini CA, DeMeester TR, Johnson LF, Skinner DB. Gastroesophageal reflux and pulmonary aspiration: incidence, functional abnormality, and results of surgical therapy. Surgery. 1979;86(1):110–9.
8. Fouad YM, Katz PO, Hatlebakk JG, Castell DO. Ineffective esophageal motility: the most common motility abnormality in patients with GERD-associated respiratory symptoms. Am J Gastroenterol. 1999;94(6):1464–7.
9. Basseri B, Conklin JL, Pimentel M, Tabrizi R, Phillips EH, Simsir SA, et al. Esophageal motor dysfunction and gastroesophageal reflux are prevalent in lung transplant candidates. Ann Thorac Surg. 2010;90(5):1630–6.
10. Suen HC, Hendrix H, Patterson GA. Special article: physiologic consequences of pneumonectomy. Consequences on the esophageal function. 1999. Chest Surg Clin N Am. 2002;12(3):587–95.
11. Davis CS, Shankaran V, Kovacs EJ, Gagermeier J, Dilling D, Alex CG, et al. Gastroesophageal reflux disease after lung transplantation: pathophysiology and implications for treatment. Surgery. 2010;148(4):737–45.
12. Fisichella PM, Jalilvand A. The role of impaired esophageal and gastric motility in end-stage lung diseases and after lung transplantation. J Surg Res. 2014;186(1):201–6.
13. Berkowitz N, Schulman LL, McGregor C, Markowitz D. Gastroparesis after lung transplantation: potential role in postoperative respiratory complications. Chest. 1995;108(6):1602–7.
14. Davis CS, Jellish WS, Fisichella PM. Laparoscopic fundoplication with or without pyloroplasty in patients with gastroesophageal reflux disease after lung transplantation: how I do it. J Gastrointest Surg. 2010;14(9):1434–41.
15. Moore JM, Vaezi MF. Extraesophageal manifestations of gastroesophageal reflux disease: real or imagined? Curr Opin Gastroenterol. 2010;26(4):389–94.
16. Chang AB, Lasserson TJ, Kiljander TO, Connor FL, Gaffney JT, Garske LA. Systematic review and meta-analysis of randomised controlled trials of gastro-oesophageal reflux interventions for chronic cough associated with gastro-oesophageal reflux. BMJ. 2006;332(7532):11–7.
17. Vaezi MF, Richter JE. Twenty-four-hour ambulatory esophageal pH monitoring in the diagnosis of acid reflux-related chronic cough. South Med J. 1997;90(3):305–11.
18. Waring JP, Lacayo L, Hunter J, Katz E, Suwak B. Chronic cough and hoarseness in patients with severe gastroesophageal reflux disease. Diagnosis and response to therapy. Dig Dis Sci. 1995;40(5):1093–7.
19. Mainie I, Tutuian R, Shay S, Vela M, Zhang X, Sifrim D, et al. Acid and non-acid reflux in patients with persistent symptoms despite acid suppressive therapy: a multicentre study using combined ambulatory impedance-pH monitoring. Gut. 2006; 55(10):1398–402.
20. Vela MF. Non-acid reflux: detection by multichannel intraluminal impedance and pH, clinical significance and management. Am J Gastroenterol. 2009;104(2):277–80.
21. Wassenaar E, Johnston N, Merati A, Montenovo M, Petersen R, Tatum R, et al. Pepsin detection in patients with laryngopharyngeal reflux before and after fundoplication. Surg Endosc. 2011;25(12):3870–6.
22. Worrell SG, DeMeester SR, Greene CL, Oh DS, Hagen JA. Pharyngeal pH monitoring better predicts a successful outcome for extraesophageal reflux symptoms after antireflux surgery. Surg Endosc. 2013;27(11):4113–8.
23. Ducoloné A, Vandevenne A, Jouin H, Grob JC, Coumaros D, Meyer C, et al. Gastroesophageal reflux in patients with asthma and chronic bronchitis. Am Rev Respir Dis. 1987;135(2):327–32.
24. Davis MV. Relationship between pulmonary disease, hiatal hernia, and gastroesophageal reflux. N Y State J Med. 1972;72(8):935–8.
25. Bowrey DJ, Peters JH, DeMeester TR. Gastroesophageal reflux disease in asthma: effects of medical and surgical antireflux therapy on asthma control. Ann Surg. 2000;231(2):161–72.
26. Bandeira CD, Rubin AS, Cardoso PFG, Moreira J da S, Machado M da M. Prevalence of gastroesophageal reflux disease in patients with idiopathic pulmonary fibrosis. J Bras Pneumol. 2009;35(12):1182–9.

27. Raghu G, Freudenberger TD, Yang S, Curtis JR, Spada C, Hayes J, et al. High prevalence of abnormal acid gastro-oesophageal reflux in idiopathic pulmonary fibrosis. Eur Respir J. 2006;27(1):136–42.

28. Salvioli B, Belmonte G, Stanghellini V, Baldi E, Fasano L, Pacilli AMG, et al. Gastro-oesophageal reflux and interstitial lung disease. Dig Liver Dis. 2006;38(12):879–84.

29. Tobin RW, Pope CE, Pellegrini CA, Emond MJ, Sillery J, Raghu G. Increased prevalence of gastroesophageal reflux in patients with idiopathic pulmonary fibrosis. Am J Respir Crit Care Med. 1998;158(6):1804–8.

30. Allaix ME, Fisichella PM, Noth I, Herbella FA, Borraez Segura B, Patti MG. Idiopathic pulmonary fibrosis and gastroesophageal reflux. Implications for treatment. J Gastrointest Surg. 2014;18(1):100–4–5.

31. Fahim A, Crooks M, Hart SP. Gastroesophageal reflux and idiopathic pulmonary fibrosis: a review. Pulm Med. 2010;2011:e634613.

32. Sweet MP, Patti MG, Leard LE, Golden JA, Hays SR, Hoopes C, et al. Gastroesophageal reflux in patients with idiopathic pulmonary fibrosis referred for lung transplantation. J Thorac Cardiovasc Surg. 2007;133(4):1078–84.

33. Hershcovici T, Jha LK, Johnson T, Gerson L, Stave C, Malo J, et al. Systematic review: the relationship between interstitial lung diseases and gastro-oesophageal reflux disease. Aliment Pharmacol Ther. 2011;34(11–12):1295–305.

34. Lee JS, Ryu JH, Elicker BM, Lydell CP, Jones KD, Wolters PJ, et al. Gastroesophageal reflux therapy is associated with longer survival in patients with idiopathic pulmonary fibrosis. Am J Respir Crit Care Med. 2011;184(12):1390–4.

35. Kilduff CE, Counter MJ, Thomas GA, Harrison NK, Hope-Gill BD. Effect of acid suppression therapy on gastroesophageal reflux and cough in idiopathic pulmonary fibrosis: an intervention study. Cough. 2014;10:4.

36. Raghu G, Yang ST-Y, Spada C, Hayes J, Pellegrini CA. Sole treatment of acid gastroesophageal reflux in idiopathic pulmonary fibrosis: a case series. Chest. 2006;129(3):794–800.

37. Raghu G, Morrow E, Collins B, Ho L, Hinojosa M, Hayes J, et al. Laparoscopic anti-reflux surgery for idiopathic pulmonary fibrosis at a single center. Eur Respir J. 2016;48(3):826–32.

38. Services UDoHaH. Organ Procurement and Transplantation Network. 2015. [Internet]. http://optntransplanthrsagov/coverage/latestdata/rptdataasp.

39. D'Ovidio F, Keshavjee S. Gastroesophageal reflux and lung transplantation. Dis Esophagus. 2006;19(5):315–20.

40. Reid KR, McKenzie FN, Menkis AH, Novick RJ, Pflugfelder PW, Kostuk WJ, et al. Importance of chronic aspiration in recipients of heart-lung transplants. Lancet. 1990;336(8709):206–8.

41. Hadjiliadis D, Duane Davis R, Steele MP, Messier RH, Lau CL, Eubanks SS, et al. Gastroesophageal reflux disease in lung transplant recipients. Clin Transpl. 2003;17(4):363–8.

42. Patti MG, Gasper WJ, Fisichella PM, Nipomnick I, Palazzo F. Gastroesophageal reflux disease and connective tissue disorders: pathophysiology and implications for treatment. J Gastrointest Surg. 2008;12(11):1900–6.

43. Zamost BJ, Hirschberg J, Ippoliti AF, Furst DE, Clements PJ, Weinstein WM. Esophagitis in scleroderma. Prevalence and risk factors. Gastroenterology. 1987;92(2):421–8.

44. Remy-Jardin M, Remy J, Wallaert B, Bataille D, Hatron PY. Pulmonary involvement in progressive systemic sclerosis: sequential evaluation with CT, pulmonary function tests, and bronchoalveolar lavage. Radiology. 1993;188(2):499–506.

45. Gasper WJ, Sweet MP, Golden JA, Hoopes C, Leard LE, Kleinhenz ME, et al. Lung transplantation in patients with connective tissue disorders and esophageal dysmotility. Dis Esophagus. 2008;21(7):650–5.

46. Tseng D, Rizvi AZ, Fennerty MB, Jobe BA, Diggs BS, Sheppard BC, et al. Forty-eight-hour pH monitoring increases sensitivity in detecting abnormal esophageal acid exposure. J Gastrointest Surg. 2005;9(8):1043–1051–1052.

47. Jobe BA, Richter JE, Hoppo T, Peters JH, Bell R, Dengler WC, et al. Preoperative diagnostic workup before antireflux surgery: an evidence and experience-based consensus of the esophageal diagnostic advisory panel. J Am Coll Surg. 2013;217(4):586–97.

48. Campos GMR, Peters JH, DeMeester TR, Öberg S, Crookes PF, Tan S, et al. Multivariate analysis of factors predicting outcome after laparoscopic Nissen fundoplication. J Gastrointest Surg. 1999;3(3):292–300.

49. Bredenoord AJ, Weusten BLAM, Timmer R, Conchillo JM, Smout AJPM. Addition of esophageal impedance monitoring to pH monitoring increases the yield of symptom association analysis in patients off PPI therapy. Am J Gastroenterol. 2006;101(3):453–9.

50. Hemmink GJM, Bredenoord AJ, Weusten BLAM, Monkelbaan JF, Timmer R, Smout AJ. Esophageal pH-impedance monitoring in patients with therapy-resistant reflux symptoms: "on" or "off" proton pump inhibitor? Am J Gastroenterol. 2008;103(10):2446–53.

51. Patel A, Sayuk GS, Gyawali CP. Acid-based parameters on pH-impedance testing predict symptom improvement with medical management better than impedance parameters. Am J Gastroenterol. 2014;109(6):836–44.

52. Zerbib F, Roman S, Ropert A, des Varannes SB, Pouderoux P, Chaput U, et al. Esophageal pH-impedance monitoring and symptom analysis in GERD: a study in patients off and on therapy. Am J Gastroenterol. 2006;101(9):1956–63.

53. Pritchett JM, Aslam M, Slaughter JC, Ness RM, Garrett CG, Vaezi MF. Efficacy of esophageal impedance/pH monitoring in patients with refractory gastroesophageal reflux disease, on and off therapy. Clin Gastroenterol Hepatol. 2009;7(7):743–8.

54. Patel A, Sayuk GS, Gyawali CP. Parameters on esophageal pH-impedance monitoring that predict outcomes of patients with gastroesophageal reflux disease. Clin Gastroenterol Hepatol. 2015;13(5):884–91.
55. Zaninotto G, DeMeester TR, Schwizer W, Johansson K-E, Cheng S-C. The lower esophageal sphincter in health and disease. Am J Surg. 1988;155(1):104–11.
56. Hill LD, Kozarek RA, Kraemer SJ, Aye RW, Mercer CD, Low DE, et al. The gastroesophageal flap valve: in vitro and in vivo observations. Gastrointest Endosc. 1996;44(5):541–7.
57. Koufman JA. The otolaryngologic manifestations of gastroesophageal reflux disease (GERD): a clinical investigation of 225 patients using ambulatory 24-hour pH monitoring and an experimental investigation of the role of acid and pepsin in the development of laryngeal injury. Laryngoscope. 1991;101(4 Pt 2 Suppl 53):1–78.
58. Spyridoulias A, Lillie S, Vyas A, Fowler SJ. Detecting laryngopharyngeal reflux in patients with upper airways symptoms: symptoms, signs or salivary pepsin? Respir Med. 2015;109(8):963–9.
59. Reder NP, Davis CS, Kovacs EJ, Fisichella PM. The diagnostic value of gastroesophageal reflux disease (GERD) symptoms and detection of pepsin and bile acids in bronchoalveolar lavage fluid and exhaled breath condensate for identifying lung transplantation patients with GERD-induced aspiration. Surg Endosc. 2014;28(6):1794–800.
60. Sereg-Bahar M, Jerin A, Jansa R, Stabuc B, Hocevar-Boltezar I. Pepsin and bile acids in saliva in patients with laryngopharyngeal reflux—a prospective comparative study. Clin Otolaryngol. 2015;40(3):234–9.
61. Katz PO, Gerson LB, Vela MF. Guidelines for the diagnosis and management of gastroesophageal reflux disease. Am J Gastroenterol. 2013;108(3):308–28; quiz 329.
62. Kahrilas PJ, Shaheen NJ, Vaezi MF, Hiltz SW, Black E, Modlin IM, et al. American Gastroenterological Association Medical Position Statement on the management of gastroesophageal reflux disease. Gastroenterology. 2008;135(4):1383–91, 1391–5.
63. Finley K, Giannamore M, Bennett M, Hall L. Assessing the impact of lifestyle modification education on knowledge and behavior changes in gastroesophageal reflux disease patients on proton pump inhibitors. J Am Pharm Assoc. 2009;49(4):544–8.
64. Ali T, Roberts DN, Tierney WM. Long-term safety concerns with proton pump inhibitors. Am J Med. 2009;122(10):896–903.
65. Heidelbaugh JJ, Kim AH, Chang R, Walker PC. Overutilization of proton-pump inhibitors: what the clinician needs to know. Ther Adv Gastroenterol. 2012;5(4):219–32.
66. Havu N. Enterochromaffin-like cell carcinoids of gastric mucosa in rats after life-long inhibition of gastric secretion. Digestion. 1986;35(Suppl 1):42–55.
67. Jianu CS, Lange OJ, Viset T, Qvigstad G, Martinsen TC, Fougner R, et al. Gastric neuroendocrine carcinoma after long-term use of proton pump inhibitor. Scand J Gastroenterol. 2012;47(1):64–7.
68. Cookson R, Flood C, Koo B, Mahon D, Rhodes M. Short-term cost effectiveness and long-term cost analysis comparing laparoscopic Nissen fundoplication with proton-pump inhibitor maintenance for gastro-oesophageal reflux disease. Br J Surg. 2005;92(6):700–6.
69. Epstein D, Bojke L, Sculpher MJ, The REFLUX trial group. Laparoscopic fundoplication compared with medical management for gastro-oesophageal reflux disease: cost effectiveness study. BMJ. 2009;339(2):b2576.
70. Spechler SJ, Lee E, Ahnen D, Goyal RK, Hirano I, Ramirez F, et al. Long-term outcome of medical and surgical therapies for gastroesophageal reflux disease: follow-up of a randomized controlled trial. JAMA. 2001;285(18):2331–8.
71. Lundell L, Miettinen P, Myrvold HE, Hatlebakk JG, Wallin L, Malm A, et al. Seven-year follow-up of a randomized clinical trial comparing proton-pump inhibition with surgical therapy for reflux oesophagitis. Br J Surg. 2007;94(2):198–203.
72. Lundell L, Miettinen P, Myrvold HE, Hatlebakk JG, Wallin L, Engström C, et al. Comparison of outcomes twelve years after antireflux surgery or omeprazole maintenance therapy for reflux esophagitis. Clin Gastroenterol Hepatol. 2009;7(12):1292–8.
73. Dallemagne B, Weerts J, Markiewicz S, Dewandre J-M, Wahlen C, Monami B, et al. Clinical results of laparoscopic fundoplication at ten years after surgery. Surg Endosc. 2006;20(1):159–65.
74. Oelschlager BK, Eubanks TR, Oleynikov D, Pope C, Pellegrini CA. Symptomatic and physiologic outcomes after operative treatment for extraesophageal reflux. Surg Endosc. 2002;16(7):1032–6.
75. Kilic A, Shah AS, Merlo CA, Gourin CG, Lidor AO. Early outcomes of antireflux surgery for United States lung transplant recipients. Surg Endosc. 2013;27(5):1754–60.
76. O'Halloran EK, Reynolds JD, Lau CL, Manson RJ, Davis RD, Palmer SM, et al. Laparoscopic Nissen fundoplication for treating reflux in lung transplant recipients. J Gastrointest Surg. 2004;8(1):132–7.
77. Hoppo T, Jarido V, Pennathur A, et al. Antireflux surgery preserves lung function in patients with gastroesophageal reflux disease and end-stage lung disease before and after lung transplantation. Arch Surg. 2011;146(9):1041–7.
78. Oleynikov D, Eubanks TR, Oelschlager BK, Pellegrini CA. Total fundoplication is the operation of choice for patients with gastroesophageal reflux disease and defective peristalsis. Surg Endosc. 2002;16(6):909–13.
79. Menezes MA, Herbella FAM, Patti MG. Laparoscopic antireflux surgery in patients with mixed connective tissue diseases. J Lap Adv Surg Tech. 2016;26(4):296–8.

Management of Airway Stenosis in the Lung Allograft: Bronchoscopy Procedures

Hardeep Singh Kalsi and Martin R. Carby

Introduction

Airway complications can occur in up to 7–18% of post-lung transplant patients and are reported to carry up to a 4% risk of mortality [1]. In this chapter, we will outline the role of interventional bronchoscopy in managing complications and the differing treatment modalities currently available.

The etiology of airway complications in lung transplant patients is varied and may manifest clinically in different ways. Complications are described as being "early" in the first 3 months or "late" in more than 3 months after surgery. There are six main types which may develop:

- Bronchial stenosis (or stricture)
- Bronchial dehiscence
- Tracheobronchomalacia
- Excessive exophytic granulation tissue
- Bronchial fistulas
- Endobronchial infections

This chapter will focus on the management of bronchial stenosis.

H. S. Kalsi · M. R. Carby (✉)
Transplant Unit, Harefield Hospital, Royal Brompton and Harefield NHS Foundation Trust, London, UK

Department of Cardiothoracic Transplantation, Harefield Hospital, Harefield, UK
e-mail: m.carby@rbht.nhs.uk

Pathology of Airway Disease

Lungs have two types of circulation: bronchial and pulmonary. Presently, reestablishment of the bronchial circulation of donor lung allografts from the recipient's systemic circulation is not routinely performed. This may lead to bronchial tissue hypoxia or ischemia and contribute to poor anastomotic healing. "Airway wall ischemia" is hypothesized to be crucial in anastomosis healing, and several factors may affect this (Box 18.1).

Over time, adaptive approaches have been made to minimize airway complications posttransplant. Early surgical approaches involving "telescoping" anastomoses have become less favorable as this may have a higher association

Box 18.1 Causes of Airway Ischemia and Hypoxia Which May Affect Tissue Healing
- Bronchial revascularization
- Method of anastomosis
- Length of donor bronchus
- Length of donor lung ventilation pre-organ harvest
- Hypovolemia
- Acute anemia
- Sepsis
- Dehydration

G. Raghu, R. G. Carbone (eds.), *Lung Transplantation*, https://doi.org/10.1007/978-3-319-91184-7_18

with bronchial stenosis or subsequent infections [2]. Omental fat grafts wrapping around anastomoses have been used in the past but are less common. Presently, "end-to-end" join is more commonly employed along with a shorter sleeve component from the donor's main bronchus as this is thought to promote better tissue healing (Fig. 18.1).

Physiologically as there is only one circulatory blood supply to the donor lungs, this results in a state of low pressure retrograde perfusion to the bronchial wall from the pulmonary circulation. Any element which may exacerbate hypoperfusion may therefore increase the incidence of poor tissue healing through decreased blood flow to the target site.

In the intensive care setting, postoperative factors such as hypotension and poor cardiac output in the context of sepsis or gross perioperative blood loss can potentially have significant downstream effects on anastomotic healing which may become apparent later on.

Bronchial stenosis is the most common complication to occur, and onset is usually between 3 and 12 months after transplantation. Stenotic lesions can be classified as being:

- Anastomotic
- Segmental non-anastomotic

A lesion can be further characterized by the degree of luminal occlusion which may be more or less than 50% of the airway diameter (Fig. 18.2).

Clinical Presentation and Spirometry

The most common symptoms that an individual may experience are wheeze, breathlessness on exertion, cough, and recurrent airway infections (in some instances halitosis). However, patients may be relatively asymptomatic for a length of time.

Spirometry or pulmonary function testing is an important tool to monitor progress in transplant recipients. It enables serial observations to be performed to assess individual response and screen for early signs of potential problems such as airway complications, infections, or possible allograft rejection.

Forced expiratory volume in 1 s (FEV1) and forced vital capacity (FVC) are the initial two objective parameters which are analyzed. In healthy newly transplant lung allografts, the FEV1/FVC ratio should be normal, i.e., 0.7. If a stenotic lesion develops, a more obstructive pattern may become apparent (Fig. 18.3a). Flow volume loops additionally provide informative detail and may demonstrate a variable intrathoracic obstruction which can develop due to a large single airway stenosis (Fig. 18.3b).

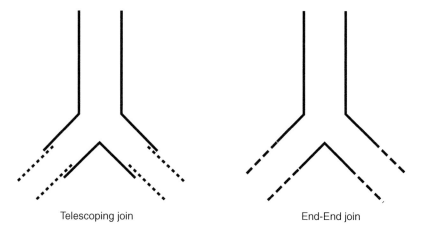

Fig. 18.1 Types of surgical anastomosis: telescoping join and end-end join

Telescoping join   End-End join

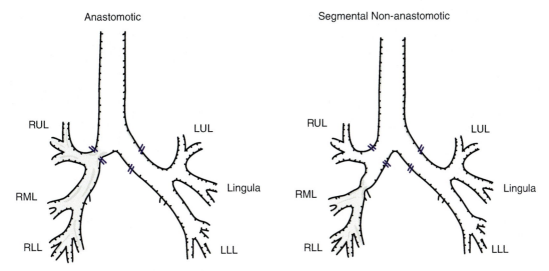

Fig. 18.2 Classification of bronchial stenosis subtype. Due to impaired airflow, secretions build up distally which may promote infection

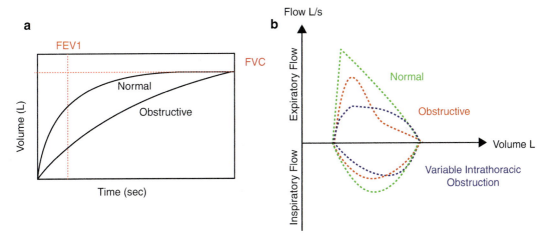

Fig. 18.3 (**a**, **b**) Pulmonary function testing in bronchial stenosis. (**a**) Spirometry curve with a conventional obstructive lung disease pattern. (**b**) Flow volume loops: during expiration, a main bronchus stenosis is exacerbated obstructing air movement out of a lung reducing gross flow

Imaging Modalities

These can be categorized into four main options:

- Chest radiography (CXR)
- Computer tomography (CT)
- Virtual bronchoscopy (VB)
- Direct visualization using fiber-optic/rigid bronchoscopy (FOB, RB) (discussed in the next section)

Chest radiography often will not demonstrate early signs of stenosis. However, recurrent infections with consolidation in the same localizing area of a lung (e.g., right middle lobe lateral segment) should raise the suspicion of a possible endobronchial luminal abnormality affecting natural airflow and movement of secretions (Fig. 18.4a, b).

In rare cases such as the "vanishing bronchus intermedius syndrome" (VIBS) in which there is

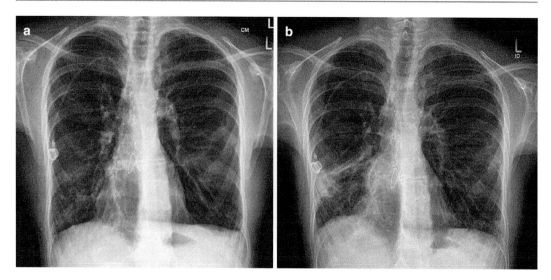

Fig. 18.4 (**a**) Lung transplant patient with cystic fibrosis and known stenosis at proximal bronchus intermedius. (**b**) Same patient presenting with RML collapse and consolidation in lateral apical segment

a gradual and eventual complete obliteration of the bronchus intermedius through progressive stenosis, a loss of lung volume may occur; in VIBS this is associated with right middle and lower lobe collapse.

CT scanning is by far the most useful and accessible noninvasive imaging tool to investigate bronchial anatomy. Posttransplant routine CT scanning is carried out in author's center before patients are discharged. It can help detect stenotic/stricturing lesions, give information as to whether airflow limitation is present, and can also assess for other potential complications such as dehiscence, fistulas, or bronchomalacia (Fig. 18.5a, b). CT scanning allows more detailed analysis of bronchial stenosis and calculation of physical dimensions. This is essential in order to guide specific measurements for potential endobronchial stenting if indicated.

Virtual bronchoscopy (VB) provides a non-invasive method of surveying the bronchial tree by generating a 3D image of the endobronchial airways using CT mapping (Fig. 18.6a, b). In one institute, the use of VB in parallel with spirometry was found to be a sensitive method of detecting the development of bronchial strictures/stenosis in both lung transplant and non-transplant patients [3]. Strong correla-

tion was seen between VB and FOB assessment outcomes. However, it may have some limitation as in the study it was found that accurate detail could only be ascertained up to the fourth division within the bronchial tree [4].

Role of Bronchoscopy

Bronchoscopy is a visual examination of the bronchial airways and an important tool used in the assessment and management of patients following lung transplantation. In most cases, a fiber-optic flexible bronchoscopy (FOB) is performed. However, in some cases rigid bronchoscopy may be required depending on clinical case characteristics and resources available.

Indications for Rigid Bronchoscopy

In the majority of cases, FOB is sufficient to allow interventions which are compatible with a 2.8 mm working channel. However, in some scenarios specific tools may be required which are not, and it is here that rigid bronchoscopy provides a key role. An experienced rigid bron-

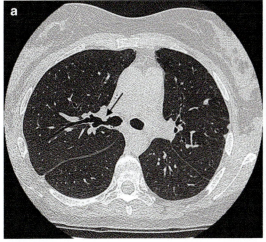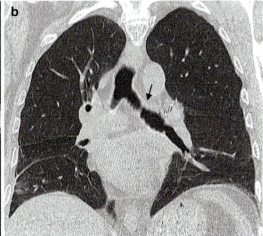

Fig. 18.5 (**a**) Lung transplant patient with alpha-1 antitrypsin deficiency, visible stenosis of right main bronchus identified on CT. (**b**) BSSLTx with previous COPD, loss of support and integrity in left main bronchus resulting in bronchomalacia

Fig. 18.6 (**a**, **b**) Virtual bronchoscopy of a lung transplant patient with a stenotic stricture. (**a**) Main trachea and carina. (**b**) Narrowed entry to the left upper lobe (LUL) seen at 11 o'clock

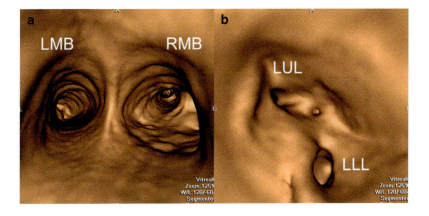

choscopist may use larger tools to perform manipulation and excision of lesions to provide more definitive and longer lasting treatment to problematic airway complications.

Furthermore, in patients who may have additional risk factors for bleeding—such as coagulopathy, chronic kidney disease, coexistent ischemic heart disease necessitating antiplatelet therapy, or known vascular structures in close proximity to a lesion—rigid bronchoscopy enables safer control and will facilitate prompt management should any potentially significant hemorrhage or airway compromise occurs. Despite this, if a significant risk or concern is anticipated, then involvement of a thoracic surgeon prior to carrying out any intervention is recommended.

Early Intervention Posttransplant

The indications for bronchoscopy may vary in the early postoperative period (Table 18.1). A low threshold to examine the airways should be held particularly as the newly transplanted lungs struggle to clear secretions effectively due to impaired or stunned mucociliary escalator function [5, 6]. Additionally, pain is an important symptom that should be managed proactively as this can impact on patient compliance with chest physiotherapy and successful airway clearance. Therefore, the early use of epidural anesthesia and topical local anesthetic applications and the input of pain management specialists and clinical psychologists can be highly beneficial.

In some centers, regular flexible bronchoscopy is performed in the intensive care setting to aid airway clearance and minimize development of superadded infections. Some transplant units may perform this routinely in a protocol-driven manner at regular intervals posttransplantation whereas other units may elect to do so according to clinical need. When bronchoscopy is carried out, samples should always be sent for analysis to guide prospective antibiotic, antiviral, or antifungal treatment in the event of any potential clinical deterioration.

In instances where persistent air leak is present as demonstrated by collateral imaging or the observed continued presence of air bubbles in a chest drain, bronchoscopy is important to rule out any anastomotic leaks, dehiscence, or fistulas which may be responsible. Lastly, in some cases bronchoscopy may be helpful to assist placement of a percutaneous tracheostomy to assist prolonged ventilator wean in an individual.

Long-Term Follow-Up

Over time, the need for bronchoscopy is guided by clinical symptoms and changes in serial spirometry. It can be used to identify complications relating to anatomical airways disease such as large airway stenosis, opportunistic infections (particularly fungal and viral), potential graft rejection or bronchiolitis obliterans syndrome (OB), and recurrent micro-aspiration (in the author's center, patients routinely undergo impedance testing to assess for potential acid reflux which over time may be damaging on allograft function). Transbronchial biopsies are essential in examining the lung parenchyma to diagnose possible allograft rejection (acute cellular (AC) or antibody-mediated (AMR)), obliterative bronchiolitis (OB), and organizing pneumonia which is not an uncommon post-infection.

Finally bronchoscopy and airway or lung sampling play a role in many research studies looking

Table 18.1 Indications for bronchoscopy early posttransplant

Procedure	Indication
Airway toilet	Removal of blood and secretions
Airway washings	Microbiology M, C, and S Fungal culture + PCR, galactomannan Viral PCR Mycobacterial culture
Histological tissue biopsy	Endobronchial: assess large airway pathology Transbronchial: assess small airways and lung parenchyma for possible rejection
Anastomosis surveillance	Assess dehiscence, stenosis, stricture, granulation Administer intervention
Tracheostomy	Provide visual assistance during placement
Research	Further understanding at cellular level

at many clinical and scientific aspects of disease in transplanted lungs.

Management of Airway Stenosis

Bronchial stenosis is the most common airway complication to occur following lung transplantation. Its incidence is thought to be 7–15% in transplant patients and associated mortality between 2 and 4% [1, 7]. While etiology may be varied, there are three main forms of airway stenosis (Fig. 18.7a–c):

- Fibrotic stricture formation due to scarring
- Transient airway slough
- Loss of supportive cartilage and connective tissue causing bronchomalacia and airway obstruction

When an airway stenosis is identified, it is important to determine whether this may be airflow limiting and thus affect effective clearance of secretions. In some instances, this may not be the case; however, in the majority of scenarios, this will develop over time. Management and choice of intervention therefore is pivotal in reestablishing adequate luminal patency and preventing short-term complications but simultaneously considering long-term implications of any treatment administered.

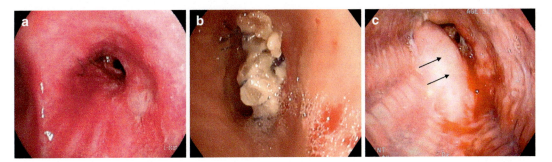

Fig. 18.7 (**a–c**) Types of stenosis. (**a**) Stenosis secondary to fibrotic stricture in the right main bronchus. (**b**) Exophytic slough obstructing the lumen of the left main bronchus. (**c**) Bronchomalacia in the left main bronchus (pre-existing stent), intermittent collapse of airway wall

Fig. 18.8 (**a–d**) Forceps/scissor removal of granulation tissue. Clockwise from top left: (**a**) Stenosis caused by slough associated with protruding surgical clip and anastomosis, small aperture into the right main bronchus (RMB). (**b**) Scissors used to dissect tissue. (**c**) Grabbing forceps used to remove slough. (**d**). Restoration of flow down the bronchus intermedius (BI) and right upper lobe (RUL)

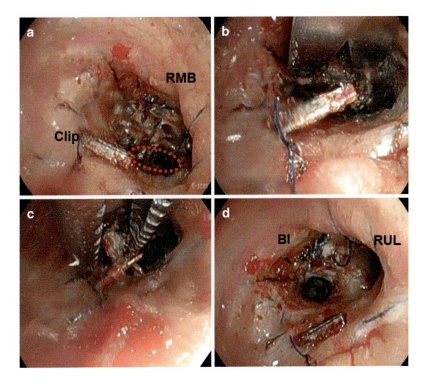

Forceps and Scissor Excision

This represents the least aggressive form of intervention and is applicable to stenosis caused by excessive granulation tissue that may form at or adjacent to bronchial anastomoses. Protrusion of suture material or surgical clips may predispose to such lesions, and in affected individual's regular maintenance, bronchoscopy may be required. The use of grabbing forceps or scissors can be performed with a flexible optical fiber bronchoscope with a 2.8 mm working channel or if required using rigid bronchoscopy (Fig. 18.8a–d).

Balloon Dilatation

The first-line treatment in many centers for stenosis is serial dilatation of the affected airway segment with a balloon catheter. This requires sequential expansion with increasing increments in the balloon size and recurrent treatments over a course of weeks to months. It is most effective in stenosis caused by fibrotic strictures alone. By stretching the endobronchial tissue circumferentially, the intended action will be to cause tears in the contracting fibrotic bands within the bronchial wall.

The balloon catheter is inserted through the working channel of a bronchoscope, and care should be taken to ensure it is not inflated while inside the channel. It should be clearly visualized on screen outside of the bronchoscope and is inflated using a pneumatic pressure syringe. Once inflated at the target site, it should be left expanded for approximately 30–60 s before deflation (Fig. 18.9a–d). The mucosa should be observed for any bleeding, and in most cases this will be mild and self-limiting. The balloon is then re-inflated to a greater size and the process repeated. Care should be taken to ensure the balloon is not inserted too distally where inflation in smaller more hazardous and friable airways may cause significant damage.

The disrupted and now shredded fibrotic bands can further be treated with cryotherapy (see later section). If the stricture has not responded despite successive attempts, then it is been unlikely that further dilatation treatment will be of any benefit. In this scenario alternatives such as endobronchial stenting may be explored.

The main complications associated with balloon dilatation are significant bleeding, hypoxia, and airway tear or complete rupture. The benefit, however, is that it can be performed under sedation in a normal bronchoscopy suite without the need for fluoroscopic or imaging guidance.

Endobronchial Stents

Placement of an endobronchial stent may be performed where balloon dilatation has failed to ameliorate fibrotic band disease (additionally it may be used in bronchomalacia). When deployed effectively, it can help maintain luminal patency and is thought to be particularly more effective with long strictures (Figs. 18.10 and 18.11a–d). CT scanning allows detailed measurements to be carried out in order to tailor the choice of stent used.

Currently two types of stents are used in clinical practice, and these are self-expanding metal stents (SEMS) which are typically composed of Nitinol (a nickel and titanium hybrid alloy) and silicone stents. The core design is based on a woven lattice-like structure to improve tensile strength and spread mechanical forces more evenly. Both can be deployed using FOB, but in

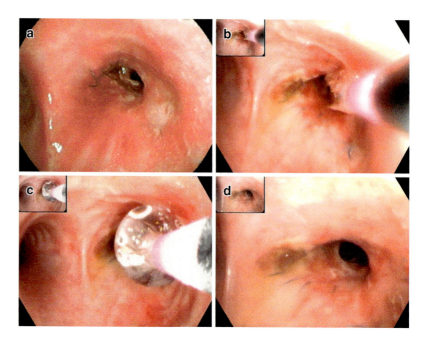

Fig. 18.9 (a–d) Balloon dilatation. Clockwise from top left: (**a**) Stenosis in the right main bronchus. (**b**) Balloon inserted carefully into the bronchus. (**c**) Balloon serially dilated to 8–9–10 mm. (**d**) Post-dilation improved luminal patency and airflow

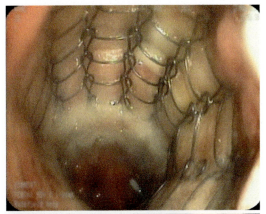

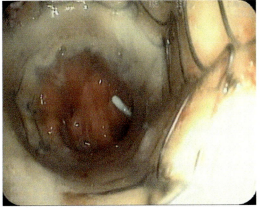

Fig. 18.10 Endobronchial stenting. Ultraflex™ (Boston Scientific, Marlborough, MA, USA) self-expanding metal stent used in author's center

some cases rigid bronchoscopy may be used depending on clinician judgment. Fluoroscopy is used to help confirm correct positioning.

Stents can be covered or uncovered depending on whether they have a sleeve-like outer coating. Uncovered stents may be preferable when treating disease which traverses a main lobar airway such as the right upper lobe (Fig. 18.11c, d). In contrast covered stents might be preferred when treating short strictures in a single airway which is prone to granulation tissue overgrowth.

There are significant risks associated with endobronchial stenting, and therefore careful consideration should be given toward patient selection. The most common are stent restenosis 10–50% (often through formation of granulation tissue which occludes the lumen) or bacterial colonization (biofouling); however, others include mal-placement, stent migration, stent fracture, airway perforation, and stent collapse [8]. Silicone stents can be removed easily as they are less likely to become incorporated in an airway wall. Despite this, they can be more prone to mucus plugging and migration when compared to SEMS.

Presently biodegradable stents have been trialed with varying results. The main apparent benefit is that they can dissolve into the airway wall within a few months [9] which may minimize some of the risks concerned with conventional stents. However, more research and experience in their use are still needed.

Cryotherapy

Often used in conjunction with balloon dilatation or sometimes with laser photoresection, cryotherapy can be used to treat residual soft tissue bands from the airway lumen or wall [10].

Equipment such as the ERBOKRYO® CA cryosurgical system employed in the author's center utilizes liquid nitrogen to freeze tissue to −80° centigrade. The probe is applied to the target site for 2–4 min at a time (Fig. 18.12a–c). Initially the appearance of a stenosis/stricture may appear unchanged. However, over the next few days to weeks, the resulting cell death and apoptosis will eventually result in the widening of the airway lumen best seen on serial bronchoscopy. Care should be taken to allow the ice crystals on the probe tip to dissolve before attempting to pull it away from the treated site; as if it adheres to the mucosal wall, then significant unintended trauma could occur upon removal.

The benefit of cryotherapy is that it selectively targets the bronchial mucosa and superficial muscle layers with little activity on underlying connective tissue and cartilage.

Laser Photoresection

This works through a mechanism of applying intense light radiation to a target site to generate heat and subsequent tissue damage. It may be

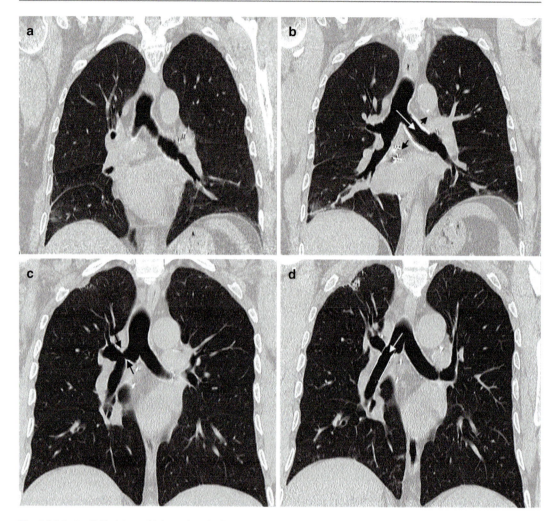

Fig. 18.11 (**a–d**) Endobronchial stenting. (**a**) Bronchomalacia of the left main bronchus. (**b**) Stent inserted resulting in good airway wall support. (**c**) Stricture in the right main bronchus. D. Stent successfully sited with good effect

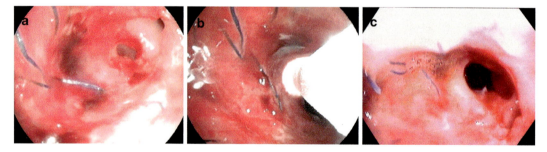

Fig. 18.12 (**a–c**) Cryotherapy applied to a stricture. (**a**) After serial balloon dilation. (**b**). Cryotherapy applied to disrupted fibrotic bands for 60 s several times. (**c**) Repeat bronchoscopy 1 week after showing improved airway patency

performed using FOB but is normally carried out with a rigid bronchoscopy and the patient under general anesthetic.

In the hands of a skilled and experienced operator, it may be used to treat airway stenoses caused by the growth of excessive fibrotic tissue leading to web-like strictures with therapeutic incisions made in a radial manner. Residual tissue which cannot be safely treated due to the risk of unwanted airway damage may be treated with cryotherapy.

There are several types of laser probes, and each one operates at a specific wavelength of light within the spectrum. Depending on the wavelength, the treatment properties may vary from coagulation, cutting, deep tissue penetration, and vaporization. Some lasers which operate within the infrared spectrum will have an additional guide light.

Care needs to be taken as an incorrect application, or misdirection could lead to significant airway perforation, hemorrhage, hypoxemia, or endobronchial fire as the laser is deployed in an oxygen-rich environment. In the case of the latter, typically it is recommended that the FiO_2 concentration should be less than 40% at the time of firing to minimize risk.

Positive Pressure Ventilation

Bronchomalacia can cause intermittent obstruction of an airway due to loss of structural integrity. Medical management involves the use of positive pressure support to splint the weakened airway open when the patient sleeps. This will often be in the form of continuous positive airway pressure ventilation (CPAP) but rarely may involve the use of noninvasive ventilation (e.g., bi-level positive airway pressure/ BIPAP) if additional hypercapnia is present, for example, in the case of obesity hypoventilation syndrome. If refractory to positive pressure ventilation, then careful consideration can be given to endobronchial stenting as mentioned previously.

Surgery

Where interventional bronchoscopy methods fail, surgery may provide a final option. In some small cases and dependent on the individual center, bronchial anastomosis reconstruction or sleeve resection may be considered.

The majority of patients, however, will often undergo a lobectomy and removal of the segment of the lung affected by a stenosis which acts as chronic foci of infection and potential sepsis (Fig. 18.13a–c). Single-photon emission computer tomography (SPECT) scanning helps to evaluate perfusion and ventilation dynamics of lung allografts in patients prior to surgery. This will often confirm that the affected section of lung is hypoventilated and contributes minimally to net gaseous exchange. Therefore in such circumstances, only relatively nonfunctional lung is being removed, and this has been proved to be an effective treatment of last resort [11].

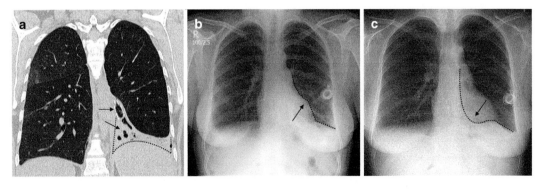

Fig. 18.13 (a–c) Surgical resection. (a) CT showing blocked endobronchial stent in the proximal left lower lobe bronchus with chronic collapse ± infection. (b). Collapse as seen on CXR with "silhouette sign." (c) Post-resection, restoration of normal diaphragm interface seen behind cardiac shadow as the left upper lobe hyperexpands

Summary

Airway complications and, in particular, bronchial stenosis post-lung transplantation are relatively common, and proactive management is advocated to prevent complications from occurring, which, in an immunosuppressed individual, could be fatal. Changes in surgical approaches aimed at minimizing bronchial complications have to some degree been effective. However, problems such as airway stenosis still occur, and, increasingly, bronchoscopic intervention is required.

The success of current treatment methods has been shown in the literature to be variable and may be dependent on individual case characteristics or simply reflect the skill of an individual operator. At present excision of tissue, balloon dilatation and stent insertion remain the most common approaches used. As survival post-lung transplant continues to increase, it is clear that bronchoscopic interventions will become more popular and necessary.

References

1. Santacruz JF, Mehta AC. Airway complications and management after lung transplantation: ischemia, dehiscence, stenosis. Proc Am Thorac Soc. 2009;6:79–93.
2. Garfein ES, McGregor CC, Galantowicz ME, Schulman LL. Deleterious effects of telescoped bronchial anastomosis in single and bilateral lung transplantation. Ann Transplant. 2000;5:5–11.
3. Shitrit D, Valdsislav P, Grubstein A, Bendayan D, Cohen M, Kramer MR. Accuracy of virtual bronchoscopy for grading tracheobronchial stenosis: correlation with pulmonary function test and fibre optic bronchoscopy. Chest. 2005;128(5):3545–50.
4. Polverosi R, Vigo M, Baron S, Rossi G. Evaluation of tracheobronchial lesions with spiral CT: comparison between virtual endoscopy and bronchoscopy. Radiol Med. 2001;102(5-6):313–9.
5. Paul A, Marelli D, Shennib H, et al. Mucociliary function in autotransplanted, allotransplanted, and sleeve respected lungs. J Thorac Cardiovasc Surg. 1989;98(4):523–8.
6. Herve P, Silbert D, Cerrina J, Simonneau G, Dartevelle P. Impairment of bronchial mucociliary clearance in long-term survivors of heart/lung and double-lung transplantation. The Paris-Sud Lung Transplant Group. Chest. 1993;103(1):59–63.
7. De Gracia J, Culebras M, Alvarez A, Catalán E, De la Rosa D, Maestre J, Canela M, Román A. Bronchoscopic balloon dilatation in the management of bronchial stenosis following lung transplantation. Respir Med. 2007;101(1):27–33.
8. J G, Fuehner T, Dierich M, Wiesner O, Simon AR, Welte T. Are metallic stents really safe? A long term analysis in lung transplant recipients. Eur Respir J. 2009;34(6):1417–22.
9. Lischke R, Pozniak J, Vondrys D, Elliott MJ. Novel biodegradable stents in the treatment of bronchial stenosis after lung transplantation. Eur J Cardiothorac Surg. 2011;40(3):619–24.
10. Fitzmaurice GJ, Redmond KC, Fitzpatrick DA, Bartosik W. Endobronchial cryotherapy facilitates end-stage treatment options in patients with bronchial stenosis: a case series. Ann Thorac Med. 2014;9(2):120–3.
11. Popov AF, Rajaruthnam D, Zych B, Bahrami T, Simon AR, Carby M, Redmond KC. Pulmonary resection for airway complication after lung transplantation in a patient with cystic fibrosis: a case report. Transplant Proc. 2011;43(10):4036–8.

Imaging of Lung Transplantation

19

Jitesh Ahuja, Siddhartha G. Kapnadak, and Sudhakar Pipavath

Introduction

Lung transplantation is a viable treatment option for end-stage lung disease. Common indications for lung transplantation are chronic obstructive pulmonary disease (COPD), idiopathic pulmonary fibrosis, cystic fibrosis, alpha-1 antitrypsin deficiency, and pulmonary arterial hypertension (PAH). Other less common indications include end-stage sarcoidosis, lymphangioleiomyomatosis (LAM), pulmonary Langerhans cell histiocytosis/granulomatosis (PLCH/G), and other interstitial lung diseases. Either single or bilateral lung transplantation can be performed. Bilateral transplantation is required for patients with suppurative lung diseases including cystic fibrosis and most patients with PAH. While suitable outcomes may be achieved with single lung transplantation for other diagnoses, there is a trend in recent years for use of bilateral transplantation, largely related to a suggestion of better long-term survival seen in registry data [1]. Specifically, according to the 2014 International Society for Heart and Lung Transplantation (ISHLT) registry report, the median survival for all adult recipients is 5.7 years, but bilateral lung recipients appear to have a better median survival than single lung recipients (7 versus 4.5 years, respectively) [1]. Overall survival after lung transplantation has improved due to refinement in surgical technique, improvement in organ procurement and preserving techniques, and advances in medical management and immunosuppression. The most common cause of mortality in first 30 days after lung transplantation is primary graft dysfunction. Infection is the most common cause of mortality in the first 6 months and chronic rejection thereafter [1].

Complications after lung transplantation are common and may have nonspecific clinical and radiologic manifestations. In addition, frequently, several of these complications may coexist and complicate their presentation. In order to reduce mortality and morbidity among lung transplant recipients, it is important to recognize these complications accurately and in time. The time point at which these complications occur relative to the date of transplant is crucial in formulating a differential diagnosis and recognizing them accurately.

In this chapter, we will describe the radiologic manifestations of various pulmonary complications occurring after lung transplantation. Complications are classified chronologically into groups based on the time from transplant:

J. Ahuja (✉) · S. Pipavath
Department of Radiology, University of Washington Medical Center, Seattle, WA, USA
e-mail: ahujaj@uw.edu; snjp@uw.edu

S. G. Kapnadak
Division of Pulmonary and Critical Care Medicine, University of Washington Medical Center, Seattle, WA, USA
e-mail: skap@uw.edu

© The Author(s) 2018
G. Raghu, R. G. Carbone (eds.), *Lung Transplantation*, https://doi.org/10.1007/978-3-319-91184-7_19

immediate (<24 h), early (24 h to 1 week), inter-mediate (8 days to 2 months), primary late (2–4 months), and secondary late (≥4 months) (Table 19.1).

Immediate Complications (<24 h)

Donor-Recipient Size Mismatch

Size mismatch between the donor lung and recipient thoracic cavity may result in mechanical complications. Most centers accept a size

Table 19.1 Post lung transplantation complications

Time of occurrence	Types of complication
Immediate (<24 h)	Donor-recipient size mismatch Hyperacute rejection
Early (>24 h to 1 week)	Primary graft dysfunction and pleural complications
Intermediate (8 days to 2 months)	Acute rejection Airway anastomotic complications: bronchial dehiscence Infections: bacterial, fungal, and viral
Primary late (2–4 months)	Infections: fungal and viral Airway anastomotic complications: bronchial stenosis
Secondary late (>4 months)	Chronic rejection Upper lobes fibrosis Organizing pneumonia PTLD Recurrence of primary disease

difference ranging from 10 to 25% [2]. If the donor lung is too large for recipient thoracic cavity, atelectasis and impaired ventilation may result. Atelectasis may be evident on immediate postoperative radiograph. On the other hand, when a small allograft lung is used in single lung transplantation for emphysema, the hyperexpanded native lung may compress the allograft, resulting in restrictive pulmonary function (Fig. 19.1a, b). Native lung volume reduction surgery performed at the time of, or after, transplantation may help prevent this complication [3].

Lung torsion is a rare but serious complication that can occur due to discrepancy in size between the recipient's enlarged thoracic cavity and donor's small lung. Imaging will show torsion of the hilar structures including vasculature and airway. It can lead to collapse of a lobe or entire lung due to airway compromise or expansible consolidated lobe due to hemorrhagic infarction. Once lung torsion is suspected, immediate surgery is indicated to avoid death from parenchymal necrosis.

Hyperacute Rejection

Hyperacute rejection is caused by the presence of preformed antibodies to donor organ-specific human leukocyte antigen (HLA) or ABO antigen. ABO matching and improved antibody detection and crossmatch techniques have made hyperacute rejection very rare after lung transplanta-

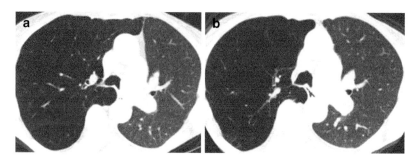

Fig. 19.1 (**a, b**) A 73-year-old woman status post left lung transplant for severe COPD. CT chest obtained 11 years after transplantation (**a**) showed hyperinflation of native right lung herniating to left hemithorax. The patient had restrictive pulmonary impairment and developed squamous cell lung cancer in the right lower lobe (not shown), for which she underwent right lower lobectomy. Post lobectomy CT (**b**) showed an improvement in hyperinflation of the right lung

tion. When present, it can lead to acute alveolar damage resulting in graft dysfunction within minutes to hours after graft reperfusion [4]. On chest radiograph, hyperacute rejection manifests as diffuse homogeneous opacification of the entire allograft. Management options include aggressive immunosuppression, plasmapheresis, or urgent retransplantation [4].

Early Complications (24 h to 1 Week)

Primary Graft Dysfunction (Ischemic Reperfusion Injury or Reperfusion Edema)

Primary graft dysfunction is a form of non-cardiogenic pulmonary edema that usually occurs by postoperative day 1, peaks in severity by day 4, and generally improves by day 7. It is diagnosed after excluding left heart failure, fluid overload, infection, and acute transplant rejection. The pathogenesis of primary graft dysfunction is multifactorial including interruption of lymphatic and bronchial circulation, donor organ ischemia, surgical trauma, denervation of donor lung, and decreased surfactant production [5].

Chest radiography and CT manifestations are nonspecific and include perihilar and lower lobe predominant ground-glass opacity, and/or consolidation, interlobular septal thickening, and peribronchial air-space opacities (Figs. 19.2 and 19.3).

Pleural Complications

Pleural complications—including pleural effusion, hemothorax, pneumothorax, and empyema—occur in 22–34% of patients after transplantation [6, 7]. Existing pleural abnormalities before lung transplantation can predispose to pleural complications. For instance, pleural infection or inflammation can result from end-stage lung diseases for which lung transplantation is required such as cystic fibrosis. Invasive procedures required to diagnose (wedge biopsy)

or treat (pleurodesis or pleural drain for pneumothorax or pleural effusion) end-stage lung disease may result in pleural abnormalities. Pneumothorax is the most common pleural complication [7]

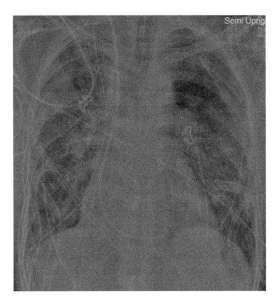

Fig. 19.2 A 43-year-old man with bilateral orthotropic lung transplant (BOLT) in 2010 for ciliary dyskinesia. Frontal chest radiograph obtained 4 days after transplantation shows diffuse lung disease, likely representing primary graft dysfunction or reperfusion pulmonary edema

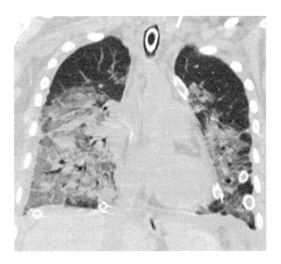

Fig. 19.3 A 30-year-old woman status post double lung transplant for cystic fibrosis. CT obtained 9 days after transplantation shows diffuse ground-glass opacity and consolidation, consistent with primary graft dysfunction. Bilateral chest tubes are in place

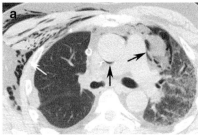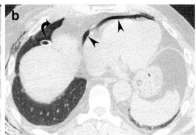

Fig. 19.4 (**a**, **b**) A 69-year-old man with single ortho-tropic lung transplant (SOLT) in 2015 for IPF. CT obtained 4 days after transplantation shows pneumomediastinum (black arrows in **a**), pneumothorax (curved arrow in **b**), pneumopericardium (arrowheads in **b**), and subcutaneous emphysema (white arrow in **a**). The bronchial anastomo-sis was intact. Right chest tube is in place. Note fibrosis in native left lung

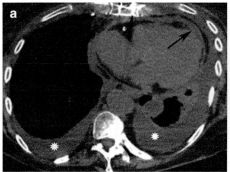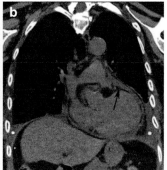

Fig. 19.5 (**a**, **b**) A 72-year-old woman with BOLT in 2013 for IPF. CT obtained 2 weeks after transplantation shows bilateral pleural effusions (asterisks **a** and **b**) with associated compressive atelectasis in lower lobes. Small pericardial effusion is also present (arrows in **a** and **b**)

(Fig. 19.4a, b). Airway anastomotic complica-tions should be suspected if pneumothorax per-sists or enlarges after the early postoperative period (>7 days after transplantation). Pleural effusion is also a common complication second-ary to increased capillary permeability and impaired lymphatic drainage of the allograft lung during the early postoperative period (Fig. 19.5a, b). Pleural fluid in the immediate postoperative period is often hemorrhagic and becomes pro-gressively less hemorrhagic by 7 days. Pleural effusion usually resolves by 2 weeks. Persistent or enlarging pleural effusion should raise suspi-cion for empyema or left heart failure. Hemothorax usually results from surgical com-plications (Fig. 19.6a, b). Persistent air leak, empyema, and hemothorax are associated with increased mortality and should be promptly rec-ognized and managed [7, 8].

Intermediate Complications (8 Days to 2 Months) and Primary Late Complications (2–4 Months)

Acute Rejection

Acute rejection usually occurs after the second postoperative week and is classically caused by cell-mediated immune response. Approximately 80% of acute rejections occur in first 3 months, and 50% of patients have at least one episode of acute rejection in the first postoperative year [9, 10]. Repeated episodes of acute rejection are considered a risk factor for the development of chronic rejection [9, 11].

When present, radiographic manifestations are nonspecific and similar to primary graft dys-function including ground-glass opacities, con-solidation, interlobular septal thickening, and

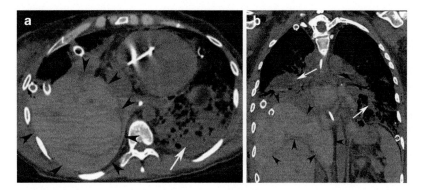

Fig. 19.6 (**a**, **b**) A 33-year-old woman with BOLT in 2015 for pulmonary arterial hypertension. CT obtained 2 days after transplantation shows high density material in right pleural space (arrowheads in **a** and **b**), consistent with hemothorax. Consolidation in both lower lobes was presumably due to aspiration (arrows)

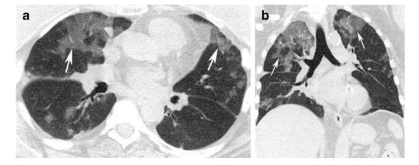

Fig. 19.7 (**a**, **b**) A 55-year-old woman with BOLT in 2013 for COPD. CT obtained 8 months after transplantation showed patchy ground-glass opacities (arrows in **a** and **b**) bilaterally. Although a nonspecific pattern, the transbronchial biopsy was consistent with A0B1 ACR with all infectious testing negative

pleural effusion (Figs. 19.7a, b, 19.8, and 19.9a, b). Radiographic improvement within 48 h of administration of intravenous corticosteroids favors the diagnosis of acute rejection [9].

Airway Anastomotic Complications

Airway anastomotic complications include bronchial dehiscence, bronchial stenosis, or bronchomalacia. Reported incidence of airway complications is approximately 15%, but there has been a decrease in the airway complication rate due to the refinement in surgical technique, improvement in immunosuppression, and donor organ preservation technique [12]. The most important factor predisposing to airway complication is donor bronchus ischemia, due to disruption of the native bronchial circulation. Recurrent

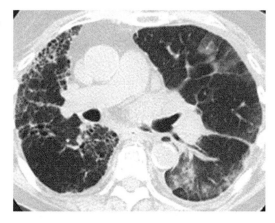

Fig. 19.8 A 69-year-old woman status post left lung transplant for chronic hypersensitivity pneumonitis. CT obtained 4 months after transplantation showed patchy ground-glass opacities in the allograft. Although a nonspecific pattern, the transbronchial biopsies revealed A2B0 acute cellular rejection. Note fibrosis in the native right lung

infection and rejection are some other contributing factors.

Bronchial dehiscence usually occurs in the first 2–4 weeks after transplantation affecting 2–3% patients [9]. CT usually shows extralumi-nal foci of air in perianastomotic region, and occasionally bronchial defects can be visualized (Figs. 19.10a–c, 19.11a, b, and 19.12a, b). Indirect signs include persistent or enlarging air leak, pneumothorax, or pneumomediastinum.

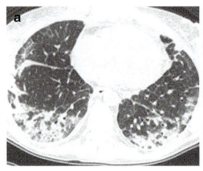
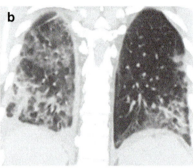

Fig. 19.9 (**a**, **b**) A 34-year-old woman status post BOLT for PAH. CT obtained 4 months after transplantation showed ground-glass opacity and consolidation bilater-ally predominantly in the lower lobes. Although a nonspe-cific pattern, transbronchial biopsies revealed A3B1R acute cellular rejection

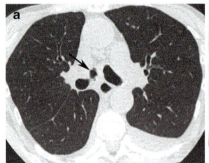
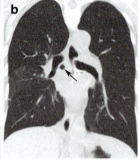
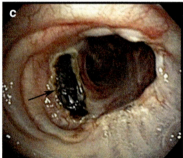

Fig. 19.10 (**a–c**) A 57-year-old woman with BOLT in 2015 for alpha-1 antitrypsin deficiency. CT obtained 6 weeks after transplantation showed small pocket of extra-luminal air (arrows in **a** and **b**) adjacent to right mainstem bronchus, consistent with bronchial anastomotic dehis-cence. This was confirmed on bronchoscopy that shows necrotic plaque on medial right mainstem bronchus (arrow in **c**)

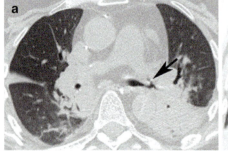
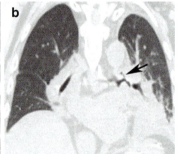

Fig. 19.11 (**a**, **b**) A 62-year-old man status post double lung transplant for sarcoidosis. CT obtained 3 weeks after transplantation shows air tracking from the left mainstem bronchus (arrows in **a** and **b**), consistent with dehiscence. Note collapse of left lower lobe

Fig. 19.12 (**a**, **b**) A 65-year-old man status post double lung transplant for IPF. CT obtained 3 weeks after transplantation showed right mainstem bronchus dehiscence (arrows in **a** and **b**) tracking into the right pleural space suggestive of bronchopleural fistula (arrowhead in **b**)

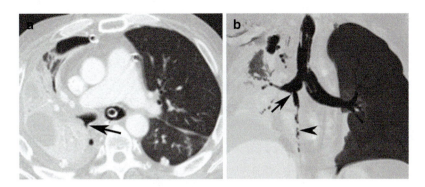

Fig. 19.13 (**a–d**) A 69-year-old man with BOLT in 2009 for IPF. Axial MinIP (**a**) shows anastomotic narrowing of right mainstem bronchus. Coronal reformation (**b**) shows narrowing of the left mainstem bronchus distal to anastomosis. Bronchoscopic images confirming narrowing of the right (**c**) and left (**d**) mainstem bronchi

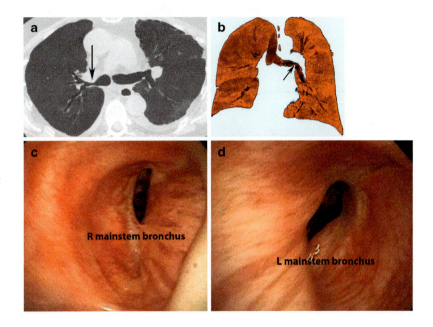

Bronchial dehiscence may resolve spontaneously or progress to bronchial stenosis.

Bronchial stenosis and bronchomalacia are late complications usually occurring at least 2–4 months after transplantation. Bronchial stenosis occurs in 10% of subjects and is usually seen at the anastomotic site or distally [13]. CT shows bronchial irregularity and focal stenosis (Figs. 19.13a–d and 19.14a, b). Management includes resection of the granulation tissue and balloon dilation with or without stenting. Bronchomalacia or transient airway narrowing can be diagnosed with bronchoscopy or CT. Inspiratory and expiratory CT images are invaluable in the diagnosis of bronchomalacia (Fig. 19.15a, b). A diagnosis is suggested when there is more than 50 (liberal) to 70% (conserva-

tive) dynamic narrowing of the airway or lunate shape of the airway on expiration.

Vascular Anastomotic Complications

Vascular anastomotic complications are uncommon. Pulmonary artery stenosis is more common than pulmonary vein stenosis. It can occur in the early or late postoperative period [14]. Contrast-enhanced CT angiogram is the best available noninvasive modality to assess narrowing or occlusion of the anastomotic site. This may cause pulmonary infarction more readily due to the absence of bronchial artery circulation in the early postoperative period. Treatment options include angioplasty and stenting.

Fig. 19.14 (**a**, **b**) A 62-year-old man with BOLT in 2014 for COPD. CT shows diffuse stenosis of bronchus intermedius (arrow in **a**). Patient underwent bronchial dilation and stenting (arrow in **b**)

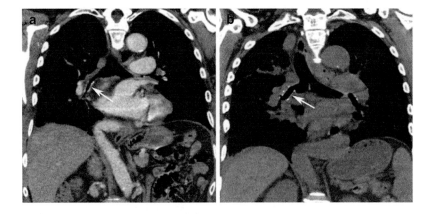

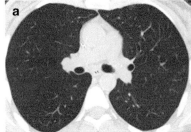 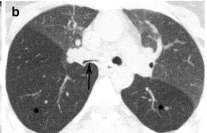

Fig. 19.15 (**a**, **b**) A 34-year-old woman with BOLT in 2006 for CF. CT during inspiration (**a**) and expiration (**b**) shows severe collapse of the bronchus intermedius during expiration (arrow in **b**) indicating bronchomalacia. Note air trapping in both lower lobes (asterisks in **b**)

Infections

Infection is the most common complication and a leading cause of morbidity and mortality after lung transplantation. Patients are at increased risk of infection because of immunosuppression, impaired mucociliary clearance, absence of cough reflex, disruption of lymphatic drainage, and direct communication between the allograft and the atmosphere.

Infectious risks vary based on factors which include the time elapsed since transplantation. Bacterial infections are the most common cause of pneumonia with incidence highest in the first 4 weeks after lung transplantation [15]. Gram-negative organisms such as *Klebsiella* species and *Pseudomonas aeruginosa* are common causative agents. Infection by gram-positive organisms including *Staphylococcus aureus* is also observed. During the first postoperative month, 35–70% recipients develop bacterial pneumonia [16]. Imaging features are similar to

the non-transplant population and include lobar or multifocal consolidation, ground-glass opacity, nodules, and pleural effusion [13, 15, 17] (Fig. 19.16a, b).

Fungal infections are caused by *Aspergillus* and less commonly by the *Candida* species. *Pneumocystis pneumonia* is uncommon these days because of routine chemoprophylaxis. Fungal infections can occur at any time but usually peak between 10 and 60 days after transplantation. These are less common but carry higher mortality compared to bacterial or viral infections. Patterns of fungal infection include angioinvasive pulmonary infection, ulcerative tracheobronchitis, and bronchial anastomosis infection [16]. CT in angioinvasive fungal infection shows ill-defined nodules or mass-like consolidation with surrounding ground-glass opacity (halo sign) indicating hemorrhage [13, 15] (Fig. 19.17a, b). On CT tracheobronchitis shows diffuse central airway wall thickening and surrounding mediastinal fat stranding. Bronchial

Fig. 19.16 (a, b) A 71-year-old man with BOLT in 2013 for COPD. CT shows bilateral peribronchial consolidation. BAL fluid grew *Pseudomonas* and MSSA

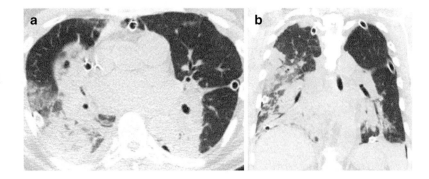

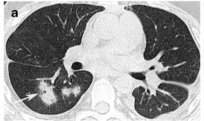
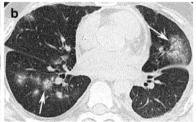

Fig. 19.17 (a, b) A 34-year-old man with BOLT in 2009 for pulmonary fibrosis after hematopoietic stem cell transplantation for acute lymphoblastic leukemia. CT shows multiple irregular nodules with peripheral ground-glass halo (arrows in **a** and **b**). BAL fluid grew *Aspergillus Fumigatus*

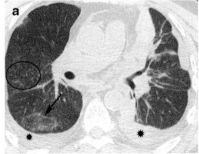
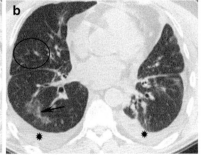

Fig. 19.18 (a, b) A 59-year-old man with BOLT in 2015 for IPF. CT shows patchy ground-glass opacity (arrows in **a** and **b**) and centrilobular nodules (circle in **a** and **b**). Viral PCR panel was positive for coronavirus and adenovirus. Note bilateral pleural effusions (asterisks in **a** and **b**)

anastomosis infection can cause bronchial dehiscence and show small foci of extra-luminal air adjacent to the airways.

Cytomegalovirus (CMV) is the most common opportunistic infection and the second most common cause of pneumonia in lung transplantation patients. CMV pneumonia usually occurs between 1 and 6 months from transplantation [13]. CMV-seronegative recipients who receive CMV-seropositive donor lungs are at increased risk for developing primary infection. CT shows varying patterns including ground-glass opacity, centrilobular nodules with tree-in-bud pattern, consolidation, and interlobular septal thickening [13, 17] (Fig. 19.18a, b). In addition to CMV, other community acquired viruses such as adenovirus, respiratory syncytial virus (RSV), and influenza and parainfluenza viruses may infect lung transplant recipients. Viral infections can predispose lung transplant recipients to obliterative bronchiolitis [18, 19], a manifestation of chronic rejection.

Secondary Late Complications (>4 Months)

Chronic Rejection

Chronic rejection is a clinicopathologic syndrome most often characterized by obliterative bronchiolitis, affecting 50% of lung transplant recipients at 5 years [20], and the term bronchiolitis obliterans syndrome (BOS) is used to describe the clinical situation. It is a major factor limiting the long-term survival in lung transplant recipients. It usually occurs 6 months after transplantation, and risk factors include prior episodes of recurrent acute rejection or infections, particularly CMV pneumonia. Obliterative bronchiolitis is the most common histologic pattern seen in BOS and manifests as eosinophilic hyaline fibrosis in respiratory bronchiolar walls with luminal occlusion [20]. Due to patchy distribution of the disease, transbronchial biopsy may be negative. In such cases diagnosis is made clinically on the basis of otherwise unexplained, persistent decrease in FEV1 indicative of small airway disease. Pulmonary function tests classically show an obstructive pattern, but combined obstruction and restriction may be seen [21]. High-resolution CT shows bronchial wall thickening, bronchiectasis, and heterogeneous areas of hyperlucent (dark) interspersed with adjacent normal lung parenchyma (mosaic attenuation) that is accentuated in exhalation images. Thus, it is very important to obtain paired inspiratory and expiratory HRCT images when chronic rejection is suspected clinically. On expiration HRCT, normal lung parenchyma becomes greyer, and hyperlucent (pathologic) lung remains dark indicating air trapping (Figs. 19.19a, b and 19.20a, b). Thus, the differentiation between normal and abnormal lung becomes more pronounced on expiration CT [13, 22].

Organizing Pneumonia Pattern

Organizing pneumonia pattern similar to patients with cryptogenic organizing pneumonia occurs in 10–28% of patients after lung transplantation and may be associated with both acute and chronic rejection [15, 23] or may represent infection. It is characterized by the presence of inflam-

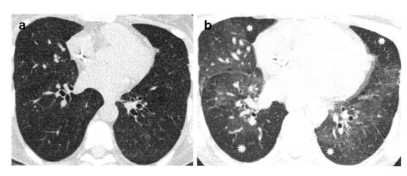

Fig. 19.19 (a, b) A 33-year-old woman with BOLT in 2007 for cystic fibrosis. CT during inspiration (a) and expiration (b) shows patchy areas of air trapping (asterisks in b), consistent with BOS

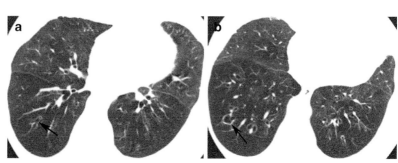

Fig. 19.20 (a, b) A 72-year-old woman with BOLT in 2013 for IPF. CT shows bronchiectasis (arrows in a and b) and mosaic attenuation, consistent with obliterative bronchiolitis indicating chronic lung allograft dysfunction of the BOS variety

matory granulation tissues within the alveoli, alveolar sacs, and ducts. It responds rapidly to high-dose corticosteroids. Bronchoscopy is often done to exclude infection before starting on high-dose corticosteroids. CT shows peripheral, peribronchovascular, or perilobular consolidation (Fig. 19.21). Frequently, peripheral arc-like consolidation with central ground-glass opacity (reverse halo/atoll sign) is seen [15, 24].

Post-transplant Lymphoproliferative Disorders (PTLD)

Post-transplant lymphoproliferative disorder is a spectrum of disease varying from benign lymphoid hyperplasia to high-grade lymphoma. It

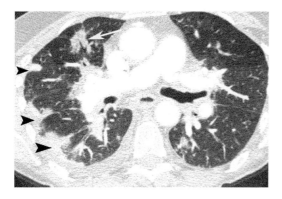

Fig. 19.21 A 59-year-old woman with BOLT in 2013 for scleroderma-associated ILD. CT shows peripheral (arrowheads) and peribronchial (arrow) consolidation. Transbronchial biopsy showed organizing pneumonia pattern without infection

typically manifests within 1 year after transplantation but can be seen from 1 month to several years after transplantation. PTLD risk is increased significantly in Epstein-Barr virus (EBV) seronegative recipients receiving lungs from seropositive donors. The other major risk factor is augmented immunosuppression. Incidence varies between 2.8 and 6% at 1 year after transplantation [25, 26]. It is more common with lung transplantation than with other solid organ transplantation. The majority of cases of PTLD is of B cell origin and associated with EBV primary infection. A much smaller proportion of PTLDs are of T cell origin, Hodgkin's type, or, rarely, plasma cell type such as multiple myeloma. These categories are more likely to be EBV-negative. EBV-associated PTLD presents early (within 1 year), usually has a benign course and is intrathoracic, whereas EBV-negative PTLD presents late (median onset 50–60 months posttransplant), generally more aggressive and extrathoracic. Early disease responds to antiviral therapy and reduction in immunosuppression. Late disease generally requires chemotherapy and radiation therapy [25]. CT shows solitary or multiple nodules with peripheral and basal predominant distribution (Figs. 19.22a, b and 19.23a, b). Mass-like consolidation and mediastinal and hilar lymphadenopathy are also commonly seen. Rarely, interlobular septal thickening can be seen. Pleural and chest wall masses with or without pleural effusion and/or pericardial effusion have been described [27, 28]. Biopsy is often needed to differentiate PTLD from infection [29, 30].

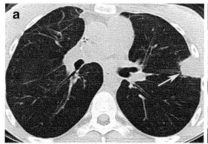
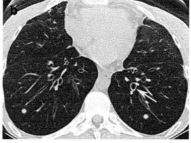

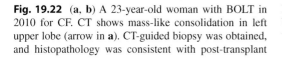

Fig. 19.22 (**a, b**) A 23-year-old woman with BOLT in 2010 for CF. CT shows mass-like consolidation in left upper lobe (arrow in **a**). CT-guided biopsy was obtained, and histopathology was consistent with post-transplant lymphoproliferative disorder (PTLD). CT also shows bronchiectasis (arrow in **b**) and air trapping, consistent with chronic lung allograft dysfunction

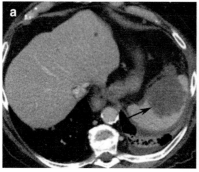
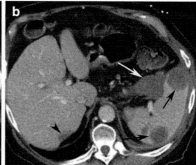

Fig. 19.23 (**a**, **b**) A 73-year-old man with BOLT in 2005 for COPD. CT shows low-density soft tissue masses in the spleen (black arrows in **a** and **b**), liver (arrowhead in **b**), and perisplenic (white arrow in **b**) region. Histopathology was consistent with PTLD

Fig. 19.24 (**a**, **b**) A 41-year-old man with BOLT in 2005 for CF. CT shows bilateral upper lung fibrosis (arrows in **a** and **b**) indicating chronic lung allograft dysfunction (CLAD) of the restrictive physiology

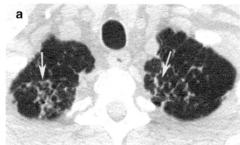
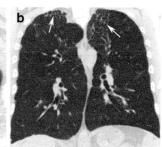

Upper Lobe Fibrosis

Upper lobe fibrosis is uncommon and occurs 1–4 years after transplantation. The exact cause for this is unknown but is described as a component of chronic allograft dysfunction (CLAD) demonstrating restrictive physiology hypothesized to be a variant of chronic rejection [21, 31]. Clinically, patients present with restrictive allograft syndrome (RAS), which is marked by restrictive pulmonary function testing and often demonstrates a more aggressive and treatment-refractory course compared to obliterative bronchiolitis. CT shows interlobular septal thickening, traction bronchiectasis, volume loss, and architectural distortion [31] (Fig. 19.24a, b).

Recurrence of Primary Disease

Recurrence of primary disease in transplanted lungs is uncommon with reported incidence of 1% [32]. Sarcoidosis is the most common disease recurring after transplantation reported in approximately 35% of patients [32, 33]. Other diseases that can recur include lymphangioleiomyomatosis (LAM), pulmonary Langerhans cell histiocytosis (PLCH), pulmonary alveolar proteinosis (PAP), and multifocal adenocarcinoma (previously bronchioloalveolar carcinoma). Recurrence of primary disease has been reported as early as 2 weeks and as late as 2 years after transplantation. The radiologic manifestations are similar to primary disease [32].

Transbronchial Biopsy Associated Complications

Bronchoscopy and transbronchial biopsy are frequently performed after lung transplantation to aide in the diagnosis of the various aforementioned complications [34]. Transbronchial biopsy itself can lead to various complications including pneumothorax, hemothorax, and pulmonary hemorrhage. Solid and cavitary nodules with surrounding ground-glass opacity may be an incidental finding in the allograft up to 1 month as a result of transbronchial biopsy in the corresponding location, and thus such a finding must be interpreted with caution and not confused with a fungal infection [35]. The temporal relationship to biopsy and location of nodules at the known biopsy sites helps distinguish these nodules from infection.

Summary

A wide spectrum of complications with overlapping radiologic findings may occur after lung transplantation. Familiarity with radiologic appearance of these complications in correlation with clinical manifestations and time course since transplantation is very helpful in the management of these patients. The threshold for performing CT should be low to detect infections in this immunocompromised population at an early stage. CT protocols should be tailored to suspected complications such as performing inspiration and expiration CT when chronic allograft dysfunction is suspected and performing CT angiogram when vascular complications are suspected. Accurate tailoring of CT protocols increases the yield of imaging and is useful in appropriate retrieval of specimens/samples from abnormal airways and pulmonary parenchyma in identifying the specific pathology. Follow-up imaging is essential and is guided by patient's clinical course and pulmonary function tests.

References

1. Yusen RD, Edwards LB, Kucheryavaya AY, Benden C, Dipchand AI, Dobbels F, et al. The registry of the International Society for Heart and Lung Transplantation: thirty-first adult lung and heart-lung transplant report--2014; focus theme: retransplantation. J Heart Lung Transplant. 2014;33(10):1009–24.
2. Frost AE. Donor criteria and evaluation. Clin Chest Med. 1997;18(2):231–7.
3. Kuno R, Kanter KR, Torres WE, Lawrence EC. Single lung transplantation followed by contralateral bullectomy for bullous emphysema. J Heart Lung Transplant. 1996;15(4):389–94.
4. Frost AE, Jammal CT, Cagle PT. Hyperacute rejection following lung transplantation. Chest. 1996;110(2):559–62.
5. Kundu S, Herman SJ, Winton TL. Reperfusion edema after lung transplantation: radiographic manifestations. Radiology. 1998;206(1):75–80.
6. Herridge MS, de Hoyos AL, Chaparro C, Winton TL, Kesten S, Maurer JR. Pleural complications in lung transplant recipients. J Thorac Cardiovasc Surg. 1995;110(1):22–6.
7. Ferrer J, Roldan J, Roman A, Bravo C, Monforte V, Pallissa E, et al. Acute and chronic pleural complications in lung transplantation. J Heart Lung Transplant. 2003;22(11):1217–25.
8. Arndt A, Boffa DJ. Pleural space complications associated with lung transplantation. Thorac Surg Clin. 2015;25(1):87–95.
9. King-Biggs MB. Acute pulmonary allograft rejection. Mechanisms, diagnosis, and management. Clin Chest Med. 1997;18(2):301–10.
10. Christie JD, Edwards LB, Aurora P, Dobbels F, Kirk R, Rahmel AO, et al. The Registry of the International Society for Heart and Lung Transplantation: twenty-sixth official adult lung and heart-lung transplantation report-2009. J Heart Lung Transplant. 2009;28(10):1031–49.
11. Knoop C, Estenne M. Acute and chronic rejection after lung transplantation. Semin Respir Crit Care Med. 2006;27(5):521–33.
12. Alvarez A, Algar J, Santos F, Lama R, Aranda JL, Baamonde C, et al. Airway complications after lung transplantation: a review of 151 anastomoses. Eur J Cardiothorac Surg. 2001;19(4):381–7.
13. Ng YL, Paul N, Patsios D, Walsham A, Chung TB, Keshavjee S, et al. Imaging of lung transplantation: review. AJR Am J Roentgenol. 2009;192(3 Suppl):S1–13, quiz S4–9.
14. Clark SC, Levine AJ, Hasan A, Hilton CJ, Forty J, Dark JH. Vascular complications of lung transplantation. Ann Thorac Surg. 1996;61(4):1079–82.
15. Krishnam MS, Suh RD, Tomasian A, Goldin JG, Lai C, Brown K, et al. Postoperative complications of lung transplantation: radiologic findings along a time continuum. Radiographics. 2007;27(4):957–74.
16. Avery RK. Infections after lung transplantation. Semin Respir Crit Care Med. 2006;27(5):544–51.
17. Collins J, Muller NL, Kazerooni EA, Paciocco G. CT findings of pneumonia after lung transplantation. AJR Am J Roentgenol. 2000;175(3):811–8.
18. Paraskeva M, Bailey M, Levvey BJ, Griffiths AP, Kotsimbos TC, Williams TP, et al. Cytomegalovirus replication within the lung allograft is associated with bronchiolitis obliterans syndrome. Am J Transplant. 2011;11(10):2190–6.
19. Collins J. Imaging of the chest after lung transplantation. J Thorac Imaging. 2002;17(2):102–12.
20. Estenne M, Maurer JR, Boehler A, Egan JJ, Frost A, Hertz M, et al. Bronchiolitis obliterans syndrome 2001: an update of the diagnostic criteria. J Heart Lung Transplant. 2002;21(3):297–310.

21. Verleden GM, Raghu G, Meyer KC, Glanville AR, Corris P. A new classification system for chronic lung allograft dysfunction. J Heart Lung Transplant. 2014;33(2):127–33.
22. Lee ES, Gotway MB, Reddy GP, Golden JA, Keith FM, Webb WR. Early bronchiolitis obliterans following lung transplantation: accuracy of expiratory thin-section CT for diagnosis. Radiology. 2000;216(2):472–7.
23. Chaparro C, Chamberlain D, Maurer J, Winton T, Dehoyos A, Kesten S. Bronchiolitis obliterans organizing pneumonia (BOOP) in lung transplant recipients. Chest. 1996;110(5):1150–4.
24. Arakawa H, Kurihara Y, Niimi H, Nakajima Y, Johkoh T, Nakamura H. Bronchiolitis obliterans with organizing pneumonia versus chronic eosinophilic pneumonia: high-resolution CT findings in 81 patients. AJR Am J Roentgenol. 2001;176(4):1053–8.
25. Reams BD, McAdams HP, Howell DN, Steele MP, Davis RD, Palmer SM. Posttransplant lymphoproliferative disorder: incidence, presentation, and response to treatment in lung transplant recipients. Chest. 2003;124(4):1242–9.
26. Paranjothi S, Yusen RD, Kraus MD, Lynch JP, Patterson GA, Trulock EP. Lymphoproliferative disease after lung transplantation: comparison of presentation and outcome of early and late cases. J Heart Lung Transplant. 2001;20(10):1054–63.
27. Carignan S, Staples CA, Muller NL. Intrathoracic lymphoproliferative disorders in the immunocompromised patient: CT findings. Radiology. 1995;197(1):53–8.
28. Dodd GD III, Ledesma-Medina J, Baron RL, Fuhrman CR. Post-transplant lymphoproliferative disorder: intrathoracic manifestations. Radiology. 1992;184(1):65–9.
29. Scarsbrook AF, Warakaulle DR, Dattani M, Traill Z. Post-transplantation lymphoproliferative disorder: the spectrum of imaging appearances. Clin Radiol. 2005;60(1):47–55.
30. Rappaport DC, Chamberlain DW, Shepherd FA, Hutcheon MA. Lymphoproliferative disorders after lung transplantation: imaging features. Radiology. 1998;206(2):519–24.
31. Konen E, Weisbrod GL, Pakhale S, Chung T, Paul NS, Hutcheon MA. Fibrosis of the upper lobes: a newly identified late-onset complication after lung transplantation? AJR Am J Roentgenol. 2003;181(6):1539–43.
32. Collins J, Hartman MJ, Warner TF, Muller NL, Kazerooni EA, McAdams HP, et al. Frequency and CT findings of recurrent disease after lung transplantation. Radiology. 2001;219(2):503–9.
33. Kazerooni EA, Jackson C, Cascade PN. Sarcoidosis: recurrence of primary disease in transplanted lungs. Radiology. 1994;192(2):461–4.
34. Boehler A, Vogt P, Zollinger A, Weder W, Speich R. Prospective study of the value of transbronchial lung biopsy after lung transplantation. Eur Respir J. 1996;9(4):658–62.
35. Kazerooni EA, Cascade PN, Gross BH. Transplanted lungs: nodules following transbronchial biopsy. Radiology. 1995;194(1):209–12.

Part IV

Lung Transplantation: Future Directions

New Horizons in Lung Transplantation

Pablo Gerardo Sanchez, Dustin M. Walters, and Michael S. Mulligan

Introduction

Lung transplantation is the preferred treatment for patients with end-stage lung disease who have exhausted other therapeutic options. Worldwide, the number of lung transplants performed annually has steadily increased over the past 30 years [1]. Despite this growth, however, the number of lungs available for transplantation fails to meet the needs of those patients on the waiting list. In the United States alone, 2394 patients were newly listed in 2013 with a waitlist mortality rate of 15.1 per 100 patient years [2]. The reported waitlist mortality greatly underestimates the actual problem because the shortfall of lungs available for transplant mandates stringent listing criteria, which could be liberalized if more organs became available.

P. G. Sanchez
Division of Cardiothoracic Surgery, Department of Surgery, University of Washington, Seattle, WA, USA
e-mail: pgsmd@uw.edu

D. M. Walters
Department of Thoracic and Cardiovascular Surgery, University of Virginia, Charlottesville, VA, USA
e-mail: dmw7f@virginia.edu

M. S. Mulligan (✉)
Department of Surgery, University of Washington, Seattle, WA, USA
e-mail: msmmd@uw.edu

The supply and demand mismatch is multifactorial, although one significant cause is the low rate of lung-specific organ utilization, which is the lowest among all transplanted organs. In current practice, only 15–20% of lungs from all potential donors are transplanted, compared to 30% of eligible hearts and 65–70% of kidneys and livers [3, 4]. The lungs, compared to other solid organs, are much more susceptible to a variety of injury mechanisms including direct trauma, aspiration, ventilator-associated pneumonia, pulmonary edema, acute lung injury from resuscitation, and neurogenic pulmonary edema. Notwithstanding this increased susceptibility, Ware et al. [5] assessed 29 pairs of lungs that were rejected for transplantation and determined that 41% would have been potentially acceptable, underscoring the challenge of assessing lungs for transplant.

Several mechanisms have been implemented to increase lung utilization and better assess organs prior to transplantation. First, donor criteria have been expanded to include conditions previously deemed unacceptable for donation. With this liberalization of donor criteria, we currently transplant lungs from older donors and those with a history of smoking, with lower PaO_2:FiO_2 ratios, and with evidence of non-reaccumulating purulent secretions on bronchoscopic examination. Use of appropriate lungs with these extended criteria has no effect on survival or other outcomes [6]. Additionally, the procurement of

© The Author(s) 2018
G. Raghu, R. G. Carbone (eds.), *Lung Transplantation*, https://doi.org/10.1007/978-3-319-91184-7_20

lungs from donors after circulatory determination of death (DCDD) has been demonstrated to be another effective means of increasing the pool of donors [7] and is associated with similar outcomes compared to donation after brain death (DBD) [7–10]. This chapter discusses evolving trends of better management of the potential donor lung, preservation techniques, and utilization of conventionally regarded as borderline or suboptimal for lung transplantation including ex vivo lung perfusion techniques to enhance the utilization of the donor lung pool that is much less than the number of people needing the suitable lung to save their lives.

Lung Donor Management

Goal-directed donor management protocols have been developed to utilize the greatest number of organs under optimal functional conditions [11, 12]. Table 20.1 summarizes recommendations made by the United Network for Organ Sharing (UNOS) for the care of cardiothoracic donors. We will focus on particular aspects of the management of the potential lung donor, such as mechanical ventilation and volume and hormonal resuscitation.

The ideal method to ventilate donors has not been determined. Historically, donors were ventilated with high tidal volumes and low positive end-expiratory pressures (PEEP) (10–15 mL/Kg and 5 cm H_2O) [13]. But recently, the benefit of using lung-protective ventilation in acute respiratory distress syndrome was translated to organ donation. A multicenter randomized clinical trial showed that a lung-protective ventilation doubles the lung utilization rate [14]. Other modes of ventilation such as airway pressure release ventilation (APRV) have been suggested [15]. We believe this practice produces misleading PaO_2 and exposes the lung to high airway pressures which can result in barotrauma.

The hemodynamic effects of brain death can also compromise lung quality. The initial hypertensive crisis can disrupt the pulmonary endothelium homeostasis by increased mechanical stress. Also, fluid resuscitation required during the

Table 20.1 United Network for Organ Sharing cardio-thoracic donor management

Echocardiogram	Done early for all donors Pulmonary artery catheter if ejection fraction <45% or high-dose inotropic support
Electrolytes	Na < 150 meq/dL K + >4.0 Correct acidosis to a pH > 7.2 with Na bicarbonate and mild-moderate hyperventilation (pCO_2 30–35 mmHg)
Ventilation	Peak airway pressures <30 cm H_2O Mild respiratory alkalosis (pCO_2 30–35 mmHg)
Hormonal resuscitation	Tri-iodothyronine (T3): 4 mcg bolus; 3 mcg/h infusion Arginine vasopressin: 1 unit bolus, 0.5–4.0 unit/h drip (titrate to SVR 800–1200) Methylprednisolone: 15 mg/kg bolus (repeat q 24 h PRN) Insulin: drip at a minimum rate of 1 unit/h (titrate to blood glucose 120–180 mg/gL) Volume resuscitation: use of colloid and avoidance of anemia important to prevent pulmonary edema – Albumin if INR and PTT normal (crystalloids may be as effective and cheaper) – Fresh frozen plasma if INR and PTT abnormal (value >1.5 × control) – Packed red blood cells to maintain PCWP 8–12 mmHg and Hgb > 10 mg/dL
Donor considered stable	Mean arterial pressure ≥ 60 mmHg CVP < 12 mmHg (ideally <6 mmHg) PCWP <12 mmHg SVR 800–1200 dynes/s/cm⁵ Left ventricular stroke work index > 15 Dopamine dosage < 10 mcg/kg/min

Data from http://unos.org/docs/Critical_Pathway.pdf

hypotensive phase can worsen gas exchange [16]. We favor a goal-directed volume repletion and the use of diuretics to regain a neutral or negative fluid balance after the initial resuscitation phase [11, 17]. Volume restrictive resuscitation protocols (CVP < 6 mmHg) do not seem to have a negative effect on kidney utilization and function. They also increase lung utilization by avoiding fluid overload and pulmonary edema and improved gas exchange [18]. The use of vasopressin or desmopressin may be required to reduce the urinary output to 100–200 mL\h in donors that develop diabetes insipidus [17].

Other hormonal therapies have also been recommended to maintain metabolic function and organ viability. The use of insulin or a dextrose solution to maintain glycemic control (glucose blood level 120–180 mg/dL), thyroxine to reduce vasopressor requirement and prevent cardiovascular collapse, and methylprednisolone to reduce inflammation and support adrenal dysfunction is part of all donor resuscitation protocols.

Other considerations when managing a potential lung donor are:

1. Performing a bronchoscopy to define airway anatomy and sampling airway secretions to define the need for directed antibiotic therapy. Donor gram stain and cultures can also be used to define antibiotic treatment post-lung transplant [19].
2. Chest X-rays. Lung infiltrates should not preclude consideration for donation. Over 50% of infiltrates seen in the initial chest X-ray resolve with appropriate donor management [20]. In addition, the contralateral lung may be successfully allocated when unilateral nonresolving infiltrates or consolidations are present.

Aggressive donor management protocols and the expansion of donor selection criteria (Table 20.2) have allowed to significantly increase the number of lung transplants without detriment to outcomes [6, 21–26].

Donation After Circulatory Death

Under clinical protocols developed and strictly applied by several experienced lung transplant programs, lungs from controlled DCDD have produced outcomes very similar to those observed

Table 20.2 Lung donor selection criteria

	Ideal donor	Extended donor
Age	20–45	18–64 no impact on PGD [21, 26]
PaO2:FiO2	>350	Initial PaO$_2$ not correlated with outcomes [23]
Smoking history	None	LTOG any smoking associated with PGD [22] UK registry small increase hazard [24]
Chest X-ray	Clear	Infiltrates clear >50% cases after adequate donor management [20]
Ventilation days	<5	–
Microbiology	Gram stain negative	Uniformly gram stains are positive [19]
Bronchoscopy	Clear	Purulent secretions are consistently present Continuous pooling during bronchoscopy may suggest pneumonia
Ischemic time	<4 h	UNOS analysis no correlation ischemic time and PGD [25]

LTOG Lung Transplant Outcomes Group, *UNOS* United Network Organ Sharing, *PGD* primary graft dysfunction, *UK* United Kingdom

with BDD. Some authors have even suggested that DCDD lungs outperform BDD lungs, due to the absence of the cardiovascular and inflammatory derangements seen in anoxic or traumatic brain death [27]. However, a recent registry analysis demonstrated that early mortality is significantly higher when using DCDD lungs from donors with head trauma, compared to those with other mechanisms of injury. The reason for this finding remains unclear [28].

Donation After Circulatory Determination of Death Protocols

DCDDs represent a unique scenario in which consent for donation and donor management occurs before the determination of death. In 2013, the American Thoracic Society, the International Society of Heart and Lung

Transplantation, the Society of Critical Care Medicine, the Association of Organ and Procurement Organizations, and the United Network of Organ Sharing published a statement based on evidence, experience, and clinical rationale [29]. This statement was tailored to provide the framework to guide the ethics and policy consideration for organ donation after controlled DCDD. In this statement, pre-circulatory death interventions such as the use of heparin, vasodilators, and diagnostic bronchoscopies were considered ethically acceptable if their use is disclosed to the donor families.

The use of systemic heparin in organ procurement has been advocated to reduce formation of intravascular thrombi, allowing more homogeneous flush distribution and better graft preservation [30]. Ethical concerns have limited the use of heparin in the setting of controlled DCDD, leading to different practices. We believe that the administration of heparin, after the decision to withdraw treatment has been agreed upon and initiated, is highly unlikely to alter outcomes (accelerate demise), at least in the absence of a contraindication such as active bleeding.

Where permitted by local regulation or practice, heparin is given before WLST [9, 31–33]. Delivery after cardiac arrest by temporary cardiac compression or by administration in the first

liter of the preservation solution has been reported [34, 35]. The Groningen group reported 35 donors in which heparin was not administered [36]. The Australian collaborative experience reported that 26 of their 72 DCDD did not receive heparin as per hospital regulations [37].

Concerns regarding the effects of normothermic ischemia on graft quality have also limited the use of DCDD lungs. Unfortunately, the metrics to define warm ischemic times remain controversial. Most centers will accept a period of 60–120 min from WLST to arrest, but the definition of when warm ischemia starts is not as clear. A recent multicenter study defined the beginning of WIT when the systolic systemic arterial blood pressure was equal or lower than 50 mmHg (Fig. 20.1) [37].

Recently a more descriptive definition divided the WIT in two phases: the *withdrawal phase*, defined as the interval between extubation (and/or withdrawal of other specific life-supporting interventions, such as inotropes or mechanical circulatory support) and onset of asystole, and the *acirculatory phase*, defined as the interval between onset of asystole and initiation of cold flush [30].

Most lung transplant centers will not consider DCDD lungs in which more than 60 min have elapsed between WLST and asystole, although

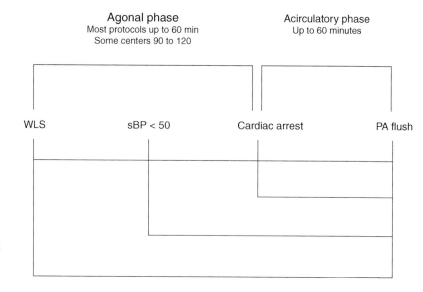

Fig. 20.1 Definition of warm ischemic times in DCDD. Definitions of warm ischemic time among lung transplant centers. *WLS* withdrawal of life support, *SBP* systolic blood pressure, *PA* pulmonary artery, *min* minutes

this criterion is based on the presumption that WIT >60 min is likely to be associated with irreversible organ injury and is not based on systematic study or scientific evidence. Few centers will accept lungs in which the donor expired within 90–120 min after WLST [28, 37].

Early and Midterm Outcomes with DCDD

Clinical experiences with DCDD lungs continue to increase. Table 20.3 summarizes early and midterm results of eight peer-reviewed reports. Two hundred and twenty-two DCDDs were transplanted into 225 recipients. Five of these reports compared DCDD to contemporary BDD outcomes. All, but one, showed no significant differences in terms of early and midterm outcomes. Puri and colleagues reported a significantly higher percentage of PGD 3 and ECMO use in lung transplant recipients of DCDD when compared to recipients of BDD—36% vs. 18% and 18% vs. 2%, respectively. Table 20.4 summarizes selected data.

In 2013 the first analysis from ISHLT DCDD registry was presented. Nine centers from North America, Europe, and Australia performed 224 lung transplants between 2003 and 2012. The 1-year survival was 89% for DCDD compared to 89% for contemporary BDD lung transplants [28]. The same year, four centers from the United Kingdom presented their DCDD experience. From 2002 to 2012, 100 lung transplants were performed using DCDD lungs.

One-year survival for recipients of DCDD lungs was 79.5% vs. 79.2% in contemporary recipients of BDD lungs. Currently DCDD lungs account for 14% of all lungs transplanted in the United Kingdom [38]. While there is growing enthusiasm for expanding DCDD lung donation in North America, in the United States, approximately 2% of all lung transplants are performed using controlled DCDDs [8].

Beyond controlled DCDD, the use of uncontrolled DCDD lungs has been proposed to further increase the supply of lungs for transplantation. The theoretical advantage to uncontrolled DCDD

donation is the potentially large number of available donor organs, which could readily overcome the deficit of lungs needed for transplantation. Uncontrolled DCD donors can enter the donation process from a variety of different means, and these potential donors have been categorized by the Maastricht classification system (Table 20.5) [39, 40]. In most cases, uncontrolled DCDD donation involves an unexpected circulatory death, for instance, a patient who suffers a cardiac arrest after acute myocardial infarction. The appeal of using lungs for transplantation from these potential donors stems from the fact that lungs will tolerate up to 90 min of warm ischemic time prior to transplantation with successful outcomes [41, 42]. During that period of warm ischemia from declaration of death until procurement, decisions can be made in conjunction with the patient's family whether to pursue transplantation.

Unfortunately, in the uncontrolled setting, organ assessment is extremely limited, almost always without imaging, bronchoscopy, and arterial blood gas data, which serve as the basis for routine determination of donor candidacy. Ex vivo lung perfusion offers the ability to carefully assess postmortem quality of lungs prior to transplantation under these circumstances.

Ex Vivo Lung Perfusion

The concept of ex vivo organ perfusion took root nearly a century ago, when Alexis Carrel and Charles Lindbergh demonstrated that animal thyroid glands could be perfused ex vivo with viability lasting several days [43]. Building on this knowledge and knowledge gained from the use of extracorporeal membranous oxygenation (ECMO) and cardiopulmonary bypass, the idea of ex vivo lung perfusion began to take shape.

In 2001, Steen and colleagues, after proof of principle animal experiments [44, 45], successfully transplanted the right lung of an uncontrolled DCDD donor after ex vivo perfusion and assessment [46]. The technique of EVLP has been refined over the ensuing years with development of acellular perfusates and specific protocols

Table 20.3 Controlled donation after circulatory death lung transplant outcomes

Group	n	PGD 3	ECMO postoperative	ICU days	Hospital days	Airway complications	30-day mortality	1-year survival
Washington University Puri et al. [34]	11	36%	18%	NR	NR	1 Required RUL sleeve	11%	88%
University Toronto Cypel et al. [25]	10	10%	10%	8.5 2–21	NR	1 Small dehiscence	0%	100%
University Groningen Van De Wauwer et al. [30]	35	24%	0%	4 3–24	32 24–66	NR	NR	91%
University Wisconsin/Loyola De Oliveira et al. [26]	18	16%	0%	4 3–8	17 15–23	5 One required Re-Tx	5%	88%
University Leuven De Vleeschauwer et al. [9]	21	≈20%	NR	7 5–19	29 23–42	None	0%	95%
Australia Collaborative eExperience Levvey et al. [31]	72	8%	NR	5 2–48	20 10–180	1 Bilateral ischemia	NR	97%
Harefield NHS Foundation Trust Harefield Hospital Zych et al. [29]	26	4%	15%	5 3–33	35 20–79	2 Endoscopic treatment	8%	88%
Cleveland Clinic Mason et al. [27]	32	3%	6%	4 NR	14 NR	6 mild necrosis 1 stenosis	3%	91%

RUL right upper lobe, *ECMO* extracorporeal membrane oxygenation, *RUL* right upper lobe, *min* minutes, *ICU* intensive care unit, *PGD* primary graft dysfunction, *NR* not reported

Table 20.4 Lung transplant outcomes. DCDD vs. BDD at the same institution

		DCDD	BDD
Washington University Puri et al. [34]	PGD 3	36%	18%
	ECMO post Tx	18%	2%
	BOS 3	10%	NR
	1-year survival	88%	NR
	Median follow-up	18 months (0–66)	29 months (NR)
University Groningen Van De Wauwer et al. [30]	PGD 3	24%	25%
	ECMO post Tx	0%	1%
	BOS-free 1 year	100%	85%
	1-year survival	91%	91%
	Median follow-up	NR	NR
University Wisconsin/Loyola De Oliveira et al. [26]	PGD 2–3	33%	26%
	ECMO post Tx	0%	6%
	BOS-free 1 year	80%	93%
	1-year survival	88%	87%
	Median follow-up	46 months (4–59)	42 months (14–86)
University Leuven De Vleeschauwer et al. [9]	PGD 3	≈20%	≈25%
	ECMO post Tx	NR	NR
	BOS-free 1 year	84%	90%
	1-year survival	95%	91%
	Median follow-up	11 months (6–23)	18 months (8–29)
Harefield NHS Foundation Trust Harefield Hospital Zych et al. [29]	PGD 3	4%	6%
	ECMO post Tx	16%	5%
	BOS-free 1 year	95%	91%
	1-year survival	88%	86%
	Median follow-up	15 months (7–27)	18 months (9–29)

PGD primary graft dysfunction, *BOS* bronchiolitis obliterans syndrome, *Tx* transplantation, *ECMO* extracorporeal membrane oxygenation, *NR* not reported, *DCDD* donation after circulatory determination of death, *BDD* brain death donation

Table 20.5 The Maastricht classification for donation after circulatory death

Category I	Patient dead on arrival to hospital	Uncontrolled
Category II	Patient survives transport to hospital but undergoes unsuccessful resuscitation	Uncontrolled
Category III	Patient awaiting circulatory death	Controlled
Category IV	Patient undergoes circulatory death after meeting brain death criteria	Uncontrolled
Category V	Patient undergoes unexpected circulatory arrest while in hospital	Uncontrolled

designed to optimize assessment and pulmonary function. As techniques have evolved, so has our understanding of EVLP and potential mechanisms of benefit. One such mechanism in the setting of brain death donation is removal of the lungs and protection from the inflammatory cytokine milieu that occurs after head injury and brain death [47, 48]. Other potential mechanisms of benefit include improvement and clearance of pulmonary edema with high oncotic perfusates and allowance for diagnostic and therapeutic bronchoscopy. EVLP can be a useful tool in the setting of DCDD, particularly uncontrolled DCDD, when there may not be sufficient opportunity to assess the quality of lungs for transplantation.

Indications for EVLP

When considering EVLP, assessment of the donor is critically important, including cause and timing of death, hospital course, and lung-specific factors including imaging, bronchoscopy, arterial blood gases, and culture results. In general, lungs from donors who meet standard criteria for lung transplantation are excluded from EVLP, and these lungs are procured, cold stored, and transported for routine transplantation.

The indications and contraindications for use of EVLP are shown in Table 20.6. In general, EVLP is considered for increased risk donors or when assessment is incomplete or limited. Indications include PaO$_2$/FiO$_2$ ratio less than 350, presence of pulmonary edema radiographically or during procurement, brain death donors with inability to fully assess lungs, and high-risk donor criteria such as massive blood transfusion. Current contraindications include pneumonia, contusions, lobar consolidation, aspiration of gastric contents, and other traumatic injuries to the lung.

ELVP Equipment

The EVLP circuit is fairly simple and essentially has two major components: (1) a circuit for perfusion and (2) a conventional ventilator. The perfusion circuit consists of a left atrial cannula, sewn directly to the left atrial cuff, which connects to a tubing that drains perfusate into a reservoir. From the reservoir, the perfusate travels through a pump and a heat/gas exchanger, followed by a leukocyte filter, and then is returned via a separate cannula to the pulmonary artery (Fig. 20.2). Importantly, the gas exchange component is a deoxygenator, allowing for assessment of pulmonary gas exchange since oxygen delivered through the conventional ventilator is

Table 20.6 Indications and contraindications of ex vivo lung perfusion (EVLP)

Indications	Contraindications
• PaO$_2$/FiO$_2$ < 350	• Pneumonia
• Radiographic pulmonary edema	• Pulmonary contusion
• Evidence of pulmonary edema during procurement	• Lobar consolidation
• DCD donation	• Aspiration
• High-risk donor factors	• Barotrauma

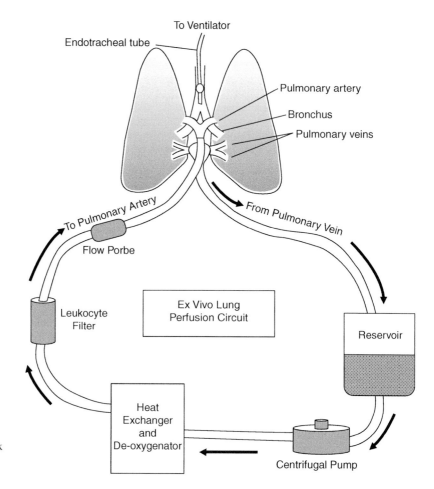

Fig. 20.2 Ex vivo lung perfusion circuit. Lungs under evaluation with acellular perfusion, using two cannulas (the pulmonary artery and left atrium). Components of the system are a hard-shell reservoir, leukocyte filter, integrated pump/heater/membrane gas exchanger (deoxygenator), gas tank for deoxygenation, and ventilator

the only source of oxygen to the system. A flow probe measures perfusate flow, allowing for tight regulation of flow through the system.

Technical Aspects of EVLP

The technical aspects of EVLP begin with the procurement of the donor lungs. In general, procurement proceeds similarly to standard DBD and DCD protocols. The main difference is that when EVLP is considered, the lungs should be harvested en bloc. The trachea should be divided high at the level of the lower neck to allow for insertion of an endotracheal tube when placed on the circuit. If the length from tracheal division to carina is not sufficient, placement of the ET tube can be challenging if not impossible. If planning on suturing the left atrium to a cuffed cannula, one should pay attention to the amount of left atrial cuff. If using a system that relies on open left atrial drainage, this matters less. Ideally, a couple centimeters of the main pulmonary artery should be left intact in order to allow for cannulation of the pulmonary artery in all cases.

Three main protocols exist for EVLP: the Toronto protocol [49], the Lund protocol [50], and the Organ Care System lung protocol [51].

General principles remain similar, although there are some differences, which will be discussed below.

The key principles for the Toronto (Fig. 20.3) protocol involve gradual rewarming of the lungs while increasing flow to 40% of the predicted donor cardiac output, protective lung ventilation, and use of a high oncotic acellular perfusate [49]. After securing cannulas within the pulmonary artery and to the left atrium and insertion of an endotracheal tube, a retrograde flush with Perfadex is performed. The cannulas are then connected to the perfusion circuit. The perfusion circuit is primed with Steen solution, methylprednisolone, heparin, and antibiotics and deaired. Flow is initiated at room temperature at only 10% of the targeted flow for the first 10 min. Flow is then increased to 20% target flow, and the temperature is set at 30 °C until the 20-min mark, at which point ventilation begins at 7 mL/kg, 5 PEEP cm H_2O, FiO_2 21%, and a respiratory rate of 7 per minute. Over the next 30 min, the flow is gradually increased to 100% targeted flow (40% predicted cardiac output), and the lungs are warmed to 37 °C. Once ventilation has begun, the deoxygenator (gas mixture 86% N_2, 8% CO_2, and 6% O_2) is set to a sweep of 1 L/min and adjusted as needed to maintain a pCO_2 between 35 and 40 mmHg.

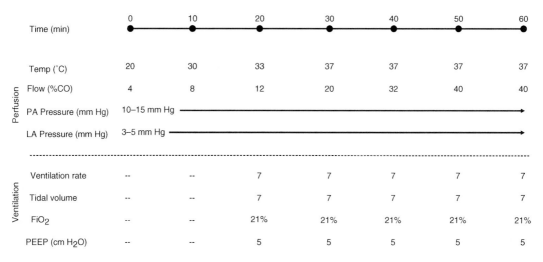

	Time (min)	0	10	20	30	40	50	60
Perfusion	Temp (°C)	20	30	33	37	37	37	37
	Flow (%CO)	4	8	12	20	32	40	40
	PA Pressure (mm Hg)	10–15 mm Hg						→
	LA Pressure (mm Hg)	3–5 mm Hg						→
Ventilation	Ventilation rate	--	--	7	7	7	7	7
	Tidal volume	--	--	7	7	7	7	7
	FiO_2	--	--	21%	21%	21%	21%	21%
	PEEP (cm H_2O)	--	--	5	5	5	5	5

Fig. 20.3 Toronto ex vivo lung perfusion protocol. Toronto's flow rates are based on the donor's calculated cardiac output (CO). Flow is initiated at 4% CO and gradually increased as the lung temperature increases, always maintaining a $P_{PA} < 15$ mmHg. Target flow is 40% CO. Ventilation and sweep gas flow (8% CO_2, 6% O_2, 86% N_2) are initiated at 32 °C. Toronto specifies a tidal volume of 7 mL/kg at a rate of 7 breaths/min on room air

During perfusion, careful attention is paid to the left atrial pressure, which is maintained at 3–5 mmHg, and this can be achieved by adjusting the height of the reservoir. Recruitment maneuvers are performed once the targeted flow, temperature, and ventilation have been reached. The Steen solution is exchanged every hour, initially with 500 mL followed by 250 mL in subsequent hours. Total perfusion time is between 4 and 6 h.

For the Toronto protocol, hourly assessments are made. Before assessment, ventilation parameters are adjusted for 5 min (10 mL/kg ventilation volume, rate 10 breaths/min, FiO2 100%). "Blood gas" analysis is performed on the perfusate. Chest radiographs are performed at the 1-h mark and every 2 h subsequently. After the 4- to 6-h perfusion time and when the lungs are deemed suitable for transplantation, the FiO2 is set at 50%, and the lungs are cooled to 15 °C. The lungs are then flushed with 500 mL Steen solution in an antegrade fashion and topically cooled with Perfadex® (XVIVO Perfusion, Göteborg, Sweden) and ice before implantation.

The Lund protocol has many similarities to the Toronto protocol, including the use of Steen for priming of the circuit; however, in the Lund protocol leukocyte, ABO compatible red blood cells are added to achieve a perfusate hematocrit of 15%. It is worth noting that no differences have been observed between acellular and cellular perfusates in terms of lung function or outcomes [52, 53]. Antibiotics, heparin, insulin, and buffer are added to the perfusate. Flow is initiated at 25 °C at a low rate (50–100 mL/min) maintaining a pulmonary arterial pressure below 20 mmHg. Flow is gradually increased toward target flow as the lungs are rewarmed maintaining low pulmonary arterial pressures and a left atrial pressure of 0 mmHg. Ventilation is begun once the temperature has reached 32 °C using a low minute ventilation of 1 L/min. The minute ventilation is increased by 1 L/min for each 1 °C temperature increase up to a final temperature of 37 °C. FiO2 is set at 100%, and respiratory rate begins low (5 breaths/min), gradually increasing to 15–20 breaths/min. The gas settings on the deoxygenator are 93% N2 and 7% CO2 with 0% oxygen. The flow of the perfusate through the circuit is likewise gradually increased toward a final target of 5–6 L/min once the lungs have warmed to 37 °C. Total reconditioning perfusion time is generally between 1 and 2 h.

Assessment on the Lund protocol begins once the temperature has reached 37 °C and target flow and ventilation have been achieved. Evaluation consists of blood gas samples drawn after 5-min intervals with gradually increasing FiO2 of 21%, 50%, and 100%. Following this laboratory assessment, a deflation test is performed, where observations are made regarding the rate and degree of deflation. Lungs are deemed acceptable for transplantation if those tests are favorable, at which point the lungs are cooled and preserved.

The third major EVLP platform is the TransMedics™ Organ Care System (Andover, MA, USA) (OCS). One unique feature of the OCS lung platform is the inherent portability of the apparatus by design. On the OCS protocol, the lungs are connected to the system at the time of procurement at the donor hospital. After procurement, an endotracheal tube is placed into the trachea, and the pulmonary artery is connected to the circuit, while the left atrium is left to openly drain. The perfusate consists of 1.5 L of Steen solution combined with red blood cells to achieve a hematocrit between 15 and 25%. Added to the perfusate are antibiotics, steroids, glucose, insulin, multivitamins, milrinone, and tris(hydroxymethyl)aminomethane (THAM). Perfusion begins at a temperature of 32 °C, which is increased to 37 °C within approximately 10 min of perfusion. Target flow is 2.5 L/min, and ventilation settings include tidal volume of 6 mL/kg donor weight, PEEP of 5 cm H_2O, and ventilation rate of 10 breaths/min. Assessments are made on the circuit, and if lungs are deemed suitable for transplantation, they are cooled before implantation.

EVLP in Donation After Circulatory Death

Concerns regarding the effects of WLST on the quality of DCDD lungs have led centers to use of EVLP to evaluate lung quality prior to transplantation [54]. Yet, others have questioned this methodology based on data demonstrating that established DCDD clinical protocols yield satisfactory outcomes without the added expense and complexity of EVLP [33, 37]. We believe that as centers extend their selection criteria and flexibilize current tolerated WIT to increase DCDD use, EVLP may prove essential by diagnostically evaluating and screening out poor quality grafts, such as the finding of a poor preservation flush, in cases in which heparin use was restricted, or donors with prolonged hypoxemia in the withdrawal phase. In addition, EVLP may recondition some grafts by decreasing pulmonary edema and removing/filtering residual thrombi.

EVLP for Reconditioning Lungs

EVLP is moving beyond its use as an assessment tool and into the realm of reconditioning lungs that are marginal and not suitable for standard transplantation. For instance, studies have already demonstrated that donor lungs affected by pulmonary edema may be successfully reconditioned with EVLP [55]. The reconditioning that occurs during EVLP is likely due to several different mechanisms. First, Steen solution, which is utilized in most perfusion protocols, has a high oncotic pressure and is therefore able to draw out edema from the pulmonary interstitium, improving oxygenation of lungs. Secondly, removal of the lungs from the brain-dead donor body importantly removes them from the inflammatory cytokine milieu that occurs after brain death and therefore may prevent further injury. Additional benefits include the ability to perform therapeutic bronchoscopy, improve atelectatic segments of lung tissue, and treat other processes such as pulmonary embolism.

Pharmacologic Therapy During EVLP

Arguably one of the greatest potential impacts of EVLP is that of pharmacologic intervention while on the EVLP circuit. Prolonged perfusion periods of 12 h or more have been demonstrated to be possible [56]. As perfusion time limits are stretched out, the potential therapeutic window expands, which may ultimately allow for treatment of pneumonia and other mechanisms of injury. In animal and human models, resolution of pulmonary edema has been demonstrated with use of beta-2 agonists [57] and addition of mesenchymal stem cells [58] or microvesicles derived from them [59]. Attempts at treating donor lungs with antibiotics while undergoing EVLP have been successful in reduction of the microbial burden [60, 61]. Models of aspiration and EVLP use have been developed [62] to better understand the injury process, and preclinical models utilizing treatment with surfactant have been shown to mitigate gastric acid-associated injury [63, 64].

Further, EVLP may be a tool for delivery of drugs to mitigate lung ischemia reperfusion injury and primary graft dysfunction. The use adenosine A_{2A} receptor agonists during EVLP has been demonstrated by the University of Virginia to attenuate lung ischemia reperfusion injury, reduce pulmonary edema, and improve graft function [65–67]. Corticosteroids [68] and plasmin [69] administration have been demonstrated to reduce ischemia reperfusion injury in a porcine lung transplant and EVLP model. Other opportunities for intervention including gene therapy and ex vivo delivery of an adenoviral vector gene encoding interleukin-10 have been demonstrated to effectively reduce lung ischemia reperfusion injury [70–72].

Clinically the Toronto, Zurich, and Edmonton groups have reported the use of fibrinolytic therapy during EVLP [73–75]. In these cases, donors initially rejected due to low oxygenation and the presence of pulmonary embolism underwent EVLP with the addition of alteplase or urokinase to the perfusate. Grafts improved during perfusion with decreasing pulmonary vascular resistance and increasing oxygenation. The recipients underwent bilateral lung transplantation and were discharged home well.

Tissue Engineering and Bioartificial Lungs

On the distant horizon, tissue engineering offers the possibility of generating new lungs using an acellular scaffolding populated with the recipient's own cells [76]. Currently this is only in experimental phases with many barriers to overcome. However, if able to be perfected, there are many obvious potential benefits, including elimination of organ shortages, expansion of recipient criteria to offer organs to an increased number of patients, decreased rejection, and obviation of the need for immunosuppression.

Portability of EVLP

The Organ Care System EVLP platform has the inherent advantage of portability, and published data have demonstrated perfusion times over 10 h with successful lung transplantation [70–72]. This offers many potential benefits for lung transplantation [77]. Organ sharing over long distances may be possible to better match donors with recipients. Additionally, there is the possibility of transportation to centralized lung reconditioning centers with increased expertise in the reconditioning process, and the timing of lung transplants may be more flexible so that they will be less disruptive to the overall flow of the operating room. Further, this may allow for earlier placement on EVLP, so that reconditioning can begin at the procurement site, rather than the destination hospital, limiting overall ischemic time. The use of portable ex vivo perfusion systems is already becoming widespread in renal transplantation with excellent results [78, 79].

Dedicated Ex Vivo Lung Perfusion Facilities

The safety of a dedicated ex vivo lung perfusion facility is currently being evaluated by the Extending Preservation and Assessment Time of Donor Lungs Using the Toronto EVLP System at a Dedicated EVLP Facility clinical trial (NCT02234128). In this trial, lungs considered high risk are procured and sent to a dedicated EVLP facility that performs the evaluation. If deemed viable during lung perfusion, the organ is packed and shipped to the transplant center.

Concerns regarding the total out-of-body time and its impact on transplant outcomes are currently under investigation using animal models [80]. Nevertheless, donors with a cold ischemic time before EVLP >10 h and EVLP time >6 h or cold ischemic time between end of EVLP and transplant >8 h are excluded from the clinical trial.

Summary

The advances in donor management, the increasing use of donors after circulatory determination of death, and the clinical translation of technologies that allow donor lung reassessment after explant have increased lung utilization without compromising lung transplant outcomes. However, the number of lungs available for transplantation continues to fail the needs of those patients on the waiting list.

References

1. Yusen RD, Edwards LB, Kucheryavaya AY, Benden C, Dipchand AI, Goldfarb SB, Levvey BJ, Lund LH, Meiser B, Rossano JW, Stehlik J, et al. The Registry of the International Society for Heart and Lung Transplantation: Thirty-second Official Adult Lung and Heart-Lung Transplantation Report—2015; Focus theme: early graft failure. J Heart Lung Transplant. 2015;34(10):1264–77.
2. Valapour M, Skeans MA, Heubner BM, Smith JM, Hertz MI, Edwards LB, Cherikh WS, Callahan ER, Snyder JJ, Israni AK, Kasiske BL. OPTN/SRTR 2013 Annual Data Report: lung. Am J Transplant. 2015;15(Suppl 2):1–28.
3. Israni AK, Zaun DA, Rosendale JD, Snyder JJ, Kasiske BL. OPTN/SRTR 2013 Annual Data Report: deceased organ donation. Am J Transplant. 2015;15(Suppl 2):1–13.
4. Klein AS, Klein AS, Messersmith EE, Ratner LE, Kochik R, Baliga PK, Ojo AO. Organ donation and utilization in the United States, 1999-2008. Am J Transplant. 2010;10(4 Pt 2):973–86.
5. Ware LB, Wang Y, Fang X, Warnock M, Sakuma T, Hall TS, Matthay M. Assessment of lungs rejected for transplantation and implications for donor selection. Lancet. 2002;360(9333):619–20.
6. Bhorade SM, Vigneswaran W, McCabe MA, Garrity ER. Liberalization of donor criteria may expand the donor pool without adverse consequence in lung transplantation. J Heart Lung Transplant. 2000;19(12):1199–204.

7. Cypel M, Levvey B, Van Raemdonck D, Erasmus M, Dark J, Love R, Mason D, Glanville AR, Chambers D, Edwards LB, Stehlik J, Hertz M, Whitson BA, Yusen RD, Puri V, Hopkins P, Snell G, Keshavjee S, International Society for Heart and Lung Transplantation. International Society for Heart and Lung Transplantation donation after circulatory death registry report. J Heart Lung Transplant. 2015;34(10):1278–82.

8. Wigfield CH, Love RB. Donation after cardiac death lung transplantation outcomes. Curr Opin Organ Transplant. 2011;16(5):462–8.

9. De Vleeschauwer SI, Wauters S, Dupont LJ, Verleden SE, Willems-Widyastuti A, Vanaudenaerde BM, Verleden GM, Van Raemdonck DE. Medium-term outcome after lung transplantation is comparable between brain-dead and cardiac-dead donors. J Heart Lung Transplant. 2011;30(9):975–81.

10. Krutsinger D, Reed RM, Blevins A, Puri V, De Oliveira NC, Zych B, Bolukbas S, Van Raemdonck D, Snell GI, Eberlein M. Lung transplantation from donation after cardiocirculatory death: a systematic review and meta-analysis. J Heart Lung Transplant. 2015;34(5):675–84.

11. Angel LF, Levine DJ, Restrepo MI, Johnson S, Sako E, Carpenter A, Calhoon J, Cornell JE, Adams SG, Chisholm GB, Nespral J, Roberson A, Levine SM. Impact of a lung transplantation donor-management protocol on lung donation and recipient outcomes. Am J Respir Crit Care Med. 2006;174(6):710–6.

12. Minambres E, Pérez-Villares JM, Chico-Fernández M, Zabalegui A, Dueñas-Jurado JM, Misis M, Mosteiro F, Rodriguez-Caravaca G, Coll E. Lung donor treatment protocol in brain dead-donors: a multicenter study. J Heart Lung Transplant. 2015;34(6):773–80.

13. Rosengard BR, Feng S, Alfrey EJ, Zaroff JG, Emond JC, Henry ML, Garrity ER, Roberts JP, Wynn JJ, Metzger RA, Freeman RB, Port FK, Merion RM, Love RB, Busuttil RW, Delmonico FL. Report of the Crystal City meeting to maximize the use of organs recovered from the cadaver donor. Am J Transplant. 2002;2(8):701–11.

14. Mascia L, Pasero D, Slutsky AS, Arguis MJ, Berardino M, Grasso S, Munari M, Boifava S, Cornara G, Della Corte F, Vivaldi N, Malacarne P, Del Gaudio P, Livigni S, Zavala E, Filippini C, Martin EL, Donadio PP, Mastromauro I, Ranieri VM. Effect of a lung protective strategy for organ donors on eligibility and availability of lungs for transplantation: a randomized controlled trial. JAMA. 2010;304(23):2620–7.

15. Hanna K, Seder CW, Weinberger JB, Sills PA, Hagan M, Janczyk RJ. Airway pressure release ventilation and successful lung donation. Arch Surg. 2011;146(3):325–8.

16. Avlonitis VS, Wigfield CH, Kirby JA, Dark JH. The hemodynamic mechanisms of lung injury and systemic inflammatory response following brain death in the transplant donor. Am J Transplant. 2005;5(4 Pt 1):684–93.

17. Rosendale JD, Kauffman HM, McBride MA, Chabalewski FL, Zaroff JG, Garrity ER, Delmonico FL, Rosengard BR. Aggressive pharmacologic donor management results in more transplanted organs. Transplantation. 2003;75(4):482–7.

18. Minambres E, Rodrigo E, Ballesteros MA, Llorca J, Ruiz JC, Fernandez-Fresnedo G, Vallejo A, González-Cotorruelo J, Arias M. Impact of restrictive fluid balance focused to increase lung procurement on renal function after kidney transplantation. Nephrol Dial Transplant. 2010;25(7):2352–6.

19. Mattner F, Kola A, Fischer S, Becker T, Haverich A, Simon A, Suerbaum S, Gastmeier P, Weissbrodt H, Strüber M. Impact of bacterial and fungal donor organ contamination in lung, heart-lung, heart and liver transplantation. Infection. 2008;36(3):207–12.

20. Bolton JS, Padia SA, Borja MC, Becker P, Orens JB, Wiener C, Yang SC, Conte JV. The predictive value and inter-observer variability of donor chest radiograph interpretation in lung transplantation. Eur J Cardiothorac Surg. 2003;23(4):484–7.

21. Baldwin MR, Peterson ER, Easthausen I, Quintanilla I, Colago E, Sonett JR, D'Ovidio F, Costa J, Diamond JM, Christie JD, Arcasoy SM, Lederer DJ. Donor age and early graft failure after lung transplantation: a cohort study. Am J Transplant. 2013;13(10):2685–95.

22. Diamond JM, Lee JC, Kawut SM, Shah RJ, Localio AR, Bellamy SL, Lederer DJ, Cantu E, Kohl BA, Lama VN, Bhorade SM, Crespo M, Demissie E, Sonett J, Wille K, Orens J, Shah AS, Weinacker A, Arcasoy S, Shah PD, Wilkes DS, Ware LB, Palmer SM, Christie JD, Lung Transplant Outcomes Group. Clinical risk factors for primary graft dysfunction after lung transplantation. Am J Respir Crit Care Med. 2013;187(5):527–34.

23. Reyes KG, Mason DP, Thuita L, Nowicki ER, Murthy SC, Pettersson GB, Blackstone EH. Guidelines for donor lung selection: time for revision? Ann Thorac Surg. 2010;89(6):1756–64; discussion 1764–5.

24. Bonser RS, Taylor R, Collett D, Thomas HL, Dark JH, Neuberger J, Cardiothoracic Advisory Group to NHS Blood and Transplant and the Association of Lung Transplant Physicians (UK). Effect of donor smoking on survival after lung transplantation: a cohort study of a prospective registry. Lancet. 2012;380(9843):747–55.

25. Hennessy SA, Hranjec T, Emaminia A, Lapar DJ, Kozower BD, Kron IL, Jones DR, Lau CL. Geographic distance between donor and recipient does not influence outcomes after lung transplantation. Ann Thorac Surg. 2011;92(5):1847–53.

26. Bittle GJ, Sanchez PG, Kon ZN, Claire Watkins A, Rajagopal K, Pierson RN 3rd, Gammie JS, Griffith BP. The use of lung donors older than 55 years: a review of the United Network of Organ Sharing database. J Heart Lung Transplant. 2013;32(8):760–8.

27. Kang CH, Anraku M, Cypel M, Sato M, Yeung J, Gharib SA, Pierre AF, de Perrot M, Waddell TK, Liu M, Keshavjee S. Transcriptional signatures in donor lungs from donation after cardiac death vs after brain

death: a functional pathway analysis. J Heart Lung Transplant. 2011;30(3):289–98.

28. Cypel M, Levvey B, Van Raemdonck D, Erasmus M, Love R, Mason D, Glanville A, Stehlik J, Herz M, Whitson B, Puri V, Dark J, Hopkins P, Snell G, Keshavjee S. Favorable outcomes of donation after cardiac death in lung transplantation: a multicenter study. J Heart Lung Transplant. 2013;32(4 Suppl):S15.

29. Gries CJ, White DB, Truog RD, Dubois J, Cosio CC, Dhanani S, Chan KM, Corris P, Dark J, Fulda G, Glazier AK, Higgins R, Love R, Mason DP, Nakagawa TA, Shapiro R, Shemie S, Tracy MF, Travaline JM, Valapour M, West L, Zaas D, Halpern SD, American Thoracic Society Health Policy Committee. An official American Thoracic Society/International Society for Heart and Lung Transplantation/Society of Critical Care Medicine/Association of Organ and Procurement Organizations/United Network of Organ Sharing Statement: ethical and policy considerations in organ donation after circulatory determination of death. Am J Respir Crit Care Med. 2013;188(1):103–9.

30. Bernat JL, D'Alessandro AM, Port FK, Bleck TP, Heard SO, Medina J, Rosenbaum SH, Devita MA, Gaston RS, Merion RM, Barr ML, Marks WH, Nathan H, O'connor K, Rudow DL, Leichtman AB, Schwab P, Ascher NL, Metzger RA, Mc Bride V, Graham W, Wagner D, Warren J, Delmonico FL. Report of a National Conference on Donation after cardiac death. Am J Transplant. 2006;6(2):281–91.

31. Cypel M, Sato M, Yildirim E, Karolak W, Chen F, Yeung J, Boasquevisque C, Leist V, Singer LG, Yasufuku K, Deperrot M, Waddell TK, Keshavjee S, Pierre A. Initial experience with lung donation after cardiocirculatory death in Canada. J Heart Lung Transplant. 2009;28(8):753–8.

32. De Oliveira NC, Osaki S, Maloney JD, Meyer KC, Kohmoto T, D'Alessandro AM, Love RB. Lung transplantation with donation after cardiac death donors: long-term follow-up in a single center. J Thorac Cardiovasc Surg. 2010;139(5):1306–15.

33. Mason DP, Brown CR, Murthy SC, Vakil N, Lyon C, Budev MM, Pettersson GB. Growing single-center experience with lung transplantation using donation after cardiac death. Ann Thorac Surg. 2012;94(2):406–11; discussion 411–2.

34. Puri V, Scavuzzo M, Guthrie T, Hachem R, Krupnick AS, Kreisel D, Patterson GA, Meyers BF. Lung transplantation and donation after cardiac death: a single center experience. Ann Thorac Surg. 2009;88(5):1609–14; discussion 1614–5.

35. Zych B, Popov AF, Amrani M, Bahrami T, Redmond KC, Krueger H, Carby M, Simon AR. Lungs from donation after circulatory death donors: an alternative source to brain-dead donors? Midterm results at a single institution. Eur J Cardiothorac Surg. 2012;42(3):542–9.

36. Van De Wauwer C, Verschuuren EA, van der Bij W, Nossent GD, Erasmus ME. The use of non-heart-beating lung donors category III can increase the donor pool. Eur J Cardiothorac Surg. 2011;39(6):e175–80; discussion e180.

37. Levvey BJ, Harkess M, Hopkins P, Chambers D, Merry C, Glanville AR, Snell GI. Excellent clinical outcomes from a national donation-after-determination-of-cardiac-death lung transplant collaborative. Am J Transplant. 2012;12(9):2406–13.

38. Thomas HL, Thomas HL, Taylor R, Simon AR, Clark SC, Dunning J, Yonan N, Banner NR, Dark JH. Donation after circulatory death lung activity in the UK—100 transplants and counting. J Heart Lung Transplant. 2013;32(4 Suppl):S15.

39. Kootstra G, Daemen JH, Oomen AP. Categories of non-heart-beating donors. Transplant Proc. 1995;27(5):2893–4.

40. Sanchez-Fructuoso AI, Prats D, Torrente J, Pérez-Contín MJ, Fernández C, Alvarez J, Barrientos A. Renal transplantation from non-heart beating donors: a promising alternative to enlarge the donor pool. J Am Soc Nephrol. 2000;11(2):350–8.

41. Gamez P, Córdoba M, Ussetti P, Carreño MC, Alfageme F, Madrigal L, Nuñez JR, Calatayud J, Ramos M, Salas C, Varela A, Lung Transplant Group of the Puerta de Hierro Hospital. Lung transplantation from out-of-hospital non-heart-beating lung donors. one-year experience and results. J Heart Lung Transplant. 2005;24(8):1098–102.

42. Greco R, Cordovilla G, Sanz E, Benito J, Criado A, Gonzalez M, De Miguel E. Warm ischemic time tolerance after ventilated non-heart-beating lung donation in piglets. Eur J Cardiothorac Surg. 1998;14(3):319–25.

43. Carrel A, Lindbergh CA. The culture of whole organs. Science. 1935;81(2112):621–3.

44. Steen S, Ingemansson R, Budrikis A, Bolys R, Roscher R, Sjöberg T. Successful transplantation of lungs topically cooled in the non-heart-beating donor for 6 hours. Ann Thorac Surg. 1997;63(2):345–51.

45. Wierup P, Andersen C, Janciauskas D, Bolys R, Sjoberg T, Steen S. Bronchial healing, lung parenchymal histology, and blood gases one month after transplantation of lungs topically cooled for 2 hours in the non-heart-beating cadaver. J Heart Lung Transplant. 2000;19(3):270–6.

46. Steen S, Sjöberg T, Pierre L, Liao Q, Eriksson L, Algotsson L. Transplantation of lungs from a non-heart-beating donor. Lancet. 2001;357(9259):825–9.

47. LaPar DJ, Rosenberger LH, Walters DM, Hedrick TL, Swenson BR, Young JS, Dossett LA, May AK, Sawyer RG. Severe traumatic head injury affects systemic cytokine expression. J Am Coll Surg. 2012;214(4):478–86; discussion 486–8.

48. Wauters S, Somers J, De Vleeschauwer S, Verbeken E, Verleden GM, van Loon J, Van Raemdonck DE. Evaluating lung injury at increasing time intervals in a murine brain death model. J Surg Res. 2013;183(1):419–26.

49. Machuca TN, Cypel M. Ex vivo lung perfusion. J Thorac Dis. 2014;6(8):1054–62.

50. Lindstedt S, Eyjolfsson A, Koul B, Wierup P, Pierre L, Gustafsson R, Ingemansson R. How to recondition ex vivo initially rejected donor lungs for clinical transplantation: clinical experience from Lund University Hospital. J Transplant. 2011;2011:754383.

51. Warnecke G, Moradiellos J, Tudorache I, Kühn C, Avsar M, Wiegmann B, Sommer W, Ius F, Kunze C, Gottlieb J, Varela A, Haverich A. Normothermic perfusion of donor lungs for preservation and assessment with the Organ Care System Lung before bilateral transplantation: a pilot study of 12 patients. Lancet. 2012;380(9856):1851–8.

52. Becker S, Steinmeyer J, Avsar M, Höffler K, Salman J, Haverich A, Warnecke G, Ochs M, Schnapper A. Evaluating acellular versus cellular perfusate composition during prolonged ex vivo lung perfusion after initial cold ischaemia for 24 hours. Transpl Int. 2016;29(1):88–97.

53. Roman M, Gjorgjimajkoska O, Neil D, Nair S, Colah S, Parmar J, Tsui S. Comparison between cellular and acellular perfusates for ex vivo lung perfusion in a porcine model. J Heart Lung Transplant. 2015;34(7):978–87.

54. Machuca TN, Machuca TN, Mercier O, Collaud S, Linacre V, Krueger T, Azad S, Singer L, Yasufuku K, de Perrot M, Pierre A, Waddell TK, Keshavjee S, Cypel M. Outcomes of lung transplantation using donation after cardiac death donors: should we use ex vivo lung perfusion? J Heart Lung Transplant. 2014;33(4 Suppl):S272.

55. Yamada T, Nakajima D, Sakamoto J, Chen F, Okamoto T, Ohsumi O, Fujinaga T, Shoji T, Sakai H, Bando T, Date H. Reconditioning of lungs with pulmonary edema in ex vivo lung perfusion circuit. J Heart Lung Transplant. 2011;30(4S):S144.

56. Cypel M, Yeung JC, Hirayama S, Rubacha M, Fischer S, Anraku M, Sato M, Harwood S, Pierre A, Waddell TK, de Perrot M, Liu M, Keshavjee S. Technique for prolonged normothermic ex vivo lung perfusion. J Heart Lung Transplant. 2008;27(12):1319–25.

57. Kondo T, Chen F, Ohsumi A, Hijiya K, Motoyama H, Sowa T, Ohata K, Takahashi M, Yamada T, Sato M, Aoyama A, Date H. beta2-Adrenoreceptor agonist inhalation during ex vivo lung perfusion attenuates lung injury. Ann Thorac Surg. 2015;100(2):480–6.

58. McAuley DF, Curley GF, Hamid UI, Laffey JG, Abbott J, McKenna DH, Fang X, Matthay MA, Lee JW. Clinical grade allogeneic human mesenchymal stem cells restore alveolar fluid clearance in human lungs rejected for transplantation. Am J Physiol Lung Cell Mol Physiol. 2014;306(9):L809–15.

59. Gennai S, Monsel A, Hao Q, Park J, Matthay MA, Lee JW. Microvesicles derived from human mesenchymal stem cells restore alveolar fluid clearance in human lungs rejected for transplantation. Am J Transplant. 2015;15(9):2404–12.

60. Andreasson A, Karamanou DM, Perry JD, Perry A, Özalp F, Butt T, Morley KE, Walden HR, Clark SC, Prabhu M, Corris PA, Gould K, Fisher AJ, Dark JH. The effect of ex vivo lung perfusion on microbial load in human donor lungs. J Heart Lung Transplant. 2014;33(9):910–6.

61. Nakajima D, Cypel M, Bonato R, Machuca TN, Iskender I, Hashimoto K, Linacre V, Chen M, Coutinho R, Azad S, Martinu T, Waddell TK, Hwang DM, Husain S, Liu M, Keshavjee S. Ex vivo perfusion treatment of infection in human donor lungs. Am J Transplant. 2016;16(4):1229–37.

62. Meers CM, Tsagkaropoulos S, Wauters S, Verbeken E, Vanaudenaerde B, Scheers H, Verleden GM, Van Raemdonck D. A model of ex vivo perfusion of porcine donor lungs injured by gastric aspiration: a step towards pretransplant reconditioning. J Surg Res. 2011;170(1):e159–67.

63. Inci I, Hillinger S, Arni S, Kaplan T, Inci D, Weder W. Reconditioning of an injured lung graft with intrabronchial surfactant instillation in an ex vivo lung perfusion system followed by transplantation. J Surg Res. 2013;184(2):1143–9.

64. Khalife-Hocquemiller T, Sage E, Dorfmuller P, Mussot S, Le Houérou D, Eddahibi S, Fadel E. Exogenous surfactant attenuates lung injury from gastric-acid aspiration during ex vivo reconditioning in pigs. Transplantation. 2014;97(4):413–8.

65. Gazoni LM, Laubach VE, Mulloy DP, Bellizzi A, Unger EB, Linden J, Ellman PI, Lisle TC, Kron IL. Additive protection against lung ischemia-reperfusion injury by adenosine A2A receptor activation before procurement and during reperfusion. J Thorac Cardiovasc Surg. 2008;135(1):156–65.

66. Stone ML, Sharma AK, Mas VR, Gehrau RC, Mulloy DP, Zhao Y, Lau CL, Kron IL, Huerter ME, Laubach VE. Ex vivo perfusion with adenosine A2A receptor agonist enhances rehabilitation of murine donor lungs after circulatory death. Transplantation. 2015;99(12):2494–503.

67. Wagner CE, Pope NH, Charles EJ, Huerter ME, Sharma AK, Salmon MD, Carter BT, Stoler MH, Lau CL, Laubach VE, Kron IL. Ex vivo lung perfusion with adenosine A2A receptor agonist allows prolonged cold preservation of lungs donated after cardiac death. J Thorac Cardiovasc Surg. 2016;151(2):538–45.

68. Martens A, Boada M, Vanaudenaerde BM, Verleden SE, Vos R, Verleden GM, Verbeken EK, Van Raemdonck D, Schols D, Claes S, Neyrinck AP. Steroids can reduce warm ischemic reperfusion injury in a porcine DCD model with EVLP evaluation. Transpl Int. 2016;29(11):1237–46.

69. Motoyama H, Chen F, Hijiya K, Kondo T, Ohsumi A, Yamada T, Sato M, Aoyama A, Bando T, Date H. Plasmin administration during ex vivo lung perfusion ameliorates lung ischemia-reperfusion injury. J Heart Lung Transplant. 2014;33(10):1093–9.

70. Fischer S, Liu M, MacLean AA, de Perrot M, Ho M, Cardella JA, Zhang XM, Bai XH, Suga M, Imai Y, Keshavjee S. In vivo transtracheal adenovirus-mediated transfer of human interleukin-10 gene to donor lungs ameliorates ischemia-reperfusion injury and improves early posttransplant graft function in the rat. Hum Gene Ther. 2001;12(12):1513–26.

71. Martins S, de Perrot M, Imai Y, Yamane M, Quadri SM, Segall L, Dutly A, Sakiyama S, Chaparro A, Davidson BL, Waddell TK, Liu M, Keshavjee S. Transbronchial administration of adenoviral-mediated interleukin-10 gene to the donor improves function in a pig lung transplant model. Gene Ther. 2004;11(24):1786–96.

72. Yeung JC, Wagnetz D, Cypel M, Rubacha M, Koike T, Chun YM, Hu J, Waddell TK, Hwang DM, Liu M, Keshavjee S. Ex vivo adenoviral vector gene delivery results in decreased vector-associated inflammation pre- and post-lung transplantation in the pig. Mol Ther. 2012;20(6):1204–11.

73. Machuca TN, Hsin MK, Ott HC, Chen M, Hwang DM, Cypel M, Waddell TK, Keshavjee S. Injury-specific ex vivo treatment of the donor lung: pulmonary thrombolysis followed by successful lung transplantation. Am J Respir Crit Care Med. 2013;188(7):878–80.

74. Inci I, Yamada Y, Hillinger S, Jungraithmayr W, Trinkwitz M, Weder W. Successful lung transplantation after donor lung reconditioning with urokinase in ex vivo lung perfusion system. Ann Thorac Surg. 2014;98(5):1837–8.

75. Luc JG, Bozso SJ, Freed DH, Nagendran J. Successful repair of donation after circulatory death lungs with large pulmonary embolus using the lung organ care system for ex vivo thrombolysis and subsequent clinical transplantation. Transplantation. 2015;99(1):e1–2.

76. Gilpin SE, Ott HC. Using nature's platform to engineer bio-artificial lungs. Ann Am Thorac Soc. 2015;12(Suppl 1):S45–9.

77. Schmack B, Weymann A, Mohite P, Garcia Saez D, Zych B, Sabashnikov A, Zeriouh M, Schamroth J, Koch A, Soresi S, Ananiadou O, De Robertis F, Karck M, Simon AR, Popov AF. Contemporary review of the organ care system in lung transplantation: potential advantages of a portable ex-vivo lung perfusion system. Expert Rev Med Devices. 2016;13(11):1035–41.

78. Cannon RM, Brock GN, Garrison RN, Smith JW, Marvin MR, Franklin GA. To pump or not to pump: a comparison of machine perfusion vs cold storage for deceased donor kidney transplantation. J Am Coll Surg. 2013;216(4):625–33; discussion 633–4.

79. Treckmann J, Moers C, Smits JM, Gallinat A, Maathuis MH, van Kasterop-Kutz M, Jochmans I, Homan van der Heide JJ, Squifflet JP, van Heurn E, Kirste GR, Rahmel A, Leuvenink HG, Pirenne J, Ploeg RJ, Paul A. Machine perfusion versus cold storage for preservation of kidneys from expanded criteria donors after brain death. Transpl Int. 2011;24(6):548–54.

80. Hsin MK, Iskender I, Nakajima D, Chen M, Kim H, dos Santos PR, Sakamoto J, Lee J, Hashimoto K, Harmantas C, Hwang D, Waddell T, Liu M, Keshavjee S, Cypel M. Extension of donor lung preservation with hypothermic storage after normothermic ex vivo lung perfusion. J Heart Lung Transplant. 2016;35(1):130–6.

Gaps and Future Directions in Lung Transplantation

21

Keith C. Meyer and Ganesh Raghu

Introduction

Significant progress has been made in clinical management of lung transplant recipients, and the scientific knowledge of lung transplantation has evolved considerably since the first transplant was performed in the United States in 1963. The first transplant recipient only survived for 19 days, but now recipients with end-stage lung disease that is progressive and refractory to non-transplant therapies can expect to survive on average for 5 years posttransplant, and the total number of patients transplanted per year now exceeds 4000 worldwide.

As lung transplantation gradually matured over the past four decades as an accepted therapy for end-stage lung disease [1, 2], many improve-

ments have been adopted that have improved posttransplant survival. These range from prudent selection of candidates to optimization of donor organ retrieval and preservation, development and refining of surgical techniques used at the time of implantation, state-of-the-art perioperative intensive care management, judicious use of effective immunosuppressive therapies, prophylactic strategies to prevent infections, and long-term posttransplant care with appropriate monitoring for diverse complications that can threaten survival of transplant recipients.

Nonetheless, projected survival of lung transplant recipients remains significantly inferior to that of recipients of most other solid organs (kidney, liver, heart). This survival gap is likely explained, in part, by the constant exposure of the lung to the ambient environment. Inhalation of pollutants or aspiration/microaspiration can predispose recipients to develop lower respiratory tract inflammation and infection, and such has been linked to development of chronic lung allograft dysfunction (CLAD), which is the main cause of allograft loss for recipients who survive beyond 1 year posttransplant. Despite these advances, a significant shortfall in the number of donor lungs available for transplant continues to persist such that risk of dying while waitlisted, especially for patients with idiopathic pulmonary fibrosis (IPF), remains unacceptably high.

K. C. Meyer (✉)
Department of Medicine, University of Wisconsin School of Medicine and Public Health,
Madison, WI, USA
e-mail: kcm@medicine.wisc.edu

G. Raghu
Division of Pulmonary, Critical Care, and Sleep Medicine, Department of Medicine University of Washington,
Seattle, WA, USA

Center for Interstitial Lung Disease, ILD, Sarcoid and Pulmonary Fibrosis Program, University of Washington Medicine, Seattle, WA, USA

Scleroderma Clinic, University of Washington Medicine, Seattle, WA, USA
e-mail: graghu@uw.edu

© The Author(s) 2018
G. Raghu, R. G. Carbone (eds.), *Lung Transplantation*, https://doi.org/10.1007/978-3-319-91184-7_21

Pretransplant Considerations and Management

While adoption and implementation of the lung allocation score (LAS) in 2005 to provide a need-based ranking system for donor lung allocation in the United States [3] have reduced the risk of death without transplant for waitlisted patients and improved the effectiveness of organ allocation and transplantation, outcomes have been reported to remain somewhat worse for recipients with very high LAS scores [4–7]. Nonetheless, a recent report indicates that recipients with higher LAS values and certain transplant indications such as idiopathic pulmonary fibrosis (IPF) or cystic fibrosis (CF) appear to receive the greatest survival benefit from lung transplantation [8], and recipients with the transplant indication of pulmonary fibrosis and very high LAS values can achieve prolonged posttransplant survival that does not differ significantly from those with lower LAS values [9]. Because patients with high or very high LAS values are at high risk of dying because a donor lung that fits their thoracic dimensions does not become available, oversized donor lungs that would otherwise match to such recipients should be considered for surgical trimming to allow such candidates the opportunity to receive a lifesaving lung transplant.

Improvements in modeling that can better predict posttransplant outcomes are needed [10, 11]. Additionally, other characteristics of potential candidates such as frailty [12] may need to be incorporated as a component of the LAS to better identify candidates at high risk of poor outcome. The presence of significant frailty may even merit consideration as a relative or absolute contraindication to that could be incorporated into a future revision of the current guideline [13] for candidate selection.

Many additional pretransplant concerns (Box 21.1) also need to be addressed and resolved as evidence accumulates in the literature in the coming years. While age is a significant factor, the presence or absence of comorbidities and relative contraindications to transplant can inform listing decisions in the context of advanced age. Other important issues include extremes of body mass index (BMI) and whether candidates can maintain adequate physical activity and participate in

Box 21.1 Key Pretransplant and Transplant Surgical Issues

Pretransplant:
- Should frailty be a criterion for determining eligibility for listing?
- Should frailty be used as a component in computing the lung allocation score (LAS)?
- Should there be an absolute upper age cutoff for transplant eligibility?
- Should there be absolute cutoffs for body mass index (BMI)?
- What should be done to screen/treat gastroesophageal reflux?
- When should listed candidates who become progressively and severely debilitated be removed from the waitlist?
- What should be done to optimize outcomes for presensitized recipients?
- Should living-related lung transplants be performed?
- Should simultaneous multi-organ transplants (heart-lung, lung-liver, lung-kidney) be performed?
- Should unilateral lobar transplants be given to elderly individuals with high operative risk?
- When should waitlisted candidates be placed on extracorporeal membrane oxygenation (ECMO) as a bridge to transplant?

Transplant Procedure:
- What operation is best for specific indications?
  - Single vs. bilateral lung
  - Lobar transplants
  - Clamshell vs. bilateral intercostal incisions for bilateral lung transplantation
- Should ex vivo lung perfusion (EVLP) be available to and/or utilized by all transplant centers?
- How should EVLP be best used to condition/salvage marginal donor lungs?
- What is the best approach to human leukocyte antigen (HLA) matching?

Box 21.1 (continued)
- Is intraoperative ECMO support superior to cardiopulmonary bypass?
- Should bronchial arterial circulation be restored when feasible?

pulmonary rehabilitation. Prompt detection and treatment of disease complications (e.g., deep vein thrombosis with/without pulmonary embolism in patients with IPF) are also required, and waitlisted candidates should be seen in the clinic frequently (e.g., every 4–6 weeks) to ensure compliance with therapies, adjust levels of supplemental oxygen as needed, and provide psychological support.

Transplantation is increasingly provided to patients receiving life support in the intensive care unit (ICU), and the use of extracorporeal membrane oxygenation (ECMO) as a bridge to transplant that can support patients with severe respiratory failure has gradually increased [14, 15]. Although outcomes for patients on either mechanical ventilation or ECMO are generally worse than outcomes for recipients who do not require such pretransplant support [14–17], ECMO may provide the only means of keeping a patient alive and can also be used to support recipients through the transplant procedure [7, 14, 15, 18–22]. Additionally, newer approaches and devices for ECMO can allow patients to be ambulatory while patients await organ offers and transplantation [23–27]. An external artificial lung (Novalung system, XENIOS AG, Heilbronn, Germany) is available for use [28–31]; this paracorporeal system, although typically not flow-assisted, can be connected to an external pump for circulatory assistance if required.

Transplant Procedure and Perioperative Management

While the vast majority of donated lungs are retrieved from brain-dead donors, the use of donation after cardiac death (DCD) donors (non-heart-beating donors who have undergone planned and controlled withdrawal of life support) has provided an additional pool of donated organs as an alternative to the traditional brain-dead donor. Not only does the use of DCD donors increase the number of lungs available for transplantation, but reports in the literature indicate that recipient outcomes are similar to those for lungs transplanted from brain-dead donors [32, 33].

Ex vivo lung perfusion (EVLP) has emerged as a technique that allows explanted donor lungs to be evaluated and reconditioned prior to recipient implantation [34, 35]. While subjected to EVLP, not only can the function of marginal/injured lungs be improved, but significant, persistent dysfunction can be identified such that implantation of lungs that appear to have an unacceptable level of dysfunction can be aborted if acceptable functional parameters cannot be met [34–40]. In addition to using EVLP to draw fluid from extravascular compartments in an edematous lung such that gas exchange can be improved and marginal lungs rendered usable [34–40], anti-inflammatory cytokines or mesenchymal stem cells could be used to facilitate injury repair, promote recovery of intercellular alveolar epithelial tight junctions, improve oxygenation, and decrease vascular resistance [41–45]. Additionally, antibiotics can be infused to suppress or eliminate donor lung infection [46], gastric acid-injured donor lungs can be potentially salvaged [47], and perfusate can be analyzed to detect biomarkers that predict high risk for early allograft dysfunction [48, 49]. With widespread implementation of EVLP, not only can ex vivo preservation times be prolonged to allow optimal organ assessment and improve donor-recipient human leukocyte antigen (HLA) matching, but the usable donor pool could be significantly expanded as donor lungs are provided to both large- and smaller-volume institutions from EVLP hubs [50–54].

While bilateral lung transplant (BLT) is considered to be the only option for septic lung disease (CF and non-CF bronchiectasis), single lung transplant (SLT) can be performed for other disease indications. International Society for Heart and Lung Transplantation (ISHLT) and United Network for Organ Sharing (UNOS) data generally support better long-term outcomes for BLTs [55–57], but conflicting data have been reported from single centers with some studies supporting better long-term survival for BLT versus SLT recipients with idiopathic pulmonary fibrosis (IPF) [58–60], while others have not detected a significant survival difference for the indication of IPF [61]. Additionally, when data are adjusted for confounders such as age [60] or pretransplant performance status [59], a significant advantage for BLT versus SLT does not persist. Although current practice is generally weighted toward a preference for BLT for younger candidates and native lung complications are avoided with BLT, SLT allows for a greater number of lungs to be offered to recipients, may diminish likelihood of dying on the waitlist if candidates are listed for BLT only [62], and may be a more appropriate operation for higher-risk and/or older age candidates. Although World Health Organization (WHO) class III pulmonary hypertension has been perceived as a contraindication to SLT, recent data do not support exclusively using BLT for such patients [63]. An evidence-based guideline or consensus statement has yet to be generated concerning which operation should be performed for patients with specific transplant indications and associated confounding factors, but appropriate use of SLT versus BLT could maximize the number of lung transplantation candidates who receive a lung transplant yet avoid a negative impact on long-term survival.

An additional and often insurmountable problem that is encountered when waitlisted patients are in dire need of transplant with very high LAS values is the issue of donor lung size and compatibility with recipient chest dimensions. Oversized donor lungs could be used in this situation and trimmed surgically to adapt a donor lung to a recipient's thoracic cavity dimensions when sizing is the only issue that would prevent such a recipient from receiving an urgently needed transplant.

Although infections remain a constant threat to lung transplant recipients, prophylactic regimens can protect recipients from specific bacterial, fungal, and viral infections. The advent of cytomegalovirus (CMV) prophylaxis has greatly reduced the impact of CMV disease on recipient survival [64, 65], and a recent, well-conducted, randomized controlled trial of prophylaxis with valganciclovir for at-risk patients (donor or recipient CMV seropositive) showed a marked reduction in CMV disease incidence for a 12-month course of valganciclovir versus a 3-month course [66]. Additional investigations further refine this and other approaches to infection prophylaxis, especially for patients who undergo transplantation for septic lung disease.

Luminex® (Austin, TX, USA) solid phase assays for HLA antibody detection have replaced complement-dependent serological techniques [67, 68], and the adoption of these assays has improved pretransplant detection and identification of antibodies (pre-sensitization) against donor HLA and allows virtual crossmatching during the allocation and match process (to avoid transplants in patients who are presensitized to donor HLA antigens) as well as the implementation of strategies to desensitize recipients perioperatively [69]. Survival of sensitized recipients has been reported to be significantly enhanced by perioperative use of plasma exchange, intravenous immune globulin, antithymocyte globulin (ATG), and mycophenolic acid [69]. By accurately predicting a donor crossmatch result, bead-based virtual crossmatching has improved access by sensitized thoracic transplant recipients to organs outside the immediate region [70, 71]. Although technical and interpretive challenges remain, solid phase antibody assays have significantly changed transplant practice and outcomes [72, 73] as various technical issues are gradually being resolved and optimal cutoff values determined. As EVLP evolves and allows more prolonged periods during which donor lungs can be maintained ex vivo, more effective donor-recipient HLA matching may become routine practice. Of note, using panel-reactive antibody (PRA) assays is problematic, and the degree of sensitization detected by PRA methods is variable and inconsistent. The newer methods described above are much more reliable.

Posttransplant Management

While posttransplant management is multifaceted and complicated, few randomized, prospective controlled trials are available to provide robust evidence for optimal recipient care. Perioperative care in the ICU requires both ventilator and circulatory support, identifying and addressing early surgical and/or medical complications, preventing and treating infectious complications, and initiating effective immunosuppressive therapies. Nearly one third of recipients will develop grade 3 primary graft dysfunction [74], and while a number of markers have been identified that correlate with increased risk of high-grade PGD [75], interventions other than supportive care have been relatively ineffective in preventing or treating PGD.

Transplant recipients are at risk for a multitude of subacute and chronic complications following successful transplantation. These include antibody-mediated and acute cellular rejection, infection, and the development of CLAD. Because up to 90% of recipients have preformed anti-HLA antibodies of which approximately one third are donor-specific antibodies (DSAs) [76], effective and carefully monitored immune suppression is essential to establish allograft immune tolerance. Other potential causes of lung allograft dysfunction include anastomotic complications or the presence of a significant degree of gastroesophageal reflux (GER), and a guideline or consensus statement is needed to guide an optimal approach to the detection and treatment of GER disease that exists pretransplant or develops de novo posttransplant [77].

The greatest threat to long-term survival for recipients who survive beyond 1 year posttransplant is CLAD [78, 79]. While delayed loss of allograft function as reflected by a persistent and/or progressive decline in the surrogate marker of forced expiratory volume in 1 s (FEV1) had been classically termed bronchiolitis obliterans syndrome (BOS) and considered indicative of the development of widespread bronchiolitis obliterans lesions that occur as a consequence of chronic rejection, recent analyses of the literature and a revision of terminology have established the entity of CLAD and its two major phenotypes of obstruc-

tive CLAD (oCLAD or obstructive BOS) and restrictive CLAD (rCLAD) or restrictive allograft syndrome (RAS) [79] as appropriate replacements for the formerly used, overarching term of BOS.

The American Thoracic Society (ATS)/European Respiratory Society (ERS)/ISHLT clinical practice guideline systematically examined available evidence for the prevention and treatment of BOS/CLAD and provided recommendations for the diagnosis and management of BOS/CLAD. Identified risk factors included PGD, various forms of alloimmune rejection (acute cellular rejection, antibody-mediated rejection, lymphocytic bronchiolitis), infections (viral, bacterial, fungal), pathologic GER, autoimmunity, and persistent bronchoalveolar lavage (BAL) neutrophilia. Although evidence from randomized controlled trials (RCTs) for preventing and treating BOS/CLAD was found to be of low or very low quality, a number of conditional recommendations were made by consensus among task force members following a comprehensive review of available publications (Box 21.2).

Box 21.2 ISHLT/ATS/ERS Clinical Practice Guidelines: Recommendations for Prevention and Treatment of BOS/CLAD[a]

1. Administer enhanced immunosuppression if acute cellular rejection ≥ grade 2 or lymphocytic bronchiolitis is found on lung biopsy.
2. Consider enhanced immunosuppression if minimal acute cellular rejection (grade 1) is found on biopsy.
3. Do not use long-term, high-dose corticosteroids to treat BOS.
4. If BOS develops while patients are on cyclosporine A as their calcineurin inhibitor, consider changing to tacrolimus.
5. Consider a trial of azithromycin for treatment of BOS.
6. If significant gastroesophageal reflux is identified in a patient who develops BOS, consider referral to an experienced surgeon for potential fundoplication to prevent reflux.
7. Consider referring recipients with end-stage BOS that is refractory to treatment for retransplantation.

[a]All are conditional recommendations with very low quality of evidence

Restrictive CLAD (RAS) can be differentiated from obstructive CLAD (BOS) on the basis of pathophysiological mechanisms, and rCLAD has a worse prognosis [80]. Both CLAD phenotypes tend to respond poorly to augmented immunosuppression or other interventions, but recent randomized clinical trials have suggested that CLAD can be prevented and/or attenuated by administering azithromycin [81, 82]. Additionally, anti-reflux surgery may provide benefit [83–89], and other approaches such as photopheresis or the administration of intravenous immune globulin (IVIG) and/or anti-CD20 antibodies may benefit recipients with either refractory acute cellular rejection or BOS if evidence of a humoral response to donor antigen (donor-specific antibody) is detected [90–92]. Another recent advance is the recognition that autoimmunity (responses directed against self-antigens including collagen V, αK1-tubulin, vimentin, and others) may play a significant role in both acute and chronic lung allograft rejection [93–98], and tolerization with oral administration of collagen V has been shown to blunt lung allograft rejection in a major histocompatibility (MHC)-mismatched animal model [99–103]. Ongoing research is greatly needed to answer many other questions concerning the pathogenesis, diagnosis, prevention, and treatment of CLAD (Box 21.3).

Monitoring recipients for evidence of lung function decline as well as monitoring for the appearance of numerous complications and comorbidities is essential to optimize posttransplant allograft function and recipient quality of life and survival. Many centers subject recipients to surveillance bronchoscopy with BAL and transbronchial biopsies (TBBs) at protocol-determined intervals to detect occult infection and/or evidence of rejection, but there is no current consensus on the use of surveillance bronchoscopy or the posttransplant timing of such. Whether recipients who are stable, are asymptomatic, and have no physiologic or imaging evidence of allograft dysfunction need periodic surveillance bronchoscopies remains unclear. Additionally, a standardized approach to the total number of TBBs that should be obtained and the optimal sites for performing TBBs for

---

Box 21.3 Chronic Lung Allograft Dysfunction (CLAD): Questions in Need of Answers

1. What are the roles and mechanisms of alloimmune and autoimmune responses in CLAD pathogenesis?
2. What is the precise role of antibody-mediated rejection in CLAD onset and progression?
3. What is the significance of the appearance of de novo anti-HLA antibodies in CLAD pathogenesis, and when and how should screening and treatment for anti-HLA/donor-specific antibodies be performed?
4. Can specific biomarkers identify and reliably predict increased risk for the development of CLAD?
5. Can biomarkers be used to detect the early (subclinical) onset of CLAD?
6. Can biomarkers be used to differentiate between the CLAD phenotypes of obstructive bronchiolitis obliterans syndrome (BOS) and restrictive allograft syndrome (RAS)?
7. Can specific CLAD phenotypes be identified that are useful for predicting prognosis and response to therapy?
8. What specific agent or combinations of posttransplant immunosuppressive agents are most likely to prevent CLAD and improve optimize allograft and patient survival?
9. Can currently available strategies facilitate prevention of CLAD?
   • Preventing PGD (e.g., role for ex vivo lung perfusion [EVLP])
   • Administration of prophylactic anti-infective agents
   • Prophylactic neo-macrolide therapy
   • Improved HLA matching at time of transplant
   • Early detection of high-risk recipients via screening for the appearance of de novo donor-specific antibodies
   • Tolerizing recipients to prevent responses to self-antigens (e.g., collagen V)

Box 21.3 (continued)

- Pretransplant fundoplication if significant GER is present
- Bronchial artery revascularization at transplant if feasible
10. Does any specific therapy significantly alter the natural history of CLAD if given when CLAD is first detected?
    - Neo-macrolides
    - Treatment of antibody-mediated rejection if detected (intravenous immunoglobulin [IVIG], plasma exchange, rituximab, etc.)
    - Extracorporeal photopheresis
    - Anti-fibrotics (e.g., pirfenidone, nintedanib, pentraxin)
    - Stem cells
11. When lung retransplantation is performed for end-stage BOS or RAS, is the retransplanted lung at increased risk for the development of significant primary graft dysfunction, acute rejection, and/or CLAD?
12. Can induction of tolerance to self-antigens (e.g., collagen V, vimentin) or strategies to augment regulatory T or B cells to promote and maintain tolerance diminish risk for CLAD?
13. Can patients who are more tolerant to their allografts (and who may therefore require less intense immunosuppression) be identified?
14. Will the use of ex vivo lung perfusion (EVLP) techniques to condition the lung allograft diminish the risk of developing CLAD?
15. What is the best approach for monitoring recipients posttransplant to detect significant occult allograft dysfunction (pulmonary function testing, imaging, bronchoscopy)?
16. What is the optimal frequency for obtaining spirometry to assist in the early detection of evolving CLAD?
17. What is the role of the lung microbiome in risk of developing CLAD, progression of CLAD, and lung allograft tolerance?

either surveillance or clinically indicated bronchoscopies does not currently exist. On the other hand, empiric treatment when evidence of evolving functional impairment is observed without tissue sampling is also problematic. Finally, there is considerable interobserver variation in the interpretation of TBB specimen histopathology even among expert pathologists. These issues need to be addressed by performing randomized clinical trials and/or the creation of consensus guidelines or statements by task forces populated by lung transplant expert panelists.

Similarly, consensus statement guidance for type and timing of lung function testing, radiologic imaging, and screening for the development of DSAs have yet to be developed but would be potentially helpful in optimizing recipient care and posttransplant outcomes. Additionally, both basic and clinical research are needed to better understand causes of lung allograft dysfunction and to identify best practices and new therapies to improve lung transplant outcomes and recipient quality of life (Box 21.4).

The Future of Lung Transplantation

Evaluation and Management of the Donor Lung

EVLP will undoubtedly revolutionize lung transplantation. EVLP could allow ex vivo maintenance of perfused and ventilated lungs that meet parameters for implantation such that enough time is available to allow better HLA matching to be performed. Moreover, resuscitation and renewal of damaged lungs or lungs with marginal function could be achieved, if required, and this could significantly expand the pool of donor lungs available for implantation. Centers that have EVLP capability will likely be established as "hubs" to which donated lungs can be taken for both observation and, if needed, repair. Reconditioning/repair would include perfusion strategies to reverse capillary leak and clear third-space edema fluid, antibiotics to clear infection, and infusion of anti-inflammatory

Box 21.4 Research Needs

1. Multicenter clinical investigations of transplant candidates and recipients to:
   - Identify risk factors and effective therapies for primary graft dysfunction (PGD).
   - Identify key risk factors for development of CLAD.
   - Evaluate therapeutic interventions to prevent and/or treat CLAD.
2. Improved animal and other laboratory models of both obstructive and restrictive phenotypes of CLAD to better understand pathogenesis and identify key mediators of airway inflammation and fibrosis
3. Additional studies of mechanisms and phenotypes of CLAD (via clinical studies/trials enrolling lung allograft recipients)
4. Guidelines for optimal testing for abnormal GER and the selection of patients (and procedure type) for antireflux surgery to prevent or treat CLAD
5. Determination of optimal approaches to allograft surveillance (e.g., the role of bronchoscopy with transbronchial biopsies in clinically stable LTX recipients, screening for de novo anti-HLA antibodies, and development of reliable tools to detect the presence of humoral rejection)

cytokines, and perfusate could be monitored for biomarkers that predict good versus marginal organ function, thereby allowing the identification of lungs that do not achieve acceptable functional parameters and avoiding implantation into waitlisted candidates to whom the lungs would be matched. EVLP hubs could then dispatch properly functioning donor lungs to satellite centers (e.g., in North America, Europe, and Australia) to be implanted into appropriately matched recipients.

Inducing Allograft Tolerance

Th17 lymphocytes that secrete interleukin-17 (IL-17), which have been linked to the pathogenesis of autoimmune disorders, have been implicated as playing key roles in acute and chronic allograft rejection [93, 94, 104–113]. Ongoing research has identified an expanded number of immune cell subsets that secrete IL-17 [113, 114], and regulatory lymphocyte subsets such as CD4+FoxP3+ T cells and B1 B cells can antagonize and suppress both allo- and autoimmune rejection responses [115–121]. As better understanding of regulatory cell mechanisms involved in immune tolerance evolves, novel approaches that harness the ability of regulatory immune cells to suppress host rejection of implanted donor tissue and inflammation may become a key aspect of posttransplant care.

Understanding the Transplanted Lung Microbiome

Investigation of the lung microbiome in health and disease is an emerging field, and the lung microbiome varies considerably among disease states [122, 123]. Additionally, bacteria, fungi, and viruses that comprise specific lung microbiomes are constantly interacting, and such interactions may be important in the development of respiratory disease states and interactions with host defense mechanisms and immune responses and regulation. Sharma and colleagues [124] have reported that microbiome signatures in the mouth, nose, proximal, and distal airways show variation with the nasal microbiome closely resembling that of the proximal and distal airways in lung transplant recipients. Additionally, myeloid-derived suppressor cell (MDSC) phenotypes predominated in proximal airways, while a preponderance of pro-inflammatory MDSCs was found in distal airways. Mouraux and colleagues [125] found correlations of pro-inflammatory bacteria (e.g., *Pseudomonas*, *Staphylococcus*, *Corynebacteria*) with expression of catabolic lung remodeling gene expression in contrast to detecting anabolic remodeling gene expression when bacteria associated with a healthy microbiome steady state (e.g., *Streptococci, Prevotella, Veillonella*) were present in BAL specimens. Indeed, a better understanding of host-microbiome interactions and the effect of such phenomena on alloimmune responses and allograft tolerance may provide important insights into injury responses and matrix remodeling in the transplanted lung.

Using Stem Cells to Prevent and Treat Lung Injury, Inflammation, and Rejection

Donor-derived mesenchymal stem cells (MSC) have been identified as potentially playing a significant role in bronchiolar fibrosis in BOS/CLAD [126–128]. However, MSC may also be capable of inhibiting function of various immune cells (T cells, B cells, NK cells, dendritic cells) and cytokine secretion [129–131]. Stem cells have been shown to reduce injury and inflammation in a number of animal models [132–143], and stem cell therapies may blunt acute ischemia-reperfusion injury and fibrotic responses to lung injury, thereby preventing or ameliorating PGD. Additionally, MSCs may be capable of promoting alveolar fluid clearance in lungs that would otherwise be rejected for transplantation due to edema and impaired gas exchange [144]. Finally, early experience using allogeneic bone marrow-derived MSCs in human lung transplant recipients with deteriorating CLAD showed slowing of the decline in FEV1 and supports the feasibility of using such therapies in patients with advanced CLAD [145].

Xenotransplantation

Lung transplantation across species may provide an alternative to allogeneic lung transplantation and could serve as a bridge to allotransplantation by allowing time for a human donor-recipient match to be made and the xenograft replaced when a human donor lung becomes available [146, 147]. However, exuberant inflammatory, immune, and coagulation responses are still to be overcome [148–150]. Nonetheless, extensive genetic engineering of pigs as a lung donor source is ongoing, and such genomic restructuring is required to prevent the acute thrombotic and severe inflammatory reactions that have occurred in various xenotransplant models including pig to primate xenotransplantation [146, 151, 152]. A combination of knocking out xenoantigens to avoid events such as triggering coagulation and inflammatory cascades and complement activation combined with pharmacologic manipulation may eventually allow transplantation of pig lungs to humans as an alternative to human-to-human lung transplantation [153].

Bioengineering Lungs

Methods have been developed to de-cellularize whole lungs to produce an intact extracellular matrix (ECM) that can be isolated, and such scaffolds can then be re-cellularized [154–157]. Although bioartificial lung grafts derived via such methods have been successfully placed orthotopically in animal models following successful re-cellularization with stem or progenitor cells and can provide gas exchange, the delayed onset of inflammation and consolidation has eventually led to loss of function [158, 159]. Nonetheless, research is ongoing to determine whether bioengineered lungs that have been adequately re-cellularized with appropriate stem cells that differentiate and replace/repopulate the more than 40 different cell types in their normal anatomic compartments can sustain function. Optimally, stem cells used to repopulate such three-dimensional scaffolds would be obtained from the prospective recipient to minimize or avoid the need for intense immunosuppression and also eliminate the risk of opportunistic infections. Although significant hurdles must yet be overcome to create a lung from a matrix scaffold repopulated with recipient-derived cells [160], biofabricated lungs may become a potential remedy to the need for lung replacement and can allow recipients with end-stage lung disease to avoid the myriad consequences of immunosuppression and infection that are inherent in current approaches to allotransplantation.

Key Points

- Recent pretransplant advances have allowed broadening of candidate eligibility and improved medical management of transplant candidates.
- EVLP has emerged as a novel tool that can expand the pool of donor lungs available for transplantation and provide the opportunity to rescue lungs with parameters indicative of impaired function that would preclude their use in the absence of EVLP availability.
- EVLP can allow prolonged ex vivo time intervals that facilitate better donor-recipient HLA matching while also monitoring biomarkers in lung perfusate that predict high risk for post-implantation dysfunction.
- CLAD represents the greatest threat to long-term allograft and patient survival following initially successful lung transplantation.
- A better understanding of CLAD etiologies and phenotypes will facilitate preemptive strategies and targeted therapies for specific forms of CLAD.
- Clinical trials that collect biosamples (e.g., plasma, serum, BAL specimens) are needed to evaluate genomic, proteomic, and metabolomic biomarkers that can be used to predict risk for CLAD or other posttransplant complications and thereby allow early detection and therapeutic interventions.
- Ongoing research and clinical trials are needed to identify novel methods to induce allograft tolerance, prevent opportunistic infection, manipulate the lung microbiome, and employ stem cell technologies.
- Although many hurdles remain, xenotransplantation and use of bioengineered lungs may become options for lung transplantation in the near future.

References

1. Kotloff RM, Thabut G. Lung transplantation. Am J Respir Crit Care Med. 2011;184(2):159–71.
2. Spahr J, Meyer K. Lung transplantation. In: Hricik D, editor. Primer on transplantation. American Society of Transplantation. 3rd ed. Oxford: Wiley-Blackwell; 2011. p. 205–37.
3. Eberlein M, Garrity ER, Orens JB. Lung allocation in the United States. Clin Chest Med. 2011;32(2):213–22.
4. Russo MJ, Iribarne A, Hong KN, et al. High lung allocation score is associated with increased morbidity and mortality following transplantation. Chest. 2010;137(3):651–7.
5. Merlo CA, Weiss ES, Orens JB, et al. Impact of U.S. Lung Allocation Score on survival after lung transplantation. J Heart Lung Transplant. 2009;28(8):769–75.
6. Weiss ES, Allen JG, Merlo CA, Conte JV, Shah AS. Lung allocation score predicts survival in lung transplantation patients with pulmonary fibrosis. Ann Thorac Surg. 2009;88(6):1757–64.
7. George TJ, Beaty CA, Kilic A, Shah PD, Merlo CA, Shah AS. Outcomes and temporal trends among high-risk patients after lung transplantation in the United States. J Heart Lung Transplant. 2012;31(11):1182–91.
8. Vock DM, Durheim MT, Tsuang WM, et al. Survival benefit of lung transplantation in the modern era of lung allocation. Ann Am Thorac Soc. 2017;14(2):172–81.
9. De Oliveira NC, Julliard W, Osaki S, et al. Lung transplantation for high-risk patients with idiopathic pulmonary fibrosis. Sarcoidosis Vasc Diffuse Lung Dis. 2016;33(3):235–41.
10. Russo MJ, Davies RR, Hong KN, et al. Who is the high-risk recipient? Predicting mortality after lung transplantation using pretransplant risk factors. J Thorac Cardiovasc Surg. 2009;138(5):1234–1238.e1.
11. Gries CJ, Rue TC, Heagerty PJ, Edelman JD, Mulligan MS, Goss CH. Development of a predictive model for long-term survival after lung transplantation and implications for the lung allocation score. J Heart Lung Transplant. 2010;29(7):731–8.
12. Hook JL, Lederer DJ. Selecting lung transplant candidates: where do current guidelines fall short? Expert Rev Respir Med. 2012;6(1):51–61.
13. Weill D, Benden C, Corris PA, et al. A consensus document for the selection of lung transplant candidates: 2014—an update from the Pulmonary Transplantation Council of the International Society for Heart and Lung Transplantation. J Heart Lung Transplant. 2015;34(1):1–15.
14. Lang G, Taghavi S, Aigner C, et al. Primary lung transplantation after bridge with extracorporeal membrane oxygenation: a plea for a shift in our paradigms for indications. Transplantation. 2012;93(7):729–36.

15. Javidfar J, Bacchetta M. Bridge to lung transplantation with extracorporeal membrane oxygenation support. Curr Opin Organ Transplant. 2012;17(5):496–502.

16. Mason DP, Thuita L, Nowicki ER, Murthy SC, Pettersson GB, Blackstone EH. Should lung transplantation be performed for patients on mechanical respiratory support? The US experience. J Thorac Cardiovasc Surg. 2010;139(3):765–73.

17. Gottlieb J, Warnecke G, Hadem J, et al. Outcome of critically ill lung transplant candidates on invasive respiratory support. Intensive Care Med. 2012;38(6):968–75.

18. Bittner HB, Lehmann S, Rastan A, et al. Outcome of extracorporeal membrane oxygenation as a bridge to lung transplantation and graft recovery. Ann Thorac Surg. 2012;94(3):942–9.

19. Nosotti M, Rosso L, Tosi D, et al. Extracorporeal membrane oxygenation with spontaneous breathing as a bridge to lung transplantation. Interact Cardiovasc Thorac Surg. 2013;16(1):55–9.

20. Ius F, Kuehn C, Tudorache I, et al. Lung transplantation on cardiopulmonary support: venoarterial extracorporeal membrane oxygenation outperformed cardiopulmonary bypass. J Thorac Cardiovasc Surg. 2012;144(6):1510–6.

21. Shafii AE, Mason DP, Brown CR, et al. Growing experience with extracorporeal membrane oxygenation as a bridge to lung transplantation. ASAIO J. 2012;58(5):526–9.

22. Javidfar J, Brodie D, Iribarne A, et al. Extracorporeal membrane oxygenation as a bridge to lung transplantation and recovery. J Thorac Cardiovasc Surg. 2012;144(3):716–21.

23. Garcia JP, Iacono A, Kon ZN, Griffith BP. Ambulatory extracorporeal membrane oxygenation: a new approach for bridge-to-lung transplantation. J Thorac Cardiovasc Surg. 2010;139(6):e137–9.

24. Shafii AE, McCurry KR. Subclavian insertion of the bicaval dual lumen cannula for venovenous extracorporeal membrane oxygenation. Ann Thorac Surg. 2012;94(2):663–5.

25. Mangi AA, Mason DP, Yun JJ, Murthy SC, Pettersson GB. Bridge to lung transplantation using short-term ambulatory extracorporeal membrane oxygenation. J Thorac Cardiovasc Surg. 2010;140(3):713–5.

26. Lowman JD, Kirk TK, Clark DE. Physical therapy management of a patient on portable extracorporeal membrane oxygenation as a bridge to lung transplantation: a case report. Cardiopulm Phys Ther J. 2012;23(1):30–5.

27. Garcia JP, Kon ZN, Evans C, et al. Ambulatory veno-venous extracorporeal membrane oxygenation: innovation and pitfalls. J Thorac Cardiovasc Surg. 2011;142(4):755–61.

28. Ricci D, Boffini M, Del Sorbo L, et al. The use of CO_2 removal devices in patients awaiting lung transplantation: an initial experience. Transplant Proc. 2010;42(4):1255–8.

29. Camboni D, Philipp A, Hirt S, Schmid C. Possibilities and limitations of a miniaturized long-term extracorporeal life support system as bridge to transplantation in a case with biventricular heart failure. Interact Cardiovasc Thorac Surg. 2009;8(1):168–70.

30. Taylor K, Holtby H. Emergency interventional lung assist for pulmonary hypertension. Anesth Analg. 2009;109(2):382–5.

31. Camboni D, Philipp A, Haneya A, et al. Serial use of an interventional lung assist device and a ventricular assist device. ASAIO J. 2010;56(3):270–2.

32. Mason DP, Thuita L, Alster JM, et al. Should transplantation be performed using donation after cardiac death? The United States experience. J Thorac Cardiovasc Surg. 2008;136(4):1061–6.

33. De Oliveira NC, Osaki S, Maloney JD, et al. Lung transplantation with donation after cardiac death donors: long-term follow-up in a single center. J Thorac Cardiovasc Surg. 2010;139(5):1306–15.

34. Cypel M, Yeung JC, Hirayama S, et al. Technique for prolonged normothermic ex vivo lung perfusion. J Heart Lung Transplant. 2008;27(12):1319–25.

35. Wierup P, Haraldsson A, Nilsson F, et al. Ex vivo evaluation of nonacceptable donor lungs. Ann Thorac Surg. 2006;81(2):460–6.

36. Cypel M, Rubacha M, Yeung J, et al. Normothermic ex vivo perfusion prevents lung injury compared to extended cold preservation for transplantation. Am J Transplant. 2009;9(10):2262–9.

37. Ingemansson R, Eyjolfsson A, Mared L, et al. Clinical transplantation of initially rejected donor lungs after reconditioning ex vivo. Ann Thorac Surg. 2009;87(1):255–60.

38. Yeung JC, Cypel M, Waddell TK, van Raemdonck D, Keshavjee S. Update on donor assessment, resuscitation, and acceptance criteria, including novel techniques—non-heart-beating donor lung retrieval and ex vivo donor lung perfusion. Thorac Surg Clin. 2009;19(2):261–74.

39. Cypel M, Yeung JC, Keshavjee S. Novel approaches to expanding the lung donor pool: donation after cardiac death and ex vivo conditioning. Clin Chest Med. 2011;32(2):233–44.

40. Cypel M, Keshavjee S. Extracorporeal lung perfusion. Curr Opin Organ Transplant. 2011;16(5):469–75.

41. Zych B, Popov AF, Stavri G, et al. Early outcomes of bilateral sequential single lung transplantation after ex-vivo lung evaluation and reconditioning. J Heart Lung Transplant. 2012;31(3):274–81.

42. Sadaria MR, Smith PD, Fullerton DA, et al. Cytokine expression profile in human lungs undergoing normothermic ex-vivo lung perfusion. Ann Thorac Surg. 2011;92(2):478–84.

43. Aigner C, Slama A, Hötzenecker K, et al. Clinical ex vivo lung perfusion—pushing the limits. Am J Transplant. 2012;12(7):1839–47.

44. Mordant P, Nakajima D, Kalaf R, et al. Mesenchymal stem cell treatment is associated

with decreased perfusate concentration of interleukin-8 during ex vivo perfusion of donor lungs after 18-hour preservation. J Heart Lung Transplant. 2016;35(10):1245–54.

45. Machuca TN, Cypel M, Bonato R, et al. Safety and efficacy of ex vivo donor lung adenoviral IL-10 gene therapy in a large animal lung transplant survival model. Hum Gene Ther. 2017;28(9):757–65.

46. Nakajima D, Cypel M, Bonato R, et al. Ex vivo perfusion treatment of infection in human donor lungs. Am J Transplant. 2016;16(4):1229–37.

47. Nakajima D, Liu M, Ohsumi A, et al. Lung lavage and surfactant replacement during ex vivo lung perfusion for treatment of gastric acid aspiration-induced donor lung injury. J Heart Lung Transplant. 2017;36(5):577–85.

48. Hsin MK, Zamel R, Cypel M, et al. Metabolic profile of ex vivo lung perfusate yields biomarkers for lung transplant outcomes. Ann Surg. 2018;267(1):196–7.

49. Hashimoto K, Cypel M, Juvet S, et al. Higher M30 and high mobility group box 1 protein levels in ex vivo lung perfusate are associated with primary graft dysfunction after human lung transplantation. J Heart Lung Transplant. 2017. pii: S1053-2498(17)31870-3 (Epub ahead of print).

50. Cypel M, Keshavjee S. Extracorporeal lung perfusion (ex-vivo lung perfusion). Curr Opin Organ Transplant. 2016;21(3):329–35.

51. Yeung JC, Cypel M, Keshavjee S. Ex-vivo lung perfusion: the model for the organ reconditioning hub. Curr Opin Organ Transplant. 2017;22(3):287–9.

52. Yeung JC, Krueger T, Yasufuku K, et al. Outcomes after transplantation of lungs preserved for more than 12 h: a retrospective study. Lancet Respir Med. 2017;5(2):119–24.

53. Hsin MK, Iskender I, Nakajima D, et al. Extension of donor lung preservation with hypothermic storage after normothermic ex vivo lung perfusion. J Heart Lung Transplant. 2016;35(1):130–6.

54. Reeb J, Keshavjee S, Cypel M. Expanding the lung donor pool: advancements and emerging pathways. Curr Opin Organ Transplant. 2015;20(5):498–505.

55. Benden C, Goldfarb SB, Edwards LB, et al. The registry of the International Society for Heart and Lung Transplantation: seventeenth official pediatric lung and heart-lung transplantation report—2014; focus theme: retransplantation. J Heart Lung Transplant. 2014;33(10):1025–33.

56. Thabut G, Christie JD, Ravaud P, et al. Survival after bilateral versus single-lung transplantation for idiopathic pulmonary fibrosis. Ann Intern Med. 2009;151(11):767–74.

57. Schaffer JM, Singh SK, Reitz BA, Zamanian RT, Mallidi HR. Single- vs double-lung transplantation in patients with chronic obstructive pulmonary disease and idiopathic pulmonary fibrosis since the implementation of lung allocation based on medical need. JAMA. 2015;313(9):936–48.

58. Mason DP, Brizzio ME, Alster JM, et al. Lung transplantation for idiopathic pulmonary fibrosis. Ann Thorac Surg. 2007;84(4):1121–8.

59. Gulack BC, Ganapathi AM, Speicher PJ, et al. What is the optimal transplant for older patients with idiopathic pulmonary fibrosis? Ann Thorac Surg. 2015;100(5):1826–33.

60. Force SD, Kilgo P, Neujahr DC, et al. Bilateral lung transplantation offers better long-term survival, compared with single-lung transplantation, for younger patients with idiopathic pulmonary fibrosis. Ann Thorac Surg. 2011;91(1):244–9.

61. De Oliveira NC, Osaki S, Maloney J, Cornwell RD, Meyer KC, et al. Lung transplant for interstitial lung disease: outcomes for single versus bilateral lung transplantation. Interact Cardiovasc Thorac Surg. 2012;14(3):263–7.

62. Nathan SD, Shlobin OA, Ahmad S, Burton NA, Barnett SD, Edwards E. Comparison of wait times and mortality for idiopathic pulmonary fibrosis patients listed for single or bilateral lung transplantation. J Heart Lung Transplant. 2010;29(10):1165–71.

63. Julliard WA, Meyer KC, De Oliveira NC, et al. The presence or severity of pulmonary hypertension does not affect outcomes for single-lung transplantation. Thorax. 2016;71(5):478–80.

64. Kotton CN, Kumar D, Caliendo AM, et al. International consensus guidelines on the management of cytomegalovirus in solid organ transplantation. Transplantation. 2010;89(7):779–95.

65. Hodson EM, Craig JC, Strippoli GF, Webster AC. Antiviral medications for preventing cytomegalovirus disease in solid organ transplant recipients. Cochrane Database Syst Rev. 2008;(2):CD003774.

66. Palmer SM, Limaye AP, Banks M, et al. Extended valganciclovir prophylaxis to prevent cytomegalovirus after lung transplantation: a randomized, controlled trial. Ann Intern Med. 2010; 152(12):761–9.

67. Murphey CL, Forsthuber TG. Trends in HLA antibody screening and identification and their role in transplantation. Expert Rev Clin Immunol. 2008;4(3):391–9.

68. Tait BD, Hudson F, Cantwell L, et al. Review article: Luminex technology for HLA antibody detection in organ transplantation. Nephrology (Carlton). 2009;14(2):247–54.

69. Tinckam KJ, Keshavjee S, Chaparro C, et al. Survival in sensitized lung transplant recipients with perioperative desensitization. Am J Transplant. 2015;15(2):417–26.

70. Zangwill SD, Ellis TM, Zlotocha J, et al. The virtual crossmatch—a screening tool for sensitized pediatric heart transplant recipients. Pediatr Transplant. 2006;10:38.

71. Tambur AR, Ramon DS, Kaufman DB, et al. Perception versus reality? Virtual crossmatch—how to overcome some of the technical and logistic limitations. Am J Transplant. 2009;9:1886.

72. Cecka JM, Kucheryavaya AY, Reinsmoen NL, Leffell MS. Calculated PRA: initial results show benefits for sensitized patients and a reduction in positive crossmatches. Am J Transplant. 2011;11:719.

73. El-Awar N, Lee J, Terasaki PI. HLA antibody identification with single antigen beads compared to conventional methods. Hum Immunol. 2005;66:989.

74. Shah RJ, Diamond JM, Cantu E, et al. Latent class analysis identifies distinct phenotypes of primary graft dysfunction after lung transplantation. Chest. 2013;144(2):616–22.

75. Morrison MI, Pither TL, Fisher AJ. Pathophysiology and classification of primary graft dysfunction after lung transplantation. J Thorac Dis. 2017;9(10):4084–97.

76. Brugière O, Suberbielle C, Thabut G, et al. Lung transplantation in patients with pretransplantation donor-specific antibodies detected by Luminex assay. Transplantation. 2013;95(5):761–5.

77. Hathorn KE, Chan WW, Lo WK. Role of gastroesophageal reflux disease in lung transplantation. World J Transplant. 2017;7(2):103–16.

78. Meyer KC, Raghu G, Verleden GM, et al. An international ISHLT/ATS/ERS clinical practice guideline: diagnosis and management of bronchiolitis obliterans syndrome. Eur Respir J. 2014;44(6):1479–503.

79. Verleden GM, Raghu G, Meyer KC, Glanville AR, Corris P. A new classification system for chronic lung allograft dysfunction. J Heart Lung Transplant. 2014;33(2):127–33.

80. Vos R, Verleden SE, Verleden GM. Chronic lung allograft dysfunction: evolving practice. Curr Opin Organ Transplant. 2015;20:483–91.

81. Vos R, Vanaudenaerde BM, Verleden SE, et al. A randomised controlled trial of azithromycin to prevent chronic rejection after lung transplantation. Eur Respir J. 2011;37(1):164–72.

82. Yates B, Murphy DM, Forrest IA, et al. Azithromycin reverses airflow obstruction in established bronchiolitis obliterans syndrome. Am J Respir Crit Care Med. 2005;172(6):772–5.

83. Gasper WJ, Sweet MP, Hoopes C, et al. Antireflux surgery for patients with end-stage lung disease before and after lung transplantation. Surg Endosc. 2008;22:495–500.

84. Hoppo T, Jarido V, Pennathur A, et al. Antireflux surgery preserves lung function in patients with gastroesophageal reflux disease and end-stage lung disease before and after lung transplantation. Arch Surg. 2011;146:1041–7.

85. Cantu E III, Appel JZ III, Hartwig MG, et al. J. Maxwell Chamberlain Memorial Paper. Early fundoplication prevents chronic allograft dysfunction in patients with gastroesophageal reflux disease. Ann Thorac Surg. 2004;78:1142–51.

86. Davis RD Jr, Lau CL, Eubanks S, et al. Improved lung allograft function after fundoplication in patients with gastroesophageal reflux disease undergoing lung transplantation. J Thorac Cardiovasc Surg. 2003;125:533–42.

87. Mertens V, Blondeau K, Pauwels A, et al. Azithromycin reduces gastroesophageal reflux and aspiration in lung transplant recipients. Dig Dis Sci. 2009;54:972–9.

88. Mertens V, Blondeau K, Van Oudenhove L, et al. Bile acids aspiration reduces survival in lung transplant recipients with BOS despite azithromycin. Am J Transplant. 2011;11:329–35.

89. Bobadilla JL, Jankowska-Gan E, Xu Q, et al. Reflux-induced collagen type v sensitization: potential mediator of bronchiolitis obliterans syndrome. Chest. 2010;138:363–70.

90. Jaksch P, Scheed A, Keplinger M, et al. A prospective interventional study on the use of extracorporeal photopheresis in patients with bronchiolitis obliterans syndrome after lung transplantation. J Heart Lung Transplant. 2012;31(9):950–7.

91. Marques MB, Schwartz J. Update on extracorporeal photopheresis in heart and lung transplantation. J Clin Apher. 2011;26(3):146–51.

92. Hachem RR, Yusen RD, Meyers BF, et al. Anti-human leukocyte antigen antibodies and preemptive antibody-directed therapy after lung transplantation. J Heart Lung Transplant. 2010; 29(9):973–80.

93. Burlingham WJ, Love RB, Jankowska-Gan E, et al. IL-17-dependent cellular immunity to collagen type V predisposes to obliterative bronchiolitis in human lung transplants. J Clin Invest. 2007;117(11):3498–506.

94. Bobadilla JL, Love RB, Jankowska-Gan E, et al. Th-17, monokines, collagen type V, and primary graft dysfunction in lung transplantation. Am J Respir Crit Care Med. 2008;177(6):660–8.

95. Saini D, Weber J, Ramachandran S, et al. Alloimmunity-induced autoimmunity as a potential mechanism in the pathogenesis of chronic rejection of human lung allografts. J Heart Lung Transplant. 2011;30(6):624–31.

96. Hachem RR, Tiriveedhi V, Patterson GA, Aloush A, Trulock EP, Mohanakumar T. Antibodies to K-α 1 tubulin and collagen V are associated with chronic rejection after lung transplantation. Am J Transplant. 2012;12(8):2164–71.

97. Takenaka M, Subramanian V, Tiriveedhi V, et al. Complement activation is not required for obliterative airway disease induced by antibodies to major histocompatibility complex class I: implications for chronic lung rejection. J Heart Lung Transplant. 2012;31(11):1214–22.

98. Sullivan JA, Jankowska-Gan E, Hegde S, et al. Th17 responses to collagen type V, kα1-tubulin, and vimentin are present early in human development and persist throughout life. Am J Transplant. 2017;17(4):944–56.

99. Yasufuku K, Heidler KM, O'Donnell PW, et al. Oral tolerance induction by type V collagen downregulates lung allograft rejection. Am J Respir Cell Mol Biol. 2001;25(1):26–34.

100. Yasufuku K, Heidler KM, Woods KA, et al. Prevention of bronchiolitis obliterans in rat lung allografts by type V collagen-induced oral tolerance. Transplantation. 2002;73(4):500–5.

101. Mizobuchi T, Yasufuku K, Zheng Y, et al. Differential expression of Smad7 transcripts identifies the

CD4+CD45RChigh regulatory T cells that mediate type V collagen-induced tolerance to lung allografts. J Immunol. 2003;171(3):1140–7.

102. Yamada Y, Sekine Y, Yoshida S, et al. Type V collagen-induced oral tolerance plus low-dose cyclosporine prevents rejection of MHC class I and II incompatible lung allografts. J Immunol. 2009;183(1):237–45.

103. Meyer KC. Diagnosis and management of bronchiolitis obliterans syndrome following lung or hematopoietic cell transplantation. Expert Rev Respir Med. 2016;10(6):599–602.

104. Vanaudenaerde BM, De Vleeschauwer SI, Vos R, et al. The role of the IL23/IL17 axis in bronchiolitis obliterans syndrome after lung transplantation. Am J Transplant. 2008;8(9):1911–20.

105. Afzali B, Lombardi G, Lechler RI, Lord GM. The role of T helper 17 (Th17) and regulatory T cells (Treg) in human organ transplantation and autoimmune disease. Clin Exp Immunol. 2007;148(1):32–46.

106. Tiriveedhi V, Takenaka M, Ramachandran S, et al. T regulatory cells play a significant role in modulating MHC class I antibody-induced obliterative airway disease. Am J Transplant. 2012;12(10):2663–74.

107. Fukami N, Ramachandran S, Takenaka M, Weber J, Subramanian V, Mohanakumar T. An obligatory role for lung infiltrating B cells in the immunopathogenesis of obliterative airway disease induced by antibodies to MHC class I molecules. Am J Transplant. 2012;12(4):867–76.

108. Serody JS, Hill GR. The IL-17 differentiation pathway and its role in transplant outcome. Biol Blood Marrow Transplant. 2012;18(1 Suppl):S56–61.

109. Shilling RA, Wilkes DS. Role of Th17 cells and IL-17 in lung transplant rejection. Semin Immunopathol. 2011;33(2):129–34.

110. Krebs R, Tikkanen JM, Ropponen JO, et al. Critical role of VEGF-C/VEGFR-3 signaling in innate and adaptive immune responses in experimental obliterative bronchiolitis. Am J Pathol. 2012;181(5):1607–20.

111. Tesar BM, Du W, Shirali AC, Walker WE, Shen H, Goldstein DR. Aging augments IL-17 T-cell alloimmune responses. Am J Transplant. 2009;9(1):54–63.

112. Vanaudenaerde BM, Dupont LJ, Wuyts WA, et al. The role of interleukin-17 during acute rejection after lung transplantation. Eur Respir J. 2006;27(4):779–87.

113. Vanaudenaerde BM, Wuyts WA, Dupont LJ, Van Raemdonck DE, Demedts MM, Verleden GM. Interleukin-17 stimulates release of interleukin-8 by human airway smooth muscle cells in vitro: a potential role for interleukin-17 and airway smooth muscle cells in bronchiolitis obliterans syndrome. J Heart Lung Transplant. 2003;22(11):1280–3.

114. Vanaudenaerde BM, Verleden SE, Vos R, et al. Innate and adaptive interleukin-17-producing lymphocytes in chronic inflammatory lung disorders. Am J Respir Crit Care Med. 2011;183(8):977–86.

115. Shi Q, Cao H, Liu J, et al. CD4+ Foxp3+ regulatory T cells induced by TGF-β, IL-2 and all-trans retinoic acid attenuate obliterative bronchiolitis in rat trachea transplantation. Int Immunopharmacol. 2011;11(11):1887–94.

116. Neujahr DC, Larsen CP. Regulatory T cells in lung transplantation—an emerging concept. Semin Immunopathol. 2011;33(2):117–27.

117. Braun RK, Molitor-Dart M, Wigfield C, et al. Transfer of tolerance to collagen type V suppresses T-helper-cell-17 lymphocyte-mediated acute lung transplant rejection. Transplantation. 2009;88(12):1341–8.

118. Jaffar Z, Ferrini ME, Girtsman TA, Roberts K. Antigen-specific Treg regulate Th17-mediated lung neutrophilic inflammation, B-cell recruitment and polymeric IgA and IgM levels in the airways. Eur J Immunol. 2009;39(12):3307–14.

119. Griffin DO, Rothstein TL. Human "orchestrator" CD11b(+) B1 cells spontaneously secrete interleukin-10 and regulate T-cell activity. Mol Med. 2012;18(9):1003–8.

120. Mauri C, Bosma A. Immune regulatory function of B cells. Annu Rev Immunol. 2012;30:221–41.

121. Li W, Bribriesco AC, Nava RG, et al. Lung transplant acceptance is facilitated by early events in the graft and is associated with lymphoid neogenesis. Mucosal Immunol. 2012;5(5):544–54.

122. Huang YJ, Charlson ES, Collman RG, Colombini-Hatch S, Martinez FD, Senior RM. The role of the lung microbiome in health and disease. A National Heart, Lung, and Blood Institute workshop report. Am J Respir Crit Care Med. 2013;187:1382–7.

123. Cui L, Morris A, Huang L, et al. The microbiome and the lung. Ann Am Thorac Soc. 2014;11(Suppl 4):S227–32.

124. Sharma NS, Wille KM, Athira S, et al. Distal airway microbiome is associated with immunoregulatory myeloid cell responses in lung transplant recipients. J Heart Lung Transplant. 2018;37(2):206–16.

125. Mouraux S, Bernasconi E, Pattaroni C, et al. Airway microbiota signals anabolic and catabolic remodeling in the transplanted lung. J Allergy Clin Immunol. 2018;141(2):718–729.e7. pii: S0091-6749(17)31102-8.

126. Lama VN, Smith L, Badri L, et al. Evidence for tissue-resident mesenchymal stem cells in human adult lung from studies of transplanted allografts. J Clin Invest. 2007;117(4):989–96.

127. Walker N, Badri L, Wettlaufer S, et al. Resident tissue-specific mesenchymal progenitor cells contribute to fibrogenesis in human lung allografts. Am J Pathol. 2011;178(6):2461–9.

128. Badri L, Murray S, Liu LX, et al. Mesenchymal stromal cells in bronchoalveolar lavage as predictors of bronchiolitis obliterans syndrome. Am J Respir Crit Care Med. 2011;183(8):1062–70.

129. De Miguel MP, Fuentes-Julián S, et al. Immunosuppressive properties of mesenchymal stem cells: advances and applications. Curr Mol Med. 2012;12(5):574–91.

130. Yi T, Song SU. Immunomodulatory properties of mesenchymal stem cells and their therapeutic applications. Arch Pharm Res. 2012;35(2):213–21.

131. Jarvinen L, Badri L, Wettlaufer S, et al. Lung resident mesenchymal stem cells isolated from human lung allografts inhibit T cell proliferation via a soluble mediator. J Immunol. 2008;181(6):4389–96.

132. Banerjee ER, Laflamme MA, Papayannopoulou T, Kahn M, Murry CE, Henderson WR Jr. Human embryonic stem cells differentiated to lung lineage-specific cells ameliorate pulmonary fibrosis in a xenograft transplant mouse model. PLoS One. 2012;7(3):e33165.

133. Sun CK, Yen CH, Lin YC, et al. Autologous transplantation of adipose-derived mesenchymal stem cells markedly reduced acute ischemia-reperfusion lung injury in a rodent model. J Transl Med. 2011;9:118.

134. Chien MH, Bien MY, Ku CC, et al. Systemic human orbital fat-derived stem/stromal cell transplantation ameliorates acute inflammation in lipopolysaccharide-induced acute lung injury. Crit Care Med. 2012;40(4):1245–53.

135. Danchuk S, Ylostalo JH, Hossain F, et al. Human multipotent stromal cells attenuate lipopolysaccharide-induced acute lung injury in mice via secretion of tumor necrosis factor-α-induced protein 6. Stem Cell Res Ther. 2011;2(3):27.

136. Saito S, Nakayama T, Hashimoto N, et al. Mesenchymal stem cells stably transduced with a dominant-negative inhibitor of CCL2 greatly attenuate bleomycin-induced lung damage. Am J Pathol. 2011;179(3):1088–94.

137. Hegab AE, Ha VL, Gilbert JL, et al. Novel stem/progenitor cell population from murine tracheal submucosal gland ducts with multipotent regenerative potential. Stem Cells. 2011;29(8):1283–93.

138. Huh JW, Kim SY, Lee JH, et al. Bone marrow cells repair cigarette smoke-induced emphysema in rats. Am J Physiol Lung Cell Mol Physiol. 2011;301(3):L255–66.

139. Firinci F, Karaman M, Baran Y, et al. Mesenchymal stem cells ameliorate the histopathological changes in a murine model of chronic asthma. Int Immunopharmacol. 2011;11(8):1120–6.

140. Chang YS, Choi SJ, Sung DK, et al. Intratracheal transplantation of human umbilical cord blood derived mesenchymal stem cells dose-dependently attenuates hyperoxia-induced lung injury in neonatal rats. Cell Transplant. 2011; 20(11–12):1843–54.

141. Toya SP, Li F, Bonini MG, et al. Interaction of a specific population of human embryonic stem cell-derived progenitor cells with CD11b+ cells ameliorates sepsis-induced lung inflammatory injury. Am J Pathol. 2011;178(1):313–24.

142. Liang OD, Mitsialis SA, Chang MS, et al. Mesenchymal stromal cells expressing heme oxygenase-1 reverse pulmonary hypertension. Stem Cells. 2011;29(1):99–107.

143. Moodley Y, Atienza D, Manuelpillai U, et al. Human umbilical cord mesenchymal stem cells reduce fibrosis of bleomycin-induced lung injury. Am J Pathol. 2009;175(1):303–13.

144. McAuley DF, Curley GF, Hamid UI, et al. Clinical grade allogeneic human mesenchymal stem cells restore alveolar fluid clearance in human lungs rejected for transplantation. Am J Physiol Lung Cell Mol Physiol. 2014;306(9):L809–15.

145. Chambers DC, Enever D, Lawrence S, et al. Mesenchymal stromal cell therapy for chronic lung allograft dysfunction: results of a first-in-man study. Stem Cells Transl Med. 2017;6(4):1152–7.

146. Cooper DK, Ekser B, Burlak C, et al. Clinical lung xenotransplantation—what donor genetic modifications may be necessary? Xenotransplantation. 2012;19(3):144–58.

147. Burdorf L, Azimzadeh AM, Pierson RN III. Xenogeneic lung transplantation models. Methods Mol Biol. 2012;885:169–89.

148. Gaca JG, Lesher A, Aksoy O, Gonzalez-Stawinski GV, Platt JL, Lawson JH, Parker W, Davis RD. Disseminated intravascular coagulation in association with pig-to-primate pulmonary xenotransplantation. Transplantation. 2002;73(11):1717–23.

149. Cantu E, Gaca JG, Palestrant D, et al. Depletion of pulmonary intravascular macrophages prevents hyperacute pulmonary xenograft dysfunction. Transplantation. 2006;81(8):1157–64.

150. Li S, Waer M, Billiau AD. Xenotransplantation: role of natural immunity. Transpl Immunol. 2009;21(2):70–4.

151. Puga Yung GL, Li Y, Borsig L, et al. Complete absence of the αGal xenoantigen and isoglobotrihexosylceramide in α1,3galactosyltransferase knock-out pigs. Xenotransplantation. 2012; 19(3):196–206.

152. Ekser B, Bianchi J, Ball S, et al. Comparison of hematologic, biochemical, and coagulation parameters in α1,3-galactosyltransferase gene-knockout pigs, wild-type pigs, and four primate species. Xenotransplantation. 2012;19(6):342–54.

153. Sahara H, Watanabe H, Pomposelli T, Yamada K. Lung xenotransplantation. Curr Opin Organ Transplant. 2017;22(6):541–8.

154. Song JJ, Ott HC. Bioartificial lung engineering. Am J Transplant. 2012;12(2):283–8.

155. Bonvillain RW, Danchuk S, Sullivan DE, et al. A nonhuman primate model of lung regeneration: detergent-mediated decellularization and initial in vitro recellularization with mesenchymal stem cells. Tissue Eng Part A. 2012;18(23–24):2437–52.

156. Price AP, England KA, Matson AM, Blazar BR, Panoskaltsis-Mortari A. Development of a decellularized lung bioreactor system for bioengineering the lung: the matrix reloaded. Tissue Eng Part A. 2010;16(8):2581–91.

157. Fritsche CS, Simsch O, Weinberg EJ, et al. Pulmonary tissue engineering using dual-compartment polymer scaffolds with integrated vascular tree. Int J Artif Organs. 2009;32(10):701–10.

158. Ott HC, Clippinger B, Conrad C, et al. Regeneration and orthotopic transplantation of a bioartificial lung. Nat Med. 2010;16(8):927–33.

159. Song JJ, Kim SS, Liu Z, et al. Enhanced in vivo function of bioartificial lungs in rats. Ann Thorac Surg. 2011;92(3):998–1005; discussion 1005–6.

160. Farré R, Otero J, Almendros I, Navajas D. Bioengineered lungs: a challenge and an opportunity. Arch Bronconeumol. 2018;54(1):31–8.

Index

© The Author(s) 2018
G. Raghu, R. G. Carbone (eds.), *Lung Transplantation*, https://doi.org/10.1007/978-3-319-91184-7